T0145242

ICSA Book Series in Statistics

The ICSA Book Series in Statistics showcases research from the International Chinese Statistical Association that has an international reach. It publishes books in statistical theory, applications, and statistical education. All books are associated with the ICSA or are authored by invited contributors. Books may be monographs, edited volumes, textbooks and proceedings.

More information about this series at http://www.springer.com/series/13402

Yinglin Xia · Jun Sun · Ding-Geng Chen

Statistical Analysis of Microbiome Data with R

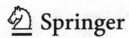 Springer

Yinglin Xia
Department of Medicine
University of Illinois at Chicago
Chicago, IL, USA

Jun Sun
Department of Medicine
University of Illinois at Chicago
Chicago, IL, USA

Ding-Geng Chen
School of Social Work
University of North Carolina
Chapel Hill, NC, USA

and

Department of Biostatistics
Gillings School of Global
    Public Health
University of North Carolina
Chapel Hill, NC, USA

and

Department of Statistics
University of Pretoria
Pretoria, South Africa

ISSN 2199-0980   ISSN 2199-0999   (electronic)
ICSA Book Series in Statistics
ISBN 978-981-13-4645-3   ISBN 978-981-13-1534-3   (eBook)
https://doi.org/10.1007/978-981-13-1534-3

This Springer imprint is published by the registered company Springer Nature Singapore Pte Ltd.
The registered company address is: 152 Beach Road, #21-01/04 Gateway East, Singapore 189721, Singapore

Yinglin Xia and Jun Sun would like to dedicate this book to their parents and parents-in-law: Qijia Xia, Xincui Wang, Zong-Xiang Sun, and Xiao-Yun Fu; and their sons: Yuxuan Xia and Jason Xia for their constant love and support.

Ding-Geng Chen would like to dedicate this book to his parents and parents-in-law who value high-education and hard-working, and to his wife, Ke, his son, John D. Chen, and his daughter, Jenny K. Chen, for their love and support.

Preface

Microbiome research and microbiome data analysis are one of the fast-growing areas in biomedical and public health research. It is evidenced and catalyzed by publications in different relevant fields of studies and methodology development, as well as large-scale projects, such as the Human Microbiome Project (HMP), the Integrative Human Microbiome Project, and Metagenomics of the Human Intestinal Tract (MetaHIT) study. By the end of 2017, HMP investigators have already published over 650 scientific papers, cited over 70,000 times (https://commonfund.nih.gov/hmp).

We are now advancing our understanding of how the microbiome impacts human health and disease, with more and more projects in microbiome funded and research and statistical methodology papers published. The masses of microbiome data generated by 16S rRNA sequencing and shotgun metagenomic sequencing via the bioinformatics pipelines (packages), promote recent major growth spurt of microbiome study. Data analysis and methodology are integral parts of microbiome research. Since microbiome data are very complicated, there is a critical need to develop all kinds of statistical methodologies for microbiome research, ranging from application to methodology, and to statistical theory.

The habit of human learning starts with the known, then processes to the unknown. Statistical analysis of microbiome data follows with the similar process. In the beginning, the researchers and statisticians used the classic statistical methods and models or borrowed them from other relevant fields, such as ecology and microarray. Later, they developed their own statistical methods and models that target one or more unique features of microbiome data. Currently, statistical methods and analysis tools for analyzing microbiome data are available from classic statistics, relevant research fields, and new developments, including visualization and characterization of structure of microbiome data sets.

Statistical tools for performing microbiome data analysis are now available in different languages and environments across different platforms, either in web-based or programming-based approaches. Obviously, R system and environment play a critical role in developing statistical tools for analyzing microbiome data.

The birth of this book is an excellent example to show how a multidisciplinary team working together to meet the need of the field. In April 2016, Dr. Jun Sun was working on a microbiome book on behalf of the American Physiological Society by Springer. She invited Dr. Yinglin Xia to contribute a book chapter on microbiome data analysis. Dr. Sun and Dr. Xia have long-time collaborations in biomedical sciences including microbiome studies. While working on the book chapter, they thought it would be a good idea to expand a brief book chapter to a comprehensive book on analyzing microbiome data. They were very happy that Dr. Ding-Geng Chen was willing to join the team and provide his expertise on statistics and microarray study. In May 2016, a book proposal on *Statistical Analysis of Microbiome Data with R* was submitted. It was well received by the peer-review and fully supported by the editors of ICSA Book Series in Statistics.

In this book, we aim to provide the step-by-step procedures to perform data analysis of microbiome data by way of the R programming language. We provide some bioinformatic and statistical foundations of data analysis because microbiome data are complicated and analysis of microbiome data is still very challenging. To strike a balance, we briefly introduce concepts, backgrounds, statistical method developments before illustrating the applications in real data.

The book was organized in this way: in the beginning three chapters, we specially provided overview and introduction of bioinformatics, features of microbiome data, and statistical analysis of microbiome data. In Chap. 4, we covered some basic skills in R programming, RStudio, ggplot2, and most often used R packages and techniques for microbiome data management and programming. In Chap. 5, we introduced classic and newly developed methods in application of hypothesis testing and power analysis of microbiome data. Chapter 6 focused on introduction of community alpha and beta measures and calculations. Chapter 7 provided most often used visualization techniques for exploratory analysis of microbiome data including graphic summary of data and clustering, ordination. Chapters 8 and 9 focused on univariate and multivariate community analysis, respectively. Many classic and newly developed methods are introduced in the application of microbiome studies. We contributed Chap. 10 to compositional analysis of microbiome data. In this chapter, we introduced basic concept, fundamental principles, brief history, procedures, and challenges of compositional data analysis. We also summarized several considerations of microbiome dataset being treated as compositional and illustrated compositional analysis of microbiome data using real data. Chapters 11 and 12 focused on count-based approaches of modeling over-dispersed and zero-inflated microbiome data, respectively. Here, we widely covered statistical methods and models of count data, including negative binomial, zero-inflated, and zero-hurdle models, and zero-inflated Beta regression model with random-effects in longitudinal setting. We also discussed the concept adjustment of model application and topics of model comparisons.

We hope the contents of these chapters and the way of organization provide a framework of statistical analysis of microbiome data. We expect this book to be used by (1) statisticians, who are working on microbiome studies, either for their own research, or for their collaborative research, such as experimental design, grant application, and data analysis; (2) researchers from microbiome and biomedical fields, such as principal investigators, clinicians, research fellows, graduate students, who are designing the studies, collecting the data; (3) researchers from other relevant or similar fields (e.g., bioinformatics, ecology, microarray, economics, etc.) and common use of statistical methods and R packages. The data and R codes used in this book are available by requesting to the first author: Yinglin Xia at yinglin.xia2007@gmail.com.

Chicago, IL, USA   Yinglin Xia
Chicago, IL, USA   Jun Sun
North Carolina, NC, USA   Ding-Geng Chen
Pretoria, South Africa
June, 2018

Acknowledgements

There are a number of people we wish to thank. We greatly appreciate those persons, who helped us from various resources and at different stages of development and writing. Thanks go to the editorial team at Springer for their enthusiasm in supporting this project and for their feedback along the way of process to publishing. Broadly, we greatly appreciate the developers of statistical methods, models, and R packages and R system and environment in general. Some of them shared their papers with us. Without their great works, the book cannot be available in current breadth and scope. We especially wish thanks to Jason for his support and proofreading of some chapters. Finally, we all wish to express our deepest appreciation to our respective families for their love, patience, and support during the writing of this book.

Contents

About the Authors

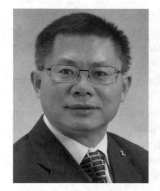

Dr. Yinglin Xia is a Research Associate Professor at the Department of Medicine, the University of Illinois at Chicago, USA. He was a Research Assistant Professor in the Department of Biostatistics and Computational Biology at the University of Rochester, Rochester, NY. Dr. Xia has worked on a variety of research projects and clinical trials in microbiome, gastroenterology, oncology, immunology, psychiatry, sleep, neuroscience, HIV, mental health, public health, social and behavioral sciences, as well as nursing caregiver. He has published more than 100 papers in peer-reviewed journals on *Statistical Methodology, Clinical Trial, Medical Statistics, Biomedical Sciences, and Social and Behavioral sciences*. He serves the editorial board of 9 scientific journals. Dr. Xia is well versed in the design and analysis in the areas of longitudinal data, mediation and moderation analyses, multilevel clustered-data, zero-inflated count data, mixed-effects model, GEE, structural equation model, meta-analysis, and ROC curve. He has successfully applied his statistical knowledge, modeling and programming skills to study designs and data analysis in biomedical research and clinical trials. He has been involved as a co-investigator or statistician in numerous NIH, CDC, and other grants. Three grants he designed on microbiome studies were funded by NIH and other funding agencies. His recent papers on microbiome data analysis are well received by peers.

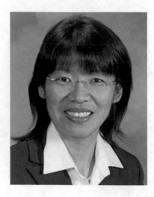

Dr. Jun Sun is a tenured Professor of Medicine at the University of Illinois at Chicago, USA. She is an elected fellow of American Gastroenterological Associate (AGA). Her research interests are host–microbiome interactions in inflammation and cancer. Her key achievements include (1) characterization of vitamin D receptor regulation of gut microbiome in intestinal homeostasis and inflammation, (2) identification of dysbiosis and intestinal dysfunction in amyotrophic lateral sclerosis (ALS), (3) characterization of bacteria in regulating intestinal stem cells, and (4) identification and characterization of the *Salmonella* effector protein AvrA in host–bacterial interactions. Dr. Sun has published over 160 scientific articles in peer-reviewed journals, including *Gut, Cell Stem Cells, Nature Genetics, JBC, American Journal of Pathology, American Journal of Physiology-GI*. She is the leading editor of three books, including a recent *Nature/Springer* book entitled *Mechanisms Underlying Host-Microbiome Interactions in Pathophysiology of Human Diseases*. This book has shown a novel theme and multiple disciplinary topics of microbiome research for broad audience. She is in the editorial board of more than 10 peer-reviewed international scientific journals. She services study sections for the NIH, American Cancer Society, and other national and international research foundations. She is the Chair-elected for the AGA microbiome section. Her research is supported by the NIH, DOD, and other research awards. Dr. Sun is a believer of scientific art and artistic science. She enjoys writing her science papers in English and poems in Chinese. She teaches her medical fellows biomedical knowledge and also the way to translate the Chinese poems. In addition to her research papers and books, her poetry collection 《让时间停留在这一刻 》 "*Let time stay still at this moment*", is published in January 2018 by Chinese Literature and History Press.

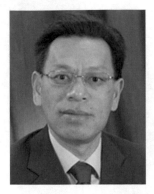

Prof. Ding-Geng Chen is a fellow of the American Statistical Association and currently the Wallace Kuralt distinguished Professor at the University of North Carolina at Chapel Hill, USA and an extraordinary Professor at University of Pretoria, South Africa. He was a Professor at the University of Rochester and the Karl E. Peace endowed eminent scholar chair in biostatistics at Georgia Southern University. He is also a senior consultant for biopharmaceuticals and government agencies with extensive expertise in clinical trial biostatistics and public health statistics. Professor Chen has written more than 150 referred publications and co-authored/co-edited 23 books on biostatistical clinical trial methodology, meta-analysis, causal-inference and data analytics, and public health statistics.

Chapter 1
Bioinformatic Analysis of Microbiome Data

In this chapter, we first introduce microbiome study and DNA sequencing in Sect. 1.1. Then we cover some basics of phylogenetics in Sect. 1.2. Next we focus on reviewing 16S rRNA sequencing and shotgun metagenomic sequencing approaches in Sects. 1.3 and 1.4 respectively. Finally, in Sect. 1.5, we briefly introduce two tools for bioinformatical analysis of 16S rRNA sequencing data. Section 1.6 is summary.

1.1 Introduction to Microbiome Study

1.1.1 What Is the Human Microbiome?

"What is it to be human?" is a fundamental topic in metaphysics, since the beginning of humans appearing on earth; this question has troubled humans until nowadays. Similarly, "what is the human microbiome?" has troubled researchers (Ursell et al. 2012) even since Lederberg's coinage of "microbiome" in 2001 (Lederberg and McCray 2001). Researchers have confused how to exactly define the human microbiome, as evidenced by interchangeably using terminologies: for example, "microbiota" and "microbiome". The term "microbiota" is referred to the microbial taxa associated with humans to signify the communities of microorganisms within a specific environment. The term "microbiome" is defined as the collection of the microbial taxa or microbes and their genes (Ursell et al. 2012; Wu et al. 2013), the entire microbial communities. Thus, if we consider these two terms differentially, "microbiota" is used to signify the communities of microorganisms, whereas "microbiome" is to signify the organisms and all of their related genomes (Wu and Lewis 2013). Depending on their origin, researchers also use specific terms, such as gut microbiome, oral microbiome, or lung microbiome. In this book, we use "microbiome" in its widest meaning: the collection of microbes or

© Springer Nature Singapore Pte Ltd. 2018
Y. Xia et al., *Statistical Analysis of Microbiome Data with R*,
ICSA Book Series in Statistics, https://doi.org/10.1007/978-981-13-1534-3_1

microorganisms that literally share our body space or inhabit an environment, creating a sort of "mini-ecosystem"(Sun and Dudeja 2018).

Although we still need to confirm whether we are born sterilely (Ley et al. 2006; Matamoros et al. 2013), it is known that we begin to be colonized with microbes at birth (Arrieta et al. 2014), or our microbiota development begins well in amniotic fluid before delivery (DiGiulio et al. 2008; DiGiulio 2012). Actually we adopt the microbiota before birth from the uterus (Mackie et al. 1999; Jimenez et al. 2005; Penders et al. 2006; Jiménez et al. 2008; Madan et al. 2012). Over the first several years of life, particularly during the first 3 years, our skin surface, oral cavity, and gut are colonized by a tremendous diversity of bacteria, archaea, fungi, and viruses (Morgan and Huttenhower 2012; Arrieta et al. 2014), until the microbiota becomes adult-like.

The largest microbial community of the human microbiome is our intestinal tract harboring up to 100 trillion (10^{14}) microbes, which are 10 times the number of human cells, and more than a 100 up to 150 times the number of the human genes (Whitman et al. 1998; Ley et al. 2006; Qin et al. 2010; Matamoros et al. 2013). The vast majority of microbes reside in colon with a density around 10^{11} to 10^{12} cells/ml (Whitman et al. 1998; Ley et al. 2006). In 2016, Sender et al. reestimated that the number of bacteria in adult colon is 3.8 x 10^{13} and the ratio of bacteria to human cells is coser 1:1 instead of 10 : 1 as previously estimated (Sender et al. 2016).

1.1.2 Microbiome Research and DNA Sequencing

Mammalian microbiome research has a long history (Sanger and Coulson 1975; Sanger et al. 1977; Goodrich et al. 2014). Historically, microbiology studies were almost entirely culture-dependent. In order to study an organism, it was necessary to grow the organism in the lab (Morgan and Huttenhower 2012). However, culture-based methods rely on the ability to grow viable organisms outside their natural habitat. It can be very difficult because many species and strains are well adapted to live in the human body. The suitable environment for microbiome is not viable in in vitro conditions. In the past, this difficulty has resulted in underestimation of the complexity of the human microbiome.

It was until 2005 with advances in DNA-sequencing technologies, such as Roche/ 454 pyrosequencing and Illumina Solexa sequencing, researchers started to analyze the DNA extracted directly from a sample rather than from individually cultured microbes (Eckburg et al. 2005). DNA Sequencing has fundamentally shifted away from classical Sanger automated sequencing to next-generation sequencing (NGS) for genome analysis (Metzker 2005, 2010; Jünemann et al. 2017).

Early in 1953, Watson and Crick solved the three-dimensional structure of DNA (Watson and Crick 1953); however, it was until 1965 that Holley et al. (1965) produced the first whole nucleic acid sequence and Sanger et al. (1965) in parallel developed a related technique (Heather and Chain 2016). The automated Sanger method is considered as a 'first-generation' technology. Although there was substantial progress during this era, the sequence reads produced by the first-generation

DNA sequencing machines are limited. The shotgun sequencing techniques have been emerged to analyze longer fragments. With the shotgun sequencing, the overlapping DNA fragments were cloned and sequenced separately, and then assembled into one long contiguous sequence (or 'contig') in silico (Staden 1979; Anderson 1981).

In 2005, 454 Life Sciences (purchased by Roche in 2007) released the pyrosequencing method (Margulies et al. 2005). Until this departure, the automated Sanger method had dominated the DNA sequencing industry for almost two decades (Metzker 2010) since Sanger developed his 'chain-termination' technique (Sanger et al. 1977) in 1977, which adventured a major breakthrough in DNA sequencing technology. The features of massively parallel analysis, high throughput, and lower cost allow a gradual shift from classical Sanger sequencing technology to NGS (Liu et al. 2012). The NGS platforms include Roche/454, Illumina/Solexa, Life/APG and Helicos BioSciences, the Polonator instrument, Pacific Biosciences. Each sequencing platform has advantages and disadvantages. For example, Roche/454 allowed the massively parallel analysis of sequencing reactions, greatly increasing the amount of DNA that can be sequenced in any one run (Margulies et al. 2005; Heather and Chain 2016). In addition, the Roche/454 technology produces long enough reads to minimize the loss in annotation (Wommack et al. 2008), to map to a reference genome easily, and has relatively fast run times (Metzker 2010). All these advantages have made Roche/454 pyrosequencing a popular choice for shotgun-sequencing metagenomics. Thus, Roche/454 platform has been recommended to apply bacterial and genome de novo assemblies, and other metagenomics applications (Metzker 2010; Liu et al. 2012). However, the Roche/454 technology has several disadvantages, such as, relatively low throughput, high reagent cost and high insertion or deletion rates in homo-polymer repeats (Metzker 2010; Thomas et al. 2012). All these disadvantages may make its technology become noncompetitive and resulted in 454 technology business shutting down by Roche in 2013 (Hollmer 2013).

Compared to Roche/454, Illumina/Solexa technology still has the limited read length, which is not sufficient for functional annotation (Wommack et al. 2008), and low multiplexing capability of samples (Metzker 2010). In Illumina/Solexa sequencing, sample loading, random scattering of clusters, sequence quality, are still technically challenging (van Dijk et al. 2014). However, Illumina/Solexa technology has several advantages, such as, offering the highest throughput, the lowest per-base costs, and successful application to metagenomics, and generalizing draft genomes from complex dataset (Liu et al. 2012; Thomas et al. 2012; van Dijk et al. 2014), high sequencing accuracy (Jünemann et al. 2017) among others. Currently, Illumina/Solexa is the most widely used platform in the field of metagenomics. It was recommended to apply to variant discovery, whole-exome capture and gene discovery in metagenomics (Metzker 2010).

The third-generation DNA sequencing methods were defined based on whether the sequencing detects single molecules, occurs in real time and does not require DNA amplification before sequencing (Schadt et al. 2010; van Dijk et al. 2014;

Heather and Chain 2016). All these characteristics simply diverge the third-generation sequencing from previous technologies.

Currently Pacific Biosciences (PacBio) leads the third-generation technology (van Dijk et al. 2014; Heather and Chain 2016). It developed its first instrument, the PacBio RS in 2010. This instrument has several advantages, such as, being capable of generating sufficiently long reads for the completing de novo genome assemblies (van Dijk et al. 2014; Heather and Chain 2016), providing detectable fluorescence, producing kinetic data, allowing for detection of modified bases and fast run times (van Dijk et al. 2014). However, it has high cost, high overall error rates, lowest throughput of all platforms, which limit its applications (van Dijk et al. 2014).

1.2 Introduction to Phylogenetics

Phylogenetics is the study of the evolutionary history and relationships among individuals or groups of organisms (e.g., species, or populations). Phylogenetics is important because it enriches our understanding of how genes, genomes, species and molecular sequences generally evolve. It provides us a tool that allows investigators to place their observations within the historical context of descent within modification and ferret out historical and proximal factors that contributes to their observations (Wiley and Lieberman 2011). From phylogenetics, we learn not only how the sequences came to be the way they are today, but also general principles that enable us to predict how they will change in the future. Thus, phylogenetic analyses are central themes in studying biodiversity, evolution, ecology, and genomes.

Human microbiome is very complicated with existing genetic and evolutionary relationships among species. The field of classification, identification and naming of biological organisms on the basis of shared characteristics is called taxonomy. Taxonomy stems from ancient Greek *taxis*, meaning 'arrangement', and *nomia*, meaning 'method'. To understand the complexity of the human microbiome, it is important to recognize the genetic and evolutionary relationships between species.

The Swedish botanist Carl Linnaeus (1707–1778) was known as the father of taxonomy, who developed a system for categorization of organisms, known as Linnaean taxonomy, and binomial nomenclature for naming organisms. Linnaeus and others ranked all living organisms into seven biological groups or levels of classification: kingdom, phylum, class, order, family, genus, and species. There are no domains in these classifications. The classification of domain is a relatively new grouping, which was first proposed by Woese et al. in 1977 (Woese and Fox 1977; Woese et al. 1990). They said, a formal or natural system of organisms should have a new taxon called "domain" above the level of kingdom. Archaea, Bacteria and Eukarya are the three domains of life.

Currently researchers agreed that all living organisms can be classified into eight major hierarchical levels, from domain (the most general) to species (the most specific) (Tyler et al. 2014). Figure 1.1 (modified from Tyler et al. 2014) shows the

Fig. 1.1 Hierarchical organization of taxonomic levels used for classifying organisms

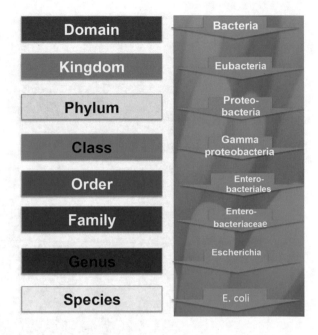

hierarchical levels of taxonomy. At each lower level, organisms are classified with their most similar characteristics. Species-level analysis provides the most precise information of life; however, higher-level analyses are also valuable, especially when species identification is challenging.

1.3   16S rRNA Sequencing Approach

Currently, there are two main approaches to sequence the uncultured microbes (Fig. 1.2): amplicon sequencing (in which only one particular gene, often 16S rRNA, is amplified and sequenced) and random shotgun sequencing. In this section, we will introduce the approach of 16S rRNA gene sequencing; in next section, we will introduce the approach of shotgun metagenomic sequencing.

1.3.1   The Advantages of 16S rRNA Sequencing

The 16S rRNA gene, sometimes called rDNA, is the conservative gene in the microbes. Lane et al. in 1985 (Lane et al. 1985) first described the use of 16S rRNA gene to identify and classify uncultured microbes in the environment. Because this gene has several desirable properties, the 16S rRNA gene sequencing has been the first metagenomics method and widely accepted. The advanced properties include:

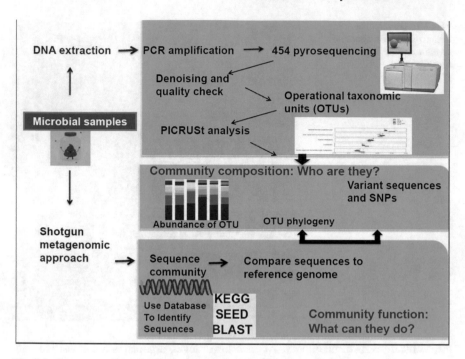

Fig. 1.2 Summary of bioinformatic methods for 16S rRNA and shotgun metagenomics

(1) The 16S rRNA gene is ubiquitous (Morgan and Huttenhower 2012) and necessary component of ribosomes translating mRNA. It presents in all bacteria and archaea (Kembel et al. 2012), whereas other commonly used marker genes are not distributed in all living organisms (Kuczynski et al. 2011). It is relatively unbiased to characterize bacterial and archaeal diversity. Although Woese and collaborators (Woese and Fox 1977; Woese et al. 1978) defined the domain Archaea more than 40 years ago, Archaea are still poorly studied with regards to their abundance and ecological role in nature (Gantner et al. 2011). Because of the advantage of 16S rRNA gene is its taxonomic coverage (Kembel et al. 2012), the domain of Archaea can be studied via 16S rRNA gene.

(2) The 16S rRNA gene contains highly conserved regions suitable for universal PCR primer design to amplify regions of interests (Schloss et al. 2011; Tyler et al. 2014). The property of highly conserved indicates that a life tree can be constructed to link together all known bacteria. It contains nine hypervariable (V) regions (V1–V9); the high variability is suitable as unique identifiers (Claesson et al. 2010) for fine level taxonomic classification. Currently, the segments of V1–V3, V4, and V4–V5 regions are most commonly used because research showed that each can provide genus-level sequence resolution, with

V1–V3 or the V1–V4 regions can provide more accurate estimates than others (Kim et al. 2011).

(3) Well-studied primer sets are available for amplifying most organisms with high specificity for bacteria (Lane et al. 1985; Weisburg et al. 1991; Sim et al. 2012). By choosing appropriate primer set according to the studied microbial community, the problem of PCR bias can be alleviated (Kuczynski et al. 2011). Using efficient computational algorithms, the chimeric reads can be readily detected (Edgar et al. 2011).

(4) Well-curated databases of reference sequences and taxonomies are available allowing sequence comparison and taxonomic assignment of organisms (Ashelford et al. 2005; Tyler et al. 2014). These databases include Ribosomal Database Project (RDP) (Cole et al. 2009), Greengenes (DeSantis et al. 2006), and SILVA (Pruesse et al. 2007).

(5) The 16S rRNA gene sequencing is also relatively cheap and simple with mature analysis pipelines.

Taken together, 16S rRNA-based sequencing remains the gold standard for sequence-based bacterial analyses. Thus, it routinely employed to profile the taxonomic content of the community.

1.3.2   Bioinformatic Analysis of 16S rRNA Sequencing Data

1.3.2.1   Processing of Samples, DNA and Library

The bioinformatic analysis of 16S rRNA sequencing starts with preparing biological samples and DNA extraction. Although variations exist, several general steps we should follow. We briefly summarize as below:

Sample Collection

Before the actual collection of the samples, we need to consider at least two things: what type of samples to be obtained and what methods to be used for collection. Depending on the specific experimental aims, the samples could be stool or tissue biopsy. The microbial profiles from these two kinds of samples may have substantial differences (Stearns et al. 2011). For collection methods, recommendations include always minimizing the level of invasiveness of the sampling procedure when designing a human study, considering recruiting barrier, and longitudinal design to detect the temporal variability of the microbial communities (Kuczynski et al. 2011). At sample collection period, a power analysis should be conducted to estimate how many samples are needed to provide sufficient power (e.g., 80%) to correctly conclude a difference between groups. We also need consider the methods of sample storage: snap frozen or preservative. DNA extractions on fresh and frozen samples can influence the structure of the microbiome, e.g., storage of samples at $-80\ °C$ versus immediate extraction of DNA from fresh samples affects the *Firmicutes* to *Bacteroidetes* ratio determined by downstream quantitative PCR analysis (Bahl et al. 2012). Although Human Microbiome Project has a recommendation manual of sample collection (NIH 2010; iHMP 2014), however, there is still no standard protocol regarding sample collection to guarantee the sample quality of microbiome data (Wu et al. 2018). We expect that researchers propose more new sample collection strategies or guidelines. For example, Vázquez-Baeza et al. recently discuss the guideline for longitudinal sampling in IBD cohorts (Vázquez-Baeza et al. 2017).

DNA Extraction

A few commercial or non-commercial kits, such as, QIAamp® DNA stool mini kit, Qiagen, FastDNA® kit, Bio 101; Nucleospin® C + T kit, Macherey-Nagal; Quantum Prep® Aquapure Genomic DNA isolation kit, Bio-Rad; and guanidium isothiocyanate/silica matrix method are available. However, which method is more effective for detecting bacterial DNA and leads to the best profile of the microbial community is still arguable (McOrist et al. 2002; Kuczynski et al. 2011) and currently no DNA extraction methods can provide a truly unbiased DNA sample (Ó Cuív et al. 2011; Yuan et al. 2012).

Library Preparation

To perform 16S rRNA sequencing, we need to prepare genomic libraries in which (fragments of) DNA or RNA molecules are fused with adapters (van Dijk et al. 2014). Then comparing genomic regions between experimental samples and reference data can be made to ensure accurately assign sequences to taxonomic groups. During library preparation, we consider which variable region of the 16S rRNA gene to be selected for sequencing (Tyler et al. 2014). As we described above, within the nine hypervariable regions, currently, the segments of V1–V3, V4, and V4–V5 regions are most commonly used.

1.3.2.2   DNA Sequencing and Quality Checking

DNA Sequencing

After DNA extraction, and library preparation, the next important step is to conduct DNA sequencing. Several next-generation sequencers are available for 16S rRNA sequencing. Among them, 454 pyrosequencing (Roche, Indianapolis, IN) and Illumina sequencing (San Diego, CA) are the commonly used sequencing technologies in microbiome studies. These two technologies offer different characteristics in levels of coverage, read length, sequence accuracy, usability, and cost, etc. (Kuczynski et al. 2011). For example, llumina sequencing can offer more coverage at a lower cost, whereas 454 pyrosequencing is able to generate longer sequences, and often increase taxonomic resolution (Tyler et al. 2014).

Quality Checking

Following sequencing, it is necessary to perform quality checking (QC). QC is referred to as pre-processing of raw sequencing reads prior to the subsequent analysis. There are two general purposes for QC: one is to improve the analysis accuracy (Schirmer et al. 2015; D'Amore et al. 2016) and another is to prevent an overestimation of the community taxa(e.g., species) diversity(Jünemann et al. 2017). Depending on the data and tools used, typically, QC includes:

(1) Detecting and removing artificial chimeric sequence. Chimeric DNA sequences often happen during PCR amplification, especially when sequencing single regions of 16S rRNA gene to estimate diversity or compare populations. Therefore, it is very critical to detect and remove chimeras to avoid confusing these undetected chimeras as novel species (Edgar et al. 2011; Edgar 2016).

(2) Filtering low quality sequences and short reads (Modolo and Lerat 2015; Jünemann et al. 2017).

(3) Denoising to reduce and correct error reads (Reeder and Knight 2010; Edgar and Flyvbjerg 2015).

Quality filtering and denoising will substantially improve the quality of sequences, thus minimizing inflation of diversity estimation and reducing spurious inferences of differences between populations.

1.3.2.3 Cluster 16S rRNA Sequences into OTUs

Two Approaches of Sequence Identification

Following quality filtering and denoising DNA sequences, to obtain datasets suitable for downstream statistical analyses, we need identify sequences by assigning them to taxonomic outcome groups.

Currently, two main approaches are phylotype-based and OTU-based methods (Schloss and Westcott 2011). As the names indicate, the phylotype-based methods directly group (i.e., assign) sequences based on their similarity to phylotypes (i.e., reference sequences), such as, assign a 16S rRNA gene sequence to the genus *Pseudomonas*; whereas OTU-based methods group sequences based on their similarity to operational taxonomic units (OTUs) (i.e., other sequences in the community).

Although phylotype-based methods have several appealing features, including easily linking a sequence to previously identified microbes, computational efficiency, and stable classification; however, the challenges with phylotype-based approach are critical: the success of assignment is highly contingent on sequencing platform and reference database (Tyler et al. 2014). For example, when reference databases are incomplete, it is impossible to analyze novel sequences detected in an experiment from previously unidentified taxonomic lineages (Schloss and Westcott 2011; Tyler et al. 2014).

OTU-based method does overcome most limitations of phylotype-based approach and has several advantages. However, it also has several limitations, such as, computationally intensive, relatively slow, and larger memory required, especially, the difficult choice of linkage method for clustering (Schloss and Westcott 2011). Currently, most published data in 16S rRNA gene sequences use OTU-based approach. Below, we will review the definition of OTU and reasons that this approach has been widely used for 16S rRNA gene sequencing studies.

Defining OTUs

An OTU is conventionally defined as containing sequences that are no more than 3% different from each other. The criterion of 3% is also used to define a species, while 5 and 20% differences are used to define genus, and phylum, respectively. Typically assigning the sequences with greater than 97% similarity to the same species, those with 95% similarity to the same genus, those with 90% similarity to the same family, and those with 80% similarity to the same phylum, although these distinctions are disputable (Stackebrandt and Goebel 1994; Bond 1995; Borneman and Triplett 1997; Hugenholtz et al. 1998; Everett et al. 1999; McCaig et al. 1999; Sait et al. 2002; Schloss and Handelsman 2004, 2005).

Why We Use OTU as Analysis Unit?

OTU has been considered an analysis unit as species level with the 16S-based sequence approach. An OTU is defined with more than 97% similarity of sequences. Thus, OTUs are sometimes considered equivalent to species. However, whether or not an OTU precisely defines a "unique" sequence remains a bioin-formatic challenge (Morgan and Huttenhower 2012). There are several related reasons:

First, these hierarchy cutoff values that are used to define the level of taxonomy have not been rigorously validated, they are simply from best fitted historical taxonomy with modern 16S rRNA gene sequencing (Schloss and Handelsman 2005). Second, OTUs are constructed independently from reference data, may contain species from multiple taxa; therefore they may not match well with true biological units (true species). Third, sample diversity estimated by OTUs has potential to be inflated (Schloss et al. 2011; Schloss and Westcott 2011; Tyler et al. 2014).

Recently gut microbiome researches have gone across OTU or species level into strain-level and try strain-level resolution to study intra-species variation, its functional role, and its relation to host health and diseases (Greenblum et al. 2015; Zhang and Zhao 2016; Ercolini 2017; Zhao et al. 2018).

Clustering to Obtain OTUs

The 97% similarity defined an OTU is a phylogenetic distance. In other words, OTUs are obtained from clustering and not from classification (Schloss and Westcott 2011). Clustering is a multivariate technique; it is used to group indi-viduals (e.g., in this case, sequences) according to relationships among the indi-viduals being grouped. The clustering algorithms commonly used in various disciplines (e.g., ecology, biology, psychology, sociology, economics) are nearest (i.e., single-linkage), furthest (i.e., complete linkage), average (i.e., average linkages), and weighted neighbor (i.e., using weighted-pair group method) (Everitt et al. 2011; Legendre and Legendre 2012). Same clustering algorithms are used to group sequences into OTU. Among them, the average neighbor algorithm was shown to produce more robust OTUs than other three algorithms (Schloss and Westcott 2011). For example, the bioinformatics tools DOTUR and MOTHUR (accelerated version of DOTUR) provide the capability to cluster sequences using either of the nearest neighbor, furthest neighbor, or average neighbor algorithms (Schloss and Handelsman 2005). QIIME uses clustering to obtain OTUs at a user-defined level of sequence similarity (e.g., 97% to approximate species-level phylotypes) through either referencing an OTU representative database (e.g., with BLAST), or purely using sequence similarity (e.g., using uclust, or mothur (Caporaso et al. 2010)). In such analysis, an OTU is generally thought of present a bacterial species (Kuczynski et al. 2012). These two OTU-based methods can both generate OTU tables to perform downstream statistical analyses.

1.3.2.4   Limitations of 16S rRNA Sequencing Approach

The 16S rRNA sequencing approach has numerous advantages, but it also has numerous disadvantages, including:

(1) Amplicon sequencing rRNA markers via PCR may miss detecting OTUs/taxa due to various biases associated with PCR, e.g., in priming and amplification (Sharpton et al. 2011; Logares et al. 2014; Sharpton 2014), which may result in substantially reducing microbial diversity in a community.
(2) 16S rRNA sequencing overestimates the community diversity or species abundance (Brown et al. 2015; Oulas et al. 2015) due to artificial sequences caused by sequencing errors and incorrectly assembled amplicons (i.e., chimeras), incorrectly assigning OTU, and the 16S locus being transferred between distantly related taxa (Acinas et al. 2004; Sharpton 2014), or variation of 16S copy number across most organisms (Kembel et al. 2012; Tyler et al. 2014). In addition, the overestimation is often difficult to identify (Wylie et al. 2012).
(3) Amplicon sequencing only discerns the taxonomic composition of the microbiome community. It cannot directly analyze the biological functions of associated taxa (Sharpton 2014).
(4) Amplicon sequencing can only analyze the taxa that taxonomically informative genetic markers are known and can be amplified. It is difficult to be used for analyzing novel or highly diverged microbes, especially viruses and fungi (Sharpton 2014).
(5) 16S rRNA sequencing approach lacks a golden standard for guiding decisions on quality control, filtering (Kembel et al. 2012), and statistical analysis and modeling (Xia and Sun 2017).

1.4   Shotgun Metagenomic Sequencing Approach

1.4.1   Definition of Metagenomics

Shotgun metagenomic sequencing is a powerful alternative to 16S rRNA sequencing for analyzing complex microbiome communities and avoids some of these limitations.

Metagenomics has been defined as "the genomic analysis of microorganisms by direct extraction and cloning of DNA from an assemblage of microorganisms" (Handelsman 2004) and a metagenome has been defined as "the entire genetic information of an ensemble of organisms, living in a common habitat" (Huson et al. 2007a, b).

The term "metagenomics is both a set of *research techniques*, comprising many related approaches and methods, and a *research field*." (National Research Council 2007) (p.13). In Greek, *meta* means "transcendent." As a research field, metage-nomics seeks to aggregately understand biology, go beyond the limits of the individual organism to "focus on the genes in the community and how genes might influence each other's activities in serving collective functions." Although indi-vidual organisms remain the research units, with metagenomics, the research will transcend individuals to focus on individuals and their genomes (National Research Council 2007) (p.13).

As a rapidly growing field of research, the aim of metagenomics is to understand the genetic diversity of a metagenome, the true diversity of microbes, their func-tions, cooperation and evolution with ideally, by identifying the (relative abun-dances of) species presented (Huson et al. 2007a, b; Huson et al. 2009). Although many other terms have been used to describe the study, "Metagenomics 2003" was used as the title of the first international conference held in Darmstadt,Germany (Riesenfeld et al. 2004).

In its approach, metagenomics refers to "computational methods that maximize understanding of the genetic composition and activities of communities" (National Research Council 2007) (p.13). Sometime, both targeted and random sequencing approaches are collectively called metagenomics (Huson et al. 2007a, b). However, most metagenomics often refers to whole-metagenome shotgun (WMS) sequencing of genomic DNA fragments from a community's metagenome (Handelsman 2001; Riesenfeld et al. 2004; Chen and Pachter 2005; Morgan and Huttenhower 2012), which exclude amplicon sequencing approach.

Metagenomic analyses have three basic tasks: taxonomic analysis, functional analysis and comparative analysis. These questions are also known as the "who are they?", "what can they do?", and "how to compare them?".

1.4.2   Advantages of Shotgun Metagenomic Sequencing

There is increasing interest in employing shotgun sequencing, rather than amplicon sequencing, to analyze microbiome samples. Because shotgun sequencing has several advantages:

(1) Shotgun metagenomics not only produces analysis data for generating hypotheses about the microbial community composition, but also provides a powerful tool to hypothesize microbial functions associated with different conditions, such as, health and disease, treatment and control, wild type and knockout. Given the functional profile, researchers can generate hypotheses on community dynamics and metabolic properties (Kuczynski et al. 2011).

In shotgun metagenomic sequencing, total DNA in a community is extracted and independently sequenced, which produces huge numbers of DNA reads that align to various genomic locations in the sample. The large available DNA reads, including non-microbes, can be sampled from taxonomically informative genomic loci (e.g., 16S), and from coding sequences (Sharpton 2014), providing insight into both microbial community structure and the functions encoded by the genomes of the microbiota (Wu and Lewis 2013). Thus, after obtaining shotgun metagenomic sequencing data, microbiome researchers can simultaneously explore two basic tasks of a microbiome study: who are they (which microorganisms are present within it) and what can they do (what each of them do)? There is an opportunity to fully characterize a community, including: (i) community composition/structure, i.e., taxonomic diversity and species relative abundance; (ii) each community member's genetic potential, including number of genes and their functionalities; (iii) intra-species and intra-population gene heterogeneity (Scholz et al. 2012; Ravin et al. 2015). Shotgun sequencing data can provide much richer data on both the organismal composition and the functional potential present in microbial communities, e.g., the metabolic potential of the community (Segata et al. 2013; Scholz et al. 2015) and characterize the genomic diversity and function of uncultured bacteria (Wrighton et al. 2012).

(2) The shotgun metagenomic sequencing is potentially unbiased (Lewandowska et al. 2015), so it has more chances to detect rare and novel viruses (Yozwiak et al. 2012; Bibby 2013; Relman 2013). It can also be used to characterize the abundance of other communities, such as, taxa and metabolic pathways (Morgan and Huttenhower 2012), plant microbiota (Vorholt 2012; Bulgarelli et al. 2013), proteins (Godzik 2011). All these highlight the validity of the approach to detect biological entities that lack ribosomal genes yet (Wu and Lewis 2013).

(3) The shotgun metagenomic sequencing approach has ability to discriminate strains of common species by gene content, which is not possible with 16S rRNA sequencing approach (Qin et al. 2010; Kuczynski et al. 2011).

1.4.3 Bioinformatic Analysis of Shotgun Metagenomic Data

Two approaches or strategies for analyzing WMS sequencing data are available: assembly-based and read-based metagenomics.

In assembly-based metagenomics, separate reads are first de novo assembled to contigs and then clustered into so-called genome bins during a binning process (Jünemann et al. 2017). Thereby, it is possible to conduct taxonomical classification and prediction of the discovered gene functions from a metagenomic sample (Ravin et al. 2015).

In read-based metagenomics, individual reads are classified with regard to taxonomy and function. Thus, it is suitable for analyzing the taxonomical composition, functions of the metagenome, and metabolic pathways (Scholz et al. 2012; Jünemann et al. 2017).

1.4.3.1 Processing of Samples, DNA and Library

Sampling

Sample processing is the first and most critical step in shotgun metagenomic sequencing studies, just like in 16S rRNA sequencing. The first element of sample processing is to convert the source nucleic acid material into a sequencing library. Typically, there are several steps:

First, to fragment long DNA or RNA molecules into a suitable size, then, to perform adapter addition. Next, to perform size selection to further enrich the desired size and to eliminate free adapters. Last, to perform PCR to select for molecules containing adapters at both ends and to generate sufficient quantities for sequencing (van Dijk et al. 2014).

The most challenges of library preparation may be the quantitative biases and the loss of material occurred during the preparation. To reduce the biases and loss of material, many algorithms have been developed and steps have been taken. The technology of direct sequencing of DNA or RNA molecules is available although it still has many challenges and limitations. In the application of this technology, we do not need library preparation or sequencing reagents. The interested readers can reference the review (van Dijk et al. 2014).

DNA Extraction

DNA extraction for metagenomic sequencing is not to target a specific genomic locus for amplification, instead it is to extract DNA from all cells in a sample (Sharpton 2014) and the obtained amounts of high-quality nucleic acids must be sufficient (Thomas et al. 2012). The resulted DNA sequence reads are aligned to various genomic locations for the myriad genomes present in the sample, including non-microbes, which can be sampled from 16S, and coding sequences that provide insight into the biological functions encoded in the genome. As a result, metagenomic data provide the opportunity to simultaneously explore two aspects of a microbial community: *who are there* and *what can they do*? (Sharpton 2014). Various robust methods for DNA extraction are available and different sample type requires specific protocols (Thomas et al. 2012).

1.4.3.2 Quality Checking

Quality Checking (QC) is important for whole metagenome shotgun (WMS) sequencing (Jünemann et al. 2017), although it is a more essential step used in 16S rRNA gene amplicon sequencing. QC in WMS sequencing shares most steps in 16S rRNA gene amplicon sequencing except for the steps specially with amplification related errors and artifacts because WMS sequencing is amplification free (Jünemann et al. 2017).

1.4.3.3 Assembly

Assembling short reads into longer, contiguous sequences ('contigs') (Staden 1979; Anderson 1981; Kunin et al. 2008) will make downstream bioinformatics analysis smoothly. There are two kinds of assemblies employed for metagenomics samples: reference-based assembly (co-assembly) and de novo assembly. Each strategy prefers to apply to biological purposes, as well as needs different effort, time and cost. The choice of using which one is based on these considerations.

Reference-based assembly performs well if the closely related reference genomes sequences are available in the metagenomic dataset; it performs poorly if the sample genome exists a large insertion, deletion, or polymorphisms, which makes the true genome of the sample different to the reference. Comparing reference-based assembly, de novo assembly typically requires larger computational resources. For example, the machines for this assembly require larger memory and run times.

How long the sequencing reads are appropriate for assembling metagenomic data? In general, long contiguous sequences not only benefits binning and classification of DNA fragments for phylogenetic or taxonomic assignment, but also make annotation easy (Thomas et al. 2012).

Many genome assemblers available for performing assembling (Jünemann et al. 2014, 2017); however, due to complexity and diversity of microbial communities, the current assembly tools have different overall performances. None of them is bias-free.

First, there are many technical problems, including: no references exist for comparing the assembling results, the complex population composition (Scholz et al. 2012), such as, large individual heterogeneity, and consequently, their genomic differences in the community, or low numbered genomes, either could challenge efficiently assembly reads into contigs, or assembled contigs only partially or limitedly represent the true genomes (Ravin et al. 2015). Second, assemblies are affected by the presence of closely related genomes. Because closely related genomes may represent genome-sized approximate repeats (Sczyrba et al. 2017). In addition, assemblies are also affected by sequencing depth. Most assemblers have limited rates of sequencing coverage; they cannot cover very-high-copy circular elements well (Sczyrba et al. 2017). Thus, the development of "metagenomic assemblers" is still at an early stage (Thomas et al. 2012).

1.4.3.4 Binning

Binning is defined as the process of sorting DNA sequences (also called reads, contigs or both) into groups that might represent an individual genome or genomes from closely related organisms (Kunin et al. 2008; Thomas et al. 2012). Mixtures of variable-length of sequence fragments originating from various organisms or individual genomes returned by contig assembly. It is a challenge for assembly to reconstruct entire genomes (Alneberg et al. 2014; Sczyrba et al. 2017). Thus, following by assembly, it is necessary to bin genome fragments.

Based on the used information, several binning algorithms have been developed. The most used ones are compositional-based binning, and purely similarity-based binning (Thomas et al. 2012). The mixture algorithms also exist, such as using both composition and similarity binning, e.g., self-organizing maps, and hierarchical clustering (Thomas et al. 2012), by coverage and composition (Alneberg et al. 2014).

Because organisms or genomes have conserved nucleotide composition, this will be reflected in sequence fragments of the genomes organisms (Thomas et al. 2012). Compositional binning algorithms are based on this fact. For example, different organisms or genomes have a certain GC or the particular abundance distribution of k-mers (Strous et al. 2012; Alneberg et al. 2014).

Unlike compositional binning, similarity-based binning uses the similarity of the gene with known genes in a reference database to classify and hence bin the sequence (Thomas et al. 2012) because the unknown DNA fragment might encode for a gene.

Both genome and taxonomic binning tools are available. Different tools have varying performances in recovering individual genome (for genome binning), sample assignment accuracy, average taxon bin completeness and purity (for taxonomic binning), analysis of low-abundance taxa (Sczyrba et al. 2017). Binning still has many challenges:

First, short reads negatively affect both composition-based and similarity-based binning. Generally, composition-based binning is not reliable for short reads, as they do not contain enough information (Thomas et al. 2012). Similarity-based binning is affected by short sequence reads. Because the short sequence reads could result in that the query sequence is only distantly related to known reference genomes (Thomas et al. 2012). If this happens, only genomes at larger taxonomic distances i.e., a very high level (e.g., phylum) of taxon can be assigned (Thomas et al. 2012; Sczyrba et al. 2017), whereas the binning contigs into a low level of taxa (e.g., species) is very challenge (Alneberg et al. 2014) if it is not possible. Second, the "chimeric" bins can be produced if the metagenomic dataset contains two or more genomes that would fall into this high taxon assignment (Thomas et al. 2012). In addition, deconvoluting strain-level diversity is challenge. It requires large samples for satisfactory performance (Sczyrba et al. 2017).

1.4.3.5 Annotation

Genome and Metagenome Functional Annotations

To gain insights beyond taxonomic composition, the sequences need to be annotated. Depending on the objective of the study, annotation can be performed on assembled contigs or unassembled reads or short contigs (Thomas et al. 2012). The former is called genome annotation and the latter is referred to as metagenome functional annotation. Many tools are available for genome annotation, such as RAST (Aziz et al. 2008), IMG (Markowitz et al. 2009). To be successfully annotated, the genome, contigs are required to be long enough.

Gene Prediction and Functional Annotation

Metagenome functional annotation of metagenomic sequences generally has two non-mutually exclusive steps: gene prediction and annotation (Sharpton 2014).

Gene prediction refers to the procedure of identifying genes of interest, protein and RNA sequences coded on the sample DNA; i.e., labeling sequences as genes or genomic elements. Functional annotation of metagenomic datasets, is to assign putative gene functions and taxonomic neighbors (Kunin et al. 2008; Thomas et al. 2012). It is very similar to genome annotation and relies on comparisons of predicted genes to existing, previously annotated sequences (Kunin et al. 2008; Scholz et al. 2012; Thomas et al. 2012).

The metagenome functional annotation targets the entire community. Thus, the tools for genome annotation have limited usage. There are many specifically developed tools for metagenome functional annotation (Kunin et al. 2008).

Many tools are available for gene prediction and functional annotation, and some of them perform well. However, less than half of metagenomic sequences can be annotated (Gilbert et al. 2010; Thomas et al. 2012) because:

(1) Gene prediction and especially functional annotation rely on comparisons to existing databases. However, both short length of metagenomic coding sequences and evolutionary distance result in low similarity to known sequences. In addition, there is no existing database to compare similarities to novel genes. Thus, both low similarity and the presence of sequence errors prevent the identification of homologs. Because novel genes without

similarities in existing databases, gene prediction and functional annotation will completely ignore them (Kunin et al. 2008).

(2) Prediction and annotation of proteins are complicated. Proteins are often fragmented and lack neighborhood context. It is even more complicated to annotate the proteins created by short-read methods, such as 454/Roche since most reads contain only fractions of proteins (Kunin et al. 2008).

(3) The biological importance of gene functions cannot be exactly understood if the gene functions are differentially represented in different communities (Kuczynski et al. 2011).

1.4.3.6 Challenges of Analyzing Shotgun Metagenomic Data

Despite aforementioned advantages, compared to targeted amplicon studies, bioinformatic analysis of shotgun metagenomic data still has challenges. First, the process of shotgun metagenomic data, including assembly, binning, gene prediction and annotation, has many technical challenges. Second, the data sets generated by metagenomic sequencing are large and complex, containing unwanted host DNA, and vulnerable to contamination. These make the bioinformatic analysis very complicated (Sharpton 2014). For example, the large and complex data make it difficult to determine the genome from which a read was derived, pose computational problems, challenge sequence alignment (Schloss and Handelsman 2008; Sharpton et al. 2011; Sharpton 2014). Thus, the unwanted host DNA needs developing molecular and bioinformatic methods to filter (Garcia-Garcerà et al. 2013; Sharpton 2014). Identifying and removing the contaminated metagenomic sequences is especially problematic, and requires particular tools to identify and filter (Schmieder and Edwards 2011). Third, the large metagenomic data sets pose even more challenges to identify the significantly different taxa between communities (Kuczynski et al. 2011). Finally, the cost of whole-genome sequencing is still high, especially in complex communities or when host DNA greatly outnumbers microbial DNA(Sharpton 2014).

1.5 Bioinformatics Data Analysis Tools

Many tools for bioinformatics data analysis have been developed to conduct 16S rRNA sequencing and shotgun metagenomic sequencing analyses. Here we briefly introduce two analysis tools for 16S rRNA sequencing data.

The widely used software packages are Quantitative Insights Into Microbial Ecology (QIIME) (Caporaso et al. 2010) (http://www.qiime.org) and mothur (Schloss et al. 2009) (http://www.mothur.org). Both packages are open source and have online tutorials and forums. They are all self-contained pipelines that can be used to analyze 16S rRNA gene sequencing data from raw sequence reads to generate OTU/abundance table, enable comparison of multiple samples and employ the use of the SILVA 16S rRNA gene reference database (Plummer et al. 2015). Due to their comprehensive features and support documentation, QIIME and mothur were reviewed as the two outstanding pipelines (Nilakanta et al. 2014). QIIME 2 was available in 2018; it is a complete redesigned and rewritten version of the QIIME microbiome analysis pipeline (https://docs.qiime2.org/2018.6/about/).

1.5.1 QIIME

QIIME is an open source bioinformatics tool designed to provide a pipeline for the process of analyzing 16S rRNA data. QIIME was developed by Knight's lab (Caporaso et al. 2010). This software is designed for the analysis of microbial ecological communities, and can be used for bacterial, archaeal, fungal, or viral sequence data (Kuczynski et al. 2012). QIIME analysis generally starts with raw sequence data (in FASTA format) from any sequencing technology, such as Illumina HiSeq, MiSeq, or 454 pyrosequencing (Kuczynski et al. 2012). QIIME scripts primarily wrap other software packages. It is implemented as a collection of command-line scripts designed to take users from raw sequence data and sample metadata through publication-quality graphics and statistics. It can analyze high-throughput data in a wide variety of ways.

1.5.2 mothur

"mothur" was initiated by Schloss and his software development team in the Department of Microbiology of Immunology at the University of Michigan. It is released in 2009 (Schloss et al. 2009). The same quality control parameters used in QIIME were used in "mothur". It is an open source software package, a command-line computer program for analyzing sequence data from microbial communities. The package is frequently used in the analysis of DNA from uncultured microbes and offers the ability to go from raw sequences to the generation of visualization tools to describe alpha and beta diversity. In any sort of phylogenetic or genotype-based community analysis, group (cluster) sequences into collections of related sequences, called *genotypes* is the first step. Most frequently, mothur was used to cluster sequences and mothur is capable of processing data generated from several DNA sequencing methods including 454 pyrosequencing, Illumina HiSeq and MiSeq, Sanger, PacBio, and IonTorrent. Thus, mothur is one of the most cited bioinformatics tool for analyzing 16S rRNA gene sequences.

1.5.3   Analyzing 16S rRNA Sequence Data Using QIIME and Mothur

In analyzing 16S rRNA gene sequence data, QIIME and mothur share many capabilities and themes, for example, quality control, clustering, classification or assigning taxonomy. Mothur has a unique step in which all sequences must be aligned to a template database and any sequences which do not overlap in the same space are removed from the analysis. Generally, QIIME and mothur conduct 16S rRNA gene sequence data analysis using following steps.

Step 1   *Quality Control or Quality Filtering.*

16S rRNA gene analysis generally begins with data pre-processing to remove or filter low number of sequences. QIIME and mothur can perform quality control or quality filtering, which is an essential step of bioinformatical analysis.

Step 2   *Pick OTUs and Assign Representative Sequences.*

The next step is OTU clustering: to pick OTUs. The most common method in QIIME is a program called uclust (Werner 2014). The OTUs are grouped based on a user-defined level of sequence similarity (e.g., 97% to approximate species-level phylotypes). The uclust and mothur perform OTU clustering purely based on sequence similarity (Caporaso et al. 2010).

OTU-picking followed by assigning representative OTU sequences into taxonomic levels (de novo OTU picking), such as family, genus, and species, by changing the sequence similarity threshold. However, to accurately assign sequences to taxonomic levels, comparison of genomic regions between experimental samples and reference data is required (Tyler et al. 2014), which is known as reference-based OTU clustering (or picking). A taxonomic identification is made by comparing the OTUs to a reference database and assigns each OTU a unique identification number (Edgar 2010; Cole et al. 2014).

Step 3   *Build OTU or Taxonomy Table.*

OTU or taxonomy table can be obtained via either QIIME or mothur. OTU table is sample by observation matrix, typically row with OTUs and columns with samples; taxonomy table typically row with OTUs and columns with taxonomy: domain, phylum, class, order, family, and genus. The number of OTUs can often be inflated for a variety of reasons. Thus, to ensure the reported number of OTUs correctly, the obtained OTU table often need to be filtered (Quince et al. 2011).

Bioinformatic analysis of 16S rRNA gene sequencing data ends with OTU table and/or Taxonomy Table. However, many tools were developed with the capabilities not only performing bioinformatic analysis, but also directly conducting basic statistical analysis. For example, QIIME can also calculate alpha and beta diversities, implement statistical tests, and visualize data (Zhang et al. 2013; Werner 2014).

1.6 Summary

In this chapter, we first briefly introduced microbiome definition, concept, phylogenetics and metagenomics, which provided the basic knowledge of microbiome study. We then comprehensively reviewed DNA Sequencing, especially the next-generation sequencing techniques; and focused on introducing both 16S rRNA sequencing and shotgun metagenomic sequencing approaches. In addition, we introduced two most commonly used bioinformatics data analysis tools: QIIME and mothur. After reading this chapter, the readers should have some basic understanding on how microbiome study is about, where and how microbiome data come from. In Chap. 2, we will introduce and describe in details the microbiome dataset structures and characteristics.

References

Acinas, S.G., L.A. Marcelino, et al. 2004. Divergence and redundancy of 16S rRNA sequences in genomes with multiple rrn operons. *Journal of Bacteriology* 186 (9): 2629–2635.

Alneberg, J., B.S. Bjarnason, et al. 2014. Binning metagenomic contigs by coverage and composition. *Nature Methods* 11: 1144.

Anderson, S. 1981. Shotgun DNA sequencing using cloned DNase I-generated fragments. *Nucleic Acids Research* 9 (13): 3015–3027.

Arrieta, M.-C., L.T. Stiemsma, et al. 2014. The intestinal microbiome in early life: Health and disease. *Frontiers in Immunology* 5: 427.

Ashelford, K.E., N.A. Chuzhanova, et al. 2005. At least 1 in 20 16S rRNA sequence records currently held in public repositories is estimated to contain substantial anomalies. *Applied and Environmental Microbiology* 71 (12): 7724–7736.

Aziz, R.K., D. Bartels, et al. 2008. The RAST server: Rapid annotations using subsystems technology. *BMC Genomics* 9.

Bahl, M.I., A. Bergström, et al. 2012. Freezing fecal samples prior to DNA extraction affects the Firmicutes to Bacteroidetes ratio determined by downstream quantitative PCR analysis. *FEMS Microbiology Letters* 329 (2): 193–197.

Bibby, K. 2013. Metagenomic identification of viral pathogens. *Trends in Biotechnology* 31 (5): 275–279.

Bond, P.L. 1995. Bacterial community structures of phosphate-removing and non-phosphate-removing activated sludges from sequencing batch reactors. *Applied and Environment Microbiology* 61: 1910–1916.

Borneman, J., and E.W. Triplett. 1997. Molecular microbial diversity in soils from eastern Amazonia: Evidence for unusual microorganisms and microbial population shifts associated with deforestation. *Applied and Environmental Microbiology* 63 (7): 2647–2653.

Brown, S.P., A.M. Veach, et al. 2015. Scraping the bottom of the barrel: Are rare high throughput sequences artifacts? *Fungal Ecology* 13: 221–225.

Bulgarelli, D., K. Schlaeppi, et al. 2013. Structure and functions of the bacterial microbiota of plants. *Annual Review of Plant Biology* 64 (1): 807–838.

Caporaso, J.G., J. Kuczynski, et al. 2010. QIIME allows analysis of high-throughput community sequencing data. *Nature Methods* 7: 335.

Chen, K., and L. Pachter. 2005. Bioinformatics for whole-genome shotgun sequencing of microbial communities. *PLoS Computational Biology* 1 (2): e24.

Claesson, M.J., Q. Wang, et al. 2010. Comparison of two next-generation sequencing technologies for resolving highly complex microbiota composition using tandem variable 16S rRNA gene regions. *Nucleic Acids Research* 38 (22): 29.

Cole, J.R., Q. Wang, et al. 2009. The ribosomal database project: Improved alignments and new tools for rRNA analysis. *Nucleic Acids Research* 37(Database issue): D141–D145.

Cole, J.R., Q. Wang, et al. 2014. Ribosomal Database Project: Data and tools for high throughput rRNA analysis. *Nucleic Acids Research* 42 (D1): D633–D642.

D'Amore, R., U.Z. Ijaz, et al. 2016. A comprehensive benchmarking study of protocols and sequencing platforms for 16S rRNA community profiling. *BMC Genomics* 17 (55): 015–2194.

DeSantis, T.Z., P. Hugenholtz, N. Larsen, M. Rojas, E.L. Brodie, K. Keller, T. Huber, D. Dalevi, P. Hu and G.L.Andersen. 2006. Greengenes, a Chimera-Checked 16S rRNA Gene Database and Workbench Compatible withARB. 72 (7): 5069–5072.

DiGiulio, D.B. 2012. Diversity of microbes in amniotic fluid. *Seminars in Fetal and Neonatal Medicine* 17 (1): 2–11.

DiGiulio, D.B., R. Romero, et al. 2008. Microbial prevalence, diversity and abundance in amniotic fluid during preterm labor: A molecular and culture-based investigation. *PLoS ONE* 3 (8): e3056.

Eckburg, P.B., E.M. Bik, et al. 2005. Diversity of the human intestinal microbial flora. *Science* 308 (5728): 1635–1638.

Edgar, R.C. 2010. Search and clustering orders of magnitude faster than BLAST. *Bioinformatics* 26.

Edgar, R. 2016. UCHIME2: Improved chimera prediction for amplicon sequencing. *bioRxiv*.

Edgar, R.C., and H. Flyvbjerg. 2015. Error filtering, pair assembly and error correction for next-generation sequencing reads. *Bioinformatics* 31 (21): 3476–3482.

Edgar, R.C., B.J. Haas, et al. 2011. UCHIME improves sensitivity and speed of chimera detection. *Bioinformatics* 27 (16): 2194–2200.

Ercolini, D. 2017. Exciting strain-level resolution studies of the food microbiome. *Microbial Biotechnology* 10 (1): 54–56.

Everett, K.D., R.M. Bush, et al. 1999. Emended description of the order Chlamydiales, proposal of Parachlamydiaceae fam. nov. and Simkaniaceae fam. nov., each containing one monotypic genus, revised taxonomy of the family Chlamydiaceae, including a new genus and five new species, and standards for the identification of organisms. *International Journal of Systematic Bacteriology* 2: 415–440.

Everitt, Brian S., Sabine Landau, et al. 2011. *Cluster analysis*. Chichester: Wiley.

Gantner, S., A. F. Andersson, L. Alonso-Sáez and S. Bertilsson (2011). Novel primers for 16S rRNA-basedarchaeal community analyses in environmental samples. *Journal of Microbiological Methods* 84 (1): 12–18.

Garcia-Garcerà, M., K. Garcia-Etxebarria, et al. 2013. A new method for extracting skin microbes allows metagenomic analysis of whole-deep skin. *PLoS ONE* 8 (9): e74914.

Gilbert, J.A., D. Field, et al. 2010. The taxonomic and functional diversity of microbes at a temperate coastal site: A 'multi-omic' study of seasonal and diel temporal variation. *PLoS ONE* 5 (11): 0015545.

Godzik, A. 2011. Metagenomics and the protein universe. *Current Opinion in Structural Biology* 21 (3): 398–403.

Goodrich, Julia K., Sara C. Di Rienzi, et al. 2014. Conducting a microbiome study. *Cell* 158 (2): 250–262.

Greenblum, S., R. Carr, et al. 2015. Extensive strain-level copy-number variation across human gut microbiome species. *Cell* 160 (4): 583–594.

Handelsman, J. 2001. *Metagenomics and microbial communities*. New York: Wiley.

Handelsman, J. 2004. Metagenomics: Application of genomics to uncultured microorganisms. *Microbiology and Molecular Biology Reviews* 68 (4): 669–685.

Heather, J.M., and B. Chain. 2016. The sequence of sequencers: The history of sequencing DNA. *Genomics* 107 (1): 1–8.

Holley, R.W., J. Apgar, et al. 1965. Structure of a ribonucleic acid. *Science* 147 (3664): 1462–1465.

Hollmer, M. 2013. Roche to close 454 life sciences as it reduces gene sequencing focus. *Fierce Biotechnology*.

Hugenholtz, P., B.M. Goebel, et al. 1998. Impact of culture-independent studies on the emerging phylogenetic view of bacterial diversity. *Journal of Bacteriology* 180 (18): 4765–4774.

Huson, D.H., A.F. Auch, et al. 2007. MEGAN analysis of metagenomic data. *Genome Research* 17 (3): 377–386.

Huson, D.H., A.F. Auch, et al. 2007. Metagenome analysis using MEGAN. In *Proceedings of the 5th Asia-Pacific Bioinformatics Conference, Volume 5 of Series on Advances in Bioinformatics and Computational Biology*, ed. D. Sankoff, L. Wang, and F. Chin.

Huson, D.H., D.C. Richter, et al. 2009. Methods for comparative metagenomics. *BMC Bioinformatics* 10 (1): S12.

iHMP 2014. The integrative human microbiome project: Dynamic analysis of microbiome-host omics profiles during periods of human health and disease. *Cell Host Microbe* 16(3): 276–289.

Jimenez, E., L. Fernandez, et al. 2005. Isolation of commensal bacteria from umbilical cord blood of healthy neonates born by cesarean section. *Current Microbiology* 51 (4): 270–274.

Jiménez, E., M.L. Marín, et al. 2008. Is meconium from healthy newborns actually sterile? *Research in Microbiology* 159 (3): 187–193.

Jünemann, S., K. Prior, et al. 2014. GABenchToB: A genome assembly benchmark tuned on bacteria and benchtop sequencers. *PLoS ONE* 9 (9): e107014.

Jünemann, S., N. Kleinbölting, et al. 2017. Bioinformatics for NGS-based metagenomics and the application to biogas research. *Journal of Biotechnology* 261: 10–23.

Kembel, S.W., M. Wu, et al. 2012. Incorporating 16S gene copy number information improves estimates of microbial diversity and abundance. *PLoS Computational Biology* 8 (10): e1002743.

Kim, M., M. Morrison, et al. 2011. Evaluation of different partial 16S rRNA gene sequence regions for phylogenetic analysis of microbiomes. *Journal of Microbiol Methods* 84 (1): 81–87.

Kuczynski, J., C.L. Lauber, et al. 2011. Experimental and analytical tools for studying the human microbiome. *Nature Reviews Genetics* 13: 47.

Kuczynski, J., J. Stombaugh, et al. 2012. Using QIIME to analyze 16S rRNA gene sequences from microbial communities. *Current Protocols in Microbiology* 1: Unit-1E.5.

Kunin, V., A. Copeland, et al. 2008. A bioinformatician's guide to metagenomics. *Microbiology and Molecular Biology Reviews: MMBR* 72 (4): 557–578.

Lane, D.J., B. Pace, et al. 1985. Rapid determination of 16S ribosomal RNA sequences for phylogenetic analyses. *Proceedings of the National Academy of Sciences of the United States of America* 82 (20): 6955–6959.

Lederberg J., and A. McCray. 2001. Ome sweet omics: a genealogical treasury of words. *The Scientist* 15: 8

Legendre, P., and L. Legendre. 2012. *Numerical ecology*. Amsterdam: Elsevier.

Lewandowska, D.W., O. Zagordi, et al. 2015. Unbiased metagenomic sequencing complements specific routine diagnostic methods and increases chances to detect rare viral strains. *Diagnostic Microbiology and Infectious Disease* 83 (2): 133–138.

Ley, R.E., D.A. Peterson, et al. 2006. Ecological and evolutionary forces shaping microbial diversity in the human intestine. *Cell* 124 (4): 837–848.

Liu, L., Y. Li, et al. 2012. Comparison of next-generation sequencing systems. *Journal of Biomedicine and Biotechnology* 2012: 11.

Logares, R., S. Sunagawa, et al. 2014. Metagenomic 16S rDNA Illumina tags are a powerful alternative to amplicon sequencing to explore diversity and structure of microbial communities. *Environmental Microbiology* 16 (9): 2659–2671.

Mackie, R.I., A. Sghir, et al. 1999. Developmental microbial ecology of the neonatal gastrointestinal tract. *American Journal of Clinical Nutrition* 69 (5): 1035S–1045S.

Madan, J.C., R.C. Salari, et al. 2012. Gut microbial colonisation in premature neonates predicts neonatal sepsis. *Archives of Disease in Childhood. Fetal and Neonatal Edition* 97 (6): F456–F462.

Margulies, M., M. Egholm, et al. 2005. Genome sequencing in open microfabricated high density picoliter reactors. *Nature* 437 (7057): 376–380.

Markowitz, V.M., K. Mavromatis, et al. 2009. IMG ER: A system for microbial genome annotation expert review and curation. *Bioinformatics* 25 (17): 2271–2278.

Matamoros, S., C. Gras-Leguen, et al. 2013. Development of intestinal microbiota in infants and its impact on health. *Trends in Microbiology* 21 (4): 167–173.

McCaig, A.E., L.A. Glover, et al. 1999. Molecular analysis of bacterial community structure and diversity in unimproved and improved upland grass pastures. *Applied and Environment Microbiology* 65 (4): 1721–1730.

McOrist, A.L., M. Jackson, et al. 2002. A comparison of five methods for extraction of bacterial DNA from human faecal samples. *Journal of Microbiological Methods* 50 (2): 131–139.

Metzker, M.L. 2005. Emerging technologies in DNA sequencing. *Genome Research* 15 (12): 1767–1776.

Metzker, M.L. 2010. Sequencing technologies—the next generation. *Nature Reviews Genetics* 11 (1): 31–46.

Modolo, L., and E. Lerat. 2015. UrQt: An efficient software for the unsupervised quality trimming of NGS data. *BMC Bioinformatics* 16 (1): 137.

Morgan, X.C., and C. Huttenhower. 2012. Human microbiome analysis. *PLOS Computational Biology* 8(12): e1002808.

National Research Council. 2007. *The new science of metagenomics: Revealing the secrets of our microbial planet*. Washington, DC: The National Academies Press.

NIH. 2010. Human microbiome project—core microbiome sampling protocol A. HMP Initiative 1: Core Microbiome Sampling Protocol A Version 9.0, 29 Mar 2010 (HMP Protocol Number: HMP-07-001).

Nilakanta, H., K.L. Drews, et al. 2014. A review of software for analyzing molecular sequences. *BMC Research Notes* 7 (1): 830.

Oulas, A., C. Pavloudi, et al. 2015. Metagenomics: Tools and insights for analyzing next-generation sequencing data derived from biodiversity studies. *Bioinformatics and Biology Insights* 9: 75–88.

Ó Cuív, P., C.D. Aguirre de Carcer, et al. 2011. The effects from DNA extraction methods on the evaluation of microbial diversity associated with human colonic tissue. *Microbial Ecology* 61(2): 353–362.

Penders, J., C. Thijs, et al. 2006. Factors influencing the composition of the intestinal microbiota in early infancy. *Pediatrics* 118 (2): 511–521.

Plummer, E, J. Twin, D.M. Bulach, S.M. Garland, and S.N. Tabrizi. 2015. A comparison of three bioinformatics pipelines for the analysis of preterm Gut Microbiota using 16S rRNA gene sequencing data. *Journal of Proteomics & Bioinformatics* 8: 283–291.

Pruesse, E., C. Quast, K. Knittel, B.M. Fuchs, W. Ludwig, J. Peplies and F.O. Glöckner. 2007. SILVA: acomprehensive online resource for quality checked and aligned ribosomal RNA sequence data compatible withARB. *Nucleic Acids Research* 35 (21): 7188–7196.

Qin, J., R. Li, et al. 2010. A human gut microbial gene catalogue established by metagenomic sequencing. *Nature* 464: 59.

Quince, C., A. Lanzen, et al. 2011. Removing noise from pyrosequenced amplicons. *BMC Bioinformatics* 12 (1): 38.

Ravin, N.V., A.V. Mardanov, et al. 2015. Metagenomics as a tool for the investigation of uncultured microorganisms. *Russian Journal of Genetics* 51 (5): 431–439.

Reeder, J., and R. Knight. 2010. Rapidly denoising pyrosequencing amplicon reads by exploiting rank-abundance distributions. *Nature Methods* 7(9): 668–669. https://doi.org/10.1038/nmeth0910-668b.

Relman, D.A. 2013. Metagenomics, infectious disease diagnostics, and outbreak investigations: Sequence first, ask questions later? *JAMA* 309 (14): 1531–1532.

Riesenfeld, C.S., P.D. Schloss, et al. 2004. Metagenomics: Genomic analysis of microbial communities. *Annual Review of Genetics* 38 (1): 525–552.

Sait, M., P. Hugenholtz, et al. 2002. Cultivation of globally distributed soil bacteria from phylogenetic lineages previously only detected in cultivation-independent surveys. *Environmental Microbiology* 4 (11): 654–666.

Sanger, F., G.G. Brownlee, et al. 1965. A two-dimensional fractionation procedure for radioactive nucleotides. *Journal of Molecular Biology* 13(2): 373–374.

Sanger, F., and A.R. Coulson. 1975. A rapid method for determining sequences in DNA by primed synthesis with DNA polymerase. *Journal of Molecular Biology* 94 (3): 441–448.

Sanger, F., S. Nicklen, et al. 1977. DNA sequencing with chain-terminating inhibitors. *Proceedings of National Academic Science United States of America* 74 (12): 5463–5467.

Schadt, E.E., S. Turner, et al. 2010. A window into third-generation sequencing. *Human Molecular Genetics* 19 (R2): 21.

Schirmer, M., U.Z. Ijaz, et al. 2015. Insight into biases and sequencing errors for amplicon sequencing with the Illumina MiSeq platform. *Nucleic Acids Research* 43 (6): 13.

Schloss, P.D., and J. Handelsman. 2004. Status of the microbial census. *Microbiology and Molecular Biology Reviews* 68 (4): 686–691.

Schloss, P.D., and J. Handelsman. 2005. Introducing DOTUR, a computer program for defining operational taxonomic units and estimating species richness. *Applied and Environment Microbiology* 71 (3): 1501–1506.

Schloss, P.D., and J. Handelsman. 2008. A statistical toolbox for metagenomics: Assessing functional diversity in microbial communities. *BMC Bioinformatics* 9 (1): 34.

Schloss, P.D., and S.L. Westcott. 2011. Assessing and improving methods used in operational taxonomic unit-based approaches for 16S rRNA gene sequence analysis. *Applied and Environment Microbiology* 77 (10): 3219–3226.

Schloss, P.D., S.L. Westcott, et al. 2009. Introducing mothur: Open-source, platform-independent, community-supported software for describing and comparing microbial communities. *Applied and Environment Microbiology* 75 (23): 7537–7541.

Schloss, P.D., D. Gevers, et al. 2011. Reducing the effects of PCR amplification and sequencing artifacts on 16S rRNA-based studies. *PLoS ONE* 6 (12): e27310.

Schmieder, R., and R. Edwards. 2011. Fast identification and removal of sequence contamination from genomic and metagenomic datasets. *PLoS ONE* 6 (3): e17288.

Scholz, M.B., C.-C. Lo, et al. 2012. Next generation sequencing and bioinformatic bottlenecks: The current state of metagenomic data analysis. *Current Opinion in Biotechnology* 23 (1): 9–15.

Scholz, M., A. Tett, et al. 2015. Computational tools for taxonomic microbiome profiling of shotgun metagenomes A2. In *Metagenomics for microbiology*, ed. I. Jacques and M.C. Rivera, 67–80. Oxford: Academic Press.

Sczyrba, A., P. Hofmann, et al. 2017. Critical assessment of metagenome interpretation—a benchmark of computational metagenomics software. *bioRxiv*.

Segata, N., D. Boernigen, et al. 2013. Computational meta'omics for microbial community studies. *Molecular Systems Biology* 9(1).

Sender, R., S. Fuchs and R. Milo. 2016. Revised estimates for the number of human and bacteria cells inthe body. *PLOS Biology* 14 (8): e1002533.

Sharpton, T.J. 2014. An introduction to the analysis of shotgun metagenomic data. *Frontiers in Plant Science* 5(209).

Sharpton, T.J., S.J. Riesenfeld, et al. 2011. PhylOTU: A high-throughput procedure quantifies microbial community diversity and resolves novel taxa from metagenomic data. *PLoS Computational Biology* 7 (1): e1001061.

Sim, K., M.J. Cox, et al. 2012. Improved detection of bifidobacteria with optimised 16S rRNA-Gene Based Pyrosequencing. *PLoS ONE* 7 (3): e32543.

Stackebrandt, E., and B.M. Goebel. 1994. *Taxonomic Note: A Place for DNA-DNA Reassociation and 16 s rRNA Sequence Analysis in the Present Species Definition in Bacteriology.*

Staden, R. 1979. A strategy of DNA sequencing employing computer programs. *Nucleic Acids Research* 6 (7): 2601–2610.

Stearns, J.C., M.D.J. Lynch, et al. 2011. Bacterial biogeography of the human digestive tract. *Scientific Reports* 1: 170.

Strous, M., B. Kraft, et al. 2012. The binning of metagenomic contigs for microbial physiology of mixed cultures. *Frontiers in Microbiology* 3: 410.

Sun, J., and P.K. Dudeja. 2018. Introduction. In *Mechanisms underlying host-microbiome interactions in pathophysiology of human diseases*, ed. J. Sun and P.K. Dudeja. New York: Springer.

Thomas, T., J. Gilbert, et al. 2012. Metagenomics—A guide from sampling to data analysis. *Microbial Informatics and Experimentation* 2 (1): 3.

Tyler, A.D., M.I. Smith, et al. 2014. Analyzing the human microbiome: A "How To" guide for physicians. *The American Journal of Gastroenterology* 109: 983.

Ursell, L.K., J.L. Metcalf, et al. 2012. Defining the human microbiome. *Nutrition Reviews* 70 (Suppl 1): S38–S44.

van Dijk, E.L., H. Auger, et al. 2014a. Ten years of next-generation sequencing technology. *Trends in Genetics* 30 (9): 418–426.

van Dijk, E.L., Y. Jaszczyszyn, et al. 2014b. Library preparation methods for next-generation sequencing: Tone down the bias. *Experimental Cell Research* 322 (1): 12–20.

Vázquez-Baeza, Y., A. Gonzalez, et al. 2017. Guiding longitudinal sampling in IBD cohorts. *Gut.*

Vorholt, J.A. 2012. Microbial life in the phyllosphere. *Nature Reviews Microbiology* 10 (12): 828–840.

Watson, J.D., and F.H. Crick. 1953. Molecular structure of nucleic acids; a structure for deoxyribose nucleic acid. *Nature* 171 (4356): 737–738.

Weisburg, W.G., S.M. Barns, et al. 1991. 16S ribosomal DNA amplification for phylogenetic study. *Journal of Bacteriology* 173 (2): 697–703.

Werner, J. 2014. *QIIME Overview Tutorial.*

Whitman, W.B., D.C. Coleman, et al. 1998. Prokaryotes: The unseen majority. *Proceedings of the National Academic Science United States of America* 95 (12): 6578–6583.

Wiley, E.O., and B.S. Lieberman. 2011. *Phylogenetics: Theory and practice of phylogenetic systematics*. Hoboken: Wiley-Blackwell.

Woese, C.R., and G.E. Fox. 1977. Phylogenetic structure of the prokaryotic domain: The primary kingdoms. *Proceedings of the National Academy of Sciences of the United States of America* 74 (11): 5088–5090.

Woese, C.R., L.J. Magrum, et al. 1978. Archaebacteria. *Journal of Molecular Evolution* 11 (3): 245–251.

Woese, C.R., O. Kandler, et al. 1990. Towards a natural system of organisms: Proposal for the domains Archaea, Bacteria, and Eucarya. *Proceedings of the National Academy of Sciences* 87 (12): 4576–4579.

Wommack, K.E., J. Bhavsar, et al. 2008. Metagenomics: Read length matters. *Applied and Environment Microbiology* 74 (5): 1453–1463.

Wrighton, K.C., B.C. Thomas, et al. 2012. Fermentation, hydrogen, and sulfur metabolism in multiple uncultivated bacterial phyla. *Science* 337 (6102): 1661–1665.

Wu, G.D., and J.D. Lewis. 2013. Analysis of the human gut microbiome and association with disease. *Clinical Gastroenterology and Hepatology* 11 (7): 774–777.

Wu, G.D., F.D. Bushmanc, et al. 2013. Diet, the human gut microbiota, and IBD. *Anaerobe* 24: 117–120.

Wu, W.-K., C.-C. Chen, et al. 2018. Optimization of fecal sample processing for microbiome study—the journey from bathroom to bench. *Journal of the Formosan Medical Association.*

Wylie, K.M., R.M. Truty, et al. 2012. Novel bacterial taxa in the human microbiome. *PLoS ONE* 7 (6): e35294.

Xia, Y., and J. Sun. 2017. Hypothesis testing and statistical analysis of microbiome. *Genes & Diseases* 4 (3): 138–148.

Yozwiak, N.L., P. Skewes-Cox, et al. 2012. virus identification in unknown tropical febrile illness cases using deep sequencing. *PLoS Neglected Tropical Diseases* 6 (2): e1485.

Yuan, S., D.B. Cohen, et al. 2012. Evaluation of methods for the extraction and purification of dna from the human microbiome. *PLoS ONE* 7 (3): e33865.

Zhang, C., and L. Zhao. 2016. Strain-level dissection of the contribution of the gut microbiome to human metabolic disease. *Genome Medicine* 8 (1): 016–0304.

Zhang, C., S. Li, et al. 2013. Structural modulation of gut microbiota in life-long calorie-restricted mice. *Nature Communications* 4: 2163.

Zhao, L., F. Zhang, et al. 2018. Gut bacteria selectively promoted by dietary fibers alleviate type 2 diabetes. *Science* 359 (6380): 1151–1156.

Chapter 2
What Are Microbiome Data?

In this chapter, we first introduce microbiome data from sources of sequencing in Sect. 2.1. Then, we describe microbiome data structure and provide several real data tables to illustrate the data structure in Sect. 2.2. The features of microbiome data are summarized in Sect. 2.3. Section 2.4 provides a real example to highlight over-dispersed and zero-inflated features of microbiome data. We describe some challenges of modeling microbiome data in Sect. 2.5. Section 2.6 is summary.

2.1 Microbiome Data

Microbiome data is generated through 16S rRNA gene sequencing and shotgun metagenomic sequencing. The bioinformatics tools include the pipeline QIIME and mothur. For example, after preprocessing the raw sequences, two ways are available to generate analyzable microbiome data (Chen et al. 2013; Li 2015). The 16S sequences are either mapped to an existing phylogenetic tree in a taxonomy-dependent way (Matsen et al. 2010) or clustered into OTUs (operational taxonomic units) according to similarity in a taxonomic-independent way (Schloss et al. 2009; Caporaso et al. 2010). The first way uses the existing phylogenetic tree structure to generate microbiome datasets, whereas the second way clusters sequence reads based on similarity level and then assigns them to different taxonomic levels. In the second way, the reads from the amplicons are clustered into OTUs, based on sequence similarity, and then OTUs are hierarchically assigned to a taxonomic tree at the kingdom, phylum, class, order, family, genus and species ranks (Liu et al. 2008; Shi and Li 2017) using available methods for accurate taxonomy assignments, including BLAST (Altschul et al. 1990), the online Greengenes (DeSantis et al. 2006) and RDP (Cole et al. 2003) classifiers, and phylogenetic tree-based and multimer clustering tree-based methods. Liu et al. compared these methods and recommended use of Greengenes or RDP classifier (Liu et al. 2008).

© Springer Nature Singapore Pte Ltd. 2018
Y. Xia et al., *Statistical Analysis of Microbiome Data with R*,
ICSA Book Series in Statistics, https://doi.org/10.1007/978-981-13-1534-3_2

The final data produced by taxonomy assignments are tables of read counts (bacterial taxa) that are assigned to nodes of a known taxonomic tree. The tables of read counts or relative abundance quantified from the read counts can be used for analyzing and modeling the microbiome composition.

2.2 Microbiome Data Structure

2.2.1 Microbiome Data Are Structured as a Phylogenetic Tree

One unique feature of microbiome data is phylogenetic tree-structured. The bacterial taxa in a community are not randomly distributed; they usually not only depend on each other, but also exist the phylogenetic relationships among bacteria, which provides insights into the evolutionary relationships among bacterial taxa: a phylogenetic tree (Chen et al. 2013). A phylogenetic tree has been defined as a ubiquitous graph in biology that describes the evolutionary relationship between a set of species (Purdom 2011) or relates all the bacterial species (Xiao et al. 2017). It consists of many levels.

The phylogenetic tree structure indicates that the relationships of taxa among diverse microbes are not only taxonomical, but also evolutionary (Koh et al. 2017, 2018). Taxa that are closer on the tree tend to have similar responses to environmental factors or have similar biological functions (Purdom 2011; Chen et al. 2013).

2.2.2 Feature-by-Sample Contingency Table

Depending on the research fields and the bioinformatics tools used to generate the high-throughput data, microbiome study and genomics generally have a data structure called feature-by-sample contingency table. The count tables typically have features as rows, and samples as columns.

In general, "features" refer to any of OTUs, genes, taxonomic levels, sequence variant, transcripts, variables, etc. "Samples" are also called replicates, subject, objects, descriptors, etc. In other fields, rows of the data matrix can be subjects, while columns can be variables. In different research fields, both rows and columns could have different names; for example, in ecology, the primary data structure is a site-by-species matrix that contains abundances, relative abundances, or the presence of species (or other taxonomic units) observed at different sampling sites. In microbiome literature, researchers often use OTU, taxon, genus, and species to refer to the features. Thus, the primary data structure in microbiome study is a taxa table or OTU table. The taxa (or OTU) table has a same data structure as a primary ecological data, but having multiple phylogenetic levels of bacterial taxa.

Table 2.1 Feature-by-sample contingency table used in microbiome, genomics, and other high-throughput data studies

Rows	Columns	Comments
Features	Samples	Used in all RNA-or DNA-sequencing experiments and contexts
OTUs (or taxa, i.e., class, genus, species)	Samples, libraries, microbiome or metagenomic samples	A feature is a species or OTU instead of a gene in the context of microbiome sequencing, DNA sequencing-based microbiome study
Genes (or tags or exons or transcripts, subsystems)	Samples, libraries	A feature is a gene in the RNA-sequencing context; the total reads per sample are called library size and sometimes referred to as depths of coverage
Observations (cases)	Variables (part of a composition)	Compositional data
Species	Sites	Ecological data

Some statistical programs may prefer data to be in the format sample-by-feature (taxon/OTU). In such cases, the rows and columns need to be transposed before analysis.

In this book, we prefer to use taxa-by-sample or sample-by-taxa to refer to microbiome data structure. However, when the feature-by-sample table is used in different context, such as in different programs and packages, we also use different names to label rows and columns. Readers should notice that we use them exchangeable. We summarize some row and column names of the feature-by-sample contingency table in Table 2.1.

2.2.3 OTU Table

Table 2.2 shows what an OTU table looks like. This is often what you will get from the 16s rRNA gene sequencing, after processing OTU picking. The table is extracted from the data sets used in our published paper (Jin et al. 2015). The table records the counts of 10 bacterial species in four extracted samples based on 16S rRNA sequencing. Table 2.3 is another version of OTU table. Each row in the OTU table corresponds to an OTU with taxa information included in the last column, while each other column corresponds to a sample.

2.2.4 Taxa Count Table

Table 2.4 is used to illustrate what a taxa count table looks like. The table is extracted from the same data sets used in the paper (Jin et al. 2015). The table

Table 2.2 An example of OTU table from 16S rRNA sequencing

Species	5_15_drySt-28F	20_12_CeSt-28F	1_11_drySt-28F	2_12_drySt-28F
Tannerella sp.	474	66	543	569
Lactococcus lactis	326	737	2297	548
Lactobacillus murinus	11	42	114	28
Lactobacillus murinus:: *Lactococcus lactis*	1	12	25	5
Parasutterella excrementihominis	1	0	1	4
Helicobacter hepaticus	87	0	0	13
Prevotella sp.	116	5	237	59
Bacteroides sp.	174	31	945	353
Barnesiella intestinihominis	8	1	0	2
Lactobacillus murinus:: *Lactobacillus* sp.	1	9	7	4

records the counts of 10 bacterial at genus level in four extracted samples based on 16S rRNA sequencing. Each row in the table corresponds to a genus while each column records a count of reads corresponding to a sample. The levels of phylum, class, family, order, and species have the same data structures.

2.2.5   Taxa Percent Table

Table 2.5 illustrates taxa percent table. As the name suggested, it has the same data structure and row and column names are same as the names in taxa count table. The values in each cell are just calculated from dividing the counts of reads in taxa count table by the total counts of reads of that taxon in the sample.

2.3   Features of Microbiome Data

Microbiome data have several features. Microbiome count data, i.e., OTU counts, taxa abundance, are naturally constrained, high dimensional, sparse with containing a large proportion of zero counts in the OTU(Taxa) table, complex covariance and correlation structures among different OTUs(taxa), and over-dispersed with large within-group heterogeneities.

Table 2.3 Another version of OTU table called sequencing OTU table

#OTU ID	10_25_drySt-28F	11_31_drySt-28F	12_32_drySt-28F	
0	0	0	0	Root
1	0	0	0	Root; Bacteria; Firmicutes; Bacilli; Lactobacillales; Streptococcaceae; Lactococcus; *Lactococcus lactis*
2	0	0	0	Root; Bacteria; Bacteroidetes; Bacteroidia
3	0	0	0	Root
4	0	0	0	Root; Bacteria; Firmicutes; Bacilli; Lactobacillales; Streptococcaceae; Lactococcus
5	0	0	0	Root; Bacteria; Firmicutes; Bacilli; Lactobacillales; Streptococcaceae; Lactococcus; *Lactococcus lactis*
6	0	0	0	Root; Bacteria; Firmicutes; Clostridia; Clostridiales; Ruminococcaceae
7	0	0	0	Root; Bacteria; Bacteroidetes; Bacteroidia
8	0	0	1	Root; Bacteria; Firmicutes; Bacilli; Lactobacillales; Streptococcaceae; Lactococcus; *Lactococcus lactis*
9	0	0	0	Root; Bacteria; Firmicutes; Bacilli; Lactobacillales; Streptococcaceae; Lactococcus; *Lactococcus lactis*

The table is also extracted from the data sets used in our paper (Jin et al. 2015). The taxa information in this table is useful (e.g., for downstream analysis)

Table 2.4 An example of taxa table from 16S rRNA sequencing

Name	5_15_drySt-28F	20_12_CeSt-28F	1_11_drySt-28F	2_12_drySt-28F
Tannerella	476	67	549	578
Lactococcus	326	737	2297	548
Lactobacillus	94	597	434	719
Parasutterella	1	0	1	4
Helicobacter	89	0	0	13
Prevotella	121	7	289	99
Bacteroides	273	34	958	377
Barnesiella	9	1	2	2
Odoribacter	1	0	22	7
Eubacterium	52	131	144	238

2.3.1   Microbiome Data Are Compositional

Microbiome count data (i.e., OTUs or taxa abundance data from 16S rRNA sequencing) are compositional with two key geometric properties. First, the total sum of all component values (sometimes called the library size) is an artifact of the sampling procedure. The library size can be affected by many factors, such as technical variability or differences in experiment-specific abundance. Second, compositional data are proportional, i.e., the distance between component values is only meaningful proportionally. The elements of the composition are non-negative and sum to unity. In Chap. 10, we will present more details of the compositional features of microbiome data.

2.3.2   Microbiome Data Are High Dimensional
and Underdetermined

Microbiome sequence data sets are high dimensional with tens of thousands of different categories. They are underdetermined, having the number of taxa or OTUs much greater than the number of samples (Kurtz et al. 2015; Tsilimigras and Fodor 2016). For example, in our murine intestinal microbiome dataset (Jin et al. 2015), there are total 8 samples (5 from VDR lockout and 3 from wild-type mice). However, there are 248 bacteria at genus rank. The high dimensionality could result in large p small n problem (Yin and Hilafu 2015), and poses statistical challenge to analyze microbiome data. In Chap. 3, we review more details of high dimensionality issues and strategies of modeling this kind of data.

Table 2.5 An example of taxa percent table from 16S rRNA sequencing

Name	5_15_drySt-28F	20_12_CeSt-28F	1_11_drySt-28F	2_12_drySt-28F
Tannerella	25.6880733944954	2.06853967273385	8.83915633553373	11.3000977517107
Lactococcus	17.5930922827847	22.7539364001235	36.9827725004025	10.7135787487781
Lactobacillus	5.12682137075014	18.8020994133992	7.39011431331509	14.154447702834 8
Parasutterella	0.0539665407447383	0	0.0161004669135405	0.0782013685239492
Helicobacter	4.80302212628171	0	0	0.273704789833822
Prevotella	6.52995143011333	0.216116085211485	0	1.93548387096774
Bacteroides	14.7328656233135	1.04970669959864	4.65303493 80132	7.3704789833822 1
Barnesiella	0.485698866702644	0.0308737264587836	15.4403477700853	0.0391006842619746
Odoribacter	0.0539665407447383	0	0.0322009338270 81	0.13685239491691 1
Eubacterium	2.80626011872639	4.04445816610065	0.35421027209789 1	4.67253176930596

2.3.3   Microbiome Data Are Over-Dispersed

Taxa count data, either taxonomy reads or OTU counts from amplicon sequencing experiments in microbiome studies or differential expression data from RNA-sequencing experiments are often over-dispersed (Xia and Sun 2017), which indicates that the variance of the counts of read is larger than what would be predicted by a pre-assumed typical multinomial regression, i.e., Poisson. The over-dispersed problem of the microbiome data is due to the facts: (1) the library sizes of DNA or RNA sequencing are widely different, and (2) OTU (taxa) count proportions vary more than expected under the posed common multinomial regression, such as Poisson model (McMurdie and Holmes 2014). In Chap. 11, we discuss microbiome data with overdispersion and model the over-dispersed microbiome data with two R packages.

2.3.4   Microbiome Data Are Often Sparse with Many Zeros

In microbiome data, sparsity is seen as the absence of many taxa across samples and zeros are generated in most experiments. Microbiome taxa abundance, especially the taxa abundance at lower taxonomic levels or OTU counts often have many zeros and right skewed (Xia and Sun 2017).

In the count data modeling, two kinds of zeros are often referred based on the sources of zeros: the sampling zeros due to sampling variability and the structural zeros above and beyond the expected zero frequency under considered model (Xia et al. 2012).

Sampling zeros are also called count zeros (Martín-Fernández et al. 2011). A count is used to record the number of times an event occurs. Count data are categorical data in which the counts represent the numbers of items falling into each of several categories (Martín-Fernández et al. 2011). Count zeros present if the event did not occur on a certain situation, but may occur in another situation. This type of zero is due to a sampling problem, because components may be unobserved due to the limited size of the sample or undetectable due to the limit of techniques. In other words, the zeros are due to insufficiently large samples (Martín-Fernández et al. 2015). The unobserved positive values may be observed with a larger number of trials or with a different sampling design. Thus, they are also called the sampling zeros.

A structural zero (Bacon-Shone 2003; van den Boogaart and Tolosana-Delgado 2013; He et al. 2014; Martín-Fernández et al. 2015; Tang et al. 2018), essential zero (Aitchison and Kay 2003; Martín-Fernández et al. 2011), genuine zeros (Martín-Fernández et al. 2015), or absolute zero (Martín-Fernández et al. 2015) is called in a given observation, when the part is not properly defined or simply cannot exist due to some deterministic reasons (van den Boogaart and Tolosana-Delgado 2013). It means that "a component which is truly zero, not something recorded as zero simply because the experimental design or the measuring instrument has not been sufficiently sensitive to detect a trace of the part" (Aitchison and Kay 2003). For example, the zeros that truly represent the absence of taxa from a particular sample belong to structural zeros (Tsilimigras and Fodor 2016).

In microbiome literature, there are rounded zeros, except sampling and structural zeros. Rounded zeros mostly appear for the continuous variables. It results from under sampling (Tsilimigras and Fodor 2016). Actually, it is not a true zero, but rather represents an observed value below a particular maximum possible rounding-off error or a below the detection value or limit (Martín-Fernández et al. 2011; van den Boogaart and Tolosana-Delgado 2013).

The reasons that many zeros exist in microbiome data may be due to structure itself and sampling (e.g., biological and technical variability) (Paulson et al. 2013). The zeros could come from structure itself. The taxa or OTUs abundance is frequently inflated with zeros because the taxa (OTUs) are subject dependent, each subject has a unique taxa/OTUs composition (Xu et al. 2015). The zero counts of taxa or OTUs are observed in a sample because the taxa (OTUs) are physically or biologically absent in the subject (structural zeros). The zero count is due to the true discovery of low-abundance taxa that are only in a few samples (Tsilimigras and Fodor 2016). For example, the most taxa (OTUs) in marker-gene studies are rare. Therefore, they are absent from a large number of samples.

Sampling results in the taxa (OTUs) unobserved or undetected in a given experiment. First, in most experiments, zeros may derive from sequencing artifacts and the highly variable sequencing depth between samples (Gloor et al. 2010; Poretsky et al. 2014; Tsilimigras and Fodor 2016). Second, zeros also occur when a given component is measured. For example, when the affected variable has a low probability of occurrence and the total number of counts is also relatively low, the component may be below the detection limit (van den Boogaart and Tolosana-Delgado 2013).

Zeros also occur in data processing. For example, microbiome data are often converted into a compositional vector of proportions by dividing the observed counts by the total number of reads. Due to the presence of rare taxa, many count zero entries may occur in the process of aligning and normalization if the known reference sequences are different or different normalization methods are used (Li 2015; Chen and Li 2016).

2.4   An Example of Over-Dispersed and Zero-Inflated Microbiome Data

Table 2.6 is an example of over-dispersed and zero-inflated taxa (OTUs) abundance data (Romero et al. 2014). The data at species rank come from case–control longitudinal study of the vaginal microbiota with 32 non-pregnant and 22 pregnant women who delivered at term (38–42 weeks). The abundance data of species have many zeros. The lowest percentage of zero is *Lactobacillus* with 14.44%, the highest is *Streptocongiccus anosus* with 73.78% zeros. Average of these 28 species

Table 2.6 Distribution of species (OTUs)

Species (OTUs)	Zero (percentage)	Median	Mean	Variance
Lactobacillus iners	15.11 (138/900)	238	1168	206E4
Lactobacillus crispatus	42.33 (381/900)	1	755.5	205E4
Atopobium vaginae	51.78 (466/900)	0	332.8	404E3
Lactobacillus	14.44 (130/900)	20	168.5	324E3
Lactobacillus jensenii	56.89 (512/900)	0	102.8	128E3
Lactobacillus gasseri	62.33 (561/900)	0	111.3	186E3
Clostridiales	58.56 (527/900)	0	49.8	22,535
Parvimonas micra	71.33 (642/900)	0	45.9	26,298
Leptotrichia amnionii	68.89 (620/900)	0	42.9	27,223
Prevotella genogroup 2	59.11 (532/900)	0	36.2	174,600
Actinomycetales	41.89 (377/900)	1	25.6	11,767
Gardnerella vaginalis	55.89 (503/900)	0	24.9	3322
Streptocongiccus anosus	73.78 (664/900)	0	18.5	30,230
Aerococcus christensenii	65.89 (593/900)	0	18.2	3710
Finegoldia magna	51.56 (464/900)	0	17.9	7606
Peptoniphilus	54.89 (494/900)	0	17.1	4050
Bifidobacteriaceae	61.11 (550/900)	0	16.6	5402
Anaerococcus	60.67 (546/900)	0	15.6	4756
Prevotella bivia	72.67 (654/900)	0	12.5	4131
Prevotella	58.56 (527/900)	0	11.8	1238
Dialister	57.33 (516/900)	0	7.7	557.6
Eggerthella	72.67 (654/900)	0	7.6	778.5
Clostridiales Family XI Incertae Sedis	67.67 (609/900)	0	6.5	682
Bacteria	66.44 (598/900)	0	5.8	553.9
Atopobium	66.33 (597/900)	0	5.8	1206
Anaerococcus vaginalis	69.11 (622/900)	0	5.8	1086
Ureaplasma	69.33 (624/900)	0	3.4	211.9
Lactobacillus vaginalis	73.33 (660/900)	0	2.7	81.3

gives 58.57% zeros. For each species, the variance is much larger than its mean (see Table 2.6), indicating overdispersion in the data.

2.5   Challenges of Modeling Microbiome Data

Microbiome data with a phylogenetic tree structure are high dimensional and underdetermined, over-dispersed and often sparse with many zeros. Modeling these kinds of feature data poses numerous challenges for traditional statistical tools. These topics are challenging to microbiome researchers and biostatisticians.

The statistical challenges include, but not limited to: (1) how to incorporate the taxa/OTUs phylogenetic tree information; (2) how to reduce dimensions and solve large p and small n problem; (3) how to handle rare taxa(OTUs); and (4) how to model the microbiome data with over-dispersion and zero-inflation. For example, the abundance of bacteria in the human gut is characterized by an increasing number of zeros at lower taxonomic levels and right skewed (Xia and Sun 2017). Zero and small values are one main source of sparsity.

Sparsity is a central challenge in the analysis of 16S rRNA-sequence data (Tsilimigras and Fodor 2016), and thus the issue of sparsity with many zeros is a central topic in analysis of microbiome data. First, sparsity with many zeros poses the critical challenges on parametric models to make accurate estimates of variance for meaningful inference and even such estimates are essentially impossible on samples that consist mostly of zeros (Tsilimigras and Fodor 2016). For example, when the taxa are sparse with many zeros, the distribution of taxa or OTUs abundance and the distribution of the taxa or OTUs occurrence probability are both skewed (Chen 2012), which results in zero inflation. Due to zero inflation, the taxa abundance with excess zeros cannot be correctly analyzed by any standard parametric model such as, a normal, binomial, Poisson, negative-binomial, and beta distributions (Martin et al. 2005). Second, sparsity with many zeros also makes nonparametric methods invalid. Nonparametric methods are based on ranks, or medians; thus, generally insensitive or more "robust" to outliers and avoid making variance estimates that can be skewed by sparse samples (Martín-Fernández et al. 2011). In the situations with many taxa having many zeros and few available samples, it will lack power to perform inference on the low-abundance taxa by using the nonparametric methods. Taking together, both traditional parametric models and nonparametric methods are not suitable for analyzing sparse microbiome data with many zeros. Therefore, analysis of sparse microbiome data with excess zeros is a real challenge. Failure to account for the excess zeros may result in biased parameter estimation and misleading inference.

2.6 Summary

In this chapter, we described and summarized the structure and features of microbiome data. We presented the OTU(taxa) tables to provide readers what the real microbiome structure and distribution look like. Microbiome data are compositional, high dimensional, underdetermined, over-dispersed, and often sparse with excess zeros. These features challenge standard statistical tools, making both parametric and non-parametric models invalid.

References

Aitchison, J., and J. Kay. 2003. Possible solution of some essential zero problems in compositional data analysis. In *Proceedings of CoDaWork'03, The 1st Compositional Data Analysis Workshop*. University of Girona, Girona (Spain). http://ima.ud.es/Activitats/CoDaWork03/.

Altschul, S.F., W. Gish, et al. 1990. Basic local alignment search tool. *Journal of Molecular Biology* 215 (3): 403–410.

Bacon-Shone, J. 2003. Modelling structural zeros in compositional data. In *Proceedings of CoDaWork'03, The 1st Compositional Data Analysis Workshop*, University of Girona, Girona (Spain). http://ima.ud.es/Activitats/CoDaWork03/.

Caporaso, J.G., J. Kuczynski, et al. 2010. QIIME allows analysis of high-throughput community sequencing data. *Nature Methods* 7.

Chen, E.Z., and H. Li. 2016. A two-part mixed-effects model for analyzing longitudinal microbiome compositional data. *Bioinformatics* 32 (17): 2611–2617.

Chen, J. 2012. Statistical methods for human microbiome data analysis. *Publicly Accessible Penn Dissertations*, Paper 497.

Chen, J., F.D. Bushman, et al. 2013. Structure-constrained sparse canonical correlation analysis with an application to microbiome data analysis. *Biostatistics* 14 (2): 244–258.

Cole, J.R., B. Chai, et al. 2003. The Ribosomal Database Project (RDP-II): Previewing a new autoaligner that allows regular updates and the new prokaryotic taxonomy. *Nucleic Acids Research* 31 (1): 442–443.

DeSantis, T.Z., P. Hugenholtz, et al. 2006. Greengenes, a chimera-checked 16S rRNA gene database and workbench compatible with ARB. *Applied and Environment Microbiology* 72 (7): 5069–5072.

Gloor, G.B., R. Hummelen, et al. 2010. Microbiome profiling by Illumina sequencing of combinatorial sequence-tagged PCR products. *PLoS One* 5.

He, H., W. Wang, et al. 2014. On the implication of structural zeros as independent variables in regression analysis: Applications to alcohol research. *Journal of Data Science (JDS)* 12 (3): 439–460.

Jin, D., S. Wu, et al. 2015. Lack of vitamin D receptor causes dysbiosis and changes the functions of the murine intestinal microbiome. *Clinical Therapeutics* 37(5): 996–1009.

Koh, H., M.J. Blaser, et al. 2017. A powerful microbiome-based association test and a microbial taxa discovery framework for comprehensive association mapping. *Microbiome* 5: 45.

Koh, H., A.E. Livanos, et al. 2018. A highly adaptive microbiome-based association test for survival traits. *BMC Genomics* 19 (1): 210.

Kurtz, Z.D., C.L. Müller, et al. 2015. Sparse and compositionally robust inference of microbial ecological networks. *PLoS Computational Biology* 11 (5): e1004226.

Li, H. 2015. Microbiome, metagenomics, and high-dimensional compositional data analysis. *Annual Review of Statistics and Its Application* 2: 73–94.

Liu, Z., T.Z. DeSantis, et al. 2008. Accurate taxonomy assignments from 16S rRNA sequences produced by highly parallel pyrosequencers. *Nucleic Acids Research* 36 (18): e120.

Martín-Fernández, J.A., J. Palarea-Albaladejo, et al. 2011. Dealing with zeros. In *Compositional data analysis*, 43–58. New York: Wiley.

Martín-Fernández, J.-A., K. Hron, et al. 2015. Bayesian-multiplicative treatment of count zeros in compositional data sets. *Statistical Modelling* 15 (2): 134–158.

Martin, T.G., B.A. Wintle, et al. 2005. Zero tolerance ecology: Improving ecological inference by modelling the source of zero observations. *Ecology Letters* 8 (11): 1235–1246.

Matsen, F.A., R.B. Kodner, et al. 2010. pplacer: Linear time maximum-likelihood and Bayesian phylogenetic placement of sequences onto a fixed reference tree. *BMC Bioinformatics* 11 (1): 538.

McMurdie, P.J., and S. Holmes. 2014. Waste not, want not: Why rarefying microbiome data is inadmissible. *PLoS Computational Biology* 10 (4): e1003531.

Paulson, J.N., O.C. Stine, et al. 2013. Differential abundance analysis for microbial marker-gene surveys. *Nature Methods* 10 (12): 1200–1202.

Poretsky, R., L.M. Rodriguez-R, et al. 2014. Strengths and limitations of 16S rRNA gene amplicon sequencing in revealing temporal microbial community dynamics. *PLoS ONE* 9 (4): e93827.

Purdom, E. 2011. Analysis of a data matrix and a graph: Metagenomic data and the phylogenetic tree. *The Annals of Applied Statistics* 5 (4): 2326–2358.

Romero, R., S.S. Hassan, et al. 2014. The composition and stability of the vaginal microbiota of normal pregnant women is different from that of non-pregnant women. *Microbiome* 2 (1): 4.

Schloss, P.D., S. L. Westcott, et al. 2009. Introducing mothur: Open-source, platform-independent, community-supported software for describing and comparing microbial communities. *Applied and Environmental Microbiology* 75.

Shi, P., and H. Li. 2017. A model for paired-multinomial data and its application to analysis of data on a taxonomic tree. *Biometrics* 73 (4): 1266–1278.

Tang, W., H. He, et al. 2018. Untangle the structural and random zeros in statistical modelings. *Journal of Applied Statistics* 45 (9): 1714–1733.

Tsilimigras, M.C.B., and A.A. Fodor. 2016. Compositional data analysis of the microbiome: Fundamentals, tools, and challenges. *Annals of Epidemiology* 26 (5): 330–335.

van den Boogaart, K.G., and R. Tolosana-Delgado. 2013. *Analyzing compositional data with R.* Berlin: Springer.

Xia, Y., and J. Sun. 2017. Hypothesis testing and statistical analysis of microbiome. *Genes & Diseases* 4 (3): 138–148.

Xia, Y., D. Morrison-Beedy, et al. 2012. Modeling count outcomes from HIV risk reduction interventions: A comparison of competing statistical models for count responses. *AIDS Research and Treatment* 2012: 11 pages.

Xiao, J., H. Cao, et al. 2017. False discovery rate control incorporating phylogenetic tree increases detection power in microbiome-wide multiple testing. *Bioinformatics* 33 (18): 2873–2881.

Xu, L., A.D. Paterson, et al. 2015. Assessment and selection of competing models for zero-inflated microbiome data. *PLoS ONE* 10 (7): e0129606.

Yin, X., and H. Hilafu. 2015. Sequential sufficient dimension reduction for large p, small n problems. *Journal of the Royal Statistical Society: Series B (Statistical Methodology)* 77 (4): 879–892.

Chapter 3
Introductory Overview of Statistical Analysis of Microbiome Data

In this chapter, we first introduce and discuss the themes and statistical hypotheses in human microbiome studies in Sect. 3.1. Then, we overview the classic statistical methods and models for microbiome studies in Sect. 3.2. In Sect. 3.3, we introduce the newly developed multivariate statistical methods. Section 3.4 introduces the compositional analysis of microbiome data. In Sect. 3.5, we discuss the longitudinal data analysis and causal inference in microbiome studies. In Sect. 3.6, we introduce some statistical packages for analyzing microbiome data. Finally, we cover the limitations of existing statistical methods and future development in Sect. 3.7.

3.1 Research Themes and Statistical Hypotheses in Human Microbiome Studies

There are mainly two themes in the current microbiome studies: (1) to characterize the relationship between microbiome features and biological, genetic, clinical or experimental conditions; and (2) to identify potential biological and environmental factors that are associated with microbiome composition. The goal of these studies is to understand mechanisms of host genetic and environmental factors that shape microbiome. Insights gained from the studies potentially contribute to the development of therapeutic strategies in modulating the microbiome composition in human diseases (Spor et al. 2011; Xia and Sun 2017).

The interactions among environment, microbiome and host are dynamic and complicated (see Fig. 3.1). To study the interactions, three general research hypotheses could be developed. Hypothesis 1 is to test the association between microbiome and host: whether the composition of the microbiome or "dysbiotic" microbiome is linked to the health or disease of host. For example, in inflammatory bowel diseases (IBD) research, we hypothesize that dysbiosis is associated with the

© Springer Nature Singapore Pte Ltd. 2018
Y. Xia et al., *Statistical Analysis of Microbiome Data with R*,
ICSA Book Series in Statistics, https://doi.org/10.1007/978-981-13-1534-3_3

Fig. 3.1 Dynamic
Interactions among
environment, microbiome and
host for the research
hypotheses in microbiome
studies

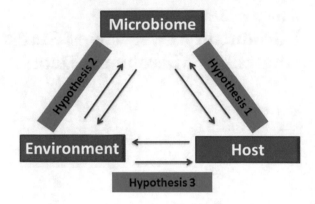

progression of the diseases (Albenberg et al. 2012; Lewis et al. 2015). In vitamin D receptor (VDR) and microbiome study, we hypothesize that lack of VDR causes dysbiosis and changes the functions of the murine intestinal microbiome (Jin et al. 2015). The hypothesis also could be on microbiome community and biological factors, such as, altered bacterial community is associated with the VDR status in intestinal epithelial cells (Wu et al. 2015).

Hypothesis 2 is to test whether microbiome is associated with environmental or biological covariates (Chen et al. 2012), whether environmental factors impact microbiome (Yassour et al. 2016), or whether an intervention has an effect on a specific microbiome composition (diversity) in health and disease. For example, we can test whether dietary interventions shape gut microbiota (Albenberg et al. 2012; Albenberg and Wu 2014), or whether a probiotic intervention impacts the composition of the human microbiota (Lahti et al. 2013). We can also hypothesize that antibiotics and diet affect gut microbial community structure (Lewis et al. 2015), nutrition influences gut microbiome composition (Backhed et al. 2015), or antibiotic treatments affect the diversity of strains of gut bacteria (Yassour et al. 2016).

Hypothesis 3 is to test the association between environment and host. To test this hypothesis, we can use the standard statistical methods and models commonly used in other biomedical sciences. For the microbiome studies, the focus is on the hypotheses 1 and 2.

In general, the null statistical hypothesis could be: there is no difference of microbiome composition in different experimental groups or genetic conditions (e.g., health and disease); or there is no difference (change) of microbiome composition in different environmental factors or with different interventions.

The core theme of these statistical hypotheses could be the same, i.e., to explore the impacts of environmental or external factors (e.g., interventions) on microbiome composition and/or richness of microbiota. However, the research topics are varying among alpha diversity (species diversity in each individual sample), bacterial richness, total number of unique operational taxonomic units (OTUs), phylogenetic diversity (the relative amount of diverse phylogenetic lineages), and species evenness in each sample (Bokulich et al. 2016).

The statistical hypothesis could be alpha diversity. For example, for antibiotic studies, we hypothesize that antibiotic treatment decreases microbial diversity (Dethlefsen et al. 2008; Jakobsson et al. 2010; Dethlefsen and Relman 2011; Nobel et al. 2015; Yassour et al. 2016), or does not decrease microbial diversity (Yassour et al. 2016); therefore, the specifically antibiotic-treated children have a less or same diverse gut microbiota (Yassour et al. 2016).

The statistical hypothesis could also be beta diversity, such as, Jaccard index of species or strains (Yassour et al. 2016) or UniFrac phylogenetic distance (Bokulich et al. 2016).

The statistical hypotheses could even be temporal microbiome community. For example, we can hypothesize that all strains are similar, the microbiome community is stable (not change over time), or compared to non-antibiotic users, antibiotic treatment make the strains less similar and less stable (Yassour et al. 2016).

To prove a scientific hypothesis, we need an appropriate statistical method. In the following two sections, we review the classical statistical tests, multivariate statistical tools, and some newly developed models and methods in analyzing microbiome data.

3.2   Classic Statistical Methods and Models in Microbiome Studies

3.2.1   Classic Statistical Tests

Many classic statistical tests are available to analyze microbiome. A hypothesis testing in microbial taxa can be performed by comparing alpha and beta diversity indices (Xia and Sun 2017). Depending on whether the data are normally or non-normally distributed, number of experimental groups, or experimental conditions, we can use a t-test, analysis of variance (ANOVA), or corresponding non-parametric test.

Two-sample t-test and its nonparametric counterpart Wilcoxon rank sum test were widely used in microbiome studies to comparing continuous variables between two groups. For example, standard t-test was used to compare alpha diversity (La Rosa et al. 2015) or population abundance (Rogosa and Sharpe 1960; Redondo-Lopez et al. 1990; Chen et al. 2012; Kim et al. 2013) between two sets of relative abundance data. Standard t-test is used even to compare the relative abundances of different phyla and genera between healthy volunteers and colorectal cancer (CRC) patients (Hillier et al. 1993; Wang et al. 2012). The non-parametric analogous Wilcoxon rank sum test (also called Mann-Whitney test) was conducted to compare alpha diversity (Yin et al. 2013), e.g., Shannon diversity (La Rosa et al. 2015), two clusters as defined by the bacterial taxonomic composition (Lewis et al. 2015). Wilcoxon rank sum test was also used to identify the differences in microbial taxa or OTUs, other nonparametric measures (Yin et al. 2013), and the relative abundances of different phyla and genera (Wang et al. 2012).

When comparing more than two groups, we choose the one-way ANOVA or its non-parametric equivalent of the Kruskal-Wallis test, depending on whether the variables are normally distributed. ANOVA was reviewed to analyze taxonomic diversity data, e.g., beta diversity (Curtis 1997), to compare proportional abundance (Sewankambo et al. 1997; Stein et al. 2013), to assess the risk model of the gut microbiome on BMI or lipids (Sewankambo et al. 1997; Kim et al. 2013), and taxonomic and functional-specific biases (Voigt et al. 2015). ANOVA test was also used to compare the functional capacity of microbiome among intestinal locations (Yang et al. 2016). Kruskal-Wallis one-way ANOVA was used to compare normalized z-score of the bacterial and fungal proportions for samples, and unequal variances of microbiome data (Gorzelak et al. 2015).

A chi-square test is usually used to compare categorical microbiome data. For example, testing a single a priori specified taxon is present at different rates across groups (La Rosa et al. 2015).

To detect differentially abundant taxa, White's research group combined several classic statistical methods and procedures to propose a statistical method, called 'Metastats' (White et al. 2009). First, the raw sequencing count (abundance data) are normalized or converted to a relative abundance data representing the proportion of each taxon to each of the individuals. Second, a two-sample non-parametrical t-test is used to analyze the differential abundance across the two treatment groups by using the Storey and Tibshirani's permutation method (Storey and Tibshirani 2003). Third, to control the false discovery rate (FDR) in multiple hypothesis testing taxa, the q-values are used to assess the significance of a test (Storey and Tibshirani 2003). Finally, to handle sparse counts, a Fisher's exact test is used to compare the differential abundance of sparsely-sampled (rare) taxa.

Metastats showed that it outperforms Student's t-test, Lu et al.'s log-linear model (Lu et al. 2005), and negative binomial (NB) model (Robinson and Smyth 2007) with simulations and real data. Actually, the proposed method is a hybrid method with combining several classic statistical methods and procedures. The statistical framework is an extension of two-sample t-test.

3.2.2 Multivariate Statistical Tools

Microbiome communities in an environmental context can be analyzed by multivariate statistical methods or models. Many statistical models and methods are available for analyzing the association of microbiome community composition and environmental covariates and outcomes. Most multivariate statistical tools used in microbiome study adopted from ecological research fields and environmental sciences (Xia and Sun 2017).

Due to high dimensionality, non-normality, and phylogenetic structure of the data, it is difficult to directly test the association of microbiome composition with potential environmental factors, using OTUs or taxa abundances. Generally, multivariate analyses first need to choose one distance measure method, and then analyze the estimated distances, in which a distance measure is defined between any of two microbiome samples.

Several tests of among-group differences are available in analyzing microbiome data: multivariate analysis of variance with permutation (PERMANOVA), and analysis of group similarities (ANOSIM), multi-response permutation procedures (MRPP), and Mantel's test (MANTEL).

PERMANOVA was proposed by Anderson and McArdle to apply the powerful ANOVA to multivariate ecological datasets (Anderson 2001; McArdle and Anderson 2001). PERMANOVA is one of most widely used nonparametric methods to fit multivariate models to microbiome data. It is a multivariate analysis of variance based on distance matrices and permutation (McArdle and Anderson 2001). Similarly as MRPP, and other multivariate analyses, PERMANOVA is generally used with one of distance measure method. For example, a PERMANOVA using unweighted UniFrac distance measure was conducted to show the composition of the gut microbiota in omnivore versus vegans (Wu et al. 2016), to assess the association with beta diversity measures (Chen et al. 2016), to test for microbial divergence among populations (Smith et al. 2015), and Bray-Curtis dissimilarity matrix (Tung et al. 2015; Yan et al. 2016).

ANOSIM is one of most widely used multivariate methods in microbiome studies. It is used to compare within- and between-group similarity (McCord et al. 2014) through a distance measure, to test the null hypothesis that the average rank similarity between samples within a group is the same as the average rank similarity between samples belonging to different groups (Giatsis et al. 2014). For example, Kelly et al. use weighted and unweighted UniFrac distances to test the strength of association with microbiome composition between treatments and among time points within treatments (Kelley et al. 2016).

In microbiome literature, the MRPP on the pairwise weighted UniFrac distance matrix was conducted to confirm the significance of the clustering (Narrowe et al. 2015), to test the factors influencing microbial communities (Degnan et al. 2012), and to compare community dissimilarities with Bray-Curtis distances (Yan et al. 2016).

Like a correlation analysis, Mantel's test was used to test association between environmental factors and host microbiome. For example, to test whether microbiome variation explains microbiome variation in host (Smith et al. 2015), the association between the host genetic distance and the variance in community beta-diversity (Sanders et al. 2014), donor microbiome and BMI (Ridaura et al. 2013), and even to identify the predictors of microbiome composition (Tung et al. 2015).

3.2.3   Over-Dispersed and Zero-Inflated Models

Taxa count data in microbiome studies, such as microbiome taxonomy reads or OTU counts from amplicon sequencing experiments or differential expression data from RNA-Seq experiments are often overdispersed and have excess zeros. In metagenomic count data, the gene-specific variability varies substantially between genes and overdispersion often occurs and affects identifying differentially abundant genes (Jonsson et al. 2017). Excess zeros also occurred in metagenomics caused by various factors, such as, the abundance of a gene that is undetectable due to the biomedical technique limit. The sampling zeros also could happen due to the large diversity between bacterial communities (Jonsson 2017).

In order to fit the microbiome count data with overdispersion and excess zeros, we often apply the negative binomial and zero inflated models. For example, a NB model was fitted to analyze microbiome abundance data (McMurdie and Holmes 2014; Xia and Sun 2017) and gut microbiome in Parkinson's disease (Yin et al. 2013). A NB model (Alekseyenko et al. 2013) was used to assess differences in sequence tag abundance and to detect differentially abundant features in clinical metagenomic samples (Van den Boogaart and Tolosana-Delgado 2013a, b).

The abundance of bacteria in the human gut is characterized by an increasing number of zeros at lower taxonomic levels and right skewed. In order to capture the characteristic of excess zeros and model the skewed microbiome data, a zero-inflated model, such as Zero-Inflated Poisson (ZIP), Zero-Inflated Negative Binomial (ZINB) or hurdle model, is needed. The appropriateness of using zero-inflated model in microbiome study was assessed by extensive simulations and a real human microbiome study (Xu et al. 2015). To capture the excess zeros and model the skewed microbiome data, Wang's research group used the hurdle model with a negative binomial distribution to analyze the species of bacteria (97% similarity threshold OTUs) (Wang et al. 2016).

In order to identify the environmental or biological covariates that are associated with different bacterial taxa while accounting for overdispersion and many zeros, Xia's research group proposed to apply an additive logistic normal multinomial regression model to link covariates to bacterial composition (counts) (Xia et al. 2013) and applied the model to analyze the association between diet and stool microbiome composition (Wu et al. 2011).

3.3 Newly Developed Multivariate Statistical Methods

In order to specifically fit multivariate data, especially microbiome data, recently, the researchers and statisticians have developed several parametric and non-parametric models. We noticed following several directions or focuses for the development of multivariate statistical methods.

3.3.1 Dirichlet-Multinomial Model

Among the parametric probability models, the multinomial and Dirichlet-multinomial distributions are the most popular ones (Holmes et al. 2012; La Rosa et al. 2012a, b). Based on Dirichlet multinomial mixtures models (Holmes et al. 2012), La Rosa and colleagues further proposed a multivariate statistic method (La Rosa et al. 2012b) for hypothesis testing and power calculations of taxonomic-based human microbiome data. The authors reparametrize the Dirichlet multinomial model to the Dirichlet multinomial mixtures to make it suitable to perform hypothesis testing across groups, based on difference between location (mean comparison) and scales (variance comparison/dispersion) (La Rosa et al. 2012a). It is implemented in R statistical software package "HMP" (La Rosa et al. 2016) using the data from the NIH Human Microbiome Project (iHMP) (Peterson et al. 2009). Its capability of performing power calculations is also attractive to researchers and statisticians when they design microbiome study and prepare for grant applications.

3.3.2 UniFrac Distance Metric Family

To compare microbial communities, multivariate analyses first need to choose one distance measure method. Numerous distance measures have been proposed (Kuczynski et al. 2010; Swenson 2011). Among them, phylogenetic distance measures, which account for the phylogenetic relationship among the taxa, are very powerful toolboxes, because they exploit the degree of divergence between different sequences.

In order to capture phylogenetic information when computing differences between microbial communities, Lozupone and Knight proposed the UniFrac distance metric in 2005. UniFrac measures the phylogenetic distance between sets of taxa in a phylogenetic tree (Lozupone and Knight 2005). The goal of the UniFrac distance metric was to enable objective comparison between microbiome samples from different conditions. In 2007, Lozupone et al. added a proportional weighting to the original UniFrac and differentiated them as unweighted UniFrac and weighted UniFrac (Lozupone et al. 2007, 2011). Since then, two versions of UniFrac are available in the microbiome literature and have been applied in thousands of research publications covering almost everything from human disease to general ecology (Lozupone et al. 2011; Smith et al. 2013). Unweighted UniFrac distance considers only species presence and absence information and counts the fraction of branch length unique to either community, and weighted UniFrac distance uses species abundance information and weights the branch length with abundance difference.

These two UniFrac distances have been become the most widely used phylogenetic distance measures. However, they have limitations: evaluated assign too much weight either to rare lineages (unweighted UniFrac distance) or to most abundant lineages (weighted UniFrac distances), thus, may not be very powerful in detecting change in moderately abundant lineages (Chen et al. 2012). Based on a variance adjusted weighted UniFrac distance (VAWUniFrac) (Chang et al. 2011), Chen et al. developed generalized UniFrac distances that extend the weighted and unweighted UniFrac distances for detecting a much wider range of biologically relevant changes in microbiome composition (Chen et al. 2012). Now, the UniFrac toolbox family has been expanded from UniFrac distances to generalized UniFrac distances. The generalized UniFrac distances were demonstrated in detecting the microbiome differences by analysis of two real human gut microbiome data sets related to linking human gut microbiome composition to long-term diet (Wu et al. 2011) and testing upper respiratory tract microbiome differences between smokers and non-smokers (Charlson et al. 2010) using PERMANOVA. Through incorporating UniFrac distances and PERMANOVA, generalized UniFrac distance measure has provided a statistical approach to test the association between microbiome composition and environmental covariates.

Two newly developed UniFrac tools were added to the UniFrac toolboxes: micropower R package (Kelly et al. 2015) and UniFrac R programs (Wong et al. 2016). In the micropower package, Kelly et al. incorporated the measures of unweighted and weighted UniFrac distances into analyses of pairwise distances and PERMANOVA to power and sample-size estimation. Under the compositional data analysis setting, Wong et al. introduced two new weightings: information UniFrac and ratio UniFrac that are not as sensitive to rarefaction and allow greater separation of outliers than classic unweighted and weighted UniFrac. The goal is to address the limitations of unweighted UniFrac's highly sensitive to rarefaction instance and to sequencing depth in uniform data sets with no clear structure or separation between groups.

3.3.3 Multivariate Bayesian Models

Multivariate Bayesian Mixed-Effects Model
Grantham et al. proposed a Bayesian mixed-effects model, called MIMIX (MIcrobiome MIXed model), for analyzing microbial taxa jointly rather than individually (Grantham et al. 2017). The capabilities of MIMIX include globally testing experimental treatment effects on microbiome composition, locally testing and estimating treatment effects on individual taxa; quantifying analysis of the microbiome heterogeneity, and characterizing the latent structure in the microbiome. MIMIX is mixed-effects model based on logistic normal multinomial (LNM) (Xia et al. 2013). As a Bayesian model, MIMIX uses Bayesian factor analysis (Rowe 2003) to capture complex dependence patterns among microbial taxa and uses continuous shrinkage Dirichlet-Laplace priors (Bhattacharya et al. 2015) to identify clusters of microbes that respond similarly to experimental conditions (Grantham et al. 2017). The authors of this model suggested that MIMIX outperform PERMANOVA with Bray-Curtis dissimilarity in detecting the presence of a significant signal and estimating sparse treatment effects in simulation study and real data (Grantham et al. 2017). However, more research studies are needed to conform the performance of this model.

Similar as Grantham et al.'s approach of jointly modeling microbial taxa abundance, Ren et al. proposed a Bayesian generalized mixed-effects regression model to account for correlations across microbial taxa and allow borrowing of information across taxa (Ren et al. 2017a). Previous multivariate approaches either assume multivariate logistic normal distributions (Xia et al. 2013; Grantham et al. 2017) or independent Dirichlet distributions (Chen and Li 2013; Wadsworth et al. 2017). The distinctions of the Bayesian nonparametric model proposed by Ren et al. lie on: (1) using a marginal Dirichlet process prior and a shrinkage prior on the latent factors to link microbial compositions and covariates while adjusting a low-dimensional space (Ren et al. 2017a; Udell and Townsend 2017), and (2) visualizing the association between covariates and microbial compositions (Ren et al. 2017b).

Multivariate Bayesian Graphical Compositional Regression
In Chap. 2, we described that microbiome composition data have the features: (a) high dimensionality; (b) sparsity with excess zero counts; (c) complex covariance structure; and (d) over-dispersed. To target the large within-group heterogeneities and potential confounders, Mao et al. proposed a Bayesian graphical regression for compositional microbiome data (Mao et al. 2017), based on a Dirichlet tree multinomial (DTM) model.
Similar as the Dirichlet-multinomial (DM) distribution, the proposed method used the DM and incorporated phylogenetic information, but directly used the phylogenetic tree as the inference tools (Wang and Zhao 2017; Tang et al. 2018). The proposed approach incorporated the DTM distribution (Dennis 1991; Wang and Zhao 2017) and graphical models under the Bayesian testing framework. DTM extends the traditional DM onto phylogenetic trees and provides more flexibility. In addition, the developed Bayesian graphical test focuses on effectively comparing group differences under the Bayesian graphical compositional regression (BGCR) framework by adjusting covariates (Mao et al. 2017). Comparing BGCR to the DTM methods (Tang et al. 2018) and to the DM test (La Rosa et al. 2012a), BGCR outperforms the other methods (Mao et al. 2017).

Bayesian Variable Selection for Multivariate Zero-Inflated Models
Jointly modeling multiple taxa is more powerful than taxon-specific univariate analysis. However, multivariate analysis of microbiome data, especially zero-inflated microbiome data with covariates is a challenge. Lee et al. proposed a Bayesian variable selection method for multivariate zero-inflated high-dimensional covariate data (Lee et al. 2017). The proposed multivariate zero-inflated Poisson (MZIP) distribution models do not require specifying the covariance structure, while incorporating a Bayesian variable selection.

3.3.4 Phylogenetic LASSO and Microbiome

The microbiome data are high-dimensional, and often have very large p and small n, which indicates that there are few data observations and many taxa, and taxa even more than data observations. In term of data matrix, p refers to the number of columns, n refers to the number of rows; then the problem large p and small n means that small n samples (data observations) contains large p taxa. Graphically, it means that there are n samples in a p dimensional space.

Statistically there are many challenges to model the high-dimensionality data (Donoho 2000; Fan and Li 2006). We need to deal with two not-excluded problems: to solve the large p and small n problem, and to work on variable section.

Typically, a larger p needs a larger n. To effectively model the high-dimensional microbiome data with large p and small n, one approach is to reduce the dimension sufficiently, i.e., reducing the dimension of predictors until the regression relationship between predictors and the response is still preserved (Li 1991; Cook 1994, 1996). In microbiome study, the covariates are also correlated or associated with each other, which adds more challenges for variable selection. Thus, a sufficient variable selection is needed (Cook 2004).

To solve the large p, small n problems, many methods have been proposed to reduce dimension of predictors (Yin and Hilafu 2015) and for variable selection. Among the methods of variable selection, several model-based penalization approaches are very useful (Yin and Hilafu 2015), including the lasso (Tibshirani 1996; Zou 2006; Zhou and Zhu 2010; Huang et al. 2012).

The 'tree-of-life' schematic, i.e., bacterial groups at different taxon levels associated a phylogeny, adds complexity to high-dimensionality data structure. Kim and his team incorporated the microbiome as a covariate in response to biological or clinical outcomes via the phylogenetic LASSO (least absolute shrinkage and selection operator) technique (Rush et al. 2016).

Similar to other variable selection methods, their variable selection method also incorporates the tree-of-life schema. The phylogenetic LASSO developed by Kim et al. has a hierarchical penalization scheme with a feasible way of grouping covariates. For example, a tree or cycles are graphically represented, respectively, based on whether or not the groupings are nested. Also, the phylogenetic LASSO uses the convex log-likelihood function (Rush et al. 2016), different from the hierarchical H-LASSO, which uses the penalized least-squares (Zhou and Zhu 2010). The algorithm of phylogenetic LASSO estimate relies on iterative adaptive reweighting. The phylogenetic LASSO can be applied to select OTUs, taxa or any other '-omic' data as covariates and then a logistic regression is used to model the response, such as, whether or not the covariates predict the fecal microbiota transplantation (FMT).

Kim et al. compared the phylogenetic LASSO to SCAD (the smoothly clipped absolute deviation) models (Xie and Huang 2009), and OLS (ordinary least squares) for the oracle model, they concluded that phylogenetic LASSO model outperformed both SCAD and OLS model based on one real clinical study.

3.4   Compositional Analysis of Microbiome Data

Much earlier in 1897, Pearson already warned that "spurious correlation" may be formed when use the ratio of two absolute measurements in the measurement of organs (Pearson 1897). Since the second half of the twentieth century, researchers in geology have known that using the standard statistical approaches to analyze composition data may make the results uninterpretable. Aitchison in the 1980s, particularly in his 1986 seminal work (Aitchison 1981, 1982, 1983, 1984, 1986), realized that every statement about a composition can be stated in terms of ratios of components and developed a set of fundamental principles, a variety of methods, operations, and tools for compositional data analysis. Of those, the logratio transformation methodology was widely accepted by statisticians and researchers in geology, ecology and other fields (Aitchison 1982; Pawlowsky-Glahn and Buccianti 2011; van den Boogaart and Tolosana-Delgado 2013a, b; Pawlowsky-Glahn et al. 2015) because with logratio transformations, the problem of a constrained sample space (the simplex) of the compositional data could be removed, and data are projected into multivariate real space. Therefore, all available standard multivariate techniques can be used again to analyze compositional data (Pawlowsky-Glahn et al. 2015). A series of publications have shown that the existing tools for compositional data analysis in geology, ecology and other fields are readily adapted and also a valid approach to analyze microbiome high-throughput sequencing data (Aitchison 1986; Pawlowsky-Glahn and Buccianti 2011; van den Boogaart and Tolosana-Delgado 2013a, b; Pawlowsky-Glahn et al. 2015; Gloor and Reid 2016; Gloor et al. 2016).

The development of methods and tools for microbiome compositional data analysis are most recent. The developing methods focus on removing the compositional constraint: all microbial relative abundances within a specimen sum to one. The constraint results in compositional data residing in a simplex rather than the Euclidean space (Aitchison 1982, 1986). To compare microbial composition appropriately, the developing methods draw inferences regarding its relative abundance of a taxon (OTU) in the ecosystem rather than the total abundance in the ecosystem from the abundance of taxa (OTUs) in the sample (Mandal et al. 2015).

To avoid "spurious correlation", Lovell et al. proposed the proportionality measure for analyzing relative data because proportionality is an appropriate correlation analysis for relative data (Lovell et al. 2015). Erb and Notredame further proposed partial proportionality, a definition adopted from partial correlations (Erb and Notredame 2016). To identify proportionally abundant taxa, a statistic for differential proportionality was proposed by Erb et al. (2017). It is equivalent to one-way ANOVA for taxon ratios.

The most representative research approaches for comparing microbiome composition are ANOVA-like differential expression (ALDEx and ALDEx2) (Fernandes et al. 2013; Gloor and Reid 2016; Gloor et al. 2016) and ANCOM (Mandal et al. 2015). Fundamentally, both approaches use the logratio transformation techniques to convert microbiome data, thus removing the compositional constraints to make the standard multivariate techniques suitable for analysis.

ANCOM is a statistical framework, which was developed to account for the compositional constraints to reduce false discoveries in detecting differences in microbial mean taxa abundance at an ecosystem level. It is based on compositional log-ratios. The authors compared ANCOM with ZIG and t-test with simulation studies and real data. They concluded that ANCOM outperforms ZIG method by substantially reducing the FDR and increasing power. The ANCOM is attractive because it makes no distributional assumptions and can be implemented in a linear model framework to adjust for covariates as well as model longitudinal data.

Compared to ANCOM, ALDEx and ALDEx2 are more comprehensive. They are applicable to nearly any type of data generated by high- throughput sequencing. They are suitable for the comparison of many different experimental designs. The statistical analyses include both two-sample and paired *t*-test, ANOVA, and non-parametric test, such as, Welch's *t* test, Wilcoxon rank sum test, Kruskal-Wallis test. They also have option to adjust *p*-values using Benjamin-Hochberg method.

3.5 Longitudinal Data Analysis and Causal Inference in Microbiome Studies

The microbiome is inherently dynamic, driven by interactions with the host and the environment, and varies over time. Thus, longitudinal microbiome data analysis provides rich information on the profile of microbiome with host and environment interactions.

The distinguishing feature of longitudinal studies is that the subjects are measured repeatedly during the study, allowing the direct assessment of changes in response variable over time (Diggle et al. 2002; Fitzmaurice et al. 2004). Longitudinal study also captures between-individual differences (heterogeneity among individuals) and within subject dynamics. It offers the opportunity to study complex biological, psychological, and behavioral hypotheses, especially those involving changes over time (Zhang et al. 2011). The advantage of longitudinal analysis is also suitable for microbiome data. It will enhance our understanding of short-and long-term trends of microbiome by intervention, such as diet, and the development and persistence of chronic diseases caused by microbiome.

3.5.1 Standard Longitudinal Models

Longitudinal designs and analyses of microbiome data have been used in various fields, including: the human infant gut microbiome in development of Type 1 diabetes (Kostic 2015). The generalized estimating equations (GEEs) and generalized linear mixed-effects model (GLMM) are the two most popular paradigms in a longitudinal setting (Zhang et al. 2011). Thus, GEE and GLMM were most likely used in microbiome studies. For example, these models were used to analyze the differences in the microbiome composition and stability between pregnant and non-pregnant women (Rome et al. 2014); the ZINB mixed-effects model was used to analyze human microbiota sequence data in esophagitis (Fang et al. 2016).

Typically, to account for over-dispersion and zero-inflated features of taxonomic abundance count data, NB or zero-inflated NB distributions were chosen to model the count data of each phylotype with random-effects to account for the correlations under the longitudinal data setting. Importantly, we need to compare the microbial relative abundance, rather than absolute counts between groups. Through adding an offset term, i.e., the log of the total number of reads, to the linear predictor function of the NB component, the absolute counts are converted to the relative abundance accounting for the variable number of reads per sample (Romero et al. 2014; Fang et al. 2016).

To treat taxa abundance as a continuous variable and model trends (linear relationships) between taxa abundance and covariates, a linear mixed-effects model with an autoregressive within subject covariance structure was used (La Rosa et al. 2014). However, this method does not explicitly handle the zero-inflation and over-dispersion in the data.

3.5.2 Newly Developed Over-Dispersed and Zero-Inflated Longitudinal Models

Zero-Inflated Gaussian Mixture Model
To address the zero-inflation and over-dispersion while identifying the bacterial taxa that are associated with covariates, several statistical models have been proposed. Paulson et al. proposed Zero-inflated Gaussian (ZIG) mixture model (Paulson et al. 2013a, b). The mixture model was designed to use a cumulative sum scaling normalization technique to correct the bias in the assessment of differential abundance introduced by total-sum normalization, and a zero-inflated Gaussian distribution mixture model to account for biases in differential abundance testing resulting from under-sampling of the microbial community. The model seeks to directly estimate the probability that an observed zero is generated from the detection distribution due to under-sampling or from the count distribution (absence of the taxonomic feature in the microbial community). ZIG mixture model log-transforms the read counts for 16S rRNA sequencing data, and then uses an empirical Bayes procedure to estimate the moderated variances. The moderated variances account for the biases because of zero counts in samples (Paulson et al. 2013a, b). This ZIG method was applied with a data from a longitudinal microbiome study (Turnbaugh et al. 2009; Paulson 2013a, b). It is implemented in the metagenomeSeq Bioconductor package. The authors used the simulation study and real data to compare ZIG to existing tools and concluded that ZIG outperforms other widely used statistical methods in the field, such as, Kruskal-Wallis test, and ZIG yields a more precise biological interpretation of the data (Paulson et al. 2013a, b). However, the extension of empirical Bayes method to a longitudinal setting was reviewed as not clear (Chen and Li 2016).

Extensions of Negative Binomial Mixed-Effects and Zero-Inflated Negative Binomial Models

Within the longitudinal setting, the negative binomial mixed-effects models (NBMMs) are the statistical model for detecting the association between the microbiome and host environmental/clinical factors for correlated microbiome count data (Zhang et al. 2017). NBMMs are based on NB model and incorporate random-effects into the fixed-effects to account for correlation among the samples. NBMMs handle over-dispersion and vary total reads via the over-dispersion parameter from NB (Zhang et al. 2017). The difference between standard NB model and NBMMs is that NBMMs are fitted via IWLS (Iterative Weighted Least Squares) algorithm. However, the models can not deal with zero-inflation.

To account for both overdispersed and excess zeros, the same authors (Zhang et al. 2016) proposed a ZINB regression for identifying differentially abundant taxa between two or more populations. The proposed ZINB uses a two-part mixtures: a NB component to account for overdispersion, and a logistic regression component to account for excess zeros. The difference between standard ZINB model and this ZINB extension lies on IWLS and EM (Expectation Maximization) algorithms utilized in the latter method. In a simulation study conducted by the authors of this method, ZINB outperforms DESeq, edgeR, and metagenomeSeq in various sparse scenarios based on AUC (Area under the Curve) estimates. Real data also suggested that the results are consistent with previous studies.

Bayesian Semiparametric Generalized Linear Regression Model

Lee and Sison-Mangus proposed a Bayesian semiparametric generalized linear regression model to investigate the association between the microbial abundance and succession change and host environmental/clinical factors, i.e., physical and biological factors (Lee and Sison-Mangus 2018). Based on the generalized linear regression model, the model uses the Laplace prior, a sparse inducing prior, to improve estimation of covariate effects on mean abundances of microbial species represented by OTUs. Similar as Zhang et al.'s NBMMs, the method specifies a NB distribution and assumes an overdispersion parameter for OTU counts. Comparing to other approaches, e.g., in Romero et al. (2014) and Zhang et al. (2017), the proposed method does not normalize OTU counts to adjust differences in sample total counts before modeling. Instead, it jointly analyzes all OTUs and simultaneously performs the normalization and estimation of covariate effects on OTU abundance.

Zero-Inflated Beta Regression Model with Random-Effects

Under the longitudinal microbiome data setting, Chen and Li proposed a two-part zero-inflated Beta regression model with random-effects (ZIBR) for testing the relationship between microbial abundance and clinical covariates (Chen and Li 2016). ZIBR treats microbiome data as compositional. The aims of ZIBR are to account for three features of microbiome compositional data: highly skewed, bounded in [0, 1), and often sparse with many zeros while considering correlations of the observations from the repeated measurements on the same subject. We will introduce the details of this method and applied it to a real longitudinal microbiome data in Chap. 12.

Differential Distribution Analysis Based on Zero-Inflated Negative Binomial Model

Chen et al. proposed a general framework of differential distribution analysis of microbiome data based on a ZINB (zero-inflated negative binomial) regression model (Chen et al. 2018). First, the count-based ZINB model has been tested to be best fit to zero-inflated and over-dispersed data (Xia et al. 2012). It was suggested statistically and biologically more appropriate for microbiome data too (Chen et al. 2018). Second, the zero-inflated model is biologically more interpretable because the assumption of mixture observed zeros, i.e., 'structural zeros' and 'sampling zeros', is more consistent with the observed human microbiome data, compared to the hurdle model (Chen et al. 2018). Previous zero-inflated models treat the dispersion as a nuisance and common parameter over all covariates (Chen and Li 2016; Fang et al. 2016; Zhang et al. 2016). In contrast, the proposed method allows covariate-dependent dispersion: the dispersion to depend on covariates such as disease condition, and addresses outliers to improve the robustness of zero-inflated models (Chen et al. 2018). To identify associated microbial taxa, the proposed method also can conduct an omnibus test of prevalence, abundance and dispersion parameters.

Mixed-Effects Dirichlet-Tree Multinomial (DTM) Model

Tang and Nicolae proposed a mixed-effect DTM model for allowing easily to use empirical Bayes shrinkage in enhancing microbial proportions inference (Tang and Nicolae 2017; Tang et al. 2018). It incorporates covariates and related taxa in microbiome studies. While considering the covariates, it focuses on prediction instead of comparison. The proposed mixed-effect DTM model has three features:

First, uses the Dirichlet-tree multinomial distribution with mixed-effects to improve the detection of phenotype-microbiome associations and prediction accuracy. By taking DTM advantages of naturally incorporating sequencing depth, over-dispersion and easily adapted to localized signals. Second, removes the unwanted covariate effects based on a mixed-effect DTM model and employs multi-scale empirical Bayes shrinkage to improve estimating microbial proportions. Third, uses random forest in incorporating shrinkage estimators (explanatory variables) as prediction tools, such as, to predict weight from microbiome.

3.5.3 Regression-Based Time Series Models

The dynamic microbiome can be analyzed via a regression-based time series model, i.e., treating the relative abundances of taxa, ecological diversity of the gut microbiota over time as a series of observations (dependent variables), and a function of time and other covariates as independent variables. For example, we can use a regression to evaluate the dependence of the human vaginal microbiome on time in the menstrual cycle and other covariates (Gajer et al. 2012; Gerber 2015), an autoregressive (AR) model to assess the tendency of the different taxonomic groups of bacteria (Palmer et al. 2007); and an infinite mixture model to treat the microbiome counts (Gupta et al. 1998).

Time-Series Clustering Method

Time-series clustering method is to group together OTUs based on similarity of their temporal profiles. It takes the approach of hypothetical OTU-level analysis, instead of averaging the OTUs (Gerber et al. 2012; Gerber 2014). For example, MC-TIMME (Microbiome Counts Trajectories Infinite Mixture Engine) is a time-series clustering algorithm developed by Gerber (2015) and Gerber et al. (2012). The non-parametric Bayesian techniques are tailored to automatically infer the temporal patterns from microbiome data and then assign OTUs in a dataset to the inferred temporal patterns (Gerber 2015).

Dynamical Systems Theory Model

Several autoregressive models have been proposed on microbial time series. The most popular ones are Lotka-Volterra (LV) models (Wilson et al. 2003; Stein et al. 2013; Fisher and Mehta 2014; Bucci et al. 2016). Stein et al. applied a dynamical systems model into microbiome time-series data (Stein et al. 2013). The model is based on generalized Lotka-Volterra (gLV) non-linear differential equations, assumes the growth of species in an ecosystem is density-bounded and modulated by other species in the system either positively or negatively. Autoregressive model also analyzes the dynamics of relative abundances of OTUs via using the gLV equations (Marino et al. 2014).

Time-Dependent Generalized Additive Models

Another dynamical systems theory model is the time-dependent generalized additive models (GAMs). The framework of GAMs is nonparametric and often preferable using in cases with little a priori information on a system (Hastie and Tibshirani 1990). GAMs have been used extensively in analyzing data of ecological time series (Moe et al. 2005; Stenseth et al. 2006; Stige et al. 2006). To capture the dynamics of the human infant gut microbiota, Trosvik et al. applied the GAMs to analyze microbiota time-series data (Trosvik et al. 2008, 2010).

Non-autoregressive Microbial Time Series Model

Gibbons and colleagues believe that there are two dynamic regimes in the human gut microbiome: external environmental fluctuations and internal processes (Gibbons et al. 2017). The external environmental fluctuations are non-autoregressive, driven by external factors (e.g., diet). In other words, most organisms function as a stable, mean-reverting behavior carrying fixed capacities and abundant taxa across individuals. The autoregressive dynamics happen occasionally when the system recovers from larger shocks. However, the external non-autoregressive fluctuations denominate the dynamics of human gut microbiome. The microbiome is a dynamically stable system, continually buffeted by internal and external forces, although the gut ecosystem is often disrupted, pushing the microbiome back to a conserved steady state. Gibbons and colleagues took a non-autoregressive approach in gut microbial time series instead of focusing on autoregressive models (e.g., Lotka-Volterra) (Gibbon et al. 2017). They used vector autoregressive models to separately model autoregressive and non-autoregressive components (Wang et al. 2015; Bose et al. 2017). VAR model is flexible and easy to be used for the analyzing stationary multivariate time series. The model assumes that the time series process with autocorrelation, cross-correlations, and serially uncorrelated or independent noise. In addition, they used continuous methods in characterizing within-host dynamics, instead of taking community state-clustering approach (Gibbons et al. 2017).

In summary, the time series approaches have been observed increasing applications in recent years. These approaches specially need be carefully designed and analyzed by appropriate analytical tools. Otherwise, the results can be extremely misleading (Gerber 2014). First, we cannot ignore the factor that the microbiome data are temporal. For example, we cannot treat the time-series data as a static time point and test them by a simple statistical procedure (e.g., t-test). We cannot treat the time-points as independent samples, which could overestimate differences between groups (Wei 2005; Guo et al. 2013; Gerber 2014). Second, we cannot average the abundances of mixed populations, especially average those abundances in sequence-based microbiome data analyses. For example, we cannot bin or aggregate two OTUs or species with opposite population dynamics. The temporal information could be lost if you aggregate OTUs or species and thus obtaining wrong microbiome profile.

3.5.4 Detecting Causality: Causal Inference and Mediation Analysis of Microbiome Data

First, microbiome may have causative effects on host. Both human and animal studies evidence the following factors: (1) studies in wild type mice (Ley et al. 2005; Samuel and Gordon 2006) and zebrafish (Rawls et al. 2004, 2006) have found a number of similarities in their microbiotic function and host interactions; and (2) the microbiota have played a role in maturation of the host immune system and even anatomical development of the intestine (Ivanov et al. 2009; Ivanov and Littman 2010).

Second, the bacterial composition (species member and abundance) of the gut microbiota is personalized (Lozupone et al. 2012; Baxter et al. 2015). Most microbiomes are strikingly divergent between distinct host species (Ley et al. 2006; Morgan and Huttenhower 2012). During the lifespan, our microbiome varies systematically across body habitats and time, can be dramatically altered transiently or long term by diseases, such as infections (Koenig et al. 2011) or medical interventions, such as antibiotics (Dethlefsen and Relman 2011; Peterfreund et al. 2012; Perez-Cobas et al. 2013). Such trends may ultimately reveal how changes of microbiome cause or prevent diseases (Costello et al. 2009). Reduced species diversity has been observed in obese humans (Ley et al. 2005, 2006); the abundance of phylum *Fusobacteria* increased significantly in the colon of colorectal cancer patients (Castellarin et al. 2012; Kostic et al. 2012). Thus, researchers in the microbiome field need understand not only the association, but also the causative functions of bacteria in human diseases (Fei and Zhao 2013; Zhao 2013; Sun and Chang 2014; Zhang and Zhao 2016).

Third, the mutual relationship between microbiome and host suggests a causal inference model, or mediation analysis and longitudinal analysis may be granted. Currently, microbiome researchers shift their emphasis from correlation to causality. However, identifying causation in microbiome studies is still rare, due to complexity in both microbiome data and statistical models. We should distinct causality from correlation and cannot directly infer causality from the relation between two variables because "correlation is neither necessary nor sufficient to establish causation" (Sugihara et al. 2012).

Mediational analysis provides the researcher with a story about a sequence of effects that leads to something (MacKinnon et al. 2007; MacKinnon 2008; Xia et al. 2012a, b). It allows us to conduct scientific investigations to explain how something comes about. Detecting the dynamic causation among microbiome, intervention and the host is very critical (Segata et al. 2012). However, to our knowledge, there are limited applications of causal inferences and mediation analysis.

3.5.5 Meta-analysis of Microbiome Data

Similar microbiome studies are often reported with inconsistent effects due to heterogeneity. Meta-analysis is designed to reduce study bias, ensure robust results, increase statistical power and improve overall biological understanding of a study effect such as a clinical trial on similar experimental conditions or treatments. The meta-analysis of microbiome studies were conducted to test the similar basic hypotheses on different conditions or treatments, such as, IBD (Walters et al. 2014) and obesity (Finucane et al. 2014; Walters et al. 2014; Sze and Schloss 2016).

Currently, web-based statistical tools and R package were available for meta-analysis of microbiome data. For example, the web-based tool "MicrobiomeAnalyst" has functions for meta-analysis (Dhariwal et al. 2017). The R package "metamicrobiomeR" was designed to perform meta-analysis across microbiome studies using random-effects models (Ho and Li 2018). The methodology for analysis of microbiome relative abundance data was developed based on zero-inflated beta GAMLSS (generalized additive models for location, scale and shape): GAMLSS-BEZI (Rigby and Stasinopoulos 2001, 2005; Stasinopoulos and Rigby 2007). It uses the GAMLSS-BEZI to estimate log (odds ratio) of relative abundances between groups and random and fixed-effects meta-analysis models to pool estimates and their standard errors to evaluate the heterogeneity and overall effects across microbiome studies.

Meta-analysis can be implemented using different algorithms or approaches, such as, combine *p*-values, effect sizes, rank orders, votes from multiple studies, or directly merge different raw data sets into a mega-data set and then consider it as a single data set. The vote approach is the simplest method of meta-analysis. It first selects differentially expressed genes or abundant taxa based on certain criteria (e.g., adjusted $p < 0.05$) for each data set; then counts the total number of detected differentially expressed genes or abundant taxa across all data sets. The vote approach should not be used except other methods cannot work out, because it is considered as statistically inefficient (Xia et al. 2013a, b). The approach of directly merge different raw data sets usually should be restricted its applications to the same or similar platform, because it ignores the inherent bias and heterogeneity of data sets from different sources (Tseng et al. 2012; Xia et al. 2013a, b).

Comparing to studies in other research field, a rigorous statistical meta-analysis of microbiome data has more challenges because the problems of individual data quality and the inherent heterogeneity of individual data sets are bigger. We should follow the guidelines of meta-analyses when design and perform meta-analyses of microbiome data (Moher et al. 2009; Sze and Schloss 2016). A rigorous statistical meta-analysis should use an appropriate underlying statistical method and a fixed-effects model or random-effects model to compare groups on the pooled data sets, in addition to concerning individual data quality and the inherent heterogeneity of individual data sets (Chen and Peace 2013). Based on this criterion, most current meta-analyses of microbiome data are not rigorous enough as the statistical meta-analysis.

Currently, most current meta-analyses of microbiome data directly merge different raw data sets into a mega-data set, then analyzed the pooled data set using usual methods i.e., alpha diversity, principal coordinate analysis (PCoA) (Lozupone et al. 2013; Adams et al. 2015; Bhute et al. 2016; Sze and Schloss 2016; Holman et al. 2017; Mancabelli et al. 2017). Other studies independently performed univariate tests on relative abundances of taxa for each data set and used a statistic method (i.e., Kruskal-Wallis test) to compare results across studies and adjust *p*-values with a correction method (i.e., the Benjamini-Hochberg false discovery rate (FDR)) (Duvallet et al. 2017). Currently the functions for meta-analysis in "MicrobiomeAnalyst" focus on visual exploration or enrichment analysis. The "MicrobiomeAnalyst" tool lacks appropriate statistical method to conduct group comparisons. Therefore, it not a rigorous statistical meta-analysis (Dhariwal et al. 2017).

From the perspective of using statistical method and model to examine overall pooled effects across studies, the approach in the metamicrobiomeR package is a rigorous statistical meta-analysis. Based on a simulation study, the authors of this package stated its three advantages: first, GAMLSS-BEZI directly and properly addresses the distribution of microbiome relative abundance data via a zero-inflated beta distribution; second, it has better power in term of detecting differential relative abundances between groups than linear model with arcsin-square root transformation (Morgan et al. 2012); and third, the estimated log (odds ratio) of relative abundances between groups are directly comparable across studies.

3.6   Introduction of Statistical Packages

Bioinformatics pipelines and R packages play a very important role in developing statistical methods and models for hypothesis testing and statistical analysis.

Bioinformatics Pipelines

QIIME (Caporaso et al. 2010) and mothur (Schloss et al. 2009) are the two popular bioinformatics pipelines. The capabilities of QIIME and mothur are comprehensive and supportive documentation, thus they were reviewed as the two outstanding pipelines (Nilakanta et al. 2014; Plummer et al. 2015). Both QIIME and mothur are self-contained that can be used to generate microbiome composition data as well as analyze 16S rRNA gene sequencing data. QIIME and mothur can perform microbiome composition and statistical analyses, including alpha and beta diversities, ANOVA, paired and two sample t-tests, adonis, ANOSIM, MRPP, PERMANOVA, PERMDISP, db-RDA, and Mantel's test (He et al. 2013; D'Argenio et al. 2014).

R Packages Adopted from Other Fields

In microbiome study, researchers and statisticians use the available standard methods and models or borrow statistical tools from other related fields to apply to their studies, especially in the early stages.

Vegan is a very important and most widely used R package (Oksanen et al. 2016), which was initially designed for community ecologists. Vegan is not self-contained. It depends on many other R packages and must be run under R statistical environment. However, vegan contains the most popular methods of multivariate analysis and tools for diversity analysis, and other potentially useful functions. Therefore, it is commonly used in analyzing ecological communities, and has been adopted to analyze microbiome data. We use vegan package to calculate diversities and other measures in Chap. 6.

DESeq (Anders and Huber 2010), DESeq 2 (Love et al. 2014), edgeR (Robinson et al. 2010) were initially developed for analyzing data of digital gene expression (Witkin and Ledger 2012) and serial analysis of gene expression (SAGE). They are useful for hypothesis testing and statistical analysis of over-dispersed count data. Both DESeq and DESeq 2 use the negative binomial distribution to test for differential expression; edgeR package implements original statistical methodology described in Robinson and Smyth (2007, 2008), Robinson et al. (2010) and McCarthy et al. (2012). We adopted them for analyzing over-dispersed microbiome count data in Chap. 11. The limma package was originally developed to detect the differential abundance of the species (Smyth 2005; Paulson et al. 2013a, b; Praveen et al. 2015).

Newly Developed R Packages for Microbiome Data

Some R packages were specially developed for microbiome data. In current years, more R packages were developed along the proposed statistical methods by microbiome researchers and statisticians. These packages have their specific capabilities to conduct hypothesis testing and statistical analysis. We will not introduce all of them because many packages have been available and new ones are still under development. Here, we select some for readers' reference. We will introduce and implement several R packages in this book.

HMP (La Rosa et al. 2016) and micropower (Kelly et al. 2015) are two R packages for conducting power and sample size calculations. We implement HMP in Chap. 5 using real microbiome data.

Among the newly developed R packages, the phyloseq package is more general statistical tools (McMurdie and Holmes 2013). First, it has integrated other available statistical packages to perform statistical hypothesis testing and analysis. For example, it integrated with or extended to DESeq, DESeq 2, edgeR packages to facilitate taxanomic diversity analysis and statistical modeling. It also contains general-purpose tools for microarray-based analysis of microbiome profiling data sets in R. Second, the phyloseq package has equipped with tools to manage microbiome data sets. For example, it has capability of importing and exporting data from other packages, even from bioinformatics pipelines, such as QIIME and mothur. Third, phyloseq has capability to perform various diversity metrics analyses. For example, after importing data into the R, one may easily perform beta diversity analysis using any or all of over 40 different ecological distance metrics; implement alpha diversity metrics; perform more sophisticated analyses, such as k-tables analysis (Thioulouse 2011) and differential analysis of microbiome data. Last, the phyloseq package has functions and tools to visualize microbiome data via barplots, boxplots, density plots, heatmaps, motion charts, and networks, and ordination and clustering.

The microbiome package conducts statistical analysis based on the phyloseq class (Lahti and Salojarvi 2014–2016). It contains general-purpose tools for microarray-based analysis of microbiome profiling data sets in R. It adds extra functionality for microbiome data sets to perform microbiota composition analysis, bi-stability analysis, calculate diversity indices and fit linear models with pairwise comparisons, and association studies. As the phyloseq package, the microbiome package has functions and tools to visualize microbiome data via barplots, boxplots, density plots, heatmaps, motion charts, networks, ordination, and clustering.

metagenomeSeq (Paulson et al. 2013a, b) is a mixture model that implements a zero-inflated Gaussian (ZIG). metagenomeSeq includes a non-parametric permutation test on t-statistics, a non-parametric Kruskal-Wallis test (Paulson 2013a, b).

R code for implementing Bayesian graphical compositional regression (BGCR) proposed by Mao et al. (2017) is freely available at https://github.com/MaStatLab/BGCR.

mBvs package implements the Bayesian variable selection method for multivariate zero-inflated high-dimensional covariate data proposed by Lee et al. (2017).

ANCOM package implements analysis of composition of microbiomes (Mandal et al. 2015). ALDEx and ALDEx2 packages implement the methods comparing microbiome composition (Fernandes et al. 2013; Gloor and Reid 2016; Gloor et al. 2016). We run ALDEx2 with real microbiome data in Chap. 10.

BhGLM package implements both methods of NBMMs and ZINB (Zhang et al. 2016, 2017).

ZIBR package implements the two-part zero-inflated Beta regression model with random-effects (Chen and Li 2016). We illustrate its use in Chap. 12.

MicrobiomeDDA implements the general framework of differential distribution analysis of microbiome data based on a ZINB (zero-inflated negative binomial) regression model (Chen et al. 2018).

metamicrobiomeR implements analysis of microbiome relative abundance data, using zero-inflated beta GAMLSS and meta-analysis across studies using random and fixed-effect models (Ho and Li 2018).

3.7   Limitations of Existing Statistical Methods and Future Development

In this chapter, we comprehensively reviewed the statistical methods and models that are currently available or have been used for analysis of microbiome data. The statistical methods and models aimed to targeting the specific features of micro-biome data, either in cross-section or longitudinal settings. These methods treat the microbiome data as relative abundance, use the raw read counts as input data sets, or develop analysis based on the data structure of phylogenetic trees.

The classical statistical methods are still widely used, while new methods have been developed over the past few years. Newly developed methods mostly targeted one or more specific features of microbiome data: high dimensionality, over-dispersion, sparsity with excess zeros, and complex covariance structure. However, the existing statistical approaches still have their limitations, including:

(a) Detecting causality and causal inference, mediation analyses are still in the infant stages. In recent years, the microbiome research has shifted the focus from correlation to causality. In ecology, how to identify causation has been discussed and a framework for identifying causation in complex ecosystems was proposed (Sugihara et al. 2012). However, suitable longitudinal and causal inference models are very limited in microbiome studies. To meet the needs of modeling the dynamic and complicated microbiome data, the statistical tools that are appropriate to analyze the causality and mediational relationship between hypothesis factors are still needed.

(b) Some studies totally ignore constraint problem or compositional nature of the microbiome data when use classical statistical methods for analyzing micro-biome proportional data. For example, Pearson correlation analysis, t-test, and ANOVA are still widely used for the analysis of microbiome data without testing the data distribution or transformation.

(c) Currently the compositional data analysis has not solved the problem of zero values. The compositional data analysis of microbiome data focused on two efforts: using log-ratio to avoid the constraint problem, and using proportionality for substituting correlation to solve the "spurious correlation" problem. Both ways lie on log-ratio transformation. Typically, a small value is added to zero read count to make log-ratio transformation definable. However, the algorithm of adding small values is not granted. Also whether or not the artificial values change the outcome is difficult to test.

(d) Count-based approaches still need to improve the capabilities of jointly modeling over-dispersion and zero-inflation. Microbiome data has been advised to treat as count data rather than compositional. The count-based models are considered as more statistically and biologically appropriate for microbiome data because this approach targets multivariate high-dimensional data structure, sparsity, over-dispersion and zero-inflation of microbiome, and it has a good concept adjustment. In recent years, several count-based models have been developed either in cross-sectional or longitudinal settings. However, some methods treat the bacterial taxa as independently and ignore the dependence among bacterial taxa; some methods have limit capabilities to deal with over-dispersion and/or zero-inflation, although they jointly model multiple bacterial taxa.

(e) The approach of phylogenetic trees seems another promise in the sense that they consider multiple levels of taxa compared to compositional and count-based approaches. However, the evolution between different levels of bacterial taxa is more complicated than in other fields (i.e., ecology). We still lack the appropriate methods or models to jointly fit multiple levels of taxa and considering the features of microbiome data, such as over-dispersion and/or zero-inflation.

In recent years, especially after we proposed this book in three years ago, great progress has been made for statistical analysis of microbiome data, evidenced by methods and models targeting the specific features of microbiome data in cross-sectional and longitudinal settings. The progress has been made from choosing standard statistical methods, borrowing them from other fields to develop its own unique methods. Some newly developed statistical methods and models are feasible and well-fitted for microbiome data. However, there are still space in developing statistical methods and models in microbiome study.

As general guideline, the focuses of new statistical methods could be in the following areas:

(a) Developing longitudinal and causal models that could enable more accurate causal inferences to fit the dynamic and complicated association among microbiome, environments and host. The prospective models should have powerful statistical tool to link changes in the microbiome to host factors (i.e., health or disease) and have capability to adjust for confounding factors to establish temporal and even causal relationships with response variables.

(b) Continuing to develop appropriate models to jointly fit and effectively account for the features of microbiome data with multivariate high-dimensional data structure, over-dispersion and sparsity with excess zeros, including statistical tools of meta-analysis.

(c) Taking into account the compositional nature of the microbiome data and fitting the microbiome data as compositional, while addressing the features of multivariate high-dimensional data structure, over-dispersion and sparsity with excess zeros.

(d) Discussing and proposing statistical models fascinating the evolution of bacteria taxa under the framework of phylogenetic trees.

These future studies need team effort involving biomedical researchers, physicians, bioinformatics experts, and biostatisticians. More mechanism-driven studies should be based on appropriate statistical design and perform analysis using the experimental models, human samples, 'omic' technologies, bioinformatic analysis, and statistic modeling (Xia and Sun 2017).

References

Adams, R.I., A.C. Bateman, et al. 2015. Microbiota of the indoor environment: A meta-analysis. *Microbiome* 3 (1): 49.

Aitchison, J. 1981. A new approach to null correlations of proportions. *Mathematical Geology* 13 (2): 175–189.

Aitchison, J. 1982. The statistical analysis of compositional data (with discussion). *Journal of the Royal Statistical Society, Series B (Statistical Methodology)* 44 (2): 139–177.

Aitchison, J. 1983. Principal component analysis of compositional data. *Biometrika* 70 (1): 57–65.

Aitchison, J. 1984. Reducing the dimensionality of compositional data sets. *Journal of the International Association for Mathematical Geology* 16 (6): 617–635.

Aitchison, J. 1986. *The statistical analysis of compositional data*. London: Chapman and Hall Ltd. Reprinted in 2003 with additional material by The Blackburn Press.

Albenberg, L.G., and G.D. Wu. 2014. Diet and the intestinal microbiome: Associations, functions, and implications for health and disease. *Gastroenterology* 146 (6): 1564–1572.

Albenberg, L.G., J.D. Lewis, et al. 2012. Food and the gut microbiota in IBD: A critical connection. *Current Opinion in Gastroenterology* 28 (4): 314–320. https://doi.org/10.1097/mog.1090b1013e328354586f.

Alekseyenko, A.V., G.I. Perez-Perez, et al. 2013. Community differentiation of the cutaneous microbiota in psoriasis. *Microbiome* 1 (1): 31.

Anders, S., and W. Huber. 2010. Differential expression analysis for sequence count data. *Genome Biology* 11 (10): R106–R106.

Anderson, M.J. 2001. A new method for non-parametric multivariate analysis of variance. *Austral Ecology* 26: 32–46.

Backhed, F., J. Roswall, et al. 2015. Dynamics and stabilization of the human gut microbiome during the first year of life. *Cell Host & Microbe* 17 (6): 852.

Baxter, N.T., J.J. Wan, et al. 2015. Intra- and interindividual variations mask interspecies variation in the microbiota of sympatric peromyscus populations. *Applied and Environment Microbiology* 81 (1): 396–404.

Bhattacharya, A., D. Pati, et al. 2015. Dirichlet–Laplace priors for optimal shrinkage. *Journal of the American Statistical Association* 110 (512): 1479–1490.

Bhute, S., P. Pande, et al. 2016. Molecular characterization and meta-analysis of gut microbial communities illustrate enrichment of prevotella and megasphaera in Indian subjects. *Frontiers in Microbiology* 7: 660.

Bokulich, N.A., J. Chung, et al. 2016. Antibiotics, birth mode, and diet shape microbiome maturation during early life. *Science Translational Medicine* 8 (343): 343ra382.

Bose, E., M. Hravnak, et al. 2017. Vector autoregressive (VAR) models and granger causality in time series analysis in nursing research: Dynamic changes among vital signs prior to cardiorespiratory instability events as an example. *Nursing Research* 66 (1): 12–19.

Bucci, V., B. Tzen, et al. 2016. MDSINE: Microbial dynamical systems inference engine for microbiome time-series analyses. *Genome Biology* 17 (1): 016–0980.

Caporaso, J.G., J. Kuczynski, et al. 2010. QIIME allows analysis of high-throughput community sequencing data. *Nature Methods* 7 (5): 335–336.

Castellarin, M., R.L. Warren, et al. 2012. Fusobacterium nucleatum infection is prevalent in human colorectal carcinoma. *Genome Research* 22 (2): 299–306.

Chang, Q., Y. Luan, et al. 2011. Variance adjusted weighted UniFrac: A powerful beta diversity measure for comparing communities based on phylogeny. *BMC Bioinformatics* 12: 118.

Charlson, E.S., J. Chen, et al. 2010. Disordered microbial communities in the upper respiratory tract of cigarette smokers. *PLoS ONE* 5 (12): e15216.

Chen, J., and H. Li. 2013. Variable selection for sparse dirichlet-multinomial regression with an application to microbiome data analysis. *The Annals of Applied Statistics* 7 (1): 418–442.

Chen, E.Z., and H. Li. 2016. A two-part mixed-effects model for analyzing longitudinal microbiome compositional data. *Bioinformatics* 32 (17): 2611–2617.

Chen, D., and K. Peace. 2013. *Applied meta-analysis with R*. New York: Chapman and Hall/CRC.

Chen, J., K. Bittinger, et al. 2012a. Associating microbiome composition with environmental covariates using generalized UniFrac distances. *Bioinformatics* 28 (16): 2106–2113.

Chen, W., F. Liu, et al. 2012b. Human intestinal lumen and mucosa-associated microbiota in patients with colorectal cancer. *PLoS ONE* 7 (6): e39743.

Chen, J., E. Ryu, et al. 2016. Impact of demographics on human gut microbial diversity in a US Midwest population. *PeerJ* 4: e1514.

Chen, J., E. King, et al. 2018. An omnibus test for differential distribution analysis of microbiome sequencing data. *Bioinformatics* 34 (4): 643–651.

Cook, R.D. 1994. On the interpretation of regression plots. *Journal of the American Statistical Association* 89 (425): 177–189.

Cook, R.D. 1996. Graphics for regressions with a binary response. *Journal of the American Statistical Association* 91 (435): 983–992.

Cook, R.D. 2004. Testing predictor contributions in sufficient dimension reduction. *The Annals of Statistics* 32 (3): 1062–1092.

Costello, E.K., C.L. Lauber, et al. 2009. Bacterial community variation in human body habitats across space and time. *Science* 326 (5960): 1694–1697.

Curtis, H. 1997. What is normal vaginal flora? *Genitourinary Medicine* 73 (3): 230.

D'Argenio, V., G. Casaburi, et al. 2014. Comparative metagenomic analysis of human gut microbiome composition using two different bioinformatic pipelines. *BioMed Research International*, 2014.

Degnan, P.H., A.E. Pusey, et al. 2012. Factors associated with the diversification of the gut microbial communities within chimpanzees from Gombe national park. *Proceedings of the National Academy of Sciences of the United States of America* 109 (32): 13034–13039.

Dennis, S.Y. 1991. On the hyper-dirichlet type 1 and hyper-liouville distributions. *Communications in Statistics—Theory and Methods* 20 (12): 4069–4081.

Dethlefsen, L., and D.A. Relman. 2011. Incomplete recovery and individualized responses of the human distal gut microbiota to repeated antibiotic perturbation. *Proceedings of the National Academy of Sciences of the United States of America* 108 (Suppl 1): 4554–4561.

Dethlefsen, L., S. Huse, et al. 2008. The pervasive effects of an antibiotic on the human gut microbiota, as revealed by deep 16S rRNA sequencing. *PLoS Biology* 6 (11): e280.

Dhariwal, A., J. Chong, et al. 2017. MicrobiomeAnalyst: a web-based tool for comprehensive statistical,visual and meta-analysis of microbiome data. *Nucleic Acids Research* 45 (W1): W180–W188

Diggle, P.J., P. Heagerty, et al. 2002. *Analysis of longitudinal data*. Oxford: Oxford University Press.

Donoho, D.L. 2000. High-dimensional data analysis: The curses and blessings of dimensionality. In *Conference on Mathematical Challenges of the 21st Century*. American Mathematical Society.

Duvallet, C., S.M. Gibbons, et al. 2017. Meta-analysis of gut microbiome studies identifies disease-specific and shared responses. *Nature Communications* 8 (1): 1784.

Erb, I., and C. Notredame. 2016. How should we measure proportionality on relative gene expression data? *Theory in Biosciences* 135: 21–36.

Erb, I., T. Quinn, et al. 2017. Differential proportionality—A normalization-free approach to differential gene expression. bioRxiv.

Fan, J., and R. Li. 2006. Statistical challenges with high dimensionality: Feature selection in knowledge discovery. In *Proceedings of the international congress of mathematicians*, vol. III, ed. M. Sanz-Sole, J. Soria, J.L. Varona, and J. Verdera, 595–622. Freiburg: European Mathematical Society.

Fang, R., B.D. Wagner, et al. 2016. Zero-inflated negative binomial mixed model: An application to two microbial organisms important in oesophagitis. *Epidemiology and Infection* 144 (11): 2447–2455.

Fei, N., and L. Zhao. 2013. An opportunistic pathogen isolated from the gut of an obese human causes obesity in germfree mice. *ISME Journal* 7 (4): 880–884.

Fernandes, A.D., J.M. Macklaim, et al. 2013. ANOVA-like differential expression (ALDEx) analysis for mixed population RNA-Seq. *PLoS ONE* 8 (7): e67019.

Finucane, M.M., T.J. Sharpton, et al. 2014. A taxonomic signature of obesity in the microbiome? Getting to the guts of the matter. *PLoS ONE* 9 (1): e84689.

Fisher, C.K., and P. Mehta. 2014. Identifying keystone species in the human gut microbiome from metagenomic timeseries using sparse linear regression. *PLoS ONE* 9 (7): e102451.

Fitzmaurice, G.M., N.M. Laird, et al. 2004. *Applied longitudinal analysis*. NJ: Wiley.

Gajer, P., R.M. Brotman, et al. 2012. Temporal dynamics of the human vaginal microbiota. *Science Translational Medicine* 4 (132): 3003605.

Gerber, G.K. 2014. The dynamic microbiome. *FEBS Letters* 588 (22): 4131–4139.

Gerber, G.K. 2015. Longitudinal microbiome data analysis. In *Metagenomics for microbiology*, ed. J. Izard and M.C. Rivera. London, UK: Elsevier Inc.

Gerber, G.K., A.B. Onderdonk, et al. 2012. Inferring dynamic signatures of microbes in complex host ecosystems. *PLoS Computational Biology* 8 (8): e1002624.

Giatsis, C., D. Sipkema, et al. 2014. The colonization dynamics of the gut microbiota in tilapia larvae. *PLoS ONE* 9 (7): e103641.

Gibbons, S.M., S.M. Kearney, et al. 2017. Two dynamic regimes in the human gut microbiome. *PLoS Computational Biology* 13 (2): e1005364.

Gloor, G.B., and G. Reid. 2016. Compositional analysis: A valid approach to analyze microbiome high-throughput sequencing data. *Canadian Journal of Microbiology* 62 (8): 692–703.

Gloor, G.B., J.R. Wu, et al. 2016. It's all relative: Analyzing microbiome data as compositions. *Annals of Epidemiology* 26 (5): 322–329.

Gorzelak, M.A., S.K. Gill, et al. 2015. Methods for improving human gut microbiome data by reducing variability through sample processing and storage of stool. *PLoS ONE* 10 (8): e0134802.

Grantham, Neal S., Brian J. Reich, et al. 2017. MIMIX: A Bayesian mixed-effects model for microbiome data from designed experiments. arXiv:1703.07747 [stat.ME].

Guo, Y., H.L. Logan, et al. 2013. Selecting a sample size for studies with repeated measures. *BMC Medical Research Methodology* 13 (1): 100.

Gupta, K., A.E. Stapleton, et al. 1998. Inverse association of H_2O_2-producing lactobacilli and vaginal Escherichia coli colonization in women with recurrent urinary tract infections. *The Journal of Infectious Diseases* 178 (2): 446–450.

Hastie, T.J., and R.J. Tibshirani. 1990. *Generalized additive models*. London: Chapman & Hall.

He, Y., B.-J. Zhou, et al. 2013. Comparison of microbial diversity determined with the same variable tag sequence extracted from two different PCR amplicons. *BMC Microbiology* 13 (1): 208.

Hillier, S.L., M.A. Krohn, et al. 1993. The normal vaginal flora, H_2O_2-producing lactobacilli, and bacterial vaginosis in pregnant women. *Clinical Infectious Diseases* 16: S273–S281.

Ho, N. T., and F. Li. 2018. MetamicrobiomeR: An R package for analysis of microbiome relative abundance data using zero-inflated beta GAMLSS and meta-analysis across studies using random effect models. bioRxiv preprint first posted online, 4 Apr 2018.

Holman, D.B., B.W. Brunelle, et al. 2017. Meta-analysis to define a core microbiota in the swine gut. *mSystems* 2 (3): e00004–e00017.

Holmes, I., K. Harris, et al. 2012. Dirichlet multinomial mixtures: Generative models for microbial metagenomics. *PLoS ONE* 7 (2): e30126.

Huang, J., P. Breheny, et al. 2012. A selective review of group selection in high-dimensional models. *Statistical Science: A Review Journal of The Institute of Mathematical Statistics* 27 (4): 481–499. https://doi.org/10.1214/1212-sts1392.

Ivanov, I.I., and D.R. Littman. 2010. Segmented filamentous bacteria take the stage. *Mucosal Immunology* 3 (3): 209–212.

Ivanov, I.I., K. Atarashi, et al. 2009. Induction of intestinal Th17 cells by segmented filamentous bacteria. *Cell* 139 (3): 485–498.

Jakobsson, H.E., C. Jernberg, et al. 2010. Short-term antibiotic treatment has differing long-term impacts on the human throat and gut microbiome. *PLoS ONE* 5 (3): e9836.

Jannicke Moe, S., A.B. Kristoffersen, et al. 2005. From patterns to processes and back: Analysing density-dependent responses to an abiotic stressor by statistical and mechanistic modelling. *Proceedings of the Royal Society B: Biological Sciences* 272 (1577): 2133–2142.

Jin, D., S. Wu, et al. 2015. Lack of vitamin D receptor causes dysbiosis and changes the functions of the murine intestinal microbiome. *Clinical Therapeutics* 37 (5): 996–1009. e1007.

Jonsson, V. 2017. *Statistical analysis and modelling of gene count data in metagenomics.* Sweden: Göteborg.

Jonsson, V., T. Osterlund, et al. 2017. Variability in metagenomic count data and its influence on the identification of differentially abundant genes. *J Comput Biol* 24 (4): 311–326.

Kanhere, M., J. He, et al. 2018. Bolus weekly vitamin D3 supplementation impacts gut and airway microbiota in adults with cystic fibrosis: A double-blind, randomized, placebo-controlled clinical trial. *Journal of Clinical Endocrinology and Metabolism* 103 (2): 564–574.

Kelley, S.T., D.V. Skarra, et al. 2016. The gut microbiome is altered in a Letrozole-induced mouse model of polycystic ovary syndrome. *PLoS ONE* 11 (1): e0146509.

Kelly, B.J., R. Gross, et al. 2015. Power and sample-size estimation for microbiome studies using pairwise distances and PERMANOVA. *Bioinformatics* 31 (15): 2461–2468.

Kim, K.A., I.H. Jung, et al. 2013. Comparative analysis of the gut microbiota in people with different levels of ginsenoside Rb1 degradation to compound K. *PLoS ONE* 8 (4): e62409.

Koenig, J.E., A. Spor, et al. 2011. Succession of microbial consortia in the developing infant gut microbiome. *Proceedings of the National Academy of Sciences of the United States of America* 1: 4578–4585.

Kostic, A.D., D. Gevers, et al. 2012. Genomic analysis identifies association of fusobacterium with colorectal carcinoma. *Genome Research* 22 (2): 292–298.

Kostic, A. D., D. Gevers, et al. 2015. The dynamics of the human infant gut microbiome in development and inprogression towards type 1 diabetes. *Cell Host & Microbe* 17 (2): 260-273

Kuczynski, J., Z. Liu, et al. 2010. Microbial community resemblance methods differ in their ability to detect biologically relevant patterns. *Nature Methods* 7 (10): 813–819.

La Rosa, P.S., J.P. Brooks, et al. 2012a. Hypothesis testing and power calculations for taxonomic-based human microbiome data. *PLoS ONE* 7 (12): e52078.

La Rosa, P.S., B. Shands, et al. 2012b. Statistical object data analysis of taxonomic trees from human microbiome data. *PLoS ONE* 7 (11): e48996.

La Rosa, P.S., B.B. Warner, et al. 2014. Patterned progression of bacterial populations in the premature infant gut. *Proceedings of the National Academy of Sciences* 111 (34): 12522–12527.

La Rosa, P.S., Y. Zhou, et al. 2015. Hypothesis testing of metagenomic data. In *Metagenomics for microbiology*, ed. J. Izard and M.C. Rivera, 81–96. Waltham, MA, USA: Academic Press.

La Rosa, Patricio S., Elena Deych, et al. 2016. HMP: Hypothesis testing and power calculations for comparing metagenomic samples from HMP. R package version 1.4.3. https://CRAN.R-project.org/package=HMP.

Lahti, L., and J. Salojarvi. 2014–2016. Microbiome R package. URL: http://microbiome.github.com.

Lahti, L., A. Salonen, et al. 2013. Associations between the human intestinal microbiota, Lactobacillus rhamnosus GG and serum lipids indicated by integrated analysis of high-throughput profiling data. *PeerJ* 1: e32.

Lee, J., and M. Sison-Mangus. 2018. A Bayesian semiparametric regression model for joint analysis of microbiome data. *Frontiers in Microbiology* 9: 522.

Lee, K.H., Brent A. Coull, et al. 2017. Bayesian variable selection for multivariate zero-inflated models: Application to microbiome count data. arXiv:1711.00157 [stat.AP].

Lewis, J.D., E.Z. Chen, et al. 2015. Inflammation, antibiotics, and diet as environmental stressors of the gut microbiome in pediatric Crohn's disease. *Cell Host & Microbe* 18 (4): 489–500.

Ley, R.E., F. Backhed, et al. 2005. Obesity alters gut microbial ecology. *Proceedings of the National Academy of Sciences of the United States of America* 102 (31): 11070–11075.

Ley, R.E., P.J. Turnbaugh, et al. 2006. Microbial ecology: Human gut microbes associated with obesity. *Nature* 444 (7122): 1022–1023.

Li, K.-C. 1991. Sliced inverse regression for dimension reduction. *Journal of the American Statistical Association* 86 (414): 316–327.

Love, M.I., W. Huber, et al. 2014. Moderated estimation of fold change and dispersion for RNA-seq data with DESeq2. *Genome Biology* 15 (12): 550.

Lovell, D., V. Pawlowsky-Glahn, et al. 2015. Proportionality: A valid alternative to correlation for relative data. *PLoS Computational Biology* 11 (3): e1004075.

Lozupone, C.A., and R. Knight. 2005. UnifFrac: A new phylogenetic method for comparing microbial communities. *Applied and Environmental Microbiology* 71 (12): 8228–8235.

Lozupone, C.A., M. Hamady, et al. 2007. Quantitative and qualitative beta diversity measures lead to different insights into factors that structure microbial communities. *Applied and Environment Microbiology* 73 (5): 1576–1585.

Lozupone, C., M.E. Lladser, et al. 2011. UniFrac: An effective distance metric for microbial community comparison. *ISME Journal* 5 (2): 169–172.

Lozupone, C.A., J.I. Stombaugh, et al. 2012. Diversity, stability and resilience of the human gut microbiota. *Nature* 489 (7415): 220–230.

Lozupone, C.A., J. Stombaugh, et al. 2013. Meta-analyses of studies of the human microbiota. *Genome Research* 23 (10): 1704–1714.

Lu, J., J.K. Tomfohr, et al. 2005. Identifying differential expression in multiple SAGE libraries: An overdispersed log-linear model approach. *BMC Bioinformatics* 6 (1): 165.

MacKinnon, D.P. 2008. *Introduction to statistical mediation analysis*. Mahwah, NJ: Erlbaum.

MacKinnon, D.P., A.J. Fairchild, et al. 2007. Mediation analysis. *Annual Review of Psychology* 58: 593–614.

Mancabelli, L., C. Milani, et al. 2017. Meta-analysis of the human gut microbiome from urbanized and pre-agricultural populations. *Environmental Microbiology* 19 (4): 1379–1390.

Mandal, S., W. Van Treuren, et al. 2015. Analysis of composition of microbiomes: A novel method for studying microbial composition. *Microbial Ecology in Health and Disease* 26: 27663.

Mao, Jialiang, Yuhan Chen, et al. 2017. Bayesian graphical compositional regression for microbiome data. arXiv:1712.04723 [stat.ME].

Marino, S., N.T. Baxter, et al. 2014. Mathematical modeling of primary succession of murine intestinal microbiota. *Proceedings of the National Academy of Sciences of the United States of America* 111 (1): 439–444.

McArdle, B.H., and M.J. Anderson. 2001. Fitting multivariate models to community data: A comment on distance based redundancy analysis. *Ecology* 82: 290–297.

McCarthy, D.J., Y. Chen, et al. 2012. Differential expression analysis of multifactor RNA-Seq experiments with respect to biological variation. *Nucleic Acids Research* 40 (10): 4288–4297.

McCord, A.I., C.A. Chapman, et al. 2014. Fecal microbiomes of non-human primates in Western Uganda reveal species-specific communities largely resistant to habitat perturbation. *American Journal of Primatology* 76 (4): 347–354.

McMurdie, P.J., and S. Holmes. 2013. Phyloseq: An R package for reproducible interactive analysis and graphics of microbiome census data. *PLoS ONE* 8 (4): e61217.

McMurdie, P.J., and S. Holmes. 2014. Waste not, want not: Why rarefying microbiome data is inadmissible. *PLoS Computational Biology* 10 (4): e1003531.

Moher, D., A. Liberati, et al. 2009. Preferred reporting items for systematic reviews and meta-analyses: The PRISMA statement. *PLOS Medicine* 6 (7): e1000097.

Morgan, X.C., and C. Huttenhower. 2012. Human microbiome analysis. *PLoS Comput Biol* 8 (12): 27. (Chapter 12).

Morgan, X.C., T.L. Tickle, et al. 2012. Dysfunction of the intestinal microbiome in inflammatory bowel disease and treatment. *Genome Biology* 13 (9): R79.

Narrowe, A.B., M. Albuthi-Lantz, et al. 2015. Perturbation and restoration of the fathead minnow gut microbiome after low-level triclosan exposure. *Microbiome* 3: 6.

Nilakanta, H., K.L. Drews, et al. 2014. A review of software for analyzing molecular sequences. *BMC Research Notes* 7 (1): 830.

Nobel, Y.R., L.M. Cox, et al. 2015. Metabolic and metagenomic outcomes from early-life pulsed antibiotic treatment. *Nature Communications* 6: 7486.

Oksanen, Jari, F. Guillaume Blanchet, et al. 2016. Vegan: Community ecology package. R package version 2.4-1. http://CRAN.R-project.org/package=vegan.

Palmer, C., E.M. Bik, et al. 2007. Development of the human infant intestinal microbiota. *PLoS Biology* 5 (7): 26.

Paulson, J.N., O.C. Stine, et al. 2013a. Differential abundance analysis for microbial marker-gene surveys. *Nature Methods* 10 (12): 1200–1202.

Paulson, J.N., O.C. Stine, et al. 2013b. Robust methods for differential abundance analysis in marker gene surveys. *Nature Methods* 10 (12): 1200–1202.

Pawlowsky-Glahn, V., and A. Buccianti. 2011. *Compositional data analysis: Theory and applications*. Chichester, UK: Wiley.

Pawlowsky-Glahn, V., J.J. Egozcue, et al. 2015. *Modeling and analysis of compositional data*. London, UK: Springer. Wiley.

Pearson, K. 1897. Mathematical contributions to the theory of evolution. On a form of spurious correlation which may arise when indices are used in the measurement of organs. *Proceedings of the Royal Society of London* LX: 489–502.

Perez-Cobas, A.E., M.J. Gosalbes, et al. 2013. Gut microbiota disturbance during antibiotic therapy: A multi-omic approach. *Gut* 62 (11): 1591–1601.

Peterfreund, G.L., L.E. Vandivier, et al. 2012. Succession in the gut microbiome following antibiotic and antibody therapies for clostridium difficile. *PLoS ONE* 7 (10): 10.

Peterson, J., S. Garges, et al. 2009. The NIH human microbiome project. *Genome Research* 19: 2317–2323.

Plummer, E., J. Twin, et al. 2015. A comparison of three bioinformatics pipelines for the analysis of preterm gut microbiota using 16S rRNA gene sequencing data. *Journal of Proteomics and Bioinformatics* 8: 283–291.

Praveen, P., F. Jordan, et al. 2015. The role of breast-feeding in infant immune system: A systems perspective on the intestinal microbiome. *Microbiome* 3 (1): 41.

Rawls, J.F., B.S. Samuel, et al. 2004. Gnotobiotic zebrafish reveal evolutionarily conserved responses to the gut microbiota. *Proceedings of the National Academy of Sciences of the United States of America* 101 (13): 4596–4601.

Rawls, J.F., M.A. Mahowald, et al. 2006. Reciprocal gut microbiota transplants from zebrafish and mice to germ-free recipients reveal host habitat selection. *Cell* 127 (2): 423–433.

Redondo-Lopez, V., R.L. Cook, et al. 1990. Emerging role of lactobacilli in the control and maintenance of the vaginal bacterial microflora. *Reviews of Infectious Diseases* 12 (5): 856–872.

Ridaura, V.K., J.J. Faith, et al. 2013. Gut microbiota from twins discordant for obesity modulate metabolism in mice. *Science* 341 (6150): 1241214.

Rigby, R., and D. Stasinopoulos. 2001. The GAMLSS project: A flexible approach to statistical modelling. In *New trends in statistical modelling: Proceedings of the 16th international workshop on statistical modelling*, ed. B. Klein and L. Korsholm, 249–256. Odense, Denmark.

Rigby, R.A., and D.M. Stasinopoulos. 2005. Generalized additive models for location, scale and shape. *Journal of the Royal Statistical Society: Series C (Applied Statistics)* 54 (3): 507–554.

Robinson, M.D., and G.K. Smyth. 2007. Moderated statistical tests for assessing differences in tag abundance. *Bioinformatics* 23 (21): 2881–2887.

Robinson, M.D., and G.K. Smyth. 2008. Small-sample estimation of negative binomial dispersion, with applications to SAGE data. *Biostatistics* 9 (2): 321–332.

Robinson, M.D., D.J. McCarthy, et al. 2010. edgeR: A bioconductor package for differential expression analysis of digital gene expression data. *Bioinformatics* 26 (1): 139–140.

Rogosa, M., and M.E. Sharpe. 1960. Species differentiation of human vaginal lactobacilli. *Journal of General Microbiology* 23: 197–201.

Romero, R., S.S. Hassan, et al. 2014. The composition and stability of the vaginal microbiota of normal pregnant women is different from that of non-pregnant women. *Microbiome* 2 (1): 4.

Rowe, D.B. 2003. *Multivariate Bayesian statistics: Models for source separation and signal unmixing*. Boca Raton, FL: CRC Press.

Rush, S., C. Lee, et al. 2016. The phylogenetic LASSO and the microbiome. arXiv:1607.08877 [stat.ML].

Samuel, B.S., and J.I. Gordon. 2006. A humanized gnotobiotic mouse model of host-archaeal-bacterial mutualism. *Proceedings of the National Academy of Sciences of the United States of America* 103 (26): 10011–10016.

Sanders, J.G., S. Powell, et al. 2014. Stability and phylogenetic correlation in gut microbiota: Lessons from ants and apes. *Molecular Ecology* 23 (6): 1268–1283.

Schloss, P.D., S.L. Westcott, et al. 2009. Introducing mothur: Open-source, platform-independent, community-supported software for describing and comparing microbial communities. *Applied and Environment Microbiology* 75 (23): 7537–7541.

Segata, N., S.K. Haake, et al. 2012. Composition of the adult digestive tract bacterial microbiome based on seven mouth surfaces, tonsils, throat and stool samples. *Genome Biology* 13 (6): 2012–2013.

Ren, Boyu, Sergio Bacallado, et al. 2017a. Bayesian nonparametric mixed effects models in microbiome data analysis. arXiv:1711.01241 [stat.ME].

Ren, Boyu, Sergio Bacallado, et al. 2017b. Bayesian nonparametric ordination for the analysis of microbial communities. arXiv:1601.05156 [stat.ME].

Sewankambo, N., R.H. Gray, et al. 1997. HIV-1 infection associated with abnormal vaginal flora morphology and bacterial vaginosis. *Lancet* 350 (9077): 546–550.

Smith, M.I., T. Yatsunenko, et al. 2013. Gut microbiomes of Malawian twin pairs discordant for kwashiorkor. *Science* 339 (6119): 548–554.

Smith, C.C., L.K. Snowberg, et al. 2015. Dietary input of microbes and host genetic variation shape among-population differences in stickleback gut microbiota. *ISME Journal* 9 (11): 2515–2526.

Smyth, G. 2005. Limma: Linear models for microarray data. In *Bioinformatics and computational biology solutions using R and bioconductor*, ed. R. Gentleman, V. Carey, S. Dudoit, and W.R. Irizarry, 397–420. New York: Springer.

Spor, A., O. Koren, et al. 2011. Unravelling the effects of the environment and host genotype on the gut microbiome. *Nature Reviews Microbiology* 9 (4): 279–290.

Stasinopoulos, D., and R. Rigby. 2007. Generalized additive models for location scale and shape (GAMLSS) in R. *Journal of Statistical Software* 23 (7): 1–46.

Stein, R.R., V. Bucci, et al. 2013. Ecological modeling from time-series inference: Insight into dynamics and stability of intestinal microbiota. *PLoS Computational Biology* 9 (12): e1003388.

Stenseth, N.C., M. Llope, et al. 2006. Seasonal plankton dynamics along a cross-shelf gradient. *Proceedings of the Royal Society B: Biological Sciences* 273 (1603): 2831–2838.

Stige, L.C., J. Stave, et al. 2006. The effect of climate variation on agro-pastoral production in Africa. *Proceedings of the National Academy of Sciences of the United States of America* 103 (9): 3049–3053.

Storey, J.D., and R. Tibshirani. 2003. Statistical significance for genomewide studies. *Proceedings of the National Academy of Sciences* 100 (16): 9440–9445.

Sugihara, G., R. May, et al. 2012. Detecting causality in complex ecosystems. *Science* 338 (6106): 496–500.

Sun, J., and E.B. Chang. 2014. Exploring gut microbes in human health and disease: Pushing the envelope. *Genes & Diseases* 1 (2): 132–139.

Swenson, N.G. 2011. Phylogenetic beta diversity metrics, trait evolution and inferring the functional beta diversity of communities. *PLoS ONE* 6 (6): e21264.

Sze, M., and P.D. Schloss. 2016. Looking for a signal in the noise: Revisiting obesity and the microbiome. biorxiv.

Tang, Y., L. Ma, et al. 2018. A phylogenetic scan test on a dirichlet-tree multinomial model for microbiome data. *The Annals of Applied Statistics* 12 (1): 1–26.

Tang, Y., and D.L. Nicolae 2017. Mixed effect Dirichlet-Tree multinomial for longitudinal microbiome data andweight prediction. arXiv:1706.06380v1 [stat.AP]. 20 Jun 2017

Thioulouse, J. 2011. Simultaneous analysis of a sequence of paired ecological tables: A comparison of several methods. *The Annals of Applied Statistics* 5 (4): 2300–2325.

Tibshirani, R. 1996. Regression shrinkage and selection via the LASSO. *Journal of the Royal Statistical Society: Series B (Methodological)* 58 (1): 267–288.

Trosvik, P., K. Rudi, et al. 2008. Characterizing mixed microbial population dynamics using time-series analysis. *ISME Journal* 2 (7): 707–715.

Trosvik, P., N.C. Stenseth, et al. 2010. Convergent temporal dynamics of the human infant gut microbiota. *ISME Journal* 4 (2): 151–158.

Tseng, G.C., D. Ghosh, et al. 2012. Comprehensive literature review and statistical considerations for microarray meta-analysis. *Nucleic Acids Research* 40 (9): 3785–3799.

Tung, J., L.B. Barreiro, et al. 2015. Social networks predict gut microbiome composition in wild baboons. *Elife* 4: e05224.

Turnbaugh, P.J., V.K. Ridaura, et al. 2009. The effect of diet on the human gut microbiome: A metagenomic analysis in humanized gnotobiotic mice. *Science Translational Medicine* 1 (6): 6ra14–16ra14.

Udell, Madeleine, and A. Townsend. 2017. Nice latent variable models have log-rank. arXiv:1705.07474 [cs.LG].

van den Boogaart, G.K., and R. Tolosana-Delgado. 2013a. *Analyzing compositional data with R.* Heidelberg: Springer.

Van den Boogaart, K.G., and R. Tolosana-Delgado. 2013b. *Analyzing compositional data with R.* London: UK, Springer.

Voigt, A.Y., P.I. Costea, et al. 2015. Temporal and technical variability of human gut metagenomes. *Genome Biology* 16: 73.

Wadsworth, W.D., R. Argiento, et al. 2017. An integrative Bayesian dirichlet-multinomial regression model for the analysis of taxonomic abundances in microbiome data. *BMC Bioinformatics* 18 (1): 94.

Walters, W.A., Z. Xu, et al. 2014. Meta-analyses of human gut microbes associated with obesity and IBD. *FEBS Letters* 588 (22): 4223–4233.

Wang, Y., X. Hu, et al. 2015. Predicting microbial interactions by using network-constrained regularization incorporating covariate coefficients and connection signs. In *2015 IEEE International Conference on Bioinformatics and Biomedicine (BIBM)*.

Wang, J., L. B. Thingholm, et al. 2016. Genome-wide association analysis identifies variation in vitamin D receptor and other host factors influencing the gut microbiota. Nature Genetics (advance online publication).

Wang, T., and H. Zhao. 2017. A dirichlet-tree multinomial regression model for associating dietary nutrients with gut microorganisms. *Biometrics* 73 (3): 792–801.

Wang, T., G. Cai, et al. 2012. Structural segregation of gut microbiota between colorectal cancer patients and healthy volunteers. *ISME Journal* 6 (2): 320–329.

Wei, W.W.S. 2005. *Time series analysis: Univariate and multivariate methods*. Boston: Pearson.

White, J.R., N. Nagarajan, et al. 2009. Statistical methods for detecting differentially abundant features in clinical metagenomic samples. *PLOS Computational Biology* 5 (4): e1000352.

Wilson, W.G., P. Lundberg, et al. 2003. Biodiversity and species interactions: Extending Lotka-Volterra community theory. *Ecology Letters* 6 (10): 944–952.

Witkin, S.S., and W.J. Ledger. 2012. Complexities of the uniquely human vagina. *Science Translational Medicine* 4 (132): 132fs11.

Wong, R.G., J.R. Wu, et al. 2016. Expanding the UniFrac toolbox. *PLoS ONE* 11 (9): e0161196.

Wu, G.D., J. Chen, et al. 2011. Linking long-term dietary patterns with gut microbial enterotypes. *Science* 334 (6052): 105–108.

Wu, S., Y.G. Zhang, et al. 2015. Intestinal epithelial vitamin D receptor deletion leads to defective autophagy in colitis. *Gut* 64 (7): 1082–1094.

Wu, G.D., C. Compher, et al. 2016. Comparative metabolomics in vegans and omnivores reveal constraints on diet-dependent gut microbiota metabolite production. *Gut* 65 (1): 63–72.

Xia, Y., and J. Sun. 2017. Hypothesis testing and statistical analysis of microbiome. *Genes & Diseases* 4 (3): 138–148.

Xia, Y., N. Lu, et al. 2012a. Statistical methods and issues in the study of suicide. In *Frontiers in suicide risk: Research, treatment and prevention*, ed. J. Lavigne and J. Kemp, 139–158. Hauppauge, New York: Nova Science.

Xia, Y., D. Morrison-Beedy, et al. 2012b. Modeling count outcomes from HIV risk reduction interventions: A comparison of competing statistical models for count responses. *AIDS Research and Treatment* 2012: 11 pages.

Xia, F., J. Chen, et al. 2013a. A logistic normal multinomial regression model for microbiome compositional data analysis. *Biometrics* 69 (4): 1053–1063.

Xia, J., C.D. Fjell, et al. 2013b. INMEX—A web-based tool for integrative meta-analysis of expression data. *Nucleic Acids Research* 41 (web server issue): W63–W70.

Xie, H., and J. Huang. 2009. SCAD-penalized regression in high-dimensional partially linear models. *The Annals of Statistics* 37 (2): 673–696.

Xu, L., A.D. Paterson, et al. 2015. Assessment and selection of competing models for zero-inflated microbiome data. *PLoS ONE* 10 (7): e0129606.

Yan, Q., J. Li, et al. 2016. Environmental filtering decreases with fish development for the assembly of gut microbiota. *Environmental Microbiology* 18 (12): 4739–4754.

Yang, H., X. Huang, et al. 2016. Uncovering the composition of microbial community structure and metagenomics among three gut locations in pigs with distinct fatness. *Scientific Reports* 6: 27427.

Yassour, M., T. Vatanen, et al. 2016. Natural history of the infant gut microbiome and impact of antibiotic treatment on bacterial strain diversity and stability. *Science Translational Medicine* 8 (343): 343ra381.

Yin, X., and H. Hilafu. 2015. Sequential sufficient dimension reduction for large p, small n problems. *Journal of the Royal Statistical Society: Series B (Statistical Methodology)* 77 (4): 879–892.

Yin, X., J. Peng, et al. 2013. Structural changes of gut microbiota in a rat non-alcoholic fatty liver disease model treated with a Chinese herbal formula. *Systematic and Applied Microbiology* 36 (3): 188–196.

Zhang, C., and L. Zhao. 2016. Strain-level dissection of the contribution of the gut microbiome to human metabolic disease. *Genome Medicine* 8 (1): 016–0304.

Zhang, H., Y. Xia, et al. 2011. Modeling longitudinal binomial responses: Implications from two dueling paradigms. *Journal of Applied Statistics* 38 (11): 2373–2390.

Zhang, X., H. Mallick, et al. 2016. Zero-inflated negative binomial regression for differential abundance testing in microbiome studies. *Journal of Bioinformatics and Genomics* 2 (2): 1–9.

Zhang, X., H. Mallick, et al. 2017. Negative binomial mixed models for analyzing microbiome count data. *BMC Bioinformatics* 18 (1): 4.

Zhao, L. 2013. The gut microbiota and obesity: From correlation to causality. *Nature Reviews Microbiology* 11 (9): 639–647.

Zhou, N., and J. Zhu. 2010. Group variable selection via a hierarchical lasso and its oracle property. *Statistics and Its Interface* 3: 557–574.

Zou, H. 2006. The adaptive lasso and its oracle properties. *Journal of the American Statistical Association* 101 (476): 1418–1429.

Chapter 4
Introduction to R, RStudio and ggplot2

In this chapter, we provide some programming and graphic skills under the environments of R, RStudio and ggplot2. In Sect. 4.1, we introduce some basic uses of R and RStudio. We also provide some useful R functions which are often used in the programming and management of microbiome data. Section 4.2 introduce the one useful R package dplyr. We use it often in the remaining chapters. In Sect. 4.3, we introduce and illustrate the ggplot2 package. This package is getting popular in recent years; the high quality graphics generated by the ggplot2 are often used in the publications of microbiome study and other research fields. We briefly summarize this chapter in Sect. 4.4.

4.1 Introduction to R and RStudio

R(R Core Team 2017) is a high-level open-source programming language and environment for statistical computing and graphics. It is a vehicle for newly developing methods of interactive data analysis. It has been rapidly developed and extended by a large collection of packages provided by researchers and volunteers.

RStudio (R Studio Team 2016) is a free and open-source integrated development environment (IDE) for R. We can check the most up-to-date citation by typing citation() at the prompt. To find the appropriate citation in the individual contributed package, type citation ("package name"), e.g., citation ("ALDEx2"). We also can check the citation from the reference manual for the package that is available on CRAN (The Comprehensive R Archive Network). To cite RStudio in publications, we can obtain the latest citation information by typing the command RStudio.Version() in a recent version of RStudio IDE.

© Springer Nature Singapore Pte Ltd. 2018
Y. Xia et al., *Statistical Analysis of Microbiome Data with R*,
ICSA Book Series in Statistics, https://doi.org/10.1007/978-981-13-1534-3_4

4.1.1   Installing R, RStudio, and R Packages

R can be downloaded from http://www.r-project.org and be installed on all three mainstream operating systems (Windows, Mac, Unix/Linux). RStudio can be downloaded from https://www.rstudio.com/products/rstudio/download3/ and can be installed on all four supported platforms (Windows, Mac, Ubuntu and Fedora). The general installation manual and introductory tutorials can be obtained from the same website. Similar to other statistical software packages, R provides a statistical framework and terminal-based interface for users to input commands for data manipulation. As an IDE, all statistical analyses and graphics can be implemented through RStudio.

R is made up of many user-written packages. The base version of R that is downloaded allows the user to get started in R, but the capabilities of base R are limited and further data analyses need to install additional packages. An R package is a collection of functions, examples, and documentation. The focus of a package is often its functionality: a special statistical methodology. We begin by illustrating some basic commands for managing R packages here in this section.

After downloading and installing R and RStudio software, an R or RStudio terminal can be started to install the required additional packages. Any package that does not appear in the installed packages matrix must be installed and loaded before its functions can be used. A package can be installed using **install.packages** ("package name").

```
> install.packages("ALDEx2")
```

In R, additional packages can also be installed from the R terminal menu "Packages" → "select the CRAN mirror" → "select repositories".

In RStudio, you can also click "Packages" → "Install" → type package name e.g., ALDEx2 in column "Packages" and choose to install from "Repository (CRAN, CRANextra)" or "Package Archive File(.zip;. tar.gz)" (if you downloaded R package in your computer) → click "Install" to install additional packages.

After installing, the packages can be loaded either in R or RStudio by the following command:

```
> library(ALDEx2)
```

Or check this package from User Library in RStudio.

To see what packages are installed, use the **installed.packages()** command. This will return a matrix with a row for each package that has been installed. Type following command display the first 5 R packages installed in your computer.

```
> installed.packages()[1:5,]
```

To see whether or not a specific package (e.g., ALDEx2) has already installed, type the command:

```
> a<-installed.packages()
> packages<-a[,1]
> is.element("ALDEx2", packages)
[1] TRUE
```

4.1.2 Set Working Directory in R

As a very important concept in R, a "working directory" is where you store your raw data, R codes and output for that specific project. You would create specific "working directory" for different projects and then you need to let R know where you like the R to read the data and the associated R programs, so you need to change your R working directory to that specific project.

In R and RStudio, the working directory of different projects can be changed. To show the working directory, we can type the getwd() command:

```
> getwd()
[1] "C:/Users/Yinglin"
```

This shows our current basic R folder. If we want to change the working directory to a specific folder for our R scripts, data and to save results in this specific folder, we can set the working directory to this folder. For example, the following R codes create a directory and a folder "Analysis" to store the R codes, raw and intermediate data files and the analysis results.

```
> setwd("E:/Home/MicrobiomeStatR/Analysis")
```

In RStudio, we can also choose "Session" → "Set Working Directory" → "To Source File Location" to set working directory. If we do not want set the working directory to source file location, we can either set it "To Files Pane Location" or "Choose Directory" from other folder. Check getwd() function again and we will find our directory has changed.

```
> getwd()
[1] "E:/Home/MicrobiomeStatR/Analysis"
```

By typing the command below, we can set working directory back to file pane folder:

```
> setwd("~/")
```

In RStudio, we can also choose "Session" → "Set Working Directory" → "To Files Pane Location" to do the same thing.

```
> getwd()
[1] "C:/Users/Yinglin"
```

If an R code file (for example, called "Rcodes.R") stored in the directory, we can use source (Rcodes.R) to access the file "Rcodes.R" and run the R codes contained in the file. The file should be a plain text file and saved with the extension. R.

Every time when we open RStudio, it goes to a default directory. We can change the default to a folder where we want our data files to be, so we do not have to do it every time. In the menu go to Tools → Global Options → Default working directory → Browse → then open a folder we want the data files to be → Select Folder.

4.1.3   Data Analysis Through RStudio

4.1.3.1   Basic Features of RStudio

RStudio allows the user to run R in a more user-friendly environment.

RStudio screen usually consists of four main panels: source editor and data viewer; environment (workspace browser) and history; R console; and files, plots, packages, help and viewer. Most panels have multiple tables with different functionalities. We briefly introduce each panel and its basic features as below.

Source editor and data viewer

This panel is located in the top left. It is a source editor for editing files and a data viewer for viewing dataframes. Its intentions and purposes are identical to every other code editor's main window. We can write R scripts here. There are several ways to create a new R script; the convenient one is to go to File → New → R Script. After the bank screen displays, we can type R commands there. To run R scripts, click on the "Run" button on the top right or leave the cursor anywhere on the line where the command is and press Ctrl-R. Output will appear in the console below. The "Source on Save" checkbox means "Load contents of file into my console's runtime every time I save the file". Checking this box makes the development flow faster by one click.

R console

The R console panel provided by RStudio is in the bottom left; its functionality is very much like most R consoles, e.g., provided by the basic RGui for Windows, where we can type commands and see output. Although we can type commands at the console, it is not really reproducible, and thus not an efficient way to manage

R scripts. We recommend readers to use source editor to write and manage their R scripts.

Environment and history

The environment and history tabs are in the top right. The **environment** tab refers to the console environment and includes all the active objects. This tab stores any object, value, function or anything we create during R session. If we click on any name of the dataset listed under "Data", the data will display on the data viewer screen left to "Data". This is where we can also import datasets manually and make them instantly available in the console.

The **history** tab keeps all the console commands we executed since the last project started. It is saved into a hidden .Rhistory file in project's folder. The history won't be saved if we did not choose to save the environment after a session. It is helpful for testing. We can save or select the commands and send them to an R script by clicking on "To Source" button or to R console by clicking on "To Console" button.

Files, plots, packages, help and viewer

The bottom right panel is the miscellaneous panel containing five separate tabs. The **files** tab shows all the files and folders in the default workspace. The **plots** tab will show all the graphs during the R session. Here we can zoom, export, configure and inspect graphs/figures. The most use is probably to export and save graphs.

The graphs can be exported and saved by choosing:

- Export → Save as Image → Save plot as Image → Image format → choose one format from: JPEG, PNG, TIFF, BMP, Metafile, SVG, EPS → Select the directory and name the graph → Save.
- Export → Save as PDF → Select the directory and name the graph → Save.
- Export → Copy to Clipboard → Copy plot to clipboard → Copy as: Bitmap or Metafile → Copy plot.

The first two options are useful when we want to create publication-quality figures or use it in a LaTeX document. The third option: copy and paste, probably is the easiest way to export a graph and is most often used in Word document.

The **packages** tab shows the list of add-ons packages installed in RStudio. To load the packages into R, we need to check them. As we introduced previously, we can also install additional packages by clicking on the "Install Packages" button. The **help** tab allows us to search the built-in documentation on R functions, datasets, and packages. The help tab can be used when we invoked the ? function. When we enter a question mark followed by the name e.g., ?data.frame in the console or run it in source editor, the information about the command name(in this case, Data Frames) will automatically open. Finally, the **viewer** is essentially RStudio's built-in browser. With RStudio, we can develop HTML documents (web pages) easily by Markdown (created by John Gruber and Aaron Swartz). The Viewer tab can show us the resulting HTML file created from an R Markdown Knit.

4.1.3.2 Illustrating Data Analysis with RStudio

In this section, we illustrate how to utilize the RStudio features to create a boxplot. The dataset hsb2demo we use is publicly available at (https://stats.idre.ucla.edu/sas/output/regression-analysis/). The data set with SAS data format was collected on 200 high schools students and are scores on various tests, including reading, writing, math, science, and social studies. The variable female is a dichotomous variable coded 1 if the student was female and 0 if male. This data set contains 200 rows and 11 variables.

The following are the variables in the columns (in order):

Column name	Description
id	Subject id
female	Gender variable
race	Race variable
ses	Socioeconomic status
schtyp	School types
prog	Programs
read	Reading score
write	Writing score
math	Math score
science	Science score
socst	Social science score

We illustrate how to create a boxplot of reading score by gender using the following main steps:

First, we download the data set and convert it to CSV format, and save it in following directory. We also set the working directory to this directory by:

Choose "Session" → "Set Working Directory" → "To Source File Location".

```
> setwd("E:/Home/MicrobiomeStatR/Analysis")
```

Next, import data in RStudio. There are several ways to import the data into R/RStudio, either through R functions or R packages; we will introduce some widely used ones in next section. Here we use the import dataset feature of RStudio. To perform this, follow the steps below.

- Click on the "Import Dataset" button in the top-right panel under the environment tab.
- Click Import Dataset dialog and choose the options (From csv....; From Excel....; From SPSS....; From SAS....; From Stata....). In this case, we choose "From csv....".
- Browse the above folder that stored the dataset hsb2demo
- Click "Open" button → Set Import Options(e.g., preferences of separator, name and other parameters) → Click "Import" button.

Now the dataset hsb2demo appears in the top-left panel for review. We can review this dataset by the View() function:

View(hsb2demo) or click the name of hsb2demo from the list of "Data" under the environment tab if it did not appear.

Then, we create a boxplot of writing scores by gender. A very useful feature of RStudio is its built-in data visualizer for R. We can create the plots and visualize them using the R functions, e.g., in this case, the boxplot() function.

```
> #Boxplot of writing score by gender
> boxplot(write ~ female,data=hsb2demo, main="High School
Students Data", xlab="Gender", ylab="Writing score by gender")
```

We copy this plot by clicking Export → Copy to Clipboard → Copy plot to clipboard → Copy as: Bitmap → Copy plot, and paste it below:

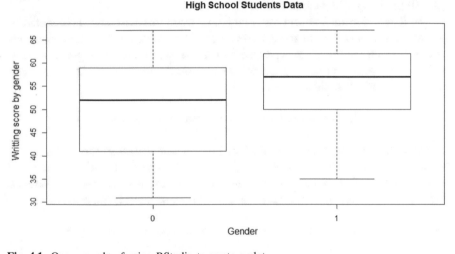

Fig. 4.1 One example of using RStudio to create a plot

If we want to create high quality of boxplot, we can use ggplot2 package, which we will introduce later. To use this package, we need install ggplot2 and load it to R/RStudio by calling library (ggplot2) or in RStudio, click Packages → check the box near to ggplot2.

4.1.4   Data Import and Export

One of critical steps for data analysis is to import data with special formats into R workspace. The most frequent data formats in microbiome study are comma separated files, Excel spreadsheets, and files generated by bioinformatics pipelines, and a variety of website data. R has functions like read.table(), read.csv() and read.csv2 (), read.delim() and other tools to import the data from the files into R workspace. Here we introduce the most often used functions and tools.

4.1.4.1   Using read.table()

First, we make a note on the argument "stringsAsFactors" before we introduce data importing functions. This is an argument to the "data.frame()" function in R, which indicates whether strings in a data frame should be treated as factor variables or as just plain strings. The argument also appears in "read.table()" and related functions because of the role these functions play in reading and converting table data to data frames. By default, "stringsAsFactors" is set to TRUE in the functions like read. table(), read.csv(), read.csv2() and read.delim() import the columns containing characters strings into R as factors. The reason for setting strings as factors is to tell R to treat categorical variables into individual dummy variables for modeling functions like lm() and glm(). However, in genomics or microbiome study, it doesn't make sense to encode the names of the genes or taxa in one column of data as factors because they are essentially just labels and not to be used in any modeling function. In this situation, we can change the "stringsAsFactors" argument into FALSE to change the default setting.

The R function read.table() reads table in a plain text with cells delimitated by one of the symbols: one or more white spaces (" "), tabs, newlines or returns. For example, when the fields are separated by commas and each row begins a name (a text format typically created by Excel), we can use the function read.table() to read the data into R workspace.

```
> tab <- read.table("genus.csv", header=TRUE,row.names=1, sep=",")
```

Where, the argument header = TRUE or T indicates that the first entry of the text file "genus.csv" should be interpreted as variable names. The argument row.names = 1 indicates that the first column should be interpreted as row names but not as a variable, and the argument sep = "," indicates that columns are separated by a comma.

```
> tab <- read.table("genus.txt", header=TRUE,row.names=1, sep="\t")
```

The argument sep = "\t" tells R that file is tab-delimited (use " " to indicate that the file is space- delimited; use "," for comma delimited in a .csv file). If a meta table(e.g., OTU table from QIIME) has a line before headers, then skip = 1 is needed to specify. If the header line starts with #, then use comment.char = "" to read them.

We can also access files in folders outside of the current folder. For example, the following read.able() link to the location of file on internet:

```
> raw<-
"https://raw.githubusercontent.com/chvlyl/PLEASE/master/1_Data
/Raw_Data/MetaPhlAn/PLEASE/G_Remove_unclassfied_Renormalized_M
erge_Rel_MetaPhlAn_Result.xls"
> tab <- read.table(raw,sep='\t',header=TRUE,row.names = 1,
check.names=FALSE,stringsAsFactors=FALSE)
```

The argument check.names = F has two reasons. One is to tell the function to ignore the duplicate entries of variables (i.e., species). For example, for microbiome data, the sample by species table can contain several species of the same name; another reason is to tell the function not to attempt to modify the names of the species so that ensure them syntactically correct (otherwise, e.g., the space in the name would be replaced by a dot).

4.1.4.2 Using read.delim()

The read.delim() function expects that input table is plain text with cells separated or delimited by tabulators.

```
> tab <- read.delim("genus.txt", header=T, row.names=1)
```

opens a tab-delimited file "genus.txt". Compared with read.delim(), we can see that read.table() offers more control in the read file type because it can read .txt or .csv files. It is a specific variant of more general function read.table().

4.1.4.3 Using read.csv() and read.csv2()

The files with *.csv format have different standards in different countries and on different platforms. In Czech the files with *.csv format have cells delimited by semicolons ";" and decimals by commas ","; while in western Europe and elsewhere the cells are delimited by commas "," and decimals are separated by dots ".". The read.csv () function reads table delimited by commas"," with decimals being dots ".". The read.csv2 () function reads table delimited by commas ";" with decimals being commas ",".

We use function read.csv () to read the csv file with separators being commas and decimals being dots as below:

```
> tab <- read.csv('table.csv', head = T, row.names = 1,
sep =',', dec = '.')
```

If the file "table.csv" has cells delimited by semicolons ";" and decimals separated commas ",", then he function read.csv2() is needed.

```
> tab <- read.csv2 ('table.csv',head = T, row.names = 1,
sep =';', dec = ',')
```

This kind of file can also be read using the read.table() function. The argument sep = ';' sets the delimiter to be semicolon, and dec = ',' sets the decimal separator to be comma.

```
> tab <- read.table (file = 'table.csv', head = T, row.names = 1,
sep =';', dec = ',')
```

4.1.4.4   Using the gdata Package

The read.xls() function of the gdata package can read spreadsheets. The function uses a module developed for the scripting language "perl", and thus requires the perl to be installed. The package is available for Windows, Mac or Linux platforms. Usually perl is already installed in Linux and Mac, but on Windows an installation of perl is required. The read.xls () function first translates the specified sheet to a comma-separated file, then calls the read.csv() function. Thus, it accepts all options of the read.csv() function. The three arguments are especially useful: the skip = and header = arguments are used to avoid misinterpreting headers and notes as data, and the as.is = TRUE argument can be used to suppress factor conversion.

```
> install.packages("gdata")
> library(gdata)
> tab <- read.xls("table.xlsx",sheet=1,header=TRUE)
```

If the perl.exe file has not been installed, then the above R code is not executable and will give an error message. If this happens, we need to download the perl.exe file and save it in a folder. In the call to read.xls, specify it as below (this is where my perl.exe is located, check yours, it might be different).

```
> tab <- read.xls("table.xlsx", sheet=1,perl="C:/Perl64/bin/perl.exe")
```

4.1.4.5   Using the XLConnect Package

Sometime, the file was saved as an Excel file. We can import directly from the *.xls file. Package **XLConnect** can read, write, and manipulate Microsoft Excel files from within R. To use this package, we install it first. Both .xls and .xlsx file formats can be used. The function readWorksheetFromFile() will open the file specified in argument file and read the sheet specified by the argument sheet. Other arguments are similar to the read.table() function.

```
> install.packages ("XLConnect")
> library (XLConnect)
> tab <- readWorksheetFromFile(file = 'table.xlsx', sheet = 1, header = T,
rownames = 1)
```

Other packages, such as xlsReadWrite, xlsx can also be used for both reading and writing to Excel files. They work in much the same way.

4.1.4.6   Using write.table() to Export Data

In microbiome study, analysis results are often exported or saved to external file. The basic tool is the function write.table(). It can write a comma separated file readable by Excel and a text file readable by Notepad.

```
> write.table(genus, file="genus_out.csv", quote=FALSE,
row.names=FALSE,sep="\t")
> write.table(genus, file="genus_out.txt", quote=FALSE,
col.names=TRUE,sep=",")
```

Where, the only required argument of write.table() is the name of a dataset or matrix. The second argument file = is used to specify the destination as either a character string to represent a file or a connection. By default, character strings are surrounded by quotes. We can use the quote = FALSE or F to suppress it. We can use the row.names = FALSE or col.names = FALSE arguments to suppress row names or column names from being written to the out file, respectively. We also have options to specify a separator other than a blank space. The sep = "\t" is used for tab-separated, the sep = "," is used for comma-separated.

Similarly to the functions read.csv() and read.csv2(), the alternative functions of write.table() are write.csv() and write.csv2(). They have appropriate options to set to produce comma-or semicolon-separated files.

4.1.5 Basic Data Manipulation

In this section, we briefly introduce some basic data handling and manipulation techniques, which are mostly associated with a data frame. A data frame is a list of vectors of equal length. Data frame is object that R handles data. It generally refers to "tabular" data: a data structure with rows representing observations, or measurements (these are sometimes called cases), and with columns containing the values of different variables (these are often called fields). In microbiome study, cases could be samples; fields could be genus, species, OTUs or any taxonomic levels. Data frames usually contain some metadata in addition to data, e.g., row and column names. The object of class data frame is the most important data structure for handling tabular statistical data in R. The default R installation comes with several data sets; here we use the famous iris data set to illustrate structure of data frame and some basic manipulations with data frame.

The iris data frame gives the measurements in centimeters of the variables sepal length and width, and petal length and width, respectively, for 50 flowers from each of 3 species of iris (*setosa*, *versicolor*, and *virginica*). Thus, it has 150 cases (rows) and 5 variables (columns) named Sepal.Length, Sepal.Width, Petal.Length, Petal. Width, and Species. For details of the data set, type help (iris) in R or RStudio.

Structure of Data Frame
We can type following R codes in R or RStudio to load the data and first several lines of data.

```
> data()
> attach(iris)
> head(iris)
  Sepal.Length Sepal.Width Petal.Length Petal.Width Species
1          5.1         3.5          1.4         0.2  setosa
2          4.9         3.0          1.4         0.2  setosa
3          4.7         3.2          1.3         0.2  setosa
4          4.6         3.1          1.5         0.2  setosa
5          5.0         3.6          1.4         0.2  setosa
6          5.4         3.9          1.7         0.4  setosa
```

Here is a table in the form of a data frame. The top row is called "header", contains the column names. Each horizontal row afterward begins with the name of the row, and then followed by the data. Each row and column of data constructs a data cell. A data cell can be retrieved by *bracket* "[]" operator: [position of row, position of column]. In other words, the coordinates begins with row position, then followed by a comma, and ends with the column position.

Create Data Frames

We can create data frames using existing data frame. Several techniques can be used to achieve it.

```
> #Create data frame using column indices
> df <- iris[,c(1,2,3)]
> head(df)
  Sepal.Length Sepal.Width Petal.Length
1          5.1         3.5          1.4
2          4.9         3.0          1.4
3          4.7         3.2          1.3
4          4.6         3.1          1.5
5          5.0         3.6          1.4
6          5.4         3.9          1.7

> # Create data frame using column indices with sequences
> df <- iris[,c(1:2,4:5)]
> head(df)
  Sepal.Length Sepal.Width Petal.Width Species
1          5.1         3.5         0.2 setosa
2          4.9         3.0         0.2 setosa
3          4.7         3.2         0.2 setosa
4          4.6         3.1         0.2 setosa
5          5.0         3.6         0.2 setosa
6          5.4         3.9         0.4 setosa

> #Create data frame using subset() and column indices
> df<- subset(iris, select=c(1,2, 4:5))
> head(df)
  Sepal.Length Sepal.Width Petal.Width Species
1          5.1         3.5         0.2 setosa
2          4.9         3.0         0.2 setosa
3          4.7         3.2         0.2 setosa
4          4.6         3.1         0.2 setosa
5          5.0         3.6         0.2 setosa
6          5.4         3.9         0.4 setosa

> # Create data frame using subset() and column names
> df <- subset(iris, select=c("Sepal.Width", "Petal.Length", "Petal.Width"))
> head(df)
  Sepal.Width Petal.Length Petal.Width
1         3.5          1.4         0.2
2         3.0          1.4         0.2
3         3.2          1.3         0.2
4         3.1          1.5         0.2
5         3.6          1.4         0.2
6         3.9          1.7         0.4
```

```
> # Create data frame by selecting  column names
> df <- iris[,c("Sepal.Width", "Petal.Length", "Petal.Width")]
> head(df)
  Sepal.Width Petal.Length Petal.Width
1         3.5          1.4         0.2
2         3.0          1.4         0.2
3         3.2          1.3         0.2
4         3.1          1.5         0.2
5         3.6          1.4         0.2
6         3.9          1.7         0.4


> #Create data frame using data.frame()
> df <- data.frame(iris$Sepal.Width, iris$Petal.Length, iris$Petal.Width)
> head(df)
  iris.Sepal.Width iris.Petal.Length iris.Petal.Width
1              3.5               1.4              0.2
2              3.0               1.4              0.2
3              3.2               1.3              0.2
4              3.1               1.5              0.2
5              3.6               1.4              0.2
6              3.9               1.7              0.4
```

We can also create data frames using c() and data.frame() manually.

```
> #Create data frame using c() manually
> Sepal.Width = c(3.5, 3.0, 3.2, 3.1,3.6,3.9)
> Petal.Length = c(1.4,1.4,1.3,1.5,1.4,1.7)
> Petal.Width = c(0.2,0.2,0.2,0.2,0.2,0.4)
> df = data.frame(Sepal.Width,Petal.Length,Petal.Width)
> df
  Sepal.Width Petal.Length Petal.Width
1         3.5          1.4         0.2
2         3.0          1.4         0.2
3         3.2          1.3         0.2
4         3.1          1.5         0.2
5         3.6          1.4         0.2
6         3.9          1.7         0.4
```

Basic Operations
We already used the head() function to preview data frame.

```
> head(iris)
```

By default, R uses a data frame as objects, sometime we need check the data set to see if it is a data frame. The attributes() print the column names (names), row names (row.names), and class, which shows whether the data set is or not a data frame.

```
> attributes(iris)
```

Alternatively, we can use class() function to check if the data set is data frame:

```
> class(iris)
[1]"data.frame"
```

We can check how many rows and columns using the dim() function:

```
> dim(iris)
[1] 150   5
```

The numbers of rows and columns can be found using the nrow() and ncol() functions.

```
> nrow(iris)
[1] 150
> ncol(iris)
[1] 5
```

The length of a vector is given by

```
> length(iris[,"Species"])
[1] 150
```

The row and column names can be found using the rownames () and colnames () functions.

```
> #check column or row names
> colnames(iris)
> rownames(iris)
```

The whole data frame can be printed using the print() function:

```
> print(iris)
```

If we just want to print the columns of interest instead of whole data frame, we can use:

```
> Species <- iris[,"Species"]
> Species
```

The cell value can be accessed by indices:

```
> iris[1,3]
[1] 1.4
```

Alternatively, the row and column names can be used instead of indices:

```
> iris["1", "Petal.Length"]
[1] 1.4
```

In contrast to indexing with positive integers, the cell values can also be accessed using negative indexing which are not part of the index vector given in brackets.

```
> head(iris[,-c(4:5)])
  Sepal.Length Sepal.Width Petal.Length
1          5.1         3.5          1.4
2          4.9         3.0          1.4
3          4.7         3.2          1.3
4          4.6         3.1          1.5
5          5.0         3.6          1.4
6          5.4         3.9          1.7
```

Check Sparsity of Microbiome Data

Some specific data manipulations are needed in microbiome study. We pick up several of them here. As we described in Chap. 2, one important feature of microbiome data is sparsity with many zeros. To check the sparsity in following table, we use the R codes below:

```
> tab=read.csv("VdrGenusCounts.csv",row.names=1,check.names=FALSE)
> #Check total zeros in the table
> sum(tab == 0)
 [1] 3103

> #Check how many non-zeros in the table
> sum(tab != 0)
 [1] 865
```

Some Functions for Graphics

This book has no intention to introduce R graphics. For introduction to R graphics, the readers can reference Chang's R Graphics Cookbook (Chang 2013); for fully exploration of ggplot2 plotting capabilities, read Teutonico's ggplot2 Essentials (Teutonico 2015); for comprehensively use of R capabilities for graphics and analysis, read Crawley's R book (Crawley 2013). However, in order to provide a background for later chapters' graphics plotting and basic knowledge for R graphics, we will briefly introduce the concept and basics of ggplot2, and two R functions for graphics: par () and layout() here.

The par () function can be used to set or query graphical parameters. Many graphical parameters are available for use; among them, the mar, and mfcol and mfrow are most often used. The sizes of the margins of the plot are measured in lines of text. The mar is used to specify the margin sizes in number of lines to plot the four sides of the plot: c (bottom, left, top, right). Be default the margin is par (mar = (c(5, 4, 4, 2) + 0.1)).

The parameters mfrow and mfcol are used to control how many graphs on the same page. To remember the names of these functions, consider them as standing for "multiple frames in rows" (mfrow) or "multiple frames in columns" (mfcol). We can obtain multiple graph panels on the same graphics device using par(mfrow), par (mfcol), par(layout), and par(fig), par(split.screen) but par(mfrow) is much the most frequently used. The mfrow have two arguments: the first is used for specifying the number of rows of graphs, and second is for number of columns of graphs per row. The default of one plot per screen is one row, one column: par(mfrow = c(1,1)).

As an alternative of mfrow () or fig (), the layout() function can be used to configure the multiple plots. By using this function, we can alter both the location and shape of multiple plotting regions independently. One syntax of the layout function is given:

layout(matrix, widths = w, heights = h)

where matrix is a matrix object specifying the location of the n figures to plot on the output device, w is a vector of column widths (with length = ncol(matrix)) and h is a vector of row heights (with length = nrow(matrix)). The function layout.show(n) plots the outlines of the *n* figures. For example, in Chap. 10, we use layout() to plot cluster dendrogram on the top of figures and a stacked bar plot on the bottom and legend on the right side. The R codes are as below:

```
> ng <- layout(matrix(c(1,3,2,3),2,2, byrow=TRUE), widths=c(5,2),
height=c(3,4))
```

We display the location of figures below:

```
> layout.show(ng)
```

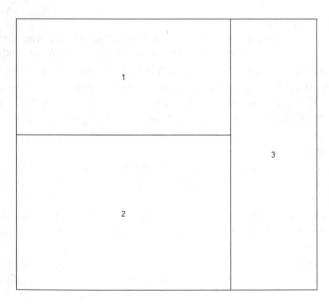

where the layout() function defines the location of the three figures: Fig. 10.3 is the cluster dendrogram, which we want to put on the top of three boxes, Fig. 10.4 is the stacked bar plot which will be located in the lower left, and Fig. 10.4's legend is to be drawn on the right side.

The readers can reference Chap. 10 for the details.

Some Options Settings

Options settings allow us to set and examine global *options* to tell R how computes and displays its results. The argument width is used to specify the maximum number of columns on a line to print with default normally 80; digits is used to control the number of significant digits to print when printing numeric values. The valid values are 0...22 with default 7. The two arguments can be used together to ensure that line breaks in the output correspond to the width of page. It is a better practice to set the same settings in R sessions, such as, when we start a new R session, we can set:

```
> options(width=65,digits=4)
```

4.1.6 Simple Summary Statistics

The most helpful function for getting an overview about R objects is summary(), which gives a collection of basic summary statistics. For example, we can use the summary() function to the iris data set:

```
> summary(iris)
  Sepal.Length    Sepal.Width     Petal.Length    Petal.Width          Species
 Min.   :4.30    Min.   :2.00    Min.   :1.00    Min.   :0.1    setosa    :50
 1st Qu.:5.10    1st Qu.:2.80    1st Qu.:1.60    1st Qu.:0.3    versicolor:50
 Median :5.80    Median :3.00    Median :4.35    Median :1.3    virginica :50
 Mean   :5.84    Mean   :3.06    Mean   :3.76    Mean   :1.2
 3rd Qu.:6.40    3rd Qu.:3.30    3rd Qu.:5.10    3rd Qu.:1.8
 Max.   :7.90    Max.   :4.40    Max.   :6.90    Max.   :2.5
```

Other functions for simply summary statistics include mean(), median(), min() and max(). They are often seen combining with the apply() function to obtain summary statistics for each dimension of a matrix or array. The usage of this function is apply (DATA, MARGIN, FUN, OPTION). Three arguments are required: data is data frame, including a matrix on which to perform the operation, margin is an index telling apply() which dimension to operate on, e.g., 1 for a matrix indicates rows, 2 indicates columns, c(1,2) indicates rows and columns. The following R codes are used to obtain the row and column means.

```
> iris_1 <- (iris[,-5])
> head(apply(iris_1, 1, mean))
[1] 2.550 2.375 2.350 2.350 2.550 2.850
> apply(iris_1, 2, mean)
Sepal.Length  Sepal.Width Petal.Length  Petal.Width
       5.843        3.057        3.758        1.199
> apply(iris_1, 2, mean,na.rm = TRUE)
Sepal.Length  Sepal.Width Petal.Length  Petal.Width
       5.843        3.057        3.758        1.199
```

The apply() and other functions for summary statistics have important applications in microbiome data. For example, the following codes use the apply() function to calculate percent abundance of each taxon (OTU) per sample:

```
> tab_perc <- apply(tab, 2, function(x){x/sum(x)})
```

Sometimes, the taxon abundance table has a taxon column at the end; in this situation, we need use −1 index to get rid of it and then calculate the percentage.

```
> tab_perc <- apply(tab[,1:ncol(tab)-1], 2, function(x){x/sum(x)})
```

For microbiome data analysis, we often need to filter taxon abundance per sample before analysis. For example, the following codes use the apply() function to get rid of the taxa in any sample with percentage less than 1%:

```
> tab_p1 <- tab[apply(tab_perc, 1, max)>0.01,]
```

The following codes are used to retain taxa (OTUs) with frequency of >0.01 in every sample:

```
> tab_p2 <- tab[apply(tab_perc, 1, min)>0.01,]
> head(tab_p2)
                5_15_drySt-28F 20_12_CeSt-28F 1_11_drySt-28F
Lactococcus                326            737           2297
Lactobacillus               94            597            434
Clostridium                130            401            597
                2_12_drySt-28F 3_13_dryst-28F 4_14_dryst-28F
Lactococcus                548           2378            471
Lactobacillus              719            322            205
Clostridium                815            203            232
```

Combining other R functions, the apply() function can also be used to filter taxa (OTUs). For example, the following codes set up a cutoff value of 1, then discard taxa (OTUs) with a mean count <=1 across all samples using the apply(), which(), and mean() functions:

```
> count <- 1
> tab_min <- data.frame(tab[which(apply(tab, 1, function(x){mean(x)})
>count),], check.names=F)
```

The following codes set up a cutoff value of 0.5, then discard taxa (OTUs) if there is a zero in half or more of the samples using the apply(), which(), and length() functions:

```
> cutoff = .5
> tab_d5 <- data.frame(tab[which(apply(tab, 1, function(x){length(which
(x!= 0))/length(x)}) > cutoff),])
```

The following codes set up a cutoff value of 500, then discard taxa (OTUs) with <500 total counts (row sum < 500) using the apply(), which(), and sum() functions:

```
> count = 500
> tab_c500 <- data.frame(tab[which(apply(tab, 1, function(x){sum(x)})
> count),])
```

4.1.7 Other Useful R Functions

In this subsection, we review some other useful functions.

Converting Data Frames
To convert the iris data frame, use t() function:

```
> #Converting data frames
> iris_t <-t(iris)
> iris_t[1:5,1:6]
             [,1]     [,2]     [,3]     [,4]     [,5]     [,6]
Sepal.Length "5.1"    "4.9"    "4.7"    "4.6"    "5.0"    "5.4"
Sepal.Width  "3.5"    "3.0"    "3.2"    "3.1"    "3.6"    "3.9"
Petal.Length "1.4"    "1.4"    "1.3"    "1.5"    "1.4"    "1.7"
Petal.Width  "0.2"    "0.2"    "0.2"    "0.2"    "0.2"    "0.4"
Species      "setosa" "setosa" "setosa" "setosa" "setosa" "setosa"
```

Sorting and Ordering Data Frames
We apply the two functions to the iris data frame and create a new data frame, then compare them as below:

```
> #Sorting and ordering data frames
> iris_2 <- (iris[,-c(3:5)])
> sorted <- sort(iris_2$Sepal.Length)
> ordered <- order(iris_2$Sepal.Length)
> new_iris<- data.frame(iris_2,sorted,ordered)
> head(new_iris)
  Sepal.Length Sepal.Width sorted ordered
1          5.1         3.5    4.3      14
2          4.9         3.0    4.4       9
3          4.7         3.2    4.4      39
4          4.6         3.1    4.4      43
5          5.0         3.6    4.5      42
6          5.4         3.9    4.6       4
```

The sort() sorted the values of Sepal.Length into ascending order. To sort into descending order, use the reverse order function rev() like this:

```
> #Sorting and ordering data frames
> rev_iris <- rev(sort(iris_2$Sepal.Length))
> head(rev_iris)
[1] 7.9 7.7 7.7 7.7 7.7 7.6
```

The numbers in this column of Sepal.Length are indices between 1 and 150. The order() returned an integer vector of indices containing the permutation that will sort the column into ascending order. The best way to understand the order() is to think that the results of x[order(x)] is identical to those of the sort(x). Thus, the following two applications of order() are same as sort(iris_2$Sepal.Length) regarding ordering column of Sepal.Length.

```
> head(iris[order(Sepal.Length),])
   Sepal.Length Sepal.Width Petal.Length Petal.Width Species
14          4.3         3.0          1.1         0.1 setosa
9           4.4         2.9          1.4         0.2 setosa
39          4.4         3.0          1.3         0.2 setosa
43          4.4         3.2          1.3         0.2 setosa
42          4.5         2.3          1.3         0.3 setosa
4           4.6         3.1          1.5         0.2 setosa

> head(iris[order(iris[,'Sepal.Length']),])
   Sepal.Length Sepal.Width Petal.Length Petal.Width Species
14          4.3         3.0          1.1         0.1 setosa
9           4.4         2.9          1.4         0.2 setosa
39          4.4         3.0          1.3         0.2 setosa
43          4.4         3.2          1.3         0.2 setosa
42          4.5         2.3          1.3         0.3 setosa
4           4.6         3.1          1.5         0.2 setosa
```

Recoding Variables Using ifelse()
The ifelse() function is very useful to recode variables based on original values, which completes two actions: to do one thing if a condition is true and another thing if the condition is false. The good thing is: while doing this, the function does for entire vectors and without using loops. For example, suppose we want to create a group based on the values of Petal.Length: if Petal.Length less than 4, then group = 1, else group = 2. The codes like this:

```
> group <- ifelse(iris$Petal.Length < 4,1,2)
```

The function can be nested. Recall, in the iris data set, there are three species: setosa, versicolor, and virginica. The following R codes create three groups for these three species:

```
> group_s <- ifelse(iris$Species %in% "setosa",1,
+                   ifelse(iris$Species %in% "versicolor",2,3))
```

Splitting a Character String Using strsplit()
The strsplit() function splits the elements of a character vector into substrings according to the chosen substring from character string. One syntax is strsplit (character string, split). Where, the first argument is a character string or vector of character strings to split, the split argument is the character substring to split the character string. If the split is an empty string (""), then the character string is split between every character. The strsplit() function outputs a list of each element of the character string that has been split. For example, one microbiome data example we used in this book has following format with rows being samples and columns being taxa. The group information is within the sample string.

```
> tab_t<-t(tab)
> head(tab_t)[1:3,c("Tannerella", "Lactococcus", "Lactobacillus")]
               Tannerella Lactococcus Lactobacillus
5_15_dryst-28F        476         326            94
20_12_CeSt-28F         67         737           597
1_11_dryst-28F        549        2297           434
```

We want to split the character string (e.g., 5_15_drySt-28F) by the character substring "_". The following codes achieve the goal:

```
> strsplit<-data.frame(row.names=rownames(tab_t),t(as.data.frame(strsplit
(rownames(tab_t),"_"))))
> head(strsplit
                  X1 X2        X3
5_15_drySt-28F    5 15  drySt-28F
20_12_CeSt-28F   20 12  CeSt-28F
1_11_drySt-28F    1 11  drySt-28F
2_12_drySt-28F    2 12  drySt-28F
3_13_drySt-28F    3 13  drySt-28F
4_14_drySt-28F    4 14  drySt-28F
```

String Pattern Matching and Replacement Using grep() and gsub()

R provides several functions for string search (or matching) and replacement based on regular expressions. The most commonly used ones are grep(), sub(), gsub(). The simple syntaxes are given: grep(pattern, string), sub(pattern, replacement, string), and gsub(pattern, replacement, string). The grep() searches for matches to pattern (its first argument) within the character vector (second argument), while both the sub() and gsub() perform replacement of matches. The argument string is a character vector. The difference between sub() and gsub() is: with sub(), the first occurrence of the regular expression is replaced, while with gsub(), all occurrences are replaced. Here we illustrate gsub() and grep().

It is noted that R treats the first argument(pattern) in sub(), gsub() and grep(), as a regular expression for effectiveness in string matching, manipulation, and R code writing and maintenance. A regular expression is to describe a pattern for a function on what and how to "match" or "match and replace" strings.

In regular expressions, the non-alphanumeric symbols/characters such as "$", "*", "+", ".", "?", "[", "^", "{", "|", "(", "\\" are called metacharacters. Metacharacters are the building blocks of regular expressions. They are specific meanings in regular expressions (Table 4.1).

To match any metacharacters in R as a regular character, we need to escape or precede them with a double backslash "\\", while match a backslash as a regular character, write four backslashes. For example, to tell the gsub() function to interpret "$" as a regular character, we precede "$" with a double backslash.

```
> re <- gsub(pattern = "\\$", replacement = ".",
"metacharacters$uses$in$regular$expressions")
> re
[1] "metacharacters.uses.in.regular.expressions"
```

Table 4.1 Some metacharacters and specific meanings in regular expression

Meta character	Meaning
"."	Matches any single alphanumeric character or symbol except for the empty string "" or a newline
"+"	Matches the preceding character one or more times
"*"	Matches the preceding character zero or more times
".*"	Matches for any character zero or more times
"?"	Matches the preceding character optional: zero or one time only
"^"	When used in a character class, to match any character but the following ones. In regular expressions, we can describe a set of characters, and call the set as a character class and denote it by square brackets
"$"	Is the instruction to match empty string at the end of a line
"|"	Allows for alternative matches, it operates like the Boolean: OR
"(", ")"	Brackets for grouping
"[", "]"	Character class brackets
"[a–z]" "[0–9]"	Character set, matches at least one of elements from the set, but no more than one unless otherwise specified. The order of the characters does not matter
"(abc)" "(123)"	Character group, matches the characters abc or 123 in that exact order

In following, the function gsub() interprets the regular expression \\.+ as: to match and replace one or more repetitions of a period.

```
> df = data.frame(how...to...interpret...metacharacters = c(1, 2),
in...regular...expressions = c(1,2))
> df
  how...to...interpret...metacharacters
1                                     1
2                                     2
  in...regular...expressions
1                          1
2                          2
> names(df) <- gsub(pattern = "\\.+", replacement = ".", x = names(df))
> names(df)
[1] "how.to.interpret.metacharacters"
[2] "in.regular.expressions"
```

Regular expressions are often seen in microbiome data manipulations. For example, the public available microbiome data set "tongue_saliva" collected both tongue and saliva samples. The tongue samples start with td_, and saliva samples start with sa_.

```
> tab_ts <- read.table("tongue_saliva.txt", header=T, row.names=1,
sep="\t")
> tab_tts <-t(tab_ts)
> rownames(tab_tts)[1:3]
[1] "td_114221" "td_111445" "td_111580"
> rownames(tab_tts)[201:203]
[1] "sa_106066" "sa_105780" "sa_103488"
```

To label these two samples with single meaningful names, e.g., "tongue" and "saliva", respectively, we can use following R codes:

```
> rownames(tab_tts) <- gsub("sa_.+", "saliva", rownames(tab_tts))
> rownames(tab_tts) <- gsub("td_.+", "tongue", rownames(tab_tts))
> rownames(tab_tts)[1:3]
[1] "tongue" "tongue" "tongue"
> rownames(tab_tts)[201:203]
[1] "saliva" "saliva" "saliva"
```

The data set "tongue_saliva" also includes a column "tax.0" presenting taxa information. We obtain them from the data set. The first lines show that the taxon names prefixed with a character and "__".

```
> tax <- tab_ts$tax.0
> tax[1:3]
[1] Root;p__Proteobacteria;c__Betaproteobacteria;o__Neisseriales;
f__Neisseriaceae;g__Neisseria
[2] Root;p__Bacteroidetes;c__Flavobacteria;o__Flavobacteriales;
f__Flavobacteriaceae;g__Capnocytophaga
[3] Root;p__Actinobacteria;c__Actinobacteria;o__Actinomycetales;
f__Actinomycetaceae;g__Actinomyces
```

To manipulate the data easily, we want to get rid of them. We can use the gsub() function to do this job:

```
> tax_1 <- gsub(".+__", "", tax)
> tax_1[1:3]
[1] "Neisseria"     "Capnocytophaga" "Actinomyces"
```

In above applications of the gsub() function, we use metacharacters in regular expressions to match the characters in the given character vector.

The grep() function also accepts a regular expression and a character string or vector of character strings. By default, it returns the indices of the elements of the strings matched by the regular expression. If the value = TRUE argument is specified, then it returns the actual strings matched by the expression.

```
> grep("[wd]", c("Sepal.Length", "Sepal.Width", "Petal.Length",
"Petal.Width","Species"))
[1] 2 4
> grep("[wd]", c("Sepal.Length", "Sepal.Width", "Petal.Length",
"Petal.Width","Species"), value = TRUE)
[1] "Sepal.Width" "Petal.Width"
```

If we want a string to be matched as is or to be interpreted literally (i.e., not as a regular expression), then use the fixed = TRUE argument.

```
> grep("Width", c("Sepal.Length", "Sepal.Width", "Petal.Length",
"Petal.Width","Species"), value = TRUE,fixed =TRUE)
[1] "Sepal.Width" "Petal.Width"
```

Using rep() and grep() to Create Group Variables in Microbiome Data
One important use of these functions in microbiome data is to create group variable based on sample information. If the readers in the beginning feel difficult to fully understand these codes, it is fine. You will find they are very useful later when you analyze your microbiome data or read other's works. We illustrate several examples below.

Use rep() to create groups

The following codes create the variable group with numerical value of 1 presenting fecal(dryST) and 2 presenting cecal(CeSt) samples:

```
> group <- data.frame(c(rep(1,length(grep("dryST", colnames(tab)))),
+                       rep(2, length(grep("CeSt", colnames(tab))))))
```

The following codes create the variable group with character value of fecal presenting dryST and cecal presenting CeSt samples:

```
> group_1 <- data.frame(c(rep("fecal",length(grep("dryST",
colnames(tab)))),rep("cecal", length(grep("CeSt", colnames(tab))))))
```

Use grep() to create groups

The following R codes use the grep() function to obtain the columns containing the two groups of fecal and cecal samples. It searches and match strings in the column headers for samples named with "drySt" or "CeSt".

```
> fecal <- grep("drySt", colnames(tab))
> cecal <- grep("CeSt", colnames(tab))
> fecal
 [1] 1 3 4 5 6 7 8 9
> cecal
 [1]  2 10 11 12 13 14 15 16
```

The above samples are not ordered in groups or experimental conditions. If the samples are ordered based on groups or experimental conditions, then we can use the rep() function to create the group variable as follows:

```
> conds <- c(rep("fecal", 8), rep("CeSt", 8))
> conds
 [1] "fecal" "fecal" "fecal" "fecal" "fecal" "fecal" "fecal"
 [8] "fecal" "CeSt"  "CeSt"  "CeSt"  "CeSt"  "CeSt"  "CeSt"
[15] "CeSt"  "CeSt"
> fecal<- colnames(tab)[grep("drySt", colnames(tab))] # fecal samples
> cecal <- colnames(tab)[grep("CeSt", colnames(tab))] # cecal samples
> df_mice <- data.frame(tab[,fecal], tab[,cecal]) # make a data frame
> head(df_mice)
                            X5_15_drySt.28F X1_11_drySt.28F X2_12_drySt.28F
Tannerella                              476             549             578
Lactococcus                             326            2297             548
Lactobacillus                            94             434             719
Lactobacillus::Lactococcus                1              25               5
Parasutterella                            1               1               4
Helicobacter                             89               0              13
                            X3_13_drySt.28F X4_14_drySt.28F X7_22_drySt.28F
Tannerella                              996             404             319
Lactococcus                            2378             471             882
Lactobacillus                           322             205             644
Lactobacillus::Lactococcus               17               1              13
Parasutterella                            2               0               0
Helicobacter                             24              32               3
```

4.2   Introduction to the dplyr Package

The dplyr package provides a set of functions for efficiently manipulating datasets in R. The package dplyr is the next generation of "plyr", focussing on only data frames. Thus it is very useful for transforming and summarizing tabular data with rows and columns, such as for microbiome data set. The dplyr package contains a set of functions ("verbs") that perform most common data manipulation tasks such as selecting specific columns, filtering for rows, re-ordering rows, adding new columns and summarizing data. The important single dplyr functions include:

- select() and rename() to select columns(variables) based on their names
- filter() to filter rows(cases) based on their values
- arrange() to re-order or arrange the rows (cases)
- mutate() and transmute() to create new columns, e.g., to add new variables that are functions of existing variables
- summarise() to summarize values
- group_by() to group observations
- sample_n() and sample_frac() to take random samples.

Also, "dplyr" contains an important function group_by() to perform another common task which is related to the "split-apply-combine" concept.

In addition, dplyr imported the pipe operator: %>% from the magrittr package. The pipe operator is very useful when we combine several functions. Generally, in R if we combine several functions, we nest them each other. The nested functions are operated from the inside to the outside. For example, in following codes, select() is nested within head(), the operator starting with selecting columns id, and write to make a new data frame, then the head() is applied to obtain the first 6 lines of the new data frame. Here we use the publicly available data set hsb2demo, which we used in Sect. 4.1.3.2 to illustrate this package.

```
> setwd("E:/Home/MicrobiomeStatR/Analysis")
> tab <- read.csv("hsb2demo.csv")
> head(tab)
   id female race ses schtyp prog read write math science socst
1  70      0    4   1      1    1   57    52   41      47    57
2 121      1    4   2      1    3   68    59   53      63    61
3  86      0    4   3      1    1   44    33   54      58    31
4 141      0    4   3      1    3   63    44   47      53    56
5 172      0    4   2      1    2   47    52   57      53    61
6 113      0    4   2      1    2   44    52   51      63    61
```

Next, we install and load dplyr.

```
> install.packages("dplyr")
> library(dplyr)
```

The pipe operator: %>%, instead of reading functions from the inside to the outside, is to read the functions from left to right. In the following R codes, we pipe the tab data frame to the select() function to select two columns (id and write), and then pipe the new data frame to the head() function which returns the head of the new data frame.

```
> tab %>%
+ select(id,write) %>%
+ head
   id write
1  70    52
2 121    59
3  86    33
4 141    44
5 172    52
6 113    52
```

Selecting Columns Using select()

The select() allows us to rapidly subset a set of columns by names using operations that usually only work on numeric variable positions:

```
> # Select columns: id, read, write and math
> head(select(tab, id, read, write, math))
   id read write math
1  70   57    52   41
2 121   68    59   53
3  86   44    33   54
4 141   63    44   47
5 172   47    52   57
6 113   44    52   51
```

To select a range of columns by name, use the ":" (colon) operator.

```
> # Select all columns between read and socst (inclusive)
> head(select(tab, read:socst))
  read write math science socst
1   57   52   41      47    57
2   68   59   53      63    61
3   44   33   54      58    31
4   63   44   47      53    56
5   47   52   57      53    61
6   44   52   51      63    61
```

To select all the columns *except* a specific column or a range of columns, use the "−" (subtraction) operator (also known as negative indexing).

```
> # Select all columns except female
> head(select(tab, -female))
   id race ses schtyp prog read write math science socst
1  70    4   1      1    1   57    52   41      47    57
2 121    4   2      1    3   68    59   53      63    61
3  86    4   3      1    1   44    33   54      58    31
4 141    4   3      1    3   63    44   47      53    56
5 172    4   2      1    2   47    52   57      53    61
6 113    4   2      1    2   44    52   51      63    61
```

```
> # Select all columns except those from female to prog (inclusive)
> head(select(tab, -(female:prog )))
   id read write math science socst
1  70   57    52   41      47    57
2 121   68    59   53      63    61
3  86   44    33   54      58    31
4 141   63    44   47      53    56
5 172   47    52   57      53    61
6 113   44    52   51      63    61
```

There are additional functions to select columns based on a specific criteria using within select(), such as starts_with(), ends_with(), matches(), contains(), and one_of(). They can help us quickly match larger blocks of variables that meet some criteria. The starts_with () is used to select all columns that start with the character string; the ends_with() to select columns that end with a character string; the matches() to select columns that match a regular expression; the contains() to select columns that match a literal string.

```
> # select all columns that start with the character string "s"
> head(select(tab, starts_with("s")))
  ses schtyp science socst
1   1      1      47    57
2   2      1      63    61
3   3      1      58    31
4   3      1      53    56
5   2      1      53    61
6   2      1      63    61
```

Selecting Rows Using filter()

The filter() allows us to select a subset of rows in a data frame. Like all single functions, the first argument is the name of data frame. The second and subsequent arguments are the variables of the data frame, selecting rows where the expression is true.

```
> #Selecting rows using filter()
> # Filter the rows for students with reading score greater than or equal 70.
> filter(tab, read >= 70)
   id female race ses schtyp prog read write math science socst
1  95      0    4   3      1    2   73    60   71      61    71
2 103      0    4   3      1    2   76    52   64      64    61
3 132      0    4   2      1    2   73    62   73      69    66
4  68      0    4   2      1    2   73    67   71      63    66
5  57      1    4   2      1    2   71    65   72      66    56
6 180      1    4   3      2    2   71    65   69      58    71
7  34      1    1   3      2    2   73    61   57      55    66
8  93      1    4   3      1    2   73    67   62      58    66
9  61      1    4   3      1    2   76    63   60      67    66
```

```
> #Filter the rows for students with both reading and math scores greater
than or equal 70
> filter(tab, read >= 70, math >= 70)
   id female race ses schtyp prog read write math science socst
1  95      0    4   3      1    2   73    60   71      61    71
2 132      0    4   2      1    2   73    62   73      69    66
3  68      0    4   2      1    2   73    67   71      63    66
4  57      1    4   2      1    2   71    65   72      66    56
```

Re-order Rows Using arrange()

The arrange() works similarly to filter() except that instead of filtering or selecting rows, it re-orders them.

```
> #Re-order by read and write
> head(arrange(tab, id, read, write))
  id female race ses schtyp prog read write math science socst
1 1      1    1   1      1    3   34    44   40      39    41
2 2      1    1   2      1    3   39    41   33      42    41
3 3      0    1   1      1    2   63    65   48      63    56
4 4      1    1   1      1    2   44    50   41      39    51
5 5      0    1   1      1    2   47    40   43      45    31
6 6      1    1   1      1    2   47    41   46      40    41

> #Use desc() to order a column in descending order
> head(arrange(tab, desc(read)))
   id female race ses schtyp prog read write math science socst
1 103    0    4   3      1    2   76    52   64      64    61
2  61    1    4   3      1    2   76    63   60      67    66
3  95    0    4   3      1    2   73    60   71      61    71
4 132    0    4   2      1    2   73    62   73      69    66
5  68    0    4   2      1    2   73    67   71      63    66
6  34    1    1   3      2    2   73    61   57      55    66
```

The pipe operator: %>% can be used with arrange() together.

```
> #To re-order rows by a particular column(female)
> tab %>% arrange(female) %>% head
   id female race ses schtyp prog read write math science socst
1  70    0    4   1      1    1   57    52   41      47    57
2  86    0    4   3      1    1   44    33   54      58    31
3 141    0    4   3      1    3   63    44   47      53    56
4 172    0    4   2      1    2   47    52   57      53    61
5 113    0    4   2      1    2   44    52   51      63    61
6  50    0    3   2      1    1   50    59   42      53    61
```

```
> #Select three columns id, gender, read from tab
> #Arrange the rows by the gender and then by read
> #Then return the head of the final data frame
> tab%>%select(id, female, read) %>%
+             arrange(female, read) %>%
+             head
    id female read
1 164      0    31
2  11      0    34
3  53      0    34
4 108      0    34
5 117      0    34
6 165      0    36


> #Filter the rows for read with score greater or equal to 70
> tab %>% select(id, female, read) %>%
+    arrange(female, read) %>%
+     filter(read >= 70)
    id female read
1  95      0    73
2 132      0    73
3  68      0    73
4 103      0    76
5  57      1    71
6 180      1    71
7  34      1    73
8  93      1    73
9  61      1    76


> #Arrange the rows for read in a descending order
> tab %>% select(id, female, read) %>%
+    arrange(female, desc(read)) %>%
+     filter(read >= 70)
    id female read
1 103      0    76
2  95      0    73
3 132      0    73
4  68      0    73
5  61      1    76
6  34      1    73
7  93      1    73
8  57      1    71
9 180      1    71
```

Create New Columns Using mutate()

Create new columns that are functions of existing columns.

```
> #Create new columns using mutate()
> #Calculate average read and write scores
> head(mutate(tab, avg_read = sum(read)/n()))
   id female race ses schtyp prog read write math science socst
1  70      0    4   1      1    1   57    52   41      47    57
2 121      1    4   2      1    3   68    59   53      63    61
3  86      0    4   3      1    1   44    33   54      58    31
4 141      0    4   3      1    3   63    44   47      53    56
5 172      0    4   2      1    2   47    52   57      53    61
6 113      0    4   2      1    2   44    52   51      63    61
   avg_read
1    52.23
2    52.23
3    52.23
4    52.23
5    52.23
6    52.23


> #To keep only the new variables, use transmute()
> head(transmute(tab,avg_read = sum(read)/n()))
   avg_read
1    52.23
2    52.23
3    52.23
4    52.23
5    52.23
6    52.23

> #Create new columns using mutate() and pipe operator
> tab %>% mutate(avg_read = sum(read/n())) %>%
+     head
   id female race ses schtyp prog read write math science socst
1  70      0    4   1      1    1   57    52   41      47    57
2 121      1    4   2      1    3   68    59   53      63    61
3  86      0    4   3      1    1   44    33   54      58    31
4 141      0    4   3      1    3   63    44   47      53    56
5 172      0    4   2      1    2   47    52   57      53    61
6 113      0    4   2      1    2   44    52   51      63    61
   avg_read
1    52.23
2    52.23
3    52.23
4    52.23
5    52.23
6    52.23
```

Summarize Values Using summarise()

The summarise() creates summary statistics for a given column in the data frame combining other summary statistics, such as, mean(), sd(), min(), max(), median(), sum(), n(), first(), last() and n_distinct(). The following codes are used to find the mean of read score.

```
> #To collapses a data frame to a single row.
> summarise(tab, avg_read = mean(read, na.rm = TRUE))
   avg_read
1    52.23
```

The following codes are used to find the mean and other summary statistics.

```
> #Create summaries of the data frame using summarise() and pipe operator
> tab %>% summarise(avg_read = mean(read),
+                        min_read = min(read),
+                        max_read = max(read),
+                        n = n())
    avg_read min_read max_read    n
1      52.23       28       76 200
```

Grouping Observations Using group_by()

This function breaks down a dataset into specified groups of rows. It splits the data frame by some variable, apply a function to the individual data frames and then combine the output. In following, we first group the total 200 observations by gender, and then get the summary statistics of reading by gender.

```
> #First group by gender, and then get the summary statistics of reading by g
ender
> by_gender <- group_by(tab, female)
> read_by_gender <- summarise(by_gender,
+                                n = n(),
+                                avg_read = mean(read, na.rm = TRUE),
+                                min_read = min(read,na.rm = TRUE),
+                                max_read = max(read,na.rm = TRUE))
> read_by_gender
# A tibble: 2 x 5
  female      n avg_read min_read max_read
   <int> <int>    <dbl>    <dbl>    <dbl>
1      0    91    52.82       31       76
2      1   109    51.73       28       76
```

The same job can be done via pipe operator.

```
> #Create summaries of the data frame using summarise() and pipe operator
> tab %>% group_by(female) %>%
+           summarise(n = n(),
+                        avg_read  = mean(read),
+                        min_read = min(read),
+                        max_read = max(read))
# A tibble: 2 x 5
  female      n avg_read min_read max_read
   <int> <int>    <dbl>    <dbl>    <dbl>
1      0    91    52.82       31       76
2      1   109    51.73       28       76
```

Randomly Sample Rows Using sample_n() and sample_frac()

```
> #Use sample_n() to sample a fixed number
> sample_n(tab, 5)
     id female race ses schtyp prog read write math science socst
183  92      1    4   3      1    1   52    67   57      63    61
156 139      1    4   2      1    2   68    59   61      55    71
184 160      1    4   2      1    2   55    65   55      50    61
47   49      0    3   3      1    3   50    40   39      49    47
85   58      0    4   2      1    3   55    41   40      44    41

> #Use sample_frac() to sample a fixed fraction
> sample_frac(tab, 0.02)
     id female race ses schtyp prog read write math science socst
38   80      0    4   3      1    2   65    62   68      66    66
160  39      1    3   3      1    2   66    67   67      61    66
127 105      1    4   2      1    2   50    41   45      44    56
130  45      1    3   1      1    3   34    35   41      29    26

> #Use replace = TRUE to perform a bootstrap sampling
> sample_n(tab, 5,replace = TRUE)
     id female race ses schtyp prog read write math science socst
11   75      0    4   2      1    3   60    46   51      53    61
180  63      1    4   1      1    1   52    65   60      56    51
182 193      1    4   2      2    2   44    49   48      39    51
103  47      1    3   1      1    2   47    46   49      33    41
96  173      1    4   1      1    1   50    62   61      63    51
```

4.3   Introduction to ggplot2

4.3.1   ggplot2 and the Grammar of Graphics

The ggplot2 package was written and maintained by Wickham (2016) to create elegant graphics for data analysis. Because its versatility, clear and consistent interface, and provides beautiful, publication-ready graphs, ggplot2 has attracted many users in the R community, and particularly in some research fields of data generated by the high-throughput sequencing technologies, such as microbiome data. This package uses the grid package to provide a series of high-level functions for creating complete plots, and extends and refines the principles of "The Grammar of Graphics" (Wilkinson 2005). The basic idea of the grammar of graphics is to independently specify plot components and combine them to build just about any kind of graphical display we want.

There are six main components in Wilkinson's grammar including: data, transformations, element, scales, guide, and coordinate system. Although the high-level components of Wickham's grammar are quite similar to those of Wilkinson's grammar; however, Wickham emphasized and named his proposed grammar of graphics as the layered grammar to differentiate from Wilkinson's grammar of graphics. The layered grammar of graphics was based on the idea of

Table 4.2 The components of the layered grammar

Layer	Descriptions
• Data • Aesthetic mappings (Aes) • Statistical transformations (Stat) • Geometric objects (Geoms) • Position adjustment (Position)	The data, mappings, statistical transformation, and geometric object, position adjustment form a layer and a plot may have multiple layers Data: are used to construct a concrete graph, consisting variables, which are stored as columns in a data frame. Data are independent from the other components and multiple datasets can be applied Mapping: the purpose of mapping is to convert data properties (typically numerical or categorical values) to aesthetic or visual properties; it is used to specify which variables to which aesthetic attributes (e.g., *x*-position, *y*-position, color, shape, size, etc.) Stat: transforms the data, typically by summarizing them in some manner (e.g., smooth line, regression line, binning or aggregating, boxplot, jitter, etc.). A stat can add new variables to the dataset. It is possible to map aesthetics to these new variables Geoms: are the geometric objects that are drawn to represent the data; each geom controls the type of plot that we create. Each geom can only display certain aesthetics (e.g., bars, lines, and points, etc.) Every geom has a default statistic, and every statistic has a default geom Position adjustment: are used to tweak the position of the geometric elements on the plot to avoid obscuring each other, e.g., in bar plots, stack or dodge (place side-by-side) the bars to avoid overlaps. In scatterplots, randomly jitter the points to reduce over-plotting
Scales	Scales: for every aesthetic attribute, there is a function, called a scale; a scale controls the mapping from data to aesthetic attributes to ensure the data values are valid for that aesthetic. Additionally, scaling is performed before statistical transformation.
Coordinate system (Coord)	Coord: maps the position of objects onto the plane of the plot. Position is often specified by two coordinates (x, y), but could be any number of coordinates Additionally, coordinate transformations occur after statistical transformation
Faceting	Faceting: is known as conditioned or trellis plots in a more general case of the plots. The faceting describes which variables should be used to split up the data, and how they should be arranged. Faceting is a powerful tool to investigate whether patterns are the same or different across conditions

building up a graphic from multiple layers of data. It defines the components of a plot as: data, aesthetic mappings, statistical transformations, geometric objects, position adjustment, scales, coordinate system and faceting, which is shown in Table 4.2.

The components of Wilkinson's grammar can be mapped to those of the layered grammar: a layer of the layered grammar is the equivalent of Wilkinson's element; the scale of the layered grammar is equivalent to the SCALE and GUIDE of Wilkinson's grammar; the coordinate system and faceting of the layered grammar

are equivalent to Wilkinson's coordinate system. However, Wilkinson's transla-
tions has no correspondence in ggplot2 (its role is played by built-in R features).

4.3.2   Simplify Specifications in Creating a Plot Using ggplot()

The algorithm of ggplot2 is simple: you provide the data, tell the ggplot2 how to
map variables to aesthetics, what graphics to use, and it takes care of the details.

In ggplot2, layers are responsible for creating the objects that we perceive on the
plot. A layer is composed of four parts: data and aesthetic mapping, a statistical
transformation (stat), a geometric object (geom), and a position adjustment
(Wickham 2010). A plot may have multiple layers. These layers are combined with
a coordinate system and transformations to generate the final plot. The following is
a plot generation process:

map variables to aesthetics → facet datasets → transform scales → compute aesthetics → train scales → map scales → render genoms.

4.3.2.1   Full Steps Without Using Defaults

In this section, we use previously used iris data set to illustrate how to create a
scatterplot with ggplot() function. We start with ggplot() to create a plot object, and
then add the other components. The full ggplot2 specification of the scatterplot of
Sepal.Length versus Sepal.Width is:

```
> library(ggplot2)
> ggplot() +
+   layer(
+      data = iris, mapping = aes(x = Sepal.Width, y = Sepal.Length),
+      geom = "point", stat = "identity", position = "identity"
+   ) +
+   scale_y_continuous() +
+   scale_x_continuous() +
+   coord_cartesian()
```

We can see that a single layer specifies the data, mapping, geom, stat, and
position, the two continuous position scales, and a Cartesian coordinate system.

4.3.2.2   To Simplify Specifications by Intelligently Using Defaults

The full specifications are very complicated; especially the layer is the most
complicated. There are two ways to simplify the grammar syntax: one is to intelligently use defaults of the grammar, which we will cover here; another is to use the

qplot() function, which we will introduce in next subsection. You can intelligently use following three kinds of defaults to simplify your codes:

(1) each geom has a default stat (and vice versa), so we only need specify either geom or stat, but not both of them. (2) do not need to specify Cartesian coordinate system, because it is the default coordinate system. (3) default scales will be added according to the aesthetic and type of variable. For example, for position, continuous values are transformed with a linear scaling, and categorical values are mapped to the integers; for color, continuous variables are mapped to a smooth path in the HCL color space, and discrete variables to evenly spaced hues with equal luminance and chroma.

Thus, we can reduce above specifications as below:

```
> ggplot() +
+   layer(
+       data = iris, mapping = aes(x = Sepal.Width, y = Sepal.Length),
+       geom = "point"
+   )
```

Typically, we can omit data =, and mapping =, instead of specifying a default dataset and mapping in the ggplot() call, and also use position-based matching in aes (x-variable, y-variable). We can also omit the layer. So the specifications can be reduced as below:

```
> ggplot(iris, aes(Sepal.Width, Sepal.Length)) +
+   geom_point()
```

When the layer is omitted, the specification for geom = "geometry" will be replaced as an according geometry function, such as, in this case, geom = "point" is replaced as geom_point(). Similar, the specification for stat = "statistic" will be replaced as an according statistic function, such as, stat = "smooth" is replaced as stat_smooth().

Any aesthetics specified in the layer will override the default. Similarly, if a dataset is specified in the layer, it will override the plot default. The following codes override the default linear-transformations, which are specified via scale_y_continuous() and scale_x_continuous(), with log-transformations using scale_x_log10 () and scale_y_log10() functions.

```
> ggplot(iris, aes(Sepal.Width, Sepal.Length)) +
+   geom_point()
> ggplot(iris, aes(Sepal.Width, Sepal.Length)) +
+   geom_point() +
+   stat_smooth(method = lm) +
+   scale_x_log10() +
+   scale_y_log10()
```

If we don't use the defaults, then the full specifications should be as below:

```
> ggplot() +
+   layer(
+     data = iris, mapping = aes(x = Sepal.Width, y = Sepal.Length),
+     geom = "point", stat = "identity", position = "identity"
+   ) +
+   layer(
+     data = iris, mapping = aes(x = Sepal.Width, y = Sepal.Length),
+     geom = "smooth", position = "identity",
+     stat = "smooth""""", method = lm
+   ) +
+   scale_y_log10() +
+   scale_x_log10() +
+   coord_cartesian()
```

The concept of the hierarchy of defaults is explained in his paper (Wickham 2010) and how to build a plot layer by layer in Chap. 5 of book (Wickham 2016).

4.3.2.3   Reduce the Amount of Typing Grammar Syntax by Using qplot()

In ggplot2, there are two main high-level functions to create a plot: qplot(), short for quick plot, and ggplot(). With qplot(), a plot is created in a way of all at once; with ggplot(), a plot is created piece-by-piece and layer functions.

The reason that ggplot2 is supplemented with qplot() is to reduce the amount of typing needed. Because even we use many defaults, the explicit grammar syntax of ggplot2 is rather verbose, which makes it difficult to rapidly experiment with different plots. It also mimics the syntax of the plot () function, making ggplot2 easier to use for who already familiar with base R graphics. For example, if use qplot() for above plot, the codes are:

```
> qplot(Sepal.Width, Sepal.Length, data = iris,
+        geom = c("point", "smooth"),
+        method = "lm", log = "xy")
```

Although qplot() is a quick and convenient for the users who are familiar with base R graphics, its limitations are obvious: since the qplot() function assumes that multiple layers will use the same data and aesthetic mappings, the method argument does not have explicit layer to apply, and the particular data transformations, the plot layout defining and controlling are also restricted. Thus, in such cases, the more advanced ggplot() functions is needed.

4.3.3 Creating a Plot Using ggplot()

4.3.3.1 Creating a Plot Layer by Layer with ggplot()

As we described in Sect. 4.3.1, the first distinct feature of the grammar of ggplot2 is layered, which means that a plot is created by at least a layer, and enhanced by adding more players to an existing plot using the ggplot() function. We described in Table 4.2 and saw in above codes, a layer combines data, aesthetic mapping, a geom (geometric object), a stat (statistical transformation), and a position adjustment. A layer is completed with a geom (geometric object), so the layers in ggplot2 are also called "geoms". Thus, in ggplot2, the plot is actually created by a geom (e.g., geom_point()) and enhanced by more geoms (e.g., geom_smooth(), etc.). One geom presents one layer of plot.

The second distinct feature of ggplot2 is that it works with a dataframe and not an individual vector. So before we use the package to create a plot, we need to convert the data to a dataframe if it is a vector. All the data supplied either to the ggplot() itself or to respective geoms to create the plot is contained within the dataframe.

In this section, we use previously used iris data set to illustrate how to create a plot layer by layer using ggplot() function. Assume that we want to create a scatterplot of Sepal. Length versus Sepal.Width.

Step 1: To initialize a basic ggplot, we start with ggplot() to create a plot object containing the data and aesthetic mapping. We name the plot object as p (Fig. 4.2).

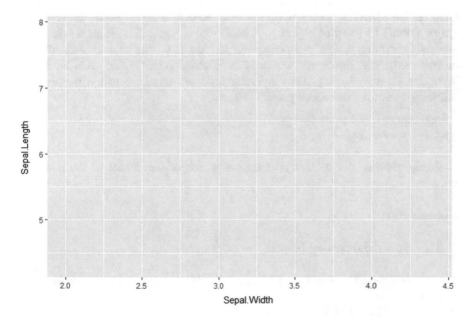

Fig. 4.2 A blank ggplot() plot object with created by data and aesthetic mapping

```
> library(ggplot2)
> p <- ggplot(iris, aes(x=Sepal.Width, y=Sepal.Length))
> # Sepal.Width and Sepal.Length are columns in iris dataframe
> p
```

Any information within the dataframe that needs for the plot should be specified inside the aes() function. In this case, we implement aesthetic mapping via the aes() function: specify x, and y variables, respectively. However, only a blank ggplot is drawn. Because so far we have only told ggplot() what dataset to use and what columns should be used for x, y axis, and color. But we haven't explicitly asked it to draw any points or a line yet. To actually draw a scatterplot or a line chart, we have to explicitly ask ggplot() by using a geom layer. The object p is an R S3 object of the class ggplot consisting data and other components containing information about this plot. We can access the details of information using the summary() function to keep track of which data was exactly used and how the variables were mapped.

```
> summary(p)
data: Sepal.Length, Sepal.Width, Petal.Length, Petal.Width,
  Species [150x5]
mapping:  x = Sepal.Width, y = Sepal.Length
faceting: <ggproto object: Class FacetNull, Facet>
```

We can see that the dataframe has 150 rows and 5 columns (variables), of those 2 variables were mapped to x and y axes respectively.

Step 2: To draw a scatterplot, we add points using a geom layer called geom_point() to the plot object p. A basic plot in ggplot2 is realized using data, aesthetic mapping and a geometry. We already have the components of data, aesthetic mapping, the component need to be added is scatterplot geom layer. The layer can be added using the + operator followed by the function defining the scatterplot with points: geom_point() (Fig. 4.3).

```
> #Add scatterplot geom (layer1)
> p1 <- p + geom_point()
```

Again, we use the summary() function to access the details of the new plot object:

```
> summary(p1)
```

This gives the following output:

```
data: Sepal.Length, Sepal.Width, Petal.Length, Petal.Width, Species
  [150x5]
mapping:  x = Sepal.Width, y = Sepal.Length
```

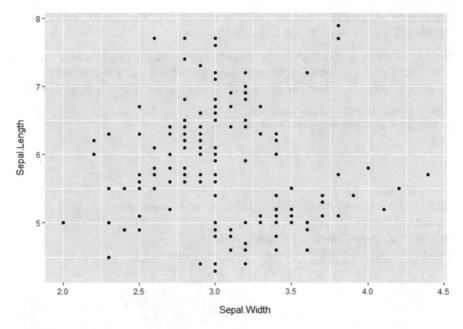

Fig. 4.3 A scatterplot created by data and aesthetic mapping and geom_point()

```
faceting: <ggproto object: Class FacetNull, Facet>
----------------------------------
geom_point: na.rm = FALSE
stat_identity: na.rm = FALSE
position_identity
```

We can see that the new plot object added the geom and stat details used.

In this plot, we create a plot object and then add a layer by the + operator to create a new plot object; alternatively we can provide all the codes together. Both options return the same results.

```
> ggplot(iris, aes(x=Sepal.Width, y=Sepal.Length)) + geom_point()
```

Like geom_point(), many other geoms are available in the ggplot2 at website (http://ggplot2.tidyverse.org/reference/). For example, except for geom_point() draws points to produce a scatterplot; geom_smooth() fits a smoother to the data and displays the smooth and its standard error; geom_boxplot() produces a box and whisker plot to summarize the distribution of a set of points; geom_path() and geom_line() draw lines between the data points. For continuous variables, geom_histogram() draws a histogram, geom_freqpoly() creates a frequency polygon, and geom_density() creates a density plot. For discrete variables, geom_bar() draws a bar chart. Here we want to add a smoothing layer.

Step 3: To draw a scatterplot with smooth curve, we add an additional geome layer called geom_smooth() to the previous plot object. For this smother plot, we set the method as lm (short for linear model) to draw the line of best fit (Fig. 4.4).

```
> #Add smoothing geom (layer2)
> p2 <- p1 + geom_smooth(method="lm")
> p2
```

```
> summary(p2)
data: Sepal.Length, Sepal.Width, Petal.Length, Petal.Width,
 Species [150x5]
mapping:  x = Sepal.Width, y = Sepal.Length
faceting: <ggproto object: Class FacetNull, Facet>
```

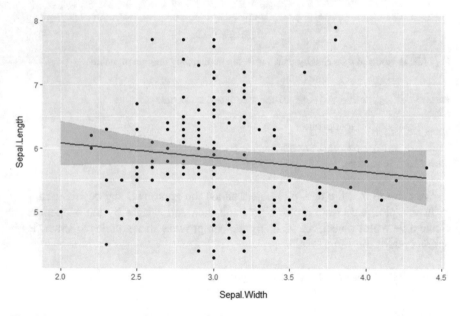

Fig. 4.4 A scatterplot created by data, aesthetic mapping, and geom_point() and geom_smooth()

```
---------------------------------
geom_point: na.rm = FALSE
stat_identity: na.rm = FALSE
position_identity

geom_smooth: na.rm = FALSE
stat_smooth: na.rm = FALSE, method = lm, formula = y ~ x, se = TRUE
position_identity
```

The output shows that an additional layer smother with linear model added to the plot object. The smother curve also has confidence bands. We can set se = FALSE to turn off the confidence bands.

```
> #set se = FALSE to turn off confidence bands
> p1 + geom_smooth(method="lm", se = FALSE)
```

4.3.3.2   Using Scales to Change the Aesthetics of a Geom Layer

The mapping from data to aesthetic attributes is controlled by the scale functions, such as in Sect. 4.3.2.1, scale_y_continuous() and scale_x_continuous() for the x-y position in the axes. The scale functions can be used to both continuous and categorical variable. For example, in continuous case, scales are used to fill histograms or density plots; in discrete case, scales are used for filling histograms or bar charts, or for scatterplots when mapping for color, size, or shape.

We need to know that the aesthetic attributes used to map to variables depend on the geom() function used. Thus, we can change the aesthetic attributes via specifying the arguments of the respective geom layer. In this case, we change the color and size of points and color of line of best fit (Fig. 4.5).

```
> p3 <- ggplot(iris, aes(x=Sepal.Width, y=Sepal.Length)) +
+ #Add scatterplot geom (layer1)
+ geom_point(col="blue", size=3) +
+ #Add smoothing geom (layer2)
+ geom_smooth(method="lm",col="red",size=2)
> p3
```

Another important application of changing color is to map different colors to the different levels of a categorical variable in source dataset. For example, in microbiome study, we often use different colors to present the different experimental groups or conditions. Since the categorical variable is in the source dataset, it must be specified within the aes() function (Fig. 4.6).

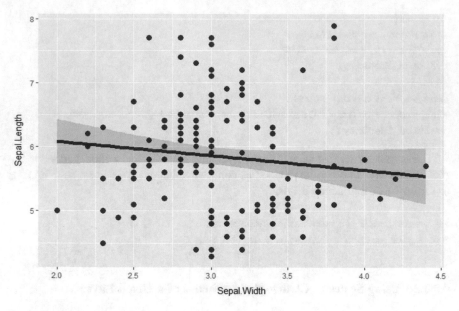

Fig. 4.5 Change the color and size of points and best fitted line

```
> p4 <- ggplot(iris, aes(x=Sepal.Width, y=Sepal.Length)) +
+   #Add scatterplot geom (layer1)
+   geom_point(aes(col=Species), size=3) +
+   #Add smoothing geom (layer2)
```

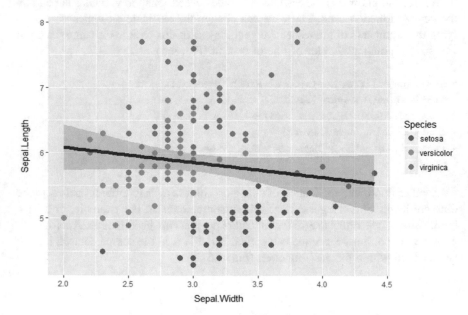

Fig. 4.6 Map the color of points based on levels of categorical variable. Three kinds of species are presented by three different colors

```
+  geom_smooth(method="lm",col="red",size=2)
> p4
```

We can see that the points in the scatterplot are presented with different colors based on species it belongs because of using aes (col = Species). Actually, in ggplot2, except for color, we can also use size, shape, stroke (thickness of boundary) and fill (fill color) to discriminate groupings in appropriate plots.

4.3.3.3   Using the Coordinate System to Adjust the Limits of X and Y Axes

The usage of the coordinate system is to adjust the mapping from coordinates to the 2D plane on the computer screen. Among the different coordinate systems available in ggplot2, the Cartesian and the polar systems are the most often used. Each coordinate system has the associated functions. For example, for Cartesian coordinate system, the coordinate functions include: coord_cartesian(xlim, ylim), coord_flip(), and coord_fixed(ratio, xlim, ylim); for polar coordinates, the function coord_polar(theta, start, direction) is often used. We can use these functions and their according arguments to adjust the attributes to display in the plot. Here we illustrate how to use the arguments xlim and ylim of coord_cartesian() to adjust the limits of X and Y axes, respectively.

In following codes, we create a new plot object p5, and change the X and Y axis limits to zoom in to the region of interest using coord_cartesian(). Then we plot this object (Fig. 4.7).

```
> p5 <- p4 + coord_cartesian(xlim=c(2.2,4.2), ylim=c(4, 7)) # zooms in
> plot(p5)
```

4.3.3.4   Adding the Labels Layer to Change the Title and Axis Labels

The plots created by ggplot2 by default do not have any title and with axis labels corresponding to the variable names used in the plot. However, in some cases, e.g., publication, we may want to add the titles to the plot and may also want to change the X and Y-axis labels. This can be done either using the labs() function in which we can specify both the axis and the title with title, x and y arguments, or using specific functions ggtitle() to change the title, and xlab() and ylab() for axis labels.

The following codes use labs() function:

```
> #Add Title and Labels using labs()
> p6 <- p5 + labs(title="Sepal width vs sepal length", subtitle="Using
```

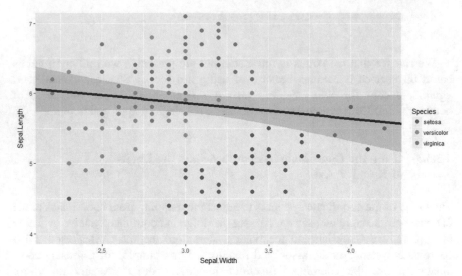

Fig. 4.7   Adjust the limits of X and Y axes using the coord_cartesian()

```
iris dataset", y="Length of Sepal", x="Width of Sepal")
> print(p6)#Or plot(p6)
```

Or

```
> plot(p6)
```

The following codes use ggtitle(), xlab() and ylab() functions:

```
> #Add Title and Labels using ggtitle(), xlab() and ylab()
> p7 <-p5 + ggtitle("Sepal width vs sepal length", subtitle="Using iris
dataset") + ylab("Length of Sepal") + xlab("Width of Sepal")
> print(p7)
```

The full scatterplot call is given using following codes:

```
> library(ggplot2)
> ggplot(iris, aes(x=Sepal.Width, y=Sepal.Length)) +
+ geom_point(aes(col=Species), size=3) +
+ geom_smooth(method="lm",col="red",size=2) +
+ coord_cartesian(xlim=c(2.2,4.2), ylim=c(4, 7)) +
+ labs(title="Sepal width vs sepal length", subtitle="Using iris
dataset",
y="Length of Sepal", x="Width of Sepal")
```

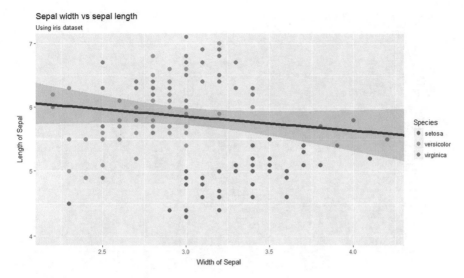

Fig. 4.8 Scatterplot with changed titles and axis labels

This generated plot is same as Fig. 4.8.

4.3.3.5 Using Faceting to Detect Patterns Across Conditions

Faceting is a powerful tool to investigate whether patterns are the same or different across conditions. The way of faceting to do so is to draw multiple plots within one figure. The functionality of faceting is similar to panels in lattice package. It is often seen in publications on microbiome study. Faceting can be performed via two main ways in ggplot2: grid faceting and wrap faceting.

Draw multiple plots in a grid using facet_grid(formula)

To create a faceting of plot, the dataset is splitted into subgroups based on two or more variables, then these subsets of dataset are used to produce subplots. The function facet_grid() is used to create the grid faceting. The syntax of the function is: facet_grid(formula).

The formula could be x ~ y, which indicates to split the plots into one row for each value of the variable x and one column for each value of the variable y. Implementing the facet_grid(x ~ y) function produces a matrix plot with rows and columns consisting the possible combinations of x and y. The formula could be x ~., which is used to split the plots by rows; implementing the facet_grid(x ~.) function splits plots with orientation by rows. The formula also could be .~ y, which is used to split the plots by columns; implementing the facet_grid(.~ y) function splits plots with orientation by columns. We illustrate facet_grid(x ~.) and

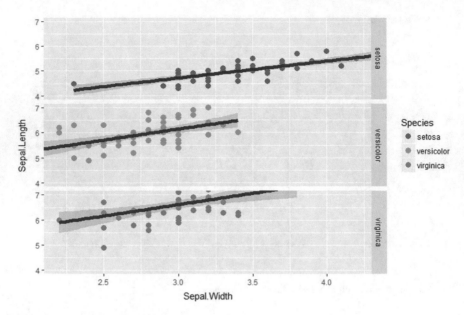

Fig. 4.9 Scatterplot with splitting plots by rows

facet_grid(. ~ y) grid faceting using previous scatterplot of sepal width versus sepal length from iris dataset, respectively.

The scatterplot has the sepal length against the sepal width for the whole dataset. We can use grid faceting to detect this relationship for different kinds of species (Figs. 4.9 and 4.10).

```
> #Spliting plots by rows
> ggplot(iris, aes(x=Sepal.Width, y=Sepal.Length)) +
+ geom_point(aes(col=Species), size=3) +
+ geom_smooth(method="lm",col="red",size=2) +
+ coord_cartesian(xlim=c(2.2,4.2), ylim=c(4, 7)) +
+ # Add Facet Grid
+ facet_grid(Species ~ .)

> #Spliting plots by columns
> ggplot(iris, aes(x=Sepal.Width, y=Sepal.Length)) +
+ geom_point(aes(col=Species), size=3) +
+ geom_smooth(method="lm",col="red",size=2) +
+ coord_cartesian(xlim=c(2.2,4.2), ylim=c(4, 7)) +
+ # Add Facet Grid
+ facet_grid(. ~ Species)
```

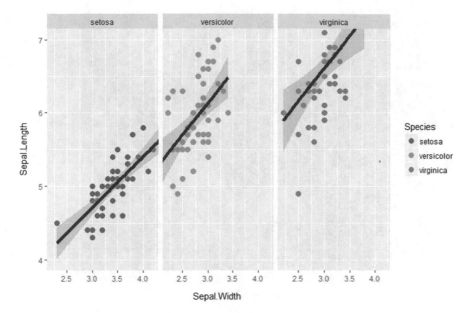

Fig. 4.10 Scatterplot with splitting plots by columns

The margin option of the facet_grid() function is very useful. It is used to create additional facets containing all the data if specifying margin = TRUE. The following codes create an additional column of all the data presenting the scatterplot for all three species (Fig. 4.11).

```
> #Spliting plots by columns
> ggplot(iris, aes(x=Sepal.Width, y=Sepal.Length)) +
+ geom_point(aes(col=Species), size=3) +
+ geom_smooth(method="lm",col="red",size=2) +
+ coord_cartesian(xlim=c(2.2,4.2), ylim=c(4, 7)) +
+ # Add Facet Grid
+ facet_grid(.~ Species, margin=TRUE)
```

If we want to split the plots based on two or more variables, we need to perform faceting for all these variables. For example, the formula . ~ y + z(facet_grid(. ~ y + z)) perform faceting for two variables with both by columns, the plots will be displayed based on one variable side by side along with the levels of another variable. This kind of visualization makes the comparison of two categorical variables very efficiently. In this formula, we can see that the additional variable z is added to y using the + operator.

Break down a large series of plots into multiple small plots using facet_wrap (formula)

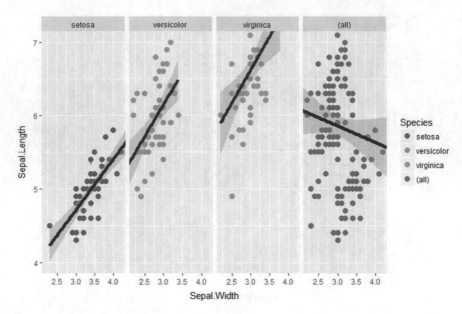

Fig. 4.11 Scatterplot with splitting plots by columns containing an additional facet for all the data

Wrap faceting produces a large series of plots into multiple small plots for individual categories. This feature makes wrap faceting especially useful to facet combinations of many levels of categorical variables. To perform wrap faceting, we use the facet_wrap(formula) function. The faceting variables can be listed as arguments in the form of facet_wrap(x ~ y + z). The variables to the left of ~ sign form the rows while those to the right form the columns. The syntax of facet_wrap(x ~ .) is used to split the plots only by x in rows and include all other subsets in the plot.

The main difference between wrap faceting and grid faceting is that with wrap faceting, it is possible to choose the number of rows and columns in the grid. We can specify them using the nrow and ncol arguments, respectively (Fig. 4.12).

```
> #Facet Wrap
> #Splitting plots by columns
> ggplot(iris, aes(x=Sepal.Width, y=Sepal.Length)) +
+ geom_point(aes(col=Species), size=3) +
+ geom_smooth(method="lm",col="red",size=2) +
+ coord_cartesian(xlim=c(2.2,4.2), ylim=c(4, 7)) +
+ #Add Facet Wrap
+ facet_wrap(~ Species, nrow=2)
```

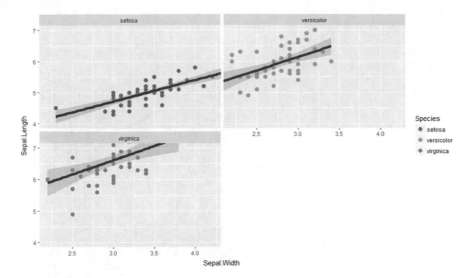

Fig. 4.12   Scatterplot with splitting plots by columns using wrap faceting

4.4   Summary

In this chapter, we introduced basic features of R, RStudio, and R Packages, as well as ggplot2. For R, RStudio, we focused on how to analyze data through R/RStudio. We also introduced some applications of R functions in microbiome data. We particularly introduced the dplyr package because it is very useful and widely used in microbiome data management. For ggplot2, we introduced the relationship of ggplot2 and the grammar of graphics. We focused on its layer feature of ggplot2, and showed how to create a plot layer by layer with the ggplot(). Overall, this chapter provides the basic statistical tools for data analysis and plots, as well as analyzing microbiome data.

References

Chang, W. 2013. *R Graphics cookbook: Practical recipes for visualizing data*. O'Reilly Media, Inc.: Sebastopol, CA, USA.
Crawley, M.J. 2013. *The R book*. Wiley: West Sussex, UK.
R Core Team. 2017. *R: A language and environment for statistical computing*. Vienna, Austria: R Core Team.
R Studio Team. 2016. *RStudio: Integrated development for R*. RStudio, Inc.: Boston.
Teutonico, D. 2015. *ggplot2 essentials*. Birmingham, UK: Packt Publishing Ltd.
Wickham, H. 2010. A layered grammar of graphics. *Journal of Computational and Graphical Statistics* 19 (1): 3–28.
Wickham, H. 2016. *ggplot2: Elegant graphics for data analysis*. New York: Springer.
Wilkinson, L. 2005. *The grammar of graphics*. New York: Springer.

Chapter 5
Power and Sample Size Calculations for Microbiome Data

In this chapter, we discuss hypothesis testing, power and sample size calculations of microbiome data with implementation in R. We begin with introduction of statistical hypothesis testing and the prerequisites for power and sample size calculations in Sect. 5.1. We then present power and sample size calculations of microbiome diversities using t-test and ANOVA in Sects. 5.2 and 5.3. In Sect. 5.4, we introduce hypothesis testing, power and sample size calculations of proportional microbiome data using parametric and nonparametric tests. In Sect. 5.5, we introduce power and sample size analyses, and effect size calculation based on a Dirichlet-multinomial model and HMP package. Section 5.6 is summary.

5.1 Hypothesis Testing and Power Analysis

5.1.1 Hypothesis Testing

The main objective of statistics is to make inferences about unknown population parameters based on the sample information: to reach conclusions on the population from the observed sample data. Statistical inferences include estimation of population parameters and hypothesis testing about population parameters. The hypothesis testing is a statistical procedure that is designed to test a statistical hypothesis. It is a major area of statistical inference in developing statistical procedures that lead to the decision on accepting or rejecting hypotheses, whereas power and sample size calculations are associated with hypothesis testing. A statistical hypothesis is an assertion or a theory concerning population, specifically about the parameters of the population distributions such as location (mean), scales (variance/dispersion). The objective of this chapter is to introduce hypothesis testing and associated power and sample size calculations in general, and specifically in microbiome study.

© Springer Nature Singapore Pte Ltd. 2018
Y. Xia et al., *Statistical Analysis of Microbiome Data with R*,
ICSA Book Series in Statistics, https://doi.org/10.1007/978-981-13-1534-3_5

5.1.1.1 Elements of a Statistical Test

There are four elements of a statistical test: (i) null hypothesis, H_0; (ii) alternative hypothesis, H_1; (iii) test statistics, and (iv) rejection region.

Every hypothesis testing procedure consists of two hypotheses. The first hypothesis is null hypothesis (denoted by H_0), a theory about the specific values of one or more population parameters. The theory is usually stated as H_0: parameter = specific value, such as $H_0 : \mu = 0.25$. The hypothesis we wish to test based upon the information contained in the sample, usually formulated with the hope that it will be rejected. The second hypothesis is known as the alternative hypothesis (denoted by H_a), a theory usually presented in a form against the null hypothesis. Typically, the null hypothesis claims that no difference or no change is achieved, whereas the alternative hypothesis declares that there is some difference or change has occurred. As a result, the null hypothesis always states that the population parameter is exactly equal to the claim value, whereas the alternative hypothesis is allowed to have several different values of the parameter. For example, in a clinical trial, if researchers want to know whether the patients with the new drug reduce less than 0.20 of the average standardized mean score compared with those received placebo 20 mm. The null hypothesis would be $H_0 : \mu \leq 0.20$ and the alternative hypothesis would be one of the following: $H_a : \mu > 0.20$, where μ denotes the average standardized mean score for the population.

The test statistic is a sample statistic used to decide whether to reject the null hypothesis. It is a function of the sample observations and some known constants upon which the statistical decision will be based. The rejection region specifies the numerical values of the test statistic for which the null hypothesis will be rejected. Specifically, it is an area of probability that tells us if our theory or hypothesis is probably true, or probably not true. Then the question is: how to choose rejection region? Briefly, rejection region is relevant to alpha level. You need to choose the alpha level you are willing to accept. For example, if you want to be 95% confident that your results are significant, you will choose a 5% alpha level (100%–95%). The "5% level" is the rejection region.

5.1.1.2 Steps for Testing Statistical Hypotheses

Statistical hypothesis testing plays a fundamental role from sample statistics to estimation of the population parameter. You can use two ways to conduct a hypothesis testing: with a critical value and with a p-value.

With a critical value, the reasoning steps are as follows:

(1) state the relevant null and alternative hypotheses because the initial research hypothesis is unknown;
(2) make the statistical assumptions of the testing sample, such as statistical independence or the distributions of the observations;

(3) choose appropriate test, and specify the relevant test statistic T;
(4) derive the distribution of the test statistic under the null hypothesis from the assumptions;
(5) select a significance level (critical region) α, typically a small value (e.g., 0.01, 0.05), which is referred to as the level of significance of the test or a probability threshold below which the null hypothesis will be rejected;
(6) compute the observed value t_{obs} of the test statistic T from the observations;
(7) decide to either reject the null hypothesis in favor of the alternative or accept it.

You can also decide either to reject or accept the null hypothesis with a p-value. If you want to use the p-value method, you need to calculate the p-value. This is the probability, under the null hypothesis, of obtaining a result equal to or more extreme than what was actually observed. If the p-value falls in the rejection region, it means you have statistically significant results; you therefore can reject the null hypothesis, and conclude that the alternative hypothesis is true. If the p-value falls outside the rejection region, it means your results cannot provide enough evidence to against the null hypothesis.

5.1.1.3 Hypothesis Testing in Microbiome Data

For microbiome community comparison, the general hypothsis tests can be written as:

(1) $H_0 : \pi_1 = \pi_0$ versus $H_A : \pi_1 \neq \pi_0$
(2) $H_0 : \pi_1 = \cdots \pi_j = \cdots = \pi_J$ versus $H_A : \pi_i \neq \pi_j$.

The above two hypothesis tests are analogous to a one sample t-test and a two sample t-test or ANOVA in classical statistics, respectively, which form the basic statistical hypothesis testing framework in microbiome study to compare:

- mean proportion of taxa to a previously specified microbiome population
- mean proportion of taxa from two sample sets
- mean proportion of taxa from more than two groups
- both mean proportion of taxa and scales cross groups.

The power and sample size calculations in microbiome study are based on the hypothesis testing framework.

As we reviewed in Chap. 2, microbiome data have unique features, but also share some common features as other research areas. Thus, the hypothesis testing and power and sample size calculations have similar setting.

For the common features of microbiome data, depending on how these data values are distributed and the number of groups to be compared, you can use a standard t-test, analysis of variance (ANOVA), or corresponding non-parametric test to the microbiome hypotheses. For the unique features of microbiome data, researchers have tried to develop appropriate statistical analysis tools including power and size calculations to better fit the data. For example, given the multivariate nature of the microbiome data structure, multivariate analysis tools are developed to take into accounts the interactions or correlations among the taxa. Among them, the HMP package uses the parametric approach based on a Dirichlet-Multinomial model of taxa counts.

5.1.2 Power Analysis and Sample Size Calculation

5.1.2.1 Importance of Power Analysis and Sample Size Calculation

The most common purpose of power analysis is to determine the minimum subjects needed to reasonably detect an effect of a given size. Additionally, power analysis is used to determine power, if an effect size and the number of subjects are available. Power analysis can also be used to compare different statistical testing procedures, such as, between a parametric and a nonparametric test of the same hypothesis.

For example, when you are planning of a study or designing an experiment for NIH grant proposal, a common question you ask is "How many subjects do we need?" The question is important because the sample size should be large enough that an effect size of scientific interest has a good opportunity to be detected if it exists.

A study with a small sample is a waste of resources in terms of time and money because the result will be invariably inconclusive. However, large sample size is also not recommended. First, it will not be useful because an effect size of scientifically little importance might also be statistically significant. Secondly, determining the appropriate sample size is important for economic reason. It is a waste of the limited available resources if an answer can be accurately found from a smaller sample. Third, in human study or randomized controlled trials, recruiting more subjects than required can be unethical. The participating patients should not be misutilized, especially, for the patients in placebo group.

5.1.2.2 Power Analysis

The power is the probability that the test correctly rejects the null hypothesis (H_0) when it is in fact false or the alternative hypothesis (H_A) is true. It can be equivalently thought of as the probability of accepting the alternative hypothesis (H_A) when it is true; that is, power is the ability of a test to detect an effect, if the effect actually exists. Thus, to understand the concept of power, we must understand the principles of hypothesis testing. The relationships among the four possible decision outcomes and their related probabilities for a statistical hypothesis test are illustrated in Table 5.1.

If the null hypothesis (H_0) is really true, there is no significant difference between (among) groups or no relationship between (among) the variables and it should not be rejected. If our decision is to retain (or fail to reject) the null

Table 5.1 Probabilities of outcomes of hypothesis testing

	Decision	
"Truth"	H_0: No difference	H_A: Difference
H_0: No difference	Pr(Correct negative) = $(1 - \alpha)$	Pr(False positive) = Pr(Type I error) = α
H_A: Difference	Pr(False negative) = Pr(Type II error) = β	Pr(Correct positive) = $(1 - \beta)$ = Power

hypothesis (H_0), we are concluding that there is no significant difference between (among) groups or no relationship between (among) the variables. We make a correct decision.

If the null hypothesis (H_0) is really false, there is a significant difference between (among) groups or a relationship between (among) the variables and it should be rejected. If our decision is to reject the null hypothesis (H_0), we are concluding that there is a significant difference between (among) groups or a relationship between (among) the variables. We again make a correct decision.

However, a Type I error (probability = α) occurs when you reject the null hypothesis when you should not have. A Type II error (probability = β) occurs when you fail to reject the null hypothesis when you should have rejected it. The power of the statistical test is defined as $1 - \beta$, which is the probability of correctly detecting the population difference; or the power of a test is generally defined as the probability of rejecting the null hypothesis when the null hypothesis is really false. The power is in general a function of the possible distributions, often determined by a parameter, under the alternative hypothesis.

There are several factors that affect power. We can informally divide these factors into the parameters that define power and methodological factors. The parameters that define power increase or decrease power in more "mechanical" way. For example, for a two-sample t-test, power depends on total sample size, ratio of group sample sizes, alpha, mean difference or effect size, standard deviation or variability. Power, effect size, sample size and alpha are four inter-related parameters that are related such that each is a function of the other three. In other words, if three of these values are fixed, the fourth is completely determined (Cohen 1988) (page 14). Thus, by increasing one, you can decrease (or increase) another: the higher the alpha is, the higher the power is (holding all the other parameters constant); the larger the effect size, the fewer subjects need (given the same power and alpha level). Though sample size calculation may vary based upon the type of study design, the basic concept remains the same.

The methodological factors include experimental design, groups, statistical procedure and model, correlation between time points, response variable, and missing data, etc. Methodological factors also affect power, through more methodological issues.

For example, repeated measures designs are virtually always more powerful than cross-sectional designs; more time points of response variable will also increase power compared to fewer data collections. The two groups with smaller effect size typically need more power to detect than those with larger effect size. Statistical procedure and model also affect power: nonparametric model may be more powerful than parametric counterpart when the assumptions of model are violated. Interaction terms often require more power than main effects to detect. Sometime, correlation between time points also affect power. A log-transformation of response variable or categorizing a continuous response variable will lead to a loss of power too because adjusting the model will lose more power than is necessary and logistic or ordinal logistic regression often requires many more subjects than does ordinary least squares regression. Finally, in general, missing data reduces power and poor imputation methods can greatly reduce power. In some statistical programs, casewise deletion is the default setting of handling missing data. Casewise deletion is one of the biggest contributors to lose of power (Graham et al. 2003; Costea et al. 2017). Therefore, when you design your study, you need to do everything possible to minimize missing data.

5.2 Power Analysis for Testing Differences in Diversity Using T-Test

5.2.1 Power Formula for Continuous Outcome

In microbiome study, the number and variety of individual taxa within a sample can be summarized using an index measure, such as the Shannon diversity index (evenness) and Chao1 index (richness). One of the fundamental objectives is to compare these species diversity across groups. The question raised by investigators is: whether there is more diversity in one group than in another. Or do the analysis results of the α-diversity from the two datasets agree with each other? Under the statistical hypothesis framework, the question can be presented:

H_0: Diversity in group 1 is no different from that of group 2
H_a: Diversity in group 1 is different from that of group 2.

The diversity measures can form the basis of the hypothesis test, power, and sample size calculations. The hypothesis tests will be presented in Chaps. 7–12. Here, we focus on power and sample size calculations.

The null hypothesis is $H_0 : \mu_1 = \mu_2$, where μ_1 and μ_2 are the true diversity means for the group 1 and group 2, respectively. The alternative hypothesis is $H_a : \mu_1 \neq \mu_2$. The null and alternative hypotheses may be rewritten as $H_0 : \mu_1 - \mu_2 = 0$ and $H_a : \mu_1 - \mu_2 = \delta \neq 0$. The goal of power analysis is to detect differences of size δ with high probability. The general power formula is given by:

$$Z_{power} = \frac{\text{test statistic}}{\text{s.e.}(\text{test statistic})} - Z_{\alpha/2} \tag{5.1}$$

For continuous endpoints, the testing statistic is mean difference δ of two groups, then

$$Z_{power} = \frac{\delta}{\text{s.e.}(\delta)} - Z_{\alpha/2} \qquad (5.2)$$

Power depends on α, δ, σ, and n. If σ known, use normal distribution in calculations, if σ needs to be estimated, use non-central t (or table).

Assume σ is known and $n_1 = n_2 = n$, then we can use the data to reform the hypothesis as below:

$$H_0 : \bar{Y}_1 - \bar{Y}_2 \sim N(0, 2\sigma^2/n)$$
$$H_a : \bar{Y}_1 - \bar{Y}_2 \sim N(\delta, 2\sigma^2/n)$$

Reject H_0 distribution if

$$\bar{Y}_1 - \bar{Y}_2 > z_{\alpha/2}\sqrt{2\sigma^2/n}$$

or

$$\bar{Y}_1 - \bar{Y}_2 < -z_{\alpha/2}\sqrt{2\sigma^2/n}$$

The power will be the Pr(Reject when H_a true). It is given below:

$$P\left(Z > z_{\alpha/2} - \delta/\sqrt{2\sigma^2/n}\right) + P\left(Z < -z_{\alpha/2} - \delta/\sqrt{2\sigma^2/n}\right) \qquad (5.3)$$

The general sample size formula for testing difference in means is as below:

$$n = \frac{2\sigma^2(Z_\beta + Z_{\alpha/2})^2}{\delta^2} \qquad (5.4)$$

where

n   Sample size in each group (assumes sizes of two groups are equal)
σ Standard deviation of the outcome variable
Z_β The z-value at desired power (typically .84 for 80% power)
$Z_{\alpha/2}$ The z-value at desired level of statistical significance (typically 1.96)
δ Effect Size (the difference in means).

If σ is unknown and needs to be estimated, and assume $n_1 = n_2 = n$, then we can reform the hypothesis as below:

Reject H_0 distribution if

$$\overline{Y}_1 - \overline{Y}_2 > t_{2(n-1),1-\alpha/2}\sqrt{2S_p^2/n}$$

$$\overline{Y}_1 - \overline{Y}_2 < t_{2(n-1),\alpha/2}\sqrt{2S_p^2/n}$$

where

$$S_p^2 = \frac{(n_1 - 1)S_1^2 + (n_2 - 1)S_2^2}{n_1 + n_2 - 2} \tag{5.5}$$

Power will be Pr(reject| H_a):

$$\frac{\overline{Y}_1 - \overline{Y}_2}{\sqrt{2S_p^2/n}} \sim t_{2(n-1)}(\delta/2\sigma^2/n) \tag{5.6}$$

where $\delta/2\sigma^2/n$ is the noncentrality parameter and the probability of rejection is computed given noncentral t distribution.

If the sample sizes in each group are imbalanced, $n_1 \neq n_2$, we can derive the sample size formula as below:

$$s.e.(\delta) = \sqrt{\frac{\sigma^2}{n_1} + \frac{\sigma^2}{n_2}} \tag{5.7}$$

Let's r = the ratio of group 2 over group 1, then $s.e.(diff) = \sqrt{\frac{\sigma^2}{n_1} + \frac{\sigma^2}{rn_1}}$. Replace it to general power formula, we obtain:

$$Z_{power} = \frac{\delta}{\sqrt{\frac{\sigma^2}{n_1} + \frac{\sigma^2}{rn_1}}} - Z_{\alpha/2} = \frac{\delta}{\sqrt{\frac{(r+1)\sigma^2}{rn_1}}} - Z_{\alpha/2}$$

$$rn_1\delta^2 = (r+1)\sigma^2(Z_{power} + Z_{\alpha/2})^2$$

We obtain sample size formula

$$n_1 = \frac{(r+1)}{r}\frac{\sigma^2(Z_{power} + Z_{\alpha/2})^2}{\delta^2} \tag{5.8}$$

If r = 1 (equal sizes of groups), then $n_1 = \frac{2\sigma^2(Z_{power} + Z_{\alpha/2})^2}{\delta^2}$.

5.2.2   Diversity Data for ALS Study

To illustrate the power analysis for testing differences in diversity using *t*-test, we compare the Shannon diversity calculated on G93A transgenic mice from an Amyotrophic lateral sclerosis (ALS) study on the impact of butyrate treatment on the fecal microbiome. G93A mice are harbor human ALS–causing SOD1 mutations that recapitulate the neuron and muscle impairment in patients with ALS. These mice are extensively used to investigate the pathomechanisms of ALS and trial therapeutics (Zhang et al. 2017). There are 9 samples in butyrate treatment and 7 G93A mutant without treatment groups. For each of the 16 mice, the Shannon diversity was calculated.

The distribution in Fig. 5.1 shows that the butyrate-treated group results in higher diversity because the histogram for this group is shifted to the right (higher diversity values) compared to the control group without butyrate (note: the vertical dashed red line labels the mean diversity for each group). In this data, the mean and standard deviation of Shannon diversity for the butyrate-treated group are 2.504 and 0.170, and for the control group without butyrate are 2.205 and 0.209. For the continuous variables, the effect size is just the difference of these two means (delta = 2.504–2.205).

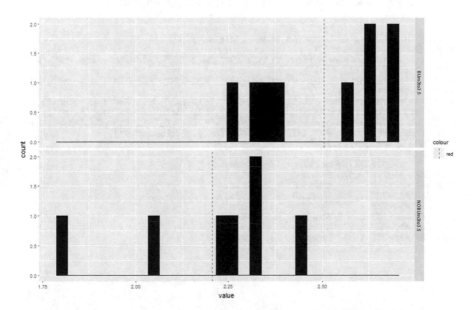

Fig. 5.1 Histograms of the Shannon diversity distributions compared on a genus level of taxa composition data from the fecal samples of ALS G93A mutant mice treated with butyrate treatment (BUm3to3.5) (upper panel) and without butyrate treatment (NOBUm3to3.5) (lower panel)

Figure 5.1 was generated by following R codes. First, we load the taxa abundance table and transpose the original taxa by sample format table into the sample by taxa format table.

```
> ##load abundance table
> abund_table=read.csv("ALSG93AGenus.csv",row.names=1,
check.names=FALSE)
> abund_table_t<-t(abund_table)
```

Then, we call diversity function from the vegan package to calculate Shannon diversity.

```
> library(vegan)
> #use the diversity function (vegan package) to calculate Shannon index
> #make a data frame of Shannon index
> H<-diversity(abund_table_t, "shannon")
> df_H<-data.frame(sample=names(H),value=H,measure=rep("Shannon",
length(H)))
```

Third, we create the variable "Group" from sample information.

```
> #Obtain grouping information from sample data
> df_H$Group <- with(df_H,
+ ifelse(as.factor(sample)%in% c("A11-28F","A12-28F","A13-28F","A14-28F","A15
-28F","A16-28F"),c("G93m1"),
+ ifelse(as.factor(sample)%in% c("A21-28F","A22-28F","A23-28F","A24-28F","A25
-28F","A26-28F"),c("WTm1"),
+ ifelse(as.factor(sample)%in% c("C11-28F","C12-28F","C13-28F"),c("G93m4"),
+ ifelse(as.factor(sample)%in% c("C21-28F","C22-28F","C23-28F"),c("WTm4"),
+ ifelse(as.factor(sample)%in% c("B11-28F","B12-28F","B13-28F","B14-28F","B15
-28F","D11-28F","D12-28F","D13-28F","D14-28F"),c("BUm3to3.5"),
+ c("NOBUm3to3.5")))))))
> df_H
            sample value measure        Group
A11-28F A11-28F 2.478 Shannon        G93m1
A12-28F A12-28F 2.162 Shannon        G93m1
A13-28F A13-28F 1.707 Shannon        G93m1
A14-28F A14-28F 2.084 Shannon        G93m1
A15-28F A15-28F 2.660 Shannon        G93m1
A16-28F A16-28F 1.971 Shannon        G93m1
A21-28F A21-28F 1.957 Shannon         WTm1
```

```
A22-28F A22-28F 1.850 Shannon         WTm1
A23-28F A23-28F 2.630 Shannon         WTm1
A24-28F A24-28F 1.768 Shannon         WTm1
A25-28F A25-28F 2.122 Shannon         WTm1
A26-28F A26-28F 1.960 Shannon         WTm1
B11-28F B11-28F 2.393 Shannon    BUm3to3.5
B12-28F B12-28F 2.677 Shannon    BUm3to3.5
B13-28F B13-28F 2.257 Shannon    BUm3to3.5
B14-28F B14-28F 2.700 Shannon    BUm3to3.5
B15-28F B15-28F 2.580 Shannon    BUm3to3.5
B21-28F B21-28F 2.262 Shannon  NOBUm3to3.5
B22-28F B22-28F 2.230 Shannon  NOBUm3to3.5
B23-28F B23-28F 2.433 Shannon  NOBUm3to3.5
B24-28F B24-28F 2.049 Shannon  NOBUm3to3.5
B25-28F B25-28F 1.814 Shannon  NOBUm3to3.5
C11-28F C11-28F 2.234 Shannon        G93m4
C12-28F C12-28F 2.271 Shannon        G93m4
C13-28F C13-28F 1.993 Shannon        G93m4
C21-28F C21-28F 1.853 Shannon        WTm4
C22-28F C22-28F 2.243 Shannon        WTm4
C23-28F C23-28F 2.195 Shannon        WTm4
D11-28F D11-28F 2.626 Shannon    BUm3to3.5
D12-28F D12-28F 2.334 Shannon    BUm3to3.5
D13-28F D13-28F 2.344 Shannon    BUm3to3.5
D14-28F D14-28F 2.625 Shannon    BUm3to3.5
D21-28F D21-28F 2.333 Shannon  NOBUm3to3.5
D22-28F D22-28F 2.312 Shannon  NOBUm3to3.5
```

The whole data set include sample data from months 1, 3, 3.5 and 4. We interest in comparisons of treatment versus not treatment during 3 to 3.5 months. So we subset the data from 3 to 3.5 months as below:

```
> library(dplyr)
> df_H_G6 <- select(df_H, Group,value)
> df_H_G93BUm3  <- filter(df_H_G6,Group=="BUm3to3.5"|Group=="NOBUm3to3.5")
> df_H_G93BUm3
          Group value
1     BUm3to3.5 2.393
2     BUm3to3.5 2.677
3     BUm3to3.5 2.257
4     BUm3to3.5 2.700
5     BUm3to3.5 2.580
6   NOBUm3to3.5 2.262
7   NOBUm3to3.5 2.230
8   NOBUm3to3.5 2.433
9   NOBUm3to3.5 2.049
10  NOBUm3to3.5 1.814
11    BUm3to3.5 2.626
12    BUm3to3.5 2.334
13    BUm3to3.5 2.344
14    BUm3to3.5 2.625
15  NOBUm3to3.5 2.333
16  NOBUm3to3.5 2.312
```

Finally, we generate Fig. 5.1 by following R codes.

```
> library(ggplot2)
> #split the plot into multiple panels
> p<-ggplot(df_H_G93BUm3, aes(x=value))+
+    geom_histogram(color="black", fill="black")+
+    facet_grid(Group ~ .)
> #Calculate the mean of each group
> ##calculate the average Shannon diversity of each group using the package
  plyr
> library(plyr)
> mu <- ddply(df_H_G93BUm3, "Group", summarise, grp.mean=mean(value))
> head(mu)
        Group grp.mean
1   BUm3to3.5    2.504
2 NOBUm3to3.5    2.205

> #add mean lines
> p+geom_vline(data=mu, aes(xintercept=grp.mean, color="red"),
+                 linetype="dashed")
```

5.2.3   Calculating Power or Sample Size Using R Function power.t.test()

To test the null hypothesis of no difference in the Shannon diversity, a *t*-test or a Wilcoxon rank sum test can be used. We leave the hypothsis testing of diversity until Chap. 7. Here, we focus on illustrating how to calculate the power or sample size using R software. In R, the function power.t.test() in basic R and the function pwr.t.test() in the pwr package can be used to conduct power analysis. We use the power.t.test. The usage of this function is shown below:

power.t.test (n = sample size, delta = effect size, sd = standard deviation, sig. level = 0.05, power = NULL, type = c("two.sample", "one.sample", "paired"), alternative = ("two.sided", "one.sided"))

where, *n* is the number of sample size per group, *delta* is true difference in means, *sd* is the standard deviation, *sig.level* is the significance level (Type I error probability), *power* is the power of test (1 minus Type II error probability), *type* is the type of *t* test, and *alternative* is one-or-two sided test.

Since the standard deviation of the mean difference is unknown, it needs to be estimated using formula in (5.5).

```
> aggregate(formula = value ~ Group,
+           data = df_H_G93BUm3,
+           FUN = var)
      Group value
1   BUm3to3.5 0.02892
2 NOBUm3to3.5 0.04349
```

```
> n1 <- 9
> n2 <-7
> s1<-sqrt(0.02892)
> s2<-sqrt(0.04349)
> s=sqrt((n1-1)*s1^2+(n2-1)*s2^2)/(n1+n2-2)
> s
[1] 0.05012
```

Now the power can be obtained from calling the power.t.test() function.

```
> power.t.test(n=2:10,delta=2.504-2.205,sd=0.05012)

    Two-sample t test power calculation

          n = 2, 3, 4, 5, 6, 7, 8, 9, 10
      delta = 0.299
         sd = 0.05012
  sig.level = 0.05
      power = 0.8324, 0.9994, 1.0000, 1.0000, 1.0000, 1.0000, 1.0000,
1.0000, 1.0000
    alternative = two.sided

NOTE: n is number in *each* group

> df_P <-data.frame(n,power)
> df_P
   n power
1  2 0.8324
2  3 0.9994
3  4 1.0000
4  5 1.0000
5  6 1.0000
6  7 1.0000
7  8 1.0000
8  9 1.0000
9 10 1.0000
```

From above power analysis, we can see that a size sample of 2 G93A mice per group, randomly assigned to butyrate treatment or no treatment control, will provide 83% power to reject the null hypothesis of no difference in the Shannon diversity in the two groups. If the sample size increases to 3 per group, the power will increase to more than 99%. We can generate power and sample size graphs to visualize the power and sample size we need to reject the null hypothesis using following R codes.

```
> n = c(2, 3, 4, 5, 6, 7, 8, 9, 10)
> power = c
(0.8324, 0.9994, 1.0000, 1.0000, 1.0000, 1.0000, 1.0000, 1.0000, 1.0000)

> power <- sapply(n, function (x) power.t.test(n=x, delta=2.504-2.205,
sd=0.05012)$power)
> plot(n, power, xlab = "Sample Size per group", ylab = "Power
to reject null",
+      main="Power curve for\n t-test with delta = 0.05",
+      lwd=2, col="red", type="l")
> abline(h = 0.90, col="blue")
```

Actually, the power and sample size calculations can be done in almost any statistical software package (e.g., in R we used power.t.test (n = 2:10, delta = 2.504–2.205, sd = 0.05012) to generate the data for Fig. 5.2).

Assume one of compared groups is a previously specified microbiome population, then the one-sample *t*-test is needed to estimate the power or sample size. The default testing of function power.t.test() is two-sample. You can specify type="one. sample" to conduct one-sample power analysis as below.

```
> power.t.test(n=2:10,delta=2.504-2.205,sd=0.05012, type = "one.sample")
```

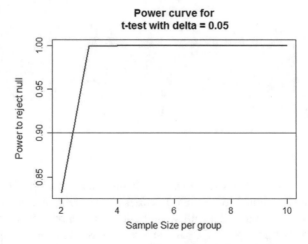

Fig. 5.2 Power of the t-test as a function of the sample size per group for effect size of 0.299 based on average Shannon diversity index of the butyrate treatment and the no treatment groups

5.3 Power Analysis for Comparing Diversity Across More than Two Groups Using ANOVA

5.3.1 Hypothesis and Theory of Power for One-Way ANOVA

For comparisons involving more than two groups, a one-way analysis of variance (ANOVA) can be used. For example, to compare the diversity in three or more groups, the hypotheses could be:

H_0 : The mean diversity in three groups are equal
H_a : Not all the diversities are equal in these three groups.

The F-tests is used in ANOVA. To calculate power for a global F test in a completely randomized design with one treatment or condition at k levels, we first need to understand and define the hypothesis. The fundamental idea for ANOVA is to partition the overall variance in diversity into a component reflecting variation among treatment groups or conditions (factor levels) and variation within treatment groups or conditions [due to measurement error (residual)] (Wu et al. 2011). For a factor α occurring at $i = 1, \ldots, K$ levels, with $j = 1, \ldots, J$ observations per level, the typical one-way ANOVA model may be expressed as

$$Y_{ij} = \mu + \alpha_i + \varepsilon_{ij} \tag{5.9}$$

In term of the statistical hypothesis framework, the hypotheses are defined as,

$$H_0 : \mu_1 = \mu_2 = \cdots = \mu_k$$
$$H_a : \mu_i \neq \mu_j \text{ for some i,j where i} \neq \text{j}$$

where, μ_i = mean of group i, k = number of groups, j = experimental units.

The F test for equality of means in a one way ANOVA assumes that the data is normal with common group variances. Also $N \geq k + 1$ and $n_i \geq 1$, where N is the total sample size and n_i is the sample size of group i. Under the null hypothesis, the distribution of the F statistic follows a central F distribution, whereas under the alternative hypothesis the distribution of the F statistic follows a noncentral F distribution with the noncentrality parameter, λ. Thus, when the null hypothesis is true, it follows a central F distribution; and when it is false, it follows a noncentral F distribution. Therefore power can be defined as the probability that the F statistic follows a noncentral distribution.

The exact power is given as,

$$\text{Power} = \Pr(F(k - 1, \ N - k, \ \lambda) \geq F_{1-\alpha}(k - 1, \ N - k)) \tag{5.10}$$

The above power defines two curves of distributions with the two hypotheses. The F-distribution under the null hypothesis defines a central F distribution, whereas the distribution under the alternative hypothesis define same F with a noncentrality parameter of λ.

R uses formula (5.10) to compute power. The noncentrality parameter λ is a key parameter in this formula. How λ is defined in R? For the balanced design, let's n = sample size of balanced groups, then λ is defined as

$$\lambda = \Delta^2 n(k) \tag{5.11}$$

where $\Delta = \frac{\sigma_\mu}{\sigma}$, is the effect size, $\sigma_\mu = \sqrt{\frac{\sum_{i=1}^{k} (\mu_i - \mu)^2}{k}}$ = between "mean" variation,

and σ = error variation. With some algebra, we get $\Delta = \frac{\sqrt{\sum_{i=1}^{k} \frac{1}{k}(\mu_i - \mu)^2}}{\sigma}$. Replace it to (5.11), we have

$$\lambda = \frac{\sum_{i=1}^{k} \frac{1}{k}(\mu_i - \mu)^2}{\sigma^2} nk,$$

with nk = N, then

$$\lambda = N\left(\frac{\sum_{i=1}^{k} \frac{1}{k}(\mu_i - \mu)^2}{\sigma^2}\right) \tag{5.12}$$

5.3.2 Calculating Power or Sample Size Using R Function pwr.avova.test()

To illustrate using the pwr.avova.test() to obtain powers with different sample sizes, we use following procedures. First, we subset data of four groups of months 1 and 4 with treatment and control.

```
> df_H_G93WTm1N4 <- filter(df_H_G6,Group%in%c("G93m1","WTm1",
"G93m4","WTm4"))
> df_H_G93WTm1N4
    Group value
1  G93m1 2.478
2  G93m1 2.162
3  G93m1 1.707
4  G93m1 2.084
5  G93m1 2.660
6  G93m1 1.971
7   WTm1 1.957
```

```
8   WTm1 1.850
9   WTm1 2.630
10  WTm1 1.768
11  WTm1 2.122
12  WTm1 1.960
13  G93m4 2.234
14  G93m4 2.271
15  G93m4 1.993
16  WTm4 1.853
17  WTm4 2.243
18  WTm4 2.195
```

Then, we get F statistic by fitting linear model.

```
> fit = lm(formula = value~Group,data=df_H_G93WTm1N4)
> anova (fit)
Analysis of Variance Table

  Response: value
            Df Sum Sq Mean Sq F value Pr(>F)
  Group      3  0.059  0.0195    0.23   0.88
  Residuals 14  1.209  0.0863
```

Finally, we call the pwr.anova.test() function from pwr package to calculate powers.

```
> library(pwr)
> pwr.anova.test(f= 0.23,k=4,n=45:55,sig.level=0.05)

Balanced one-way analysis of variance power calculation

          k = 4
          n = 45, 46, 47, 48, 49, 50, 51, 52, 53, 54, 55
          f = 0.23
  sig.level = 0.05
      power = 0.7276, 0.7383, 0.7486, 0.7586, 0.7683, 0.7777, 0.7868,
0.7956, 0.8041, 0.8123, 0.8202

NOTE: n is number in each group
```

The results above show that 52 samples are needed for each group to obtain 80% based on the effect sizes detected in this pilot study using ANOVA test.

5.4   Power Analysis for Comparing a Taxon of Interest Across Groups

5.4.1   Hypothesis and Basic Power and Sample Size Formulas for Comparing Proportions

In microbiome data sets, 0 indicates a taxon is absent in the sample and 1 means the taxon presents in the sample. Such binary data can be easily transformed to proportion. If the research is interesting to the abundance of a specific taxon, then a Chi-square test can be used to compare the proportions across groups. The hypothesis for comparing a single specified taxon across groups will be:

H_0: Percentage of the specified taxon in group 1 is no different from that of group 2
H_a: Percentage of the specified taxon in group 1 is different from that of group 2.

Equation (5.4) can be easily modified to test taxon proportions. When we test taxon proportions, we are assessing whether the proportion P_1 responding to a one group (e.g., treatment) is different from the proportion P_2 responding to another group (e.g., control). This is equivalent to the null hypothesis $H_0 : P_1 - P_2 = 0$ versus the alternative hypothesis $H_a : P_1 - P_2 = \delta \neq 0$.

Equation (5.13) is modified from Eq. (5.4) to test difference in proportions:

$$n = \frac{2(\bar{p})(1 - \bar{p})(Z_\beta + Z_{\alpha/2})^2}{(p_1 - p_2)^2} \tag{5.13}$$

where

n	Sample size in each group (assumes sizes of two groups are equal)
$(\bar{p})(1 - \bar{p})$	A measure of variability (similar to standard deviation)
Z_β	The z-value at desired power (typically .84 for 80% power)
$Z_{\alpha/2}$	The z-value at desired level of statistical significance (typically 1.96)
$p_1 - p_2$	Effect Size (the difference in proportions).

In general, when outcome is binary, the sample size that needs is given as follows.

$$n = \frac{r + 1}{r} \frac{\bar{p}(1 - \bar{p})(Z_\beta + Z_{\alpha/2})^2}{(p_1 - p_2)^2} \tag{5.14}$$

Similarly in continuous cases, the imbalanced sample size formula for two groups of proportions can be derived. If $n_1 \neq n_2$, then the ratio between the sample sizes of the two groups is $r = \frac{n_1}{n_2}$. The test statistic is constructed as:

$$z = \frac{P_1 - P_2}{\sqrt{\frac{P_1(1-P_1)}{n_1} + \frac{P_2(1-P_2)}{n_2}}} \tag{5.15}$$

which is asymptotically normally distributed and therefore the σ in Eq. (5.4) can be replaced by

$$\sigma = \sqrt{\frac{P_1(1-P_1)}{n_1} + \frac{P_2(1-P_2)}{n_2}}$$

The formulas that are used to compute sample size and power are given below, respectively:

$$n_1 = rn_2 \text{ and } n_2 = \left(\frac{P_1(1-P_1)}{r} + P_2(1-P_2)\right)\left(\frac{z_{1-\alpha/2} + z_{1-\beta}}{P_1 - P_2}\right)^2, \tag{5.16}$$

$$1 - \beta = \Phi(z - z_{1-\alpha/2}) + \Phi(-z - z_{1-\alpha/2}). \tag{5.17}$$

where

- $r = \frac{n_1}{n_2}$ is the matching ratio
- Φ is the standard Normal distribution function
- Φ^{-1} is the standard Normal quantile function
- α is Type I error
- β is Type II error
- $1 - \beta$ is power.

5.4.2   Power Analysis Using R Function power.prop.test()

In our ALS study (Zhang et al. 2017), we find that treatment with oral 2% sodium butyrate for 2.5 months was associated with significant enhancement of the abundance of the butyrate-producing bacteria Butyrivibrio fibrisolvens in the species level. We are interested to compare whether this taxon is present at different rates between treatment and control groups. In order to design future study, we want to calculate sample size to ensure that the study has sufficient power to detect effect size based on this pilot study.

In this section, we illustrate function power.prop.test() to conduct power analysis using our ALS G93A mice data, In Sect. 5.4.3, we will illustrate the χ^2 test and Fisher's exact test. We transform the abundance count data of Butyrivibrio

Table 5.2 Distribution of the rate of Butyrivibrio fibrisolvens between butyrate treatment and control from ALS G93A mice data set

Group	Presence	Absence	Total
Butyrate	9 (100%)	0 (0%)	9
Control	4 (57%)	3 (43%)	7

fibrisolvens into a binary variable to indicate present and absent of species Butyrivibrio fibrisolvens. We summarize the transformed data in Table 5.2.

The following R codes load abundance table.

```
abund_table_Spe=read.csv("ALSG93AButyrivibrioSpecies.csv",row.names=1,
check.names=FALSE)
```

The original abundance data is a count table with species for row and sample for column. The following transpose function "t()" transposes this species count table into sample for row and species for column.

```
> abund_table_Spe<-t(abund_table_Spe)
```

The grouping information can be obtained from the sample identifiers.

```
> grouping<-data.frame(row.names=rownames(abund_table_Spe),t(as.data.
frame(strsplit(rownames(abund_table_Spe),"-"))))
```

The 9 samples labled as "B11","B12","B13","B14", "B15","D11","D12", "D13", and "D14" were randomly assigned to butyrate treatment group, other 7 samples were assigned to control group.

The following R codes are used to create a group variable to present the grouping information.

```
> grouping$Group <-
with(grouping,ifelse(as.factor(X1)%in%c("B11","B12","B13","B14",
"B15","D11","D12","D13","D14"),c("Butyrate"), c("Control")))
```

After the species abundance table and grouping information table are combined into one data frame, the data are ready to be analyzed.

```
> Butyrivibrio_G <-cbind(abund_table_Spe, grouping)
> rownames(Butyrivibrio_G)<-NULL
> Butyrivibrio_G
   Butyrivibrio  X1  X2       Group
1            14 B11 28F Butyrate
2            39 B12 28F Butyrate
3            18 B13 28F Butyrate
4            41 B14 28F Butyrate
5            19 B15 28F Butyrate
6             0 B21 28F  Control
7            16 B22 28F  Control
8             1 B23 28F  Control
9             8 B24 28F  Control
10            0 B25 28F  Control
11           78 D11 28F Butyrate
12            4 D12 28F Butyrate
13           17 D13 28F Butyrate
14           94 D14 28F Butyrate
15            1 D21 28F  Control
16            0 D22 28F  Control
```

The count of Butyrivibrio fibrisolvens with 0 is coded as "Absent", otherwise as "Present".

```
> Butyrivibrio_G$Present <- ifelse((Butyrivibrio_G$Butyrivibrio > 0),
"Present","Absent")
> Butyrivibrio_G
   Butyrivibrio  X1  X2       Group Present
1            14 B11 28F Butyrate Present
2            39 B12 28F Butyrate Present
3            18 B13 28F Butyrate Present
4            41 B14 28F Butyrate Present
5            19 B15 28F Butyrate Present
6             0 B21 28F  Control  Absent
7            16 B22 28F  Control Present
8             1 B23 28F  Control Present
9             8 B24 28F  Control Present
10            0 B25 28F  Control  Absent
11           78 D11 28F Butyrate Present
12            4 D12 28F Butyrate Present
13           17 D13 28F Butyrate Present
14           94 D14 28F Butyrate Present
15            1 D21 28F  Control Present
16            0 D22 28F  Control  Absent
```

The data are summarized as 2×2 contingency table.

```
> library(MASS) # load the MASS package
> tbl = table(Butyrivibrio_G$Group, Butyrivibrio_G$Present)
> tbl               # the contingency table

            Absent Present
  Butyrate       0       9
  Control        3       4
```

The above table shows the distribution of the proportion–4 (57%) out of 7 control samples had Butyrivibrio fibrisolvens, while 9 (100%) out of 9 Butyrate treatment samples did. The following plain R codes are used to implement the sample size and power calculations using above formulas in (5.16) and (5.17).

```
> p1=1.0
> p2=0.57
> r=1
> alpha=0.05
> beta=0.20
> (n2=(p1*(1-p1)/r+p2*(1-p2))*((qnorm(1-alpha/2)+qnorm(1-beta))/
(p1-p2))^2)
[1] 10.4
> ceiling(n2)
[1] 11
> z=(p1-p2)/sqrt(p1*(1-p1)/n2/r+p2*(1-p2)/n2)
> (Power=pnorm(z-qnorm(1-alpha/2))+pnorm(-z-qnorm(1-alpha/2)))
[1] 0.8
```

However, the convenient way is to use following R function power.prop.test. You can specify multiple samples to test the powers.

```
> power.prop.test(n=10:20, p1=1, p2=.57, sig.
level=0.05, power=NULL, alternative=c("one.sided"), strict = FALSE)

Two-sample comparison of proportions power calculation

              n = 10, 11, 12, 13, 14, 15, 16, 17, 18, 19, 20
             p1 = 1
             p2 = 0.57
      sig.level = 0.05
          power = 0.7928, 0.8290, 0.8596, 0.8852, 0.9065, 0.9242, 0.9387, 0.9
506, 0.9603, 0.9682, 0.9746
    alternative = one.sided

NOTE: n is number in *each* group
```

The results show that 11 samples in each group can obtain 83% power to detect the effect sizes based on our pilot study.

5.4.3   Power Analysis Using χ^2 Test and Fisher Exact Test

5.4.3.1   Theory of Power for a χ^2 Test for Comparing Proportions

The hypotheses for testing proportions of microbiome composition can also be tested by a chi squared statistic. The χ^2 test statistic is defined as,

$$X^2 = \sum_{i=1}^{n} \frac{(E_i - O_i)^2}{E_i} \tag{5.18}$$

where

O_i an observed frequency
E_i an expected (theoretical) frequency, asserted by the null hypothesis
n   the number of possible outcomes of each event

Similar as the distribution of the F statistic, the distribution of the χ^2-statistic follows a central chi square distribution when the null hypothesis is true. When it's false it follows a noncentral chi squared distribution with the noncentrality parameter, λ. Thus essentially power for chi square distribution is the probability that the data comes from a noncentral chi squared distribution.

Basically, the χ^2 distribution defines two curves: one follows a central χ^2 distribution under null hypothesis; the other follows a noncentral χ^2 distribution with the noncentrality parameter, λ. The chi square value with a probability of 0.05 under the null hypothesis is represented with a vertical line. If the χ^2 statistic falls into the left of the line, then it indicates it came from the null distribution and if it is on the right of the line, then it came from the alternative distribution. The area under the alternative hypothesis curve to the right of the line represents the power of the test. For example, in microbiome study, we assume the proportions from group 1 or condition 1 follows a central χ^2 distribution, while group 2 or condition 2 follows a noncentral χ^2 distribution.

Chi-Squared Power in R use this expression,

$$\text{Power} = \Pr(\chi^2(df, \lambda) \geq \chi^2_{1-\alpha}(df)) \tag{5.19}$$

The noncentrality parameter, λ, is defined as,

$$\lambda = \Delta^2 N$$

where

$\Delta = \sqrt{\sum_{i=1}^{n} \frac{(p_{1i}-p_{0i})^2}{p_{0i}}}$ effect size
N   total sample size

5.4.3.2 Implementing Power Analysis Using the Function pwr.chisq. test()

To find the sample size required for a specified power, R finds an N that will satisfy Eq. (5.19).

In this section, we illustrate power analysis using χ^2 test and Fisher exact test using our Butyrivibrio fibrisolvens present/absent data from ALS G93A mice data set. To conduct power analysis, we first need to estimate the effect size. For continuous measures, such as in Shannon diversity case, the effect size is just calculated as the difference in means. With categorical data, there are several measures can be used as the effect size including Cramer's V (Phi coefficient φ), odds ratio and relative risk (Cohen 1988). You can choose one based on your interest of study. Here we use Cramer's V, which is a measure of association for nominal variables. Effectively it is the Pearson chi-square statistic rescaled to have values between 0 and 1.

This measure of Cramer's V is defined as

$$V = \sqrt{\frac{\varphi^2}{t}} = \sqrt{\frac{\chi^2}{Nt}}\varphi \tag{5.20}$$

where χ^2 is the Pearson chi-square when the null hypothesis is true, N is the total sample size, t is the smaller of the number of rows minus one or the number of columns minus one. If r is the number of rows, and c is the number of columns, then t = minimum (r − 1, c − 1).

For a 2 × 2 contingency table, of course, this is just the square root of chi-square divided by the number of observations, which is equal to the phi coefficient φ. The Cramer's V can be estimated by using function cramersV from lsr package.

```
> library(lsr)
> cramersV(tbl)
[1] 0.3833
```

Given the Cramer's V, now we can use the function pwr.chisq.test() from the pwr package to conduct the power analysis.

```
> library(pwr)
> pwr.chisq.test(w = 0.3833, N = 45:60, df = 1, sig.
level = 0.05, power = NULL)

    Chi squared power calculation

w = 0.3833
N = 45, 46, 47, 48, 49, 50, 51, 52, 53, 54, 55, 56, 57, 58, 59, 60
df = 1
sig.level = 0.05
power = 0.7295, 0.7388, 0.7479, 0.7567, 0.7652, 0.7735, 0.7815,
```

```
0.7893, 0.7969, 0.8042, 0.8113, 0.8182, 0.8248, 0.8313, 0.8375, 0.8435
```

NOTE: N is the number of observations

The results show that 54 samples are needed in each group to correctly reject the null hypothesis with 80% power based on χ^2 test and using Cramer's V (Phi coefficient φ) as effect size.

5.4.3.3   Implementing Power Analysis Using the Functions power.fisher.test() and power.exact.test()

If the cell values are small (<5) in the contingency table, Chi-squared test may be incorrect, a Fisher exact test is applied. Thus, we illustrate two recently developed R power functions power.fisher.test() and power.exact.test() from the statmod and Exact packages, respectively. Compared with pwr.chisq.test(), both versions of Fisher tests have less flexibility to specify multiple samples in one test. In the following example, we use same proportions (p1 = 1.0, p2 = 0.57) from contingency table, and 15 samples for each group to estimate the power.

```
> library(statmod)
> power.fisher.test(1.0,0.57,15,15,alpha=0.05, nsim=1000)
[1] 0.844
```

The following R codes use the power.exact.test function to calculate power for unconditional exact test.

```
> library(Exact)
> power.exact.test(1.0, 0.57, 15, 15, method="Fisher")
$power
[1] 0.8454

$alternative
[1] "two.sided"

$method
[1] "fisher"
```

The results show that 15 samples are needed in each group to correctly reject the null hypothesis with 84% power based on the Fisher exact test.

5.5 Comparing the Frequency of All Taxa Across Groups Using Dirichlet-Multinomial Model

5.5.1 Multivariate Hypothesis Testing and Dirichlet-Multinomial Model

The above approach of comparing a taxon of interest is an univariate 'one-taxon-at-a-time' analysis. Because microbiome data have multivariate structure, we often conduct comparison of multiple taxa by comparing the abundances of each taxon across groups separately and then adjust for multiple comparisons. The univariate approach is generally less powerful than multivariate approaches because it does not take into account the interactions that exist between taxa, whereas the multivariate approaches jointly modeling microbial taxa abundance (La Rosa et al. 2012, 2015; Boyu Ren et al. 2017; Grantham et al. 2017). Microbiome researchers have made effort to develop statistical methods to conduct multivariate hypotheses concerning the effects of treatments or experimental factors on whole assemblages of bacterial taxa, and in estimating sample sizes for such experiments. Under the multivariate hypothesis testing framework to compare microbiome populations, one of the null hypotheses can be:

H_0: The different treatments or experimental factors have no different effects on whole community of taxa.
H_a: The different treatments or experimental factors do have different effects on whole community of taxa.

One of multivariate statistic methods is the Dirichlet-Multinomial distribution; it has been shown to model for microbiome data well (Holmes et al. 2012). La Rosa and colleagues reparameterize the Dirichlet multinomial model to make it suitable to perform hypothesis testing across groups based on difference between location (mean comparison) as well as scales (variance comparison/dispersion) (La Rosa et al. 2012). The motheds have capabilities to perform parameter estimation, multivariate hypothesis testing, power and sample size calculation. In this chapter, we first introduce reparameterized Dirichlet multinomial model; then focus on calculating power and sample size using the HMP Package.

Consider a set of microbiome samples measured on P subjects with K distinct taxa at an arbitrary level (e.g., phylum, class, etc.) identified across all samples. Let x_{ik}, $i = 1, \ldots, P$; $k = 1, \ldots, K$ be the number of reads in subject i for taxon k, and let x_i be the taxa count vector obtained from sample i. When taxon k is not in sample i, then x_{ik} is 0. Let $N_{i.} = \sum_{k=1}^{K} x_{ik}$ be the total number of sequence reads in sample i, $N_{.k} = \sum_{i=1}^{P} x_{ik}$ be the total number of sequence reads for taxon k across all samples, and sum of them be the total number of sequences over all samples and taxa.

The count data with this kind of structure is generally analyzed by a multinomial distribution. However, its appropriateness of using multinomial distribution assumes that the true frequency of each category is the same across all samples (La Rosa et al. 2012). In addition, the multinomial model can result in an increased Type I Error when the data present overdispersion. Thus, it is not appropriate to use the multinomial distribution to model microbiome count data because each taxon in microbiome data is not the same across all samples due to sample variabilities.

To fit microbiome taxon count data with this data structure, La Rosa et al. reparameterized the Dirichlet-multinomial distribution (La Rosa et al. 2012). It is characterized by two set of parameters: π and θ (Tvedebrink 2010):

$$\pi = \{\pi_j, j = 1,\ldots, K\}, \quad 0 \le \pi_j \le 1, \tag{5.21}$$

where, $\{\pi_j\}$ = mean proportion of taxa j. That is, is a vector of the expected taxa frequencies, or the vector of relative abundances, $\sum \pi_j = 1$. Each element of the vector could be OTU, species, genus or any other rank in the microbial taxonomy.

$$P(X_i = x_i; \pi, \theta) = \frac{N_{i.}!}{x_{i1}!\ldots x_{ik}!} = \frac{\Pi_{j=1}^{K}\Pi_{r=1}^{x_{ij}}\{\pi_j(1-\theta) + (r-1)\theta\}}{\Pi_{r=1}^{N_{i.}}(1-\theta) + (r-1)\theta} \tag{5.22}$$

where, θ is the overdispersion parameter, or the measure of dispersion. It measures the within-sample excess of variability with respect to a multinomial distribution; with $\theta \ge 0$ suggesting overdispersion.

Compared to the multinomial distribution, the parameterization of Dirichlet-multinomial distribution makes it suitable to perform hypothesis testing across groups based on difference between locations by comparisons of π vectors as well as scales by comparison of θ values. For example, for two-groups of comparisons (i.e., controls and cases), the null hypothesis: $\pi_1 = \pi_2$ expresses equality of community composition. It was proposed to test the null hypothesis using the generalized Wald test of Koehler and Wilson (1986) and La Rosa et al. (2012).

As Dirichlet-multinomial, the reparameted Dirichlet-multinomial model can be used to analyze both taxa composition and rank abundance distributions (RAD) data. These two approaches are called "taxa composition data analysis" and "rank abundance distributions data analysis", respectively (La Rosa et al. 2012). Two approaches have different focuses: one is community composition (what bacteria are there); another is community structure (such as richness and diversity).

5.5.2 Power and Sample Size Calculations Under Dirichlet-Multinomial Model

In Sect. 5.1, we discussed that several factors affect power including the parameters that define power and methodological factors. Power and sample size in Dirichlet multinomial model depend on the probability model parameters, the hypothesis being tested, and the effect size. The simulation study conducted by La Rosa et al (2012) showed that the effect size, overdispersion, and sample size influence power. The power goes up with increasing the effect size or increasing sample size, decreasing overdispersion. In some examples the number of reads also impacts power, with holding effect size, overdispersion, and sample size constant, power increases as the number of reads increases. In summary, statistical power is impacted by the number of samples per treatment (sample size or replication level) and number of sequence reads per sample (sequencing depth) (Kristin et al. 2015), and overdispersion.

For simplicity, let us consider the problem of comparing microbiome samples of taxa frequencies between two experimental groups, such as butyrate-treated versus without butyrate-treated mice. For comparing taxa frequencies to a previously specified microbiome population, more than two groups, and other hypothesis testing, the interested readers are encouraged to refer to the original articles (La Rosa et al. 2012). For comparison of π across two groups, assume that the model parameters π and θ are known for each group, the testing hypothesis is formed as:

$H_0 : \pi_1 = \pi_2$ versus the alternative $H_A : \pi_1 \neq \pi_2$

The effect size is defined by how far apart the vector of taxa frequencies π_1 and π_2 are from each other. As we mentioned in Sect. 5.4.3.2, there are several ways to measure the effect size. One of them is a Cramer's V in (5.20). With the microbiome data structure in Table 5.3, row r is the number of groups being compared, and column c is the total number of taxa. From the formula, Cramer's V depends on the sample size and number of reads. To reduce the influence of the sample size and number of reads, La Rosa et al. proposed a modified Cramer's φ criterion(La Rosa et al. 2012, 2015), which ranges from 0, denoting the taxa frequencies are the same in both groups, to 1, denoting the taxa frequencies are maximally different.

$$\varphi_m = \sqrt[2]{\frac{\chi^2}{\chi^2 \max}}, \tag{5.23}$$

where χ^2_{max} is the Chi-square statistic for the maximum difference between the taxa frequency means being compared, which is achieved when taxa in each group are

Table 5.3 Power calculations (based on alpha = 0.05) using the Dirichlet-multinomial model to compare the expected taxa frequencies of the Buty versus the NoButy populations, using as a reference the taxa frequencies obtained from the 10 samples

Samples	Reads				
	500 (%)	1000 (%)	2000 (%)	5000 (%)	10,000 (%)
5	3.50	10.99	24.58	43.66	53.95
10	98.8	99.9	99.9	100	100
15	100	100	100	100	100

non-overlapping across groups. In the case of comparing two groups, and there is no overdispersion $\chi^2_{max} = N$, then φ_m reduce to the Cramer's φ criterion.

5.5.3 Power and Size Calculations Using HMP Package

HMP is a R package developed for hypothesis testing and power calculations to compare metagenomic samples originally from HMP (La Rosa et al. 2016). Power and sample size calculations can be done either by using the asymptotic distributions of the statistics or by means of Monte-Carlo simulation implemented via HMP package. Here, we illustrate power and sample size calculations by Monte-Carlo simulation using our ALS G93A mice example.

5.5.3.1 Preparing Data Sets for Use of HMP Package

First, install and call HMP package.

```
> install.packages("HMP",repo="http://cran.r-project.org", dep=TRUE)
> library(HMP)
```

Then set work directory and load taxa abundance data sets.

```
> setwd("F:/Home/MicrobiomeStatR/Analysis")
> Buty=read.csv("ALSG93A3.5mButyrateGenus.csv",row.names=1,
check.names=FALSE)
> NOButy=read.csv("ALSG93A3.5mNoButyrateGenus.csv",row.names=1,
check.names=FALSE)
```

The original data sets have the format of taxa by sample. As shown in Table 5.3, the reparameterized Dirichlet multinomial model and HMP package need the data sets to have sample by taxa format. Therefore, we use the t() function to transpose the original data sets into the data sets with sample by taxa formats.

```
> head(Buty)
                        B11-28F B12-28F B13-28F B14-28F B15-28F
Lactococcus                  17     204       8       7       4
Tannerella                  646     170     670     421     548
Barnesiella                   6       2      12       8      21
Bacteroides                 604     406     436     260     443
Hydrogenoanaerobacterium      1       0       7       1       0
Clostridium                 179     398     564     400     737
> head(NOButy)
                        B21-28F B22-28F B23-28F B24-28F B25-28F
Lactococcus                  52      21       0       9       1
Tannerella                  787     756     395    1266    1111
Barnesiella                  12      21       8      24      17
Bacteroides                 130     241     192     228     315
Hydrogenoanaerobacterium      0       0       0       0       1
Clostridium                 458     344     418     167     334
```

```
> Buty_t <- t(Buty)
> NOButy_t<-t(NOButy)
> head(Buty_t)
        Lactococcus Tannerella Barnesiella Bacteroides
B11-28F          17        646           6         604
B12-28F         204        170           2         406
B13-28F           8        670          12         436
B14-28F           7        421           8         260
B15-28F           4        548          21         443
> head(NOButy_t)
        Lactococcus Tannerella Barnesiella Bacteroides
B21-28F          52        787          12         130
B22-28F          21        756          21         241
B23-28F           0        395           8         192
B24-28F           9       1266          24         228
B25-28F           1       1111          17         315
```

The following codes check the number of taxa and the number of sample in each data set.

```
> ncol(Buty_t)  # for the number of taxa
[1] 196
> nrow(Buty_t)  # for the number of samples
[1] 5
> ncol(NOButy_t)  # for the number of taxa
[1] 196
> nrow(NOButy_t)  # for the number of samples
[1] 5
```

5.5.3.2 Power and Size Calculations Using Taxa Composition Data Analysis

The function MC.Xdc.statistics() uses simulation and likelihood ratio test to provide the power and size of the several sample Dirichlet-Multinomial parameter test comparison. Here, we compare two sample sets of "Buty" and "NOButy".

One sample syntax is like this:

MC.Xdc.statistics(group.Nrs, numMC = 1000, alphap, type = "ha", siglev = 0.05, est = "mom")

where, *group.Nrs* is used for specifying the number of reads/sequence depth for each sample in a group. *numMC* is used for specifying the number of Monte-Carlo experiments. In practice at least 1000 should be specified.

If alphap is used for computing size of the test statistics (Type I error), i.e., when type = "hnull" is specified, then alphap specifies the matrix where rows are vectors of alpha parameters for the reference group. Such as, the following codes: alphap <- fit_Buty $gamma specifies the "Buty" gamma matrix for the reference group.

If alphap is used for computing power of the test statistics (Type II error), i.e., the default, or when type = " ha" is specified, then alphap represents the matrix consisting of vectors of alpha parameters for each taxa in each group. Such as, the following codes: alphap <- rbind(fit_Buty$gamma, fit_NOButy$gamma) specifies both "Buty" and "NOButy" gamma matrice for each taxa in each group.

If type = "hnull", then the size of the test statistics is computed; If type = "ha", then the power of the test statistics is computed, which is also the default.

siglev is used for specifying the significance level for size of the test or power calculation. The default is 0.05.

est is used for specifying the type of parameter estimator to be used with the Likelihood-ratio-test statistics, 'mle' or 'mom'. Default value is 'mom'. The authors of HMP package notes that 'mle' will take much longer time to run and is not optimal for small sample sizes, while the result from 'mom' is more conservative in small sample case.

First, get a list of Dirichlet-multinomial parameters(i.e., loglik, gamma, pi and theta) for the data using the function DM.MoM().

```
> fit_Buty <- DM.MoM(Buty_t);fit_NOButy <- DM.MoM(NOButy_t)
> fit_Buty
```

Second, set up the number of Monte-Carlo experiments, here we use 1000, the minimum value recommneted in practice and generate the number of reads per sample.

```
> numMC <- 1000
> ##The first number is the number of reads and the second is the number of
samples or subjects
> nrsGrp1 <- rep(1000, 10)
> nrsGrp2 <- rep(1000, 10)
> group_Nrs <- list(nrsGrp1, nrsGrp2)
```

Third, compute size of the test statistics (Type I error).

```
> alphap <- fit_Buty $gamma
> pval1 <- MC.Xdc.statistics(group_Nrs, numMC, alphap, "hnull")
```

```
> pval1
[1] 0.000999
```

Finally, Compute power of the test statistics (Type II error).

```
> alphap <- rbind(fit_Buty$gamma, fit_NOButy$gamma)
> pval2 <- MC.Xdc.statistics(group_Nrs, numMC, alphap)
> pval2
[1] 0.999
```

Table 5.3 shows a power analysis to compare the taxa frequencies of the Buty versus the NOButy populations using 5% significance level based on the Dirichlet-multinomial parameters obtained from the Buty and NOButy 10 sample dataset. Each entry represents the power achieved for the specified number of samples, and number of reads at 0.05 significance level. For example, for number of samples = 10, and number of reads per sample = 500, the study has 98.8% power to detect the effect size observed in the data. The results show that the power is impacted by increasing the number of reads when samples are small (in this case, 5); but is not impacted by increasing the number of reads when larger size of samples is achieved (in this case, 10). The results also indicate that when sufficient samples are achieved, increasing sample size does not increase power.

5.5.3.3   Power and Size Calculations Using Rank Abundance Distributions Data Analysis

Several Sample RAD-Probability Mean Test Comparison With Known Reference Vector of Proportions
The function MC.Xmc.statistics() use simulation and the generalized Wald-type statistics to provide the power and size of the several sample RAD-probability mean test comparison with known reference vector of proportions. Here, again we compare two sample sets of "Buty" and "NOButy".
One sample syntax is like this:

   MC.Xmc.statistics(group.Nrs, numMC = 1000, pi0, group.pi, group.theta, type = "ha", siglev = 0.05)

   where, group.Nrs, numMC, type and siglev are defined as in MC.Xdc.statistics() fnction.

   pi0 is the RAD-probability mean vector. If group.pi = "hnull", then this argument is ignored; if group.pi = "ha", then it specifies a matrix where each row is a vector pi values for each group. Group.theta is a vector of overdispersion values for each group.

   The technical challenges for analyzing rare taxa are low convergence rates and less precise test statistics. To improve the convergence rates and accurate estimates, in microbiome studies, one way is to get rid off the less frequent taxa, such as in any sample with percentage less than 1%; another way is to combine all less frequent taxa, such as, weighted average across all groups with less than 1% into one taxon called "other" (La Rosa et al. 2012). We did not use these techniques in above taxa composition data analysis when call MC.Xdc.statistics()function. Here, we use the Data.filter() function to order taxa in order of decreasing abundance and collapse less-abundant taxa into one category labeling as "Other".

One sample syntax is like this:

Data.filter(data, order.type = "sample", minReads = 1000, numTaxa = 10, perTaxa = NULL)

where, data is a matrix of taxonomic counts(columns) for each sample(rows).

If order.type = "sample", then rank taxa based on its taxonomic frequency;if order.type = "data", then rank taxa based on cumulative taxonomic counts across all samples (default). Let's minReads = one read cut-off value, then the samples with a total number of reads less than this read cut-off value will be deleted. The arguments numTaxa and perTaxa, only one should be specified in one call. The argument numTaxa is used to specify the number of taxa to keep, while collapsing the other (less abundant) taxa into "Other" category. The argument perTaxa is used to combine percentage of data to keep, while collapsing the remaining taxa.

First, order taxa in order of decreasing abundance and collapse less-abundant taxa into "Other" category using the Data.filter() function.

```
> filter_Buty<- Data.filter(Buty_t, "sample", 1000, 10)
> head(filter_Buty)
                                                    Other
B11-28F 646 604 265 196 179 159 103 53 52 32         261
B12-28F 406 398 312 242 204 170 102 82 50 45         382
B13-28F 670 564 436 110  65  62  59 58 47 39         266
B14-28F 421 400 260 149 111  67  64 58 49 48         421
B15-28F 737 548 443 281 214  97  94 69 59 53         476
```

```
> filter_NOButy<- Data.filter(NOButy_t, "sample", 1000, 10)
> head(filter_NOButy)
                                                    Other
B21-28F  787 458 231 130 114 110  67 61 52 35         220
B22-28F  973 756 344 312 241 151 145 56 40 38         256
B23-28F  418 395 192 165  80  42  41 37 36 34         238
B24-28F 1266 425 402 228 167 142 113 54 42 25         178
B25-28F 1111 334 315 102  59  53  43 35 22 19         133
```

Second, get a list of Dirichlet-multinomial parameters(i.e., loglik, gamma, pi and theta) for the data using the function DM.MoM().

```
> fit_Buty <- DM.MoM(Buty_t);fit_NOButy <- DM.MoM(NOButy_t)
```

```
> fit_Buty$pi
0.23155 0.20212 0.13796 0.07863 0.06215 0.04462 0.03393 0.02573
                Other
0.02066 0.01745 0.14520
```

```
> fit_NOButy$pi
0.36373 0.18909 0.11850 0.07482 0.05278 0.03977 0.03266 0.01940
                    Other
0.01533 0.01206 0.08185

> fit_Buty$theta
[1] 0.007523
> fit_NOButy$theta
[1] 0.01615
```

Third, set up the number of Monte-Carlo experiments, here we use 1000, the minimum value recommneted in practice and generate the number of reads per sample.

```
> numMC <- 1000
> #The first number is the number of reads and
> #the second is the number of subjects
> nrsGrp1 <- rep(1000, 10);nrsGrp2 <- rep(1000, 10)
> group_Nrs <- list(nrsGrp1, nrsGrp2)
```

Fourth, set up the values of the vector of taxa frequencies (taxa proportion) and overdispersion parameters for each group.

```
> pi0 <- fit_Buty$pi
> group_theta <- c(0.007523, 0.01615)
```

Fifth, compute size of the test statistics (Type I error).

```
> pval1 <- MC.Xmc.statistics
(group_Nrs, numMC, pi0, group.theta=group_theta, type="hnull")
> pval1
[1] 0.08492
```

Finally, compute power of the test statistics (Type II error).

```
> group_pi <- rbind(fit_Buty$pi, fit_NOButy$pi)
> pval2 <- MC.Xmc.statistics
(group_Nrs, numMC, pi0, group_pi, group_theta)
> pval2
[1] 0.999
```

Table 5.4 shows the power analysis results of rank abundance distributions (RAD) data analysis using the function MC.Xmc.statistics(). The RAD data analysis achieved a higher power to detect the effect size comparing to taxa composition data analysis. For example, with only 5 samples per group, 500 reads per sample,

Table 5.4 Power calculations (based on alpha = 0.05) using the Dirichlet-multinomial model to compare the ranked expected taxa frequencies from the Buty and the NoButy populations, using as a reference the taxa frequencies obtained from the 10 samples

	Reads				
Samples	500 (%)	1000 (%)	2000 (%)	5000 (%)	10,000 (%)
3	70.63	73.03	75.12	72.53	76.52
5	89.61	92.61	92.21	92.61	94.01
10	99.9	99.9	99.9	99.9	99.9

we can achieve 89.61% power. Actually, comparing to the taxa composition data analysis, the RAD data analysis approach decreases power because the information in the data is lost when the taxa labels are ignored (La Rosa et al. 2012). The higher power achieved in this case is because the RAD data analysis reduced the 196 taxa to 11 taxa including 1 "pooled less frequently abundant taxa".

Several Sample RAD-Probability Mean Test Comparison With Unknown Vector of Proportion

The function MC.Xmcupo.statistics() use simulation and the generalized Wald-type statistics to provide the power and size of the several sample RAD probability mean test comparisons without reference vector of proportions. Here, again we compare two sample sets of "Buty" and "NOButy".

One sample syntax is like this:

MC.Xmcupo.statistics(group.Nrs, numMC = 1000, pi0, group.pi, group.theta, type = "ha", siglev = 0.05)

where, group.Nrs, numMC, type, siglev, pi0, group.pi, and group.theta are defined as in the fnction MC.Xmc.statistics().

The function MC.Xmcupo.statistics() runs at the same way as the function MC.Xmc.statistics().

```
> ##Generate the number of reads per sample
> ##The first number is the number of reads and the second is the number of
Samples or subjects
> nrsGrp1 <- rep(1000, 10);nrsGrp2 <- rep(1000, 10)
> group_Nrs <- list(nrsGrp1, nrsGrp2)

> pi0 <- fit_Buty$pi
> group_theta <- c(0.007523, 0.01615)
> ##Computing size of the test statistics (Type I error)
> group_theta <- c(fit_Buty$theta, fit_NOButy$theta)
> pval1 <- MC.Xmcupo.statistics
(group_Nrs, numMC, pi0, group.theta=group_theta, type="hnull")
> pval1
[1] 0.004995
> ##Computing Power of the test statistics (Type II error)
```

Table 5.5 Power calculations (based on alpha = 0.05) using the Dirichlet-multinomial model to compare the ranked expected taxa frequencies from the Buty and the NoButy populations, without using a reference vector of proportions

Samples	Reads				
	500 (%)	1000 (%)	2000 (%)	5000 (%)	10,000 (%)
3	18.88	21.88	22.28	25.37	24.08
5	38.16	45.25	49.45	51.85	50.85
10	87.91	92.31	94.81	95.9	95.2

```
> group_pi <- rbind(fit_Buty$pi, fit_NOButy$pi)
> pval2 <- MC.Xmcupo.statistics(group_Nrs, numMC, group.pi=-
group_pi, group.theta=group_theta)
> pval2
[1] 0.9231
```

Table 5.5 shows the power analysis results of rank abundance distributions (RAD) data analysis using the function MC.Xmcupo.statistics(). The powers achieved by the function MC.Xmcupo.statistics () is smaller than those by the function MC.Xmc.statistics() due to without using a reference vector of proportions.

5.5.4   Effect Size Calculation Using HMP Package

HMP Package has the capability to calculate effect size. Here, we illustrate the effect size calculation, using the function Xmcupo.effectsize(), which computes the Cramer's Phi and Modified Cramer's Phi Criterion for the test statistic Xmcupo.sevsample(). The interested readers can reference the HMP package to conduct hypothesis testing, using the function Xmcupo.sevsample(). Here, we focus on the effect size calculation.

The syntax is:

Xmcupo.effectsize(group.data)

where, group.data is a list where each element is a matrix of taxonomic counts (columns) for each sample(rows).

```
> ##Combine the data sets into a single list
> group_data <- list(filter_Buty, filter_NOButy)
> effect <- Xmcupo.effectsize(group_data)
> effect
          Chi-Squared              Cramer Phi Modified-Cramer Phi
             20.97915                 0.02899              0.15208
              P value
              0.02124
```

The effect sizes observed in the RAD data analysis based on the test statistic Xmcupo.sevsample are 0.03 for Cramer Phi, 0.15 for Modified-Cramer Phi, respectively.

5.6 Summary

This chapter focused on power and sample size calculations for microbiome data. Both univariate and multivariate analysis approaches were introduced. For univariate analysis approach, we introduced and illustrated parametric and non-pararemetric tests and models; for multivariate analysis approach, the focus was on power and sample size calculations using the parametric Dirichlet-multinomial model. Both statistical theory and the associated R packages were introduced in each analysis.

We started with introducing the elements of hypothesis testing and power analysis, and forming hypothesis testing and power analysis with microbiome data. Second, we divided four sections to separately cover power and sample size analyses for testing differences in diversity using t-test; comparing diversity across more than two groups using ANOVA; comparing a taxon of interest across groups; and comparing the frequency of all taxa across groups using Dirichlet-multinomial model.

Microbiome power analysis is very important for study design of microbiome studies. The hypothesis testing methods and models are limited in literature, especially rare for appropriate multivariate models. Except those we illustrated in this chapter, we also found a few other metheds appeared in research papers (Kelly et al. 2015; Mattiello et al. 2016). We do not intend to further discuss them due to lack of detail documents or only available in web-based application.

References

Boyu, Ren, Sergio, Bacallado, et al. 2017. Bayesian nonparametric ordination for the analysis of microbial communities. arXiv:1601.05156 [stat.ME].

Cohen, J. 1988. *Statistical power analysis for the behavioral sciences*. Hillsdale, New Jersey: Lawrence Erlbaum Associates.

Costea, P.I., G. Zeller, et al. 2017. Towards standards for human fecal sample processing in metagenomic studies. *Nat Biotech*. Advance online publication.

Graham, J.W., P.E. Cumsille, et al. 2003. *Methods for handling missing data*. Handbook of Psychology, vol. 2, ed. J.A. Schinka and W.F. Velicer, 87–114. New York: Wiley.

Hart, M.M., A. Kristin, et al. 2015. Navigating the labyrinth: A guide to sequence-based, community ecology of arbuscular mycorrhizal fungi. *New Phytologist* 207 (1): 235–247.

Holmes I, Harris K, et al. 2012 Dirichlet multinomial mixtures: Generative models for microbial metagenomics. *PLoS One* 7: e30126.

Kelly, B.J., R. Gross, et al. 2015. Power and sample-size estimation for microbiome studies using pairwise distances and PERMANOVA. *Bioinformatics* 31 (15): 2461–2468.

Koehler, K.J., and J.R. Wilson. 1986. Chi-square tests for comparing vectors of proportions for several cluster samples. *Communications in Statistics—Theory and Methods* 15 (10): 2977–2990.

La Rosa, P.S., J.P. Brooks, et al. 2012. Hypothesis testing and power calculations for taxonomic-based human microbiome data. *PLoS ONE* 7 (12): e52078.

La Rosa, P.S., Y. Zhou, et al. 2015. Hypothesis testing of metagenomic data. In *Metagenomics for microbiology*, ed. J. Izard and M.C. Rivera, 81–96. Waltham, MA, USA: Academic Press.

Mattiello, F., B. Verbist, et al. 2016. A web application for sample size and power calculation in case-control microbiome studies. *Bioinformatics* 32 (13): 2038–2040.

Neal, S., Grantham, Brian J. Reich, et al. (2017). MIMIX: A Bayesian mixed-effects model for microbiome data from designed experiments. arXiv:1703.07747 [stat.ME].

Tvedebrink, T. 2010. Overdispersion in allelic counts and θ-correction in forensic genetics. *Theoretical Population Biology* 78 (3): 200–210.

Wu, G.D., J. Chen, et al. (2011). Linking long-term dietary patterns with gut microbial enterotypes. *Science* 334.

Zhang, Y.-G., S. Wu, et al. 2017. Target intestinal microbiota to alleviate disease progression in amyotrophic lateral sclerosis. *Clinical Therapeutics* 39 (2): 322–336.

Zhernakova, A., A. Kurilshikov, et al. 2016. Population-based metagenomics analysis reveals markers for gut microbiome composition and diversity. *Science* 352 (6285): 565–569.

Chapter 6
Community Diversity Measures and Calculations

In this chapter, we use a real microbiome data set to introduce community diversity measures and their calculations. We introduce $Vdr^{-/-}$ mice data set in Sect. 6.1. The concepts of alpha, beta and gamma diversities are covered in Sect. 6.2. In Sects. 6.3 and 6.4, we introduce some common used alpha and beta diversity measures and calculations, respectively. Section 6.5 is a brief summary of this chapter.

6.1 $Vdr^{-/-}$ Mice Data Set

Murine intestinal microbiome data (Jin et al. 2015) are generated from fecal and cecal stool of vitamin D receptor knockout ($Vdr^{-/-}$) and wild-type (WT) mice with 454 pyrosequencing. The whole data sets include 5 samples of $Vdr^{-/-}$ mice and 3 samples of WT mice from both fecal and cecal locations. The overall purpose of this study is to explore whether VDR status regulates the composition and functions of the intestinal bacterial community. The null hypothesis is that Vdr status and intestinal location is not associated with taxonomic alterations of the bacterial community in the gut. The post sequencing data have six levels of taxa, including phylum, class, family, order, genus, and species. For better differentiation from sample to sample, we analyze the intestinal microbiota at the genus level in this chapter.

6.2 Introduction to Community Diversities

Analyses of community diversities are widely used in community microbiome study. Throughout this book, we use the term diversity to mean richness, or the number of types, and various diversity indices. For clarity, we will often refer to species or genus as the measured unit of diversity, but our discussion can be applied

© Springer Nature Singapore Pte Ltd. 2018
Y. Xia et al., *Statistical Analysis of Microbiome Data with R*,
ICSA Book Series in Statistics, https://doi.org/10.1007/978-981-13-1534-3_6

to operational taxonomic units (OTUs) or any level of taxa. Most diversity methods assume that data are counts of individuals. Three levels of diversity (alpha diversity, beta diversity and gamma diversity) have become central to community ecology (Whittaker 1967, 1969). In microbiome study, alpha diversity and beta diversity are commonly used. In Chap. 7, the alpha and beta diversity measures will be explored with various plots and clustering and ordination techniques. Chapters 8 and 9 will focus on hypothesis testing of alpha diversity and beta diversity.

6.2.1   Alpha Diversity

Whittaker (1960) introduced and divided diversity into various components. The best known distinct components are alpha diversity and the beta diversity.

Alpha diversity as one of the basic diversity indices is defined as diversity in one spot or sample. It acts like a summary statistic of a single population (Morgan and Huttenhower 2012). Although several slightly different definitions of alpha diversity have been used, such as Whittaker himself used the term for both the species diversity in a single subunit and the mean species diversity in a collection of subunits (Whittaker 1960, 1972), alpha diversity is used for local diversity. In microbiome study, alpha diversity is referred to as diversity within a single sample or within a community.

6.2.2   Beta Diversity

One important purpose of microbiome study is to determine whether the microbiome communities can be classified together or need to be separated in their bacteria, to differentiate treatment from control, healthy from disease, genetic deficiency from wild type. The questions of community classification lead us to measure the *similarity* between two community samples (beta-diversity). The concept of "similarity" or beta-diversity and its measures mainly come from ecology and other fields.

Beta diversity was originally defined by Whittaker as a measure of change in diversity across environmental gradients; in other words, it is the rate of change in species composition from one community to another along gradients (Whittaker 1960). Hence, it reflects species replacement as one moves across space or time (Magurran 2004). Beta diversity is also known as 'species turnover'. In general, beta diversity evaluates differences between two or more local assemblages or between local and regional assemblages (Koleff et al. 2003; Lozupone and Knight 2008), thus allowing us to elucidate how much diversity is unique to a local assemblage, or describe how many taxa are shared between communities. The microbiome researchers adopted the concept and techniques from these studies.

6.2.3 Gamma Diversity

In ecological literature, there is another extreme diversity called gamma diversity, the diversity of a region or a landscape that contains several communities. In microbiome literature, gamma diversity is rarely used. Thus, in this book, we focus on alpha and beta diversities. However, simply describing the relationship among alpha, beta and gamma diversities may be helpful for understanding alpha and beta diversities. Practically, alpha diversity can be considered to be the diversity of the individual sample or observation, and gamma diversity to be the diversity of all sample combined, whereas beta diversity is a measure of how distinct the sampling units are along gradients.

6.3 Alpha Diversity Measures and Calculations

Alpha diversity is one of the essential concepts in ecology, biological and micro-biome community. The fundamental questions encountered by researchers are: how many species present? When you speak this way, you are describing the richness of community. How many species are truly there? When you talk this way, you are talking about diversity of community. And when you ask how even are each species relatively to each other? You want to know the evenness of community. Community diversity indices combine species richness and abundance into a single value of evenness. Communities that are numerically dominated by one or a few species exhibit low evenness while communities where abundance is distributed equally among species exhibit high evenness (Gotelli 2008). In microbiome literature, Chao 1 index (Chao 1984), which is qualitative species-based measures, Shannon (or Shannon-Wiener) index (Shannon 1948; Shannon and Weaver 1949) and Simpson's index (Simpson 1949), which are quantitative species-based measures, have been most widely applied. The Chao 1 index and number of taxa, Shannon-Wiener Diversity, Simpson Diversity, Pielou's Evenness indices will be introduced in Sects. 6.3.1, 6.3.2, 6.3.3 and 6.3.4, respectively. All these four indices are made into a dataframe and combined together in Sect. 6.3.5.

6.3.1 Chao 1 Richness Index and Number of Taxa

Species richness estimators estimate the total number of species present in a sample or community. This is the oldest and the simplest concept of species diversity. Two non-parametric estimators of species richness for presence/absence data were developed by Anne Chao and are called 'Chao 1' and 'Chao 2' in the literature

(Colwell and Coddington 1994). They are very similar in concept. Chao 1 index is based upon the number of rare classes (i.e., OTUs) found in a sample (Chao 1984). It is commonly used in ecology and microbiome studies. The formula is given as below:

$$S_{Chao1} = S_{obs} + \frac{n_1^2}{2n_2} \tag{6.1}$$

where S_{Chao1} is the estimated number of species, S_{obs} is the number of species observed in total, n_1 is the number of singleton taxa (taxa represented by a single read in that community), such as number of species represented only once in the samples (unique species), and n_2 is the number of doubleton taxa, such as number of species represented only twice in the samples. Chao (1984) noted that this index is particularly useful for data sets skewed toward the low-abundance classes, as is likely to be the case with microbiome data. However, from above formula, we can see if the number of singleton taxa n_1 is larger, that is, a sample contains many singletons; in such case, it is likely that more undetected OTUs exist, and then the Chao 1 index will estimate greater species richness than it would for a sample without rare OTUs.

Further to above Chao 1 measure in (6.1), Chao also derived a closed-form solution for the variance of S_{Chao1} (Chao 1987):

$$Var(S_{Chao1}) = n_2 \left(\frac{m^4}{4} + m^3 + \frac{m^2}{2} \right), \tag{6.2}$$

where $m = \frac{n_1}{n_2}$. This formula estimates the precision of Chao1 from multiple samples.

The alpha diversity is calculated based on raw abundance data. The data structure should be rows for samples and columns for taxa (such as, genera, species). Alpha diversity can be calculated by several R packages. Here, we will use the ecological R package called vegan (for "vegetation analysis") to estimate the four most often used alpha indices in the microbiome literature: number of taxa, Chao1 richness, Shannon evenness and Simpson index using the $Vdr^{-/-}$ mice data set.

First, let us read the genus count abundance data into R and load vegan package.

```
> options(width=65,digits=4)
> abund_table=read.csv("VdrGenusCounts.csv",row.names=1,
check.names=FALSE)
> library(vegan)
```

The following print of few lines shows that the data structure is taxa (in these case, genera) by sample format.

```
> head(abund_table)
                          5_15_dryst-28F 20_12_Cest-28F
Tannerella                           476             67
Lactococcus                          326            737
Lactobacillus                         94            597
Lactobacillus::Lactococcus             1             12
Parasutterella                         1              0
Helicobacter                          89              0
```

The data table needs to be transformed into samples by taxa (genera) before calculating various diversities.

```
> abund_table<-t(abund_table)
> head(abund_table)
                Tannerella Lactococcus Lactobacillus
5_15_dryst-28F         476         326            94
20_12_Cest-28F          67         737           597
1_11_dryst-28F         549        2297           434
2_12_dryst-28F         578         548           719
3_13_dryst-28F         996        2378           322
4_14_dryst-28F         404         471           205
...
```

The extremely simple function specnumber can be used to find the number of species or any taxa. Here the function specnumber() is used to calculate the number of genera.

```
> num_genera <- specnumber(abund_table)
> num_genera
 5_15_dryst-28F 20_12_Cest-28F  1_11_dryst-28F  2_12_dryst-28F
             52             52              65              76
 3_13_dryst-28F  4_14_dryst-28F  7_22_dryst-28F  8_23_dryst-28F
             60             44              40              59
 9_24_dryst-28F 19_11_Cest-28F 21_13_Cest-28F 22_14_Cest-28F
             52             37              42              46
23_15_Cest-28F 25_22_Cest-28F 26_23_Cest-28F 27_24_Cest-28F
             54             48              70              68
```

Adding up the number of taxa (genera in this case) present in the samples is the simplest way to estimate diversity. However, this method ignores the identity of the taxa (genera in this case) and their abundances, two very different communities might be identical. For example, the following two communities are the same based on the number of taxa counted or taxon richness (both have 5 taxa), but obviously they are different communities.

Taxon	Community I	Community II
A	10	5
B	1	5
C	1	5
D	1	5
E	1	5

We can also estimate the number of genera and Chao1 index in our $Vdr^{-/-}$ mice data set using estimateR() function. We will get the observed number of genera in each sample, and the estimated number of Chao1 estimator. Please note that Chao1 index can be only calculated on integer counts. Thus, in case of only relative abundances available, we need to transform all counts to integers. In $Vdr^{-/-}$ mice data set, the read already has integer counts, so we do not need transform here.

```
> index=estimateR(abund_table)
> index
            5_15_dryst-28F 20_12_Cest-28F 1_11_dryst-28F
S.obs               52.000         52.000         65.000
S.chao1             94.750         59.800         77.000
se.chao1            28.108          5.793          7.959
S.ACE               77.282         63.759         78.082
se.ACE               4.682          4.145          4.232
            2_12_dryst-28F 3_13_dryst-28F 4_14_dryst-28F
S.obs               76.000         60.000         44.000
S.chao1            103.273         85.667         55.143
se.chao1            14.582         14.700          8.227
S.ACE              107.093         93.093         56.428
se.ACE               5.545          5.889          3.637
            7_22_dryst-28F 8_23_dryst-28F 9_24_dryst-28F
S.obs               40.000         59.000         52.000
S.chao1             62.750         67.667         80.500
se.chao1            16.685          6.413         17.929
S.ACE               61.256         73.286         77.312
se.ACE               4.617          4.400          4.553
            19_11_Cest-28F 21_13_Cest-28F 22_14_Cest-28F
S.obs               37.000         42.000         46.000
S.chao1             52.167         55.000         59.000
se.chao1            10.850          9.628          9.629
S.ACE               53.477         52.857         57.695
se.ACE               3.641          3.438          3.812
            23_15_Cest-28F 25_22_Cest-28F 26_23_Cest-28F
S.obs               54.000         48.000         70.000
S.chao1             60.875         51.000        112.857
se.chao1             5.564          2.863         23.947
S.ACE               64.287         54.193        104.126
se.ACE               4.090          3.448          5.506
            27_24_Cest-28F
S.obs               68.000
S.chao1             78.059
se.chao1             6.176
S.ACE               93.628
se.ACE               5.435
```

From the above matrix, we can see that function estimate R generates 5 indices, in which chao1 is listed as second row. Thus we can extract Chao 1 index using the following R codes:

```
> chao1_genus=estimateR(abund_table)[2,]
> chao1_genus
5_15_dryst-28F 20_12_Cest-28F 1_11_dryst-28F 2_12_dryst-28F
         94.75          59.80          77.00         103.27
3_13_dryst-28F 4_14_dryst-28F 7_22_dryst-28F 8_23_dryst-28F
         85.67          55.14          62.75          67.67
9_24_dryst-28F 19_11_Cest-28F 21_13_Cest-28F 22_14_Cest-28F
         80.50          52.17          55.00          59.00
23_15_Cest-28F 25_22_Cest-28F 26_23_Cest-28F 27_24_Cest-28F
         60.88          51.00         112.86          78.06
```

6.3.2 Shannon-Wiener Diversity Index

One of the most popular measures of species diversity is Shannon-Wiener diversity index, labeled as H'. It considers the differences in proportion or abundance of each species. This index is based on information theory, measures the uncertainty: How difficult would it be to predict correctly the species of the next individual collected? The formula of Shannon index is:

$$H' = -\sum_{i=1}^{S} p_i \ln p_i, \tag{6.3}$$

where p_i is the proportion of individuals (or relative abundance) of species i in the community and S is the total number of species present so that $\sum_{i=1}^{S} p_i = 1$. Information theory is to measure the amount of uncertainty, so that the larger the value of H', the greater the uncertainty. The Shannon-Wiener measure H' increases with the number of species in the community and in theory can reach very large values. In practice for biological communities H' does not seem to exceed 5.0 (Washington 1984). Shannon's index "gives more importance" to less common categories (for example, rare species, in microbiome studies). Strictly speaking, the Shannon-Wiener measure of information content should be used only on random samples drawn from a large community in which the total number of species is known (Pielou 1966).

We can use the diversity function in the vegan package to calculate Shannon-Wiener diversity. Alternatively, we can use plain R codes based on above formula. Here we show both approaches. First, let's use the diversity() function, the R codes are listed as below.

```
> shannon_genus <- diversity(abund_table,index="shannon",MARGIN=1)
> shannon_genus
5_15_drySt-28F 20_12_CeSt-28F 1_11_drySt-28F 2_12_drySt-28F
         2.461          2.340          2.228          2.734
3_13_drySt-28F 4_14_drySt-28F 7_22_drySt-28F 8_23_drySt-28F
         2.077          2.467          1.777          2.000
9_24_drySt-28F 19_11_CeSt-28F 21_13_CeSt-28F 22_14_CeSt-28F
         1.972          1.345          2.016          1.955
23_15_CeSt-28F 25_22_CeSt-28F 26_23_CeSt-28F 27_24_CeSt-28F
         1.614          1.959          2.271          2.002
```

The default index of diversity function is Shannon index, so the index="shannon" can be omitted.

```
> shannon_genus <- diversity(abund_table,MARGIN=1)
> shannon_genus
5_15_drySt-28F 20_12_CeSt-28F 1_11_drySt-28F 2_12_drySt-28F
         2.461          2.340          2.228          2.734
3_13_drySt-28F 4_14_drySt-28F 7_22_drySt-28F 8_23_drySt-28F
         2.077          2.467          1.777          2.000
9_24_drySt-28F 19_11_CeSt-28F 21_13_CeSt-28F 22_14_CeSt-28F
         1.972          1.345          2.016          1.955
23_15_CeSt-28F 25_22_CeSt-28F 26_23_CeSt-28F 27_24_CeSt-28F
         1.614          1.959          2.271          2.002
```

Since the Shannon index calculation is relative to rows. The argument MARGIN=1 can be omitted also.

```
> shannon_genus <- diversity(abund_table)
> shannon_genus
5_15_drySt-28F 20_12_CeSt-28F 1_11_drySt-28F 2_12_drySt-28F
         2.461          2.340          2.228          2.734
3_13_drySt-28F 4_14_drySt-28F 7_22_drySt-28F 8_23_drySt-28F
         2.077          2.467          1.777          2.000
9_24_drySt-28F 19_11_CeSt-28F 21_13_CeSt-28F 22_14_CeSt-28F
         1.972          1.345          2.016          1.955
23_15_CeSt-28F 25_22_CeSt-28F 26_23_CeSt-28F 27_24_CeSt-28F
         1.614          1.959          2.271          2.002
```

Now we will illustrate the calculation by plan R codes using the formula of Shannon-Wiener diversity Index. Since in above formula p_i is the proportion of individuals (or relative abundance) of species i in the community, we use decostand () function in vegan package to convert count data in each sample into proportions.

```
> # use decostand to convert data into proportions
> abund_table_total<-decostand(abund_table, MARGIN=1, method="total")
```

The augments of MARGIN = 1 mean "rows", MARGIN = 2 mean "columns" of the matrix-like object data (in this case, abund_table); method = "total" means to divide by margin total (MARGIN = 1 is also the default). By applying function decostand, we obtained the proportion of individuals in the samples that belong to each gene. We then can use Shannon-Wiener index formula to calculate the index as below.

```
> # multiply that matrix X a natural log transformed matrix - p*ln(p)
> abund_table_p_lnp<-abund_table_total*log(abund_table_total)
> # sum values by sample and multiply by -1
> rowSums(abund_table_p_lnp,na.rm=TRUE)*-1
5_15_drySt-28F 20_12_CeSt-28F 1_11_drySt-28F 2_12_drySt-28F
         2.461          2.340          2.228          2.734
3_13_drySt-28F 4_14_drySt-28F 7_22_drySt-28F 8_23_drySt-28F
         2.077          2.467          1.777          2.000
9_24_drySt-28F 19_11_CeSt-28F 21_13_CeSt-28F 22_14_CeSt-28F
         1.972          1.345          2.016          1.955
23_15_CeSt-28F 25_22_CeSt-28F 26_23_CeSt-28F 27_24_CeSt-28F
         1.614          1.959          2.271          2.002
```

We can see that these two approaches obtain the same results.

6.3.3   Simpson Diversity Index

Simpson in 1949 (Simpson 1949) proposed a new concept of diversity which combines two separate ideas, species richness and evenness. The new non-parametric measure of diversity states that diversity is inversely related to the probability that two individuals picked at random belong to the same species. Actually, the new defined concept of diversity is about species heterogeneity (Good 1953) although in ecological literature this concept is synonymous with diversity (Hurlbert 1971). For an infinite population the formula of Simpson index is given by:

$$D = 1 - \sum_{i=1}^{S} p_i^2 \qquad (6.4)$$

where p_i is the proportion of individuals (or relative abundance) of species i in the community. Simpson's index ranges from 0 (low diversity) to almost 1. In contrary to the Shannon's index, Simpson's diversity index "gives more importance" to more common species.

Since heterogeneity contains both species richness and evenness, it was natural for researchers to try to separately measure the evenness component from richness. The null hypothesis of evenness is all species in a hypothetical community are equally common. However, most communities contain a few dominant species and many species that are relatively uncommon. Evenness measures attempt to quantify this unequal representation against the null hypothesis. As the independent measures of species richness, many different measures of evenness (or equitability) have been proposed in the literature. In microbiome literature, two evenness measures have been used.

The definition of Simpson's index of evenness is obtained from reciprocal of Simpson's index. The Simpson's original index is given by:

$$D_O = \sum_{i=1}^{S} p_i^2 \qquad (6.5)$$

The inverse Simpson index is given by:

$D_I = \frac{1}{\sum_{i=1}^{S} p_i^2}$, which is the reciprocal of Simpson's original index ($1/D_O$), where p_i is the proportion of species i in the community. Simpson's index of evenness is defined as

$$E = \frac{1}{S \sum_{i=1}^{S} p_i^2}, \qquad (6.6)$$

where S is the number of species in the sample. This index ranges from 0 to 1 and is relatively unaffected by the rare species in the sample.

We can use either diversity() function in the vegan package or plain R function to calculate Simpson's index. The following R codes use the diversity() function.

```
> simp_genus <- diversity(abund_table, "simpson")
> simp_genus
5_15_drySt-28F 20_12_CeSt-28F 1_11_drySt-28F 2_12_drySt-28F
        0.8645          0.8649          0.8125          0.9097
3_13_drySt-28F 4_14_drySt-28F 7_22_drySt-28F 8_23_drySt-28F
        0.7916          0.8859          0.7423          0.7890
9_24_drySt-28F 19_11_CeSt-28F 21_13_CeSt-28F 22_14_CeSt-28F
        0.7695          0.5717          0.8139          0.8020
23_15_CeSt-28F 25_22_CeSt-28F 26_23_CeSt-28F 27_24_CeSt-28F
        0.6687          0.7649          0.8546          0.7845
```

The following R codes use Simpson index formula to calculate the index. The count data need to be converted into proportions before using this formual.

```
> ##using plain R functions
> #use decostand to convert data into proportions
> abund_table_total<-decostand(abund_table, MARGIN=1, method="total")
> # square the proportions
> abund_table_total_p2<-abund_table_total^2
> # get the row sums
> 1-rowSums(abund_table_total_p2, na.rm=TRUE)
5_15_drySt-28F 20_12_CeSt-28F 1_11_drySt-28F 2_12_drySt-28F
        0.8645          0.8649          0.8125          0.9097
3_13_drySt-28F 4_14_drySt-28F 7_22_drySt-28F 8_23_drySt-28F
        0.7916          0.8859          0.7423          0.7890
9_24_drySt-28F 19_11_CeSt-28F 21_13_CeSt-28F 22_14_CeSt-28F
        0.7695          0.5717          0.8139          0.8020
23_15_CeSt-28F 25_22_CeSt-28F 26_23_CeSt-28F 27_24_CeSt-28F
        0.6687          0.7649          0.8546          0.7845
```

The inverse Simpson index can be calculated by specifying the method "invsimpson" or "inv" as below. The interested readers can easily obtain the Simpson's index of evenness using above formula in (6.6).

```
> inv_simp <- diversity(abund_table, "invsimpson")
> inv_simp
5_15_drySt-28F 20_12_CeSt-28F 1_11_drySt-28F 2_12_drySt-28F
         7.379           7.401           5.335          11.069
3_13_drySt-28F 4_14_drySt-28F 7_22_drySt-28F 8_23_drySt-28F
         4.797           8.765           3.881           4.739
9_24_drySt-28F 19_11_CeSt-28F 21_13_CeSt-28F 22_14_CeSt-28F
         4.338           2.335           5.373           5.051
23_15_CeSt-28F 25_22_CeSt-28F 26_23_CeSt-28F 27_24_CeSt-28F
         3.019           4.254           6.877           4.640
```

6.3.4   Pielou's Evenness Index

The most common evenness is Pielou's evenness:

$$J = \frac{H'}{\log(S)},\tag{6.7}$$

where H' is Shannon-Weiner diversity and S is the total number of species observed in a sample.

Many diversity indices, such as Simpson's diversity, Shannon-Weiner diversity incorporate evenness. However, it has been shown that the diversity indices which concentrate totally on evenness are fraught with problems, including dependence on species counts (McCune and Grace 2002). A particular problem with Pielou's index is that it is a ratio of a relatively stable index, H', and one that is strongly dependent on sample size, S.

Pielou index can be calculated using specnumber() and diversity() functions based on its formula we introduced above as below.

```
> ##using specnumber and diversity functions
> S <- specnumber(abund_table)
> H<-diversity(abund_table, "shannon")
> J <- H/log(S)
> J
5_15_dryST-28F 20_12_CeST-28F 1_11_dryST-28F 2_12_dryST-28F
        0.6228         0.5921         0.5337         0.6314
3_13_dryST-28F 4_14_dryST-28F 7_22_dryST-28F 8_23_dryST-28F
        0.5074         0.6519         0.4818         0.4904
9_24_dryST-28F 19_11_CeST-28F 21_13_CeST-28F 22_14_CeST-28F
        0.4991         0.3724         0.5394         0.5107
23_15_CeST-28F 25_22_CeST-28F 26_23_CeST-28F 27_24_CeST-28F
        0.4047         0.5060         0.5345         0.4745
```

Besides the above indices, within a community, several other estimators including the Abundance-based Coverage Estimator (ACE) (Chao and Lee 1992; Chao et al. 1993), and Jackknife (Heltshe and Forrester 1983) measures can be found for calculating alpha diversity of taxa expected within a single population. However, we do not discuss them in details and the interested readers can explore them in the ecological and microbiome literatures.

6.3.5 Make a Dataframe of Diversity Indices

We can make a dataframe for number of genera using the following R codes.

```
> #make a dataframe of number of genera
> N <- specnumber(abund_table)
> df_N <-data.frame(sample=names(N),value=N,measure=rep("Number",
length(N)))
```

The following R codes are used to make a dataframe for Chao 1 index.

```
> #make a dataframe of Chao1 richness
> CH=estimateR(abund_table)[2,]
> df_CH <-data.frame(sample=names(CH),value=CH,measure=rep("Chao1",
length(CH)))
```

The following R codes are used to make a dataframe for Shannon index.

```
> #make a dataframe of Shannon evenness
> H<-diversity(abund_table, "shannon")
> df_H<-data.frame(sample=names(H),value=H,measure=rep("Shannon",
length(H)))
```

The following R codes are used to make a dataframe for Simpson index.

```
> #make a dataframe of Simpson index
> df_simp<-data.frame(sample=names(simp_genus),value=simp_genus,
measure=rep("Simpson",length(simp_genus)))
```

The following R codes are used to make a dataframe for Pielou index.

```
> #make a dataframe of Pielou index
> df_J<-data.frame(sample=names(J),value=J,measure=rep("Pielou",
length(J)))
```

We can combine all the dataframes together for future use.

```
> df<-rbind(df_N,df_CH,df_H,df_simp,df_J)
> rownames(df)<-NULL
> df
            sample      value measure
1   5_15_dryst-28F    52.0000  Number
2  20_12_CeSt-28F     52.0000  Number
3   1_11_dryst-28F    65.0000  Number
4   2_12_dryst-28F    76.0000  Number
5   3_13_dryst-28F    60.0000  Number
6   4_14_dryst-28F    44.0000  Number
7   7_22_dryst-28F    40.0000  Number
8   8_23_dryst-28F    59.0000  Number
9   9_24_dryst-28F    52.0000  Number
10 19_11_CeSt-28F     37.0000  Number
11 21_13_CeSt-28F     42.0000  Number
12 22_14_CeSt-28F     46.0000  Number
13 23_15_CeSt-28F     54.0000  Number
14 25_22_CeSt-28F     48.0000  Number
15 26_23_CeSt-28F     70.0000  Number
16 27_24_CeSt-28F     68.0000  Number
17  5_15_dryst-28F    94.7500  Chao1
18 20_12_CeSt-28F     59.8000  Chao1
19  1_11_dryst-28F    77.0000  Chao1
20  2_12_dryst-28F   103.2727  Chao1
21  3_13_dryst-28F    85.6667  Chao1
22  4_14_dryst-28F    55.1429  Chao1
23  7_22_dryst-28F    62.7500  Chao1
24  8_23_dryst-28F    67.6667  Chao1
25  9_24_dryst-28F    80.5000  Chao1
26 19_11_CeSt-28F     52.1667  Chao1
27 21_13_CeSt-28F     55.0000  Chao1
28 22_14_CeSt-28F     59.0000  Chao1
29 23_15_CeSt-28F     60.8750  Chao1
30 25_22_CeSt-28F     51.0000  Chao1
31 26_23_CeSt-28F    112.8571  Chao1
32 27_24_CeSt-28F     78.0588  Chao1
33  5_15_dryst-28F     2.4607  Shannon
34 20_12_CeSt-28F      2.3397  Shannon
35  1_11_dryst-28F     2.2280  Shannon
36  2_12_dryst-28F     2.7344  Shannon
37  3_13_dryst-28F     2.0773  Shannon
38  4_14_dryst-28F     2.4668  Shannon
39  7_22_dryst-28F     1.7772  Shannon
40  8_23_dryst-28F     1.9996  Shannon
41  9_24_dryst-28F     1.9720  Shannon
42 19_11_CeSt-28F      1.3448  Shannon
43 21_13_CeSt-28F      2.0161  Shannon
44 22_14_CeSt-28F      1.9554  Shannon
45 23_15_CeSt-28F      1.6145  Shannon
46 25_22_CeSt-28F      1.9588  Shannon
47 26_23_CeSt-28F      2.2708  Shannon
48 27_24_CeSt-28F      2.0022  Shannon
49  5_15_dryst-28F     0.8645  Simpson
50 20_12_CeSt-28F      0.8649  Simpson
51  1_11_dryst-28F     0.8125  Simpson
52  2_12_dryst-28F     0.9097  Simpson
53  3_13_dryst-28F     0.7916  Simpson
54  4_14_dryst-28F     0.8859  Simpson
55  7_22_dryst-28F     0.7423  Simpson
56  8_23_dryst-28F     0.7890  Simpson
57  9_24_dryst-28F     0.7695  Simpson
58 19_11_CeSt-28F      0.5717  Simpson
59 21_13_CeSt-28F      0.8139  Simpson
60 22_14_CeSt-28F      0.8020  Simpson
61 23_15_CeSt-28F      0.6687  Simpson
62 25_22_CeSt-28F      0.7649  Simpson
63 26_23_CeSt-28F      0.8546  Simpson
```

```
64 27_24_CeSt-28F    0.7845 Simpson
65 5_15_dryСt-28F    0.6228 Pielou
66 20_12_CeSt-28F    0.5921 Pielou
67 1_11_dryСt-28F    0.5337 Pielou
68 2_12_dryСt-28F    0.6314 Pielou
69 3_13_dryСt-28F    0.5074 Pielou
70 4_14_dryСt-28F    0.6519 Pielou
71 7_22_dryСt-28F    0.4818 Pielou
72 8_23_dryСt-28F    0.4904 Pielou
73 9_24_dryСt-28F    0.4991 Pielou
74 19_11_CeSt-28F    0.3724 Pielou
75 21_13_CeSt-28F    0.5394 Pielou
76 22_14_CeSt-28F    0.5107 Pielou
77 23_15_CeSt-28F    0.4047 Pielou
78 25_22_CeSt-28F    0.5060 Pielou
79 26_23_CeSt-28F    0.5345 Pielou
80 27_24_CeSt-28F    0.4745 Pielou
```

6.4   Beta Diversity Measures and Calculations

Ecologists have proposed a number of beta diversity indices (Whittaker 1969; Wilson and Mohler 1983; Oksanen and Tonteri 1995). In the literature of animal and plant ecology, there are more than two dozen measures of similarity available (Koleff et al. 2003). All commonly used indices can be found using betadiver() function in the BiodiversityR package. We can check the definitions of beta diversities through the BiodiversityR package. First, we load "BiodiversityR":

```
> library(BiodiversityR)
```

Then call function betadiver() to obtain the following 24 definitions of beta diversities.

```
> betadiver(help=TRUE)
1 "w" = (b+c)/(2*a+b+c)
2 "-1" = (b+c)/(2*a+b+c)
3 "c" = (b+c)/2
4 "wb" = b+c
5 "r" = 2*b*c/((a+b+c)^2-2*b*c)
6 "I" = log(2*a+b+c) - 2*a*log(2)/(2*a+b+c) -
((a+b)*log(a+b) + (a+c)*log(a+c)) / (2*a+b+c)
7 "e" = exp(log(2*a+b+c) - 2*a*log(2)/(2*a+b+c) -
((a+b)*log(a+b) + (a+c)*log(a+c)) / (2*a+b+c))-1
8 "t" = (b+c)/(2*a+b+c)
9 "me" = (b+c)/(2*a+b+c)
```

```
10 "j" = a/(a+b+c)
11 "sor" = 2*a/(2*a+b+c)
12 "m" = (2*a+b+c)*(b+c)/(a+b+c)
13 "-2" = pmin(b,c)/(pmax(b,c)+a)
14 "co" = (a*c+a*b+2*b*c)/(2*(a+b)*(a+c))
15 "cc" = (b+c)/(a+b+c)
16 "g" = (b+c)/(a+b+c)
17 "-3" = pmin(b,c)/(a+b+c)
18 "l" = (b+c)/2
19 "19" = 2*(b*c+1)/(a+b+c)/(a+b+c-1)
20 "hk" = (b+c)/(2*a+b+c)
21 "rlb" = a/(a+c)
22 "sim" = pmin(b,c)/(pmin(b,c)+a)
23 "gl" = 2*abs(b-c)/(2*a+b+c)
24 "z" = (log(2)-log(2*a+b+c)+log(a+b+c))/log(2)
```

The beta diversity indices are grouped into two broad classes of similarity measures: *binary* similarity coefficients and *quantitative* similarity coefficients. When only measure of presence/absence data are available for the species in a community, then the *binary* similarity coefficients are used; whereas when some measures of relative abundance also be available for each species, the *quantitative* similarity coefficients will be applied.

The methods of estimating alpha is fairly straightforward, but the measurement of beta diversity has been controversial (Ellison 2010). Some beta diversity measures are designed solely to determine whether communities are significantly different, others are measures of distance between pairs of communities that satisfy the requirements of a distance metric. For example, the widely used are the Jaccard and Bray-Curtis coefficients for measuring the distance between communities based on the species that they contain (Lozupone and Knight 2008). The key point to selection of the proper measure of beta diversity is based on microbiome hypothesis testing and the methods that must be tailored to the hypothesis, rather than vice versa.

Beta diversity is calculated by using a similarity or dissimilarity (distance) measure to represent the relationships of samples. In this chapter, we are going to calculate three matrices: Bray-Curtis dissimilarity measure, Jaccard index and

Sørensen index of dissimilarity. Of which, the first two are particularly widely applied matrices in ecology and microbiome studies. Beta diversities can be estimated by using vegan, BiodiversityR, or other packages.

6.4.1   Binary Similarity Coefficients: Jaccard and Sørensen Indices

The coefficients (or association) of presence-absence binary data can be calculated using a 2 × 2 contingency table.

		Sample A	
		No. of species present	No. of species absent
Sample B	No. of species present	a	b
	No. of species absent	c	d

where
a—Number of species in sample A and sample B (joint occurrences)
b—Number of species in sample B but not in sample A
c—Number of species in sample A but not in sample B
d—Number of species absent in both samples (zero-zero matches).

There are more than 20 binary similarity measures now in the literature. The most often used similarity coefficients for binary data are Jaccard and Sørensen's indices. The Jaccard's Index is given below:

$$S_j = \frac{a}{a+b+c} \tag{6.8}$$

where

S_j Jaccard's similarity coefficient as defined in above presence-absence matrix
a Number of species in sample A and sample B (joint occurrences)
b Number of species in sample B but not in sample A
c Number of species in sample A but not in sample B.

Jaccard's dissimilarity coefficient $1 - S_j$ is modified from this similarity. Jaccard's dissimilarity measure can be calculated using the vegdist function() in vegan package as below.

```
> jaccard<-vegdist(abund_table, "jaccard")
> jaccard
```

	5_15_dryST-28F	20_12_CeST-28F	1_11_dryST-28F
20_12_CeST-28F	0.8039		
1_11_dryST-28F	0.7400	0.6718	
2_12_dryST-28F	0.6922	0.5042	0.5446
3_13_dryST-28F	0.7331	0.7132	0.3389
4_14_dryST-28F	0.4332	0.6329	0.6574
7_22_dryST-28F	0.6446	0.5992	0.6849
8_23_dryST-28F	0.7869	0.7471	0.5800
9_24_dryST-28F	0.7487	0.6143	0.4521
19_11_CeST-28F	0.8928	0.6920	0.8269
21_13_CeST-28F	0.8538	0.5078	0.8173
22_14_CeST-28F	0.8452	0.5406	0.7148
23_15_CeST-28F	0.9191	0.7695	0.6632
25_22_CeST-28F	0.7788	0.4398	0.7354
26_23_CeST-28F	0.8887	0.6313	0.6920
27_24_CeST-28F	0.8382	0.6362	0.5679

	2_12_dryST-28F	3_13_dryST-28F	4_14_dryST-28F
20_12_CeST-28F			
1_11_dryST-28F			
2_12_dryST-28F			
3_13_dryST-28F	0.6542		
4_14_dryST-28F	0.5829	0.6344	
7_22_dryST-28F	0.6626	0.7043	0.5887
8_23_dryST-28F	0.6771	0.5933	0.7670
9_24_dryST-28F	0.6080	0.3821	0.6850
19_11_CeST-28F	0.7607	0.8507	0.7886
21_13_CeST-28F	0.6660	0.8293	0.7172
22_14_CeST-28F	0.5680	0.7760	0.6855
23_15_CeST-28F	0.7650	0.6908	0.8714
25_22_CeST-28F	0.6664	0.7795	0.6645
26_23_CeST-28F	0.6264	0.7623	0.8249
27_24_CeST-28F	0.6370	0.6436	0.7723

	7_22_dryST-28F	8_23_dryST-28F	9_24_dryST-28F
20_12_CeST-28F			
1_11_dryST-28F			
2_12_dryST-28F			
3_13_dryST-28F			
4_14_dryST-28F			
7_22_dryST-28F			
8_23_dryST-28F	0.6976		
9_24_dryST-28F	0.6071	0.4739	
19_11_CeST-28F	0.8658	0.9062	0.8651
21_13_CeST-28F	0.7476	0.8625	0.7909
22_14_CeST-28F	0.7045	0.8215	0.7451
23_15_CeST-28F	0.8234	0.6406	0.5969
25_22_CeST-28F	0.4669	0.7841	0.7051
26_23_CeST-28F	0.7542	0.5303	0.6093
27_24_CeST-28F	0.7456	0.6846	0.5728

	19_11_CeSt-28F	21_13_CeSt-28F	22_14_CeSt-28F
20_12_CeSt-28F			
1_11_drySt-28F			
2_12_drySt-28F			
3_13_drySt-28F			
4_14_drySt-28F			
7_22_drySt-28F			
8_23_drySt-28F			
9_24_drySt-28F			
19_11_CeSt-28F			
21_13_CeSt-28F	0.6707		
22_14_CeSt-28F	0.7354	0.5814	
23_15_CeSt-28F	0.8863	0.8704	0.7662
25_22_CeSt-28F	0.7855	0.6228	0.5749
26_23_CeSt-28F	0.8346	0.7917	0.6969
27_24_CeSt-28F	0.5743	0.7752	0.7249

	23_15_CeSt-28F	25_22_CeSt-28F	26_23_CeSt-28F
20_12_CeSt-28F			
1_11_drySt-28F			
2_12_drySt-28F			
3_13_drySt-28F			
4_14_drySt-28F			
7_22_drySt-28F			
8_23_drySt-28F			
9_24_drySt-28F			
19_11_CeSt-28F			
21_13_CeSt-28F			
22_14_CeSt-28F			
23_15_CeSt-28F			
25_22_CeSt-28F	0.7921		
26_23_CeSt-28F	0.6223	0.7188	
27_24_CeSt-28F	0.6779	0.7430	0.6331

Sørensen's index (1948) is very similar to the Jaccard measure, which is given below:

$$S_S = \frac{2a}{2a+b+c} \tag{6.9}$$

where S_S = Sørensen's similarity coefficient.

This index can also be modified to a coefficient of *dissimilarity:* $1 - S_S$. The Sørensen and Jaccard coefficients are thought as very closely correlated (Baselga and Orme 2012). The range of all similarity coefficients for binary data is supposed to be 0 (no similarity) to 1 (complete similarity). In fact, this is not true for all coefficients. The Sørensen index of dissimilarity can be calculated for all samples using vegan function vegdist() with binary data:

```
> Sørensen<-vegdist(abund_table,binary=TRUE)
> Sørensen
```

	5_15_dryST-28F	20_12_CeSt-28F	1_11_drySt-28F
20_12_CeSt-28F	0.4808		
1_11_dryST-28F	0.4188	0.4017	
2_12_dryST-28F	0.4219	0.3750	0.2908
3_13_dryST-28F	0.3393	0.3750	0.3120
4_14_dryST-28F	0.3542	0.4583	0.3394
7_22_dryST-28F	0.4130	0.5435	0.4095
8_23_dryST-28F	0.3514	0.3874	0.2742
9_24_dryST-28F	0.3269	0.4423	0.3333
19_11_CeSt-28F	0.5506	0.3933	0.5098
21_13_CeSt-28F	0.5106	0.4043	0.4766
22_14_CeSt-28F	0.4898	0.3878	0.5135
23_15_CeSt-28F	0.3774	0.4528	0.5126
25_22_CeSt-28F	0.4600	0.3400	0.4690
26_23_CeSt-28F	0.4918	0.4098	0.4222
27_24_CeSt-28F	0.4333	0.4167	0.4286

	2_12_dryST-28F	3_13_dryST-28F	4_14_dryST-28F
20_12_CeSt-28F			
1_11_dryST-28F			
2_12_dryST-28F			
3_13_dryST-28F	0.3382		
4_14_dryST-28F	0.3667	0.3077	
7_22_dryST-28F	0.5000	0.3800	0.3810
8_23_dryST-28F	0.3185	0.3445	0.3592
9_24_dryST-28F	0.3438	0.3036	0.3125
19_11_CeSt-28F	0.5044	0.5464	0.6049
21_13_CeSt-28F	0.4576	0.4510	0.4651
22_14_CeSt-28F	0.4590	0.4906	0.4444
23_15_CeSt-28F	0.4923	0.4737	0.4898
25_22_CeSt-28F	0.5000	0.5000	0.5217
26_23_CeSt-28F	0.4384	0.4769	0.5263
27_24_CeSt-28F	0.3889	0.4219	0.4821

	7_22_dryST-28F	8_23_dryST-28F	9_24_dryST-28F
20_12_CeSt-28F			
1_11_dryST-28F			
2_12_dryST-28F			
3_13_dryST-28F			
4_14_dryST-28F			
7_22_dryST-28F			
8_23_dryST-28F	0.3939		
9_24_dryST-28F	0.4130	0.2973	
19_11_CeSt-28F	0.5844	0.4583	0.5056
21_13_CeSt-28F	0.5122	0.4455	0.4468
22_14_CeSt-28F	0.4419	0.5048	0.4286
23_15_CeSt-28F	0.5532	0.4336	0.3774
25_22_CeSt-28F	0.4773	0.4019	0.4400
26_23_CeSt-28F	0.5273	0.3023	0.4262
27_24_CeSt-28F	0.4815	0.3858	0.3667

	19_11_CeSt-28F	21_13_CeSt-28F	22_14_CeSt-28F
20_12_CeSt-28F			
1_11_dryST-28F			
2_12_dryST-28F			
3_13_dryST-28F			
4_14_dryST-28F			
7_22_dryST-28F			
8_23_dryST-28F			
9_24_dryST-28F			
19_11_CeSt-28F			
21_13_CeSt-28F	0.3671		
22_14_CeSt-28F	0.4940	0.3182	
23_15_CeSt-28F	0.4505	0.3958	0.4000
25_22_CeSt-28F	0.4824	0.4000	0.4255

	23_15_CeSt-28F	25_22_CeSt-28F	26_23_CeSt-28F
26_23_CeSt-28F	0.4206	0.4107	0.4655
27_24_CeSt-28F	0.4667	0.4727	0.4035
20_12_CeSt-28F			
1_11_dryST-28F			
2_12_dryST-28F			
3_13_dryST-28F			
4_14_dryST-28F			
7_22_dryST-28F			
8_23_dryST-28F			
9_24_dryST-28F			
19_11_CeSt-28F			
21_13_CeSt-28F			
22_14_CeSt-28F			
23_15_CeSt-28F			
25_22_CeSt-28F	0.3529		
26_23_CeSt-28F	0.4194	0.3898	
27_24_CeSt-28F	0.4262	0.3621	0.3913

6.4.2   Distance (Dissimilarity) Coefficients: Bray-Curtis Index

For microbiome abundance data, the measures of distance coefficients are not really distances. They actually measure "*dissimilarity*". The simplest case of distance coefficients is two species in two community samples. The *smaller* the distance, the *more similar* the two communities are. When a distance coefficient is zero, communities are identical. However, since the measures are distance coefficients (although are not really distances), they can be visualized. This visualization feature is intuitively appealing to the microbiome researchers. Measures of dissimilarity include Euclidian distance, Manhattan, and Bray-Curtis measures.

The Euclidian distance can be measured by the following formula:

$$d_{jk} = \sqrt{\sum_{i=1}^{n} \left(X_{ij} - X_{ik}\right)^2} \tag{6.10}$$

where

d_{jk} Euclidean distance between samples j and k
X_{ij} Number of individuals of species i in sample j
X_{ik} Number of individuals of species i in sample k
n Total number of species in samples.

The Manhattan measure is one of the simplest metric functions. The formula of Manhattan is given by:

$$d_M(j, k) = \sum_{i=1}^{n} \left|X_{ij} - X_{ik}\right| \tag{6.11}$$

where

$d_M(j,k)$ Manhattan distance between samples j and k
X_{ij}, X_{ik} Number of individuals in species i in each sample (j, k)
n Total number of species in samples.

The Bray-Curtis dissimilarity, named after J. Roger Bray and John T. Curtis (Bray and Curtis 1957), is a statistic measure used to quantify the compositional dissimilarity between two different samples, based on counts at each sample. Bray-Curtis dissimilarity comes from Euclidean distance. As defined by Bray and Curtis, the index of dissimilarity is given as follow.

$$BC = \frac{\sum_{i=1}^{n} |X_{ij} - X_{ik}|}{\sum_{i=1}^{n} (X_{ij} + X_{ik})} \tag{6.12}$$

where

BC Bray-Curtis measure of dissimilarity
X_{ij}, X_{ik} Number of individuals in species i in each sample (j, k)
n Total number of species in samples.

Bray-Curtis measure is the standardized Manhattan metric (Bray and Curtis 1957) so that it has a range from 0 (similar) to 1 (dissimilar). One feature of the Bray-Curtis measure is that it ignores cases in which the species is absent in both community samples, and it is dominated by the abundant species so that rare species add very little to the value of the coefficient.

The best known index of beta diversity is based on the ratio of total number of species in a collection of samples S and the average richness per one sample $\bar{\alpha}$ (Tuomisto 2010):

$$\beta = S/\bar{\alpha} - 1 \tag{6.13}$$

Subtraction of one means that $\beta = 0$ when there are no excess species or no heterogeneity between samples. As we can see from above formula, S increases with the number of samples even in the case that samples are all subsets of the same community. This really causes problem in ecology and also in microbiome studies. Thus, Whittaker suggested using pairwise comparison of samples to find the index (Whittaker 1960). The new index called the Sørensen index of dissimilarity can be expressed as:

$$\beta = \frac{a+b+c}{(2a+b+c)/2} - 1 = \frac{b+c}{2a+b+c} \tag{6.14}$$

where

a = Number of shared species in two samples
b and c = Numbers of species unique to each sample, respectively
$\bar{\alpha} = (2a+b+c)/2$, the average richness per one sample
S = a + b + c

Bray-Curtis dissimilarity measure can be calculated using the vegdist() function in vegan package as below.

```
> bray<-vegdist(abund_table, "bray")
> bray
                 5_15_dryst-28F 20_12_Cest-28F 1_11_dryst-28F
20_12_Cest-28F       0.6720
1_11_dryst-28F       0.5873          0.5058
2_12_dryst-28F       0.5293          0.3371          0.3742
3_13_dryst-28F       0.5786          0.5542          0.2041
4_14_dryst-28F       0.2765          0.4629          0.4896
7_22_dryst-28F       0.4756          0.4277          0.5208
8_23_dryst-28F       0.6487          0.5963          0.4084
9_24_dryst-28F       0.5984          0.4433          0.2921
19_11_Cest-28F       0.8064          0.5290          0.7049
21_13_Cest-28F       0.7449          0.3403          0.6910
22_14_Cest-28F       0.7320          0.3704          0.5562
23_15_Cest-28F       0.8503          0.6254          0.4961
25_22_Cest-28F       0.6377          0.2819          0.5816
26_23_Cest-28F       0.7997          0.4613          0.5291
27_24_Cest-28F       0.7215          0.4664          0.3966
                 2_12_dryst-28F 3_13_dryst-28F 4_14_dryst-28F
20_12_Cest-28F
1_11_dryst-28F
2_12_dryst-28F
3_13_dryst-28F       0.4861
4_14_dryst-28F       0.4114          0.4645
7_22_dryst-28F       0.4955          0.5436          0.4172
8_23_dryst-28F       0.5119          0.4217          0.6220
9_24_dryst-28F       0.4368          0.2362          0.5210
19_11_Cest-28F       0.6138          0.7401          0.6510
21_13_Cest-28F       0.4992          0.7083          0.5591
22_14_Cest-28F       0.3966          0.6340          0.5214
23_15_Cest-28F       0.6194          0.5276          0.7720
25_22_Cest-28F       0.4997          0.6387          0.4976
26_23_Cest-28F       0.4560          0.6159          0.7019
27_24_Cest-28F       0.4674          0.4745          0.6291
                 7_22_dryst-28F 8_23_dryst-28F 9_24_dryst-28F
20_12_Cest-28F
1_11_dryst-28F
2_12_dryst-28F
3_13_dryst-28F
4_14_dryst-28F
7_22_dryst-28F
8_23_dryst-28F       0.5356
9_24_dryst-28F       0.4359          0.3105
19_11_Cest-28F       0.7634          0.8284          0.7623
21_13_Cest-28F       0.5969          0.7582          0.6541
22_14_Cest-28F       0.5438          0.6970          0.5938
23_15_Cest-28F       0.6998          0.4713          0.4254
25_22_Cest-28F       0.3046          0.6449          0.5445
26_23_Cest-28F       0.6055          0.3608          0.4381
27_24_Cest-28F       0.5944          0.5204          0.4013
                 19_11_Cest-28F 21_13_Cest-28F 22_14_Cest-28F
20_12_Cest-28F
1_11_dryst-28F
2_12_dryst-28F
3_13_dryst-28F
4_14_dryst-28F
7_22_dryst-28F
8_23_dryst-28F
9_24_dryst-28F
19_11_Cest-28F
21_13_Cest-28F       0.5046
22_14_Cest-28F       0.5815          0.4099
23_15_Cest-28F       0.7958          0.7705          0.6211
25_22_Cest-28F       0.6467          0.4522          0.4034
```

	23_15_CeSt-28F	25_22_CeSt-28F	26_23_CeSt-28F
26_23_CeSt-28F	0.7161	0.6553	0.5347
27_24_CeSt-28F	0.4028	0.6330	0.5686
20_12_CeSt-28F			
1_11_drySt-28F			
2_12_drySt-28F			
3_13_drySt-28F			
4_14_drySt-28F			
7_22_drySt-28F			
8_23_drySt-28F			
9_24_drySt-28F			
19_11_CeSt-28F			
21_13_CeSt-28F			
22_14_CeSt-28F			
23_15_CeSt-28F			
25_22_CeSt-28F	0.6558		
26_23_CeSt-28F	0.4517	0.5610	
27_24_CeSt-28F	0.5128	0.5911	0.4632

As seen above, all Bray-Curtis, Jaccard and Sørensen are in distance format matrix, which only has values in the lower triangle of the matrix. After we obtain beta diversity indices, we can conduct hypothesis testing and statistical analysis on them. Typically these dissimilarity matrixes can be analyzed by a multivariate technique and hypothesis testing using a multivariate analysis of variances, such as nonparametric MANOVA, multi-response permutation procedure (MRPP) or analysis of similarities (ANOSIM). We will cover these contents in Chaps. 7 and 9.

6.5   Summary

In this chapter, we introduced community diversities: alpha, beta and gamma indices. The focus was given to the alpha and beta diversities and their calculations. Microbiome study often starts with estimation of Chao 1 and Shannon diversities. Beta diversity has been applied to two conceptual models: the change in species richness over an ecological gradient (multiplicative model) (Whittaker 1972) and simply to measure variation among samples within a study area (additive model) (Anderson et al. 2011). Beta diversity can be seen as species turnover or as variation in species composition (Anderson et al. 2011). The two conceptual models have been linked to two different definitions of beta diversity.

The calculations were illustrated using $Vdr^{-/-}$ mice data set. The readers can use these methods and the associated R codes to analyze their own study. The measurements of alpha and beta diversities are the bases of hypothesis testing of microbiome community study.

References

Anderson, M.J., T.O. Crist, et al. 2011. Navigating the multiple meanings of beta diversity: A roadmap for the practicing ecologist. *Ecology Letters* 14 (1): 19–28.

Baselga, A., and Orme C.D.L. 2012. betapart: An R package for the study of beta diversity. *Methods in Ecology and Evolution* 3: 808–812.

Bray, J.R., and J.T. Curtis. 1957. An ordination of upland forest communities of southern Wisconsin. *Ecological Monographs* 27: 325–349.

Chao, A. 1984. Nonparametric estimation of the number of classes in a population. *Scandinavian Journal of Statistics* 11: 265–270.

Chao, A. 1987. Estimating the population size for capture-recapture data with unequal catchability. *Biometrics* 43: 783–791.

Chao, A., and S.-M. Lee. 1992. Estimating the number of classes via sample coverage. *Journal of American Statistical Association* 87: 210–217.

Chao, A., M.-C. Ma, et al. 1993. Stopping rules and estimation for recapture debugging with unequal failure rates. *Biometrics* 43: 783–791.

Colwell, R.K., and J.A. Coddington. 1994. Estimating terrestrial biodiversity through extrapolation. *Philosophical Transactions of the Royal Society of London. Series B, Biological sciences* 345 (1311): 101–118.

Ellison, A.M. 2010. Partitioning diversity. *Ecology* 91 (7): 1962–1963.

Good, I. 1953. The population frequencies of species and the estimation of population parameters. *Biometrika* 40: 237–264.

Gotelli, N.J. 2008. A primer of ecology. Sunderland, MA: Sinauer Associates, Inc.

Heltshe, J., and N. Forrester. 1983. Estimating species richness using the jackknife procedure. *Biometrics* 39: 1–11.

Hurlbert, S.H. 1971. The non-concept of species diversity: A critique and alternative parameters. *Ecology* 52: 577–589.

Jin, D., S. Wu, et al. 2015. Lack of vitamin D receptor causes dysbiosis and changes the functions of the murine intestinal microbiome. *Clinical Therapeutics* 37 (5): 996–1009. e1007.

Koleff, P., K. Gaston, et al. 2003. Measuring beta diversity for presence-absence data. *Journal of Animal Ecology* 72: 367–382.

Lozupone, C.A., and R. Knight. 2008. Species divergence and the measurement of microbial diversity. *FEMS Microbiology Reviews* 32 (4): 557–578.

Magurran, A.E. 2004. *Measuring biological diversity*. Oxford: Blackwell Publishing.

McCune, B., and J.B. Grace. 2002. Analysis of ecological communities. MJM Press.

Morgan, X.C., and C. Huttenhower. 2012. Chapter 12: Human microbiome analysis. *PLoS Computational Biology* 8 (12): e1002808.

Oksanen, J., and T. Tonteri. 1995. Rate of compositional turnover along gradients and total gradient length. *Journal of Vegetation Science* 6 (6): 815–824.

Pielou, E.C. 1966. The measurement of diversity in different types of biological collections. *Journal of Theoretical Biology* 13: 131–144.

Shannon, C.E. 1948. A mathematical theory of communication. *Bell System Technical Journal* 27 (379–423): 623–656.

Shannon, C.E., and W. Weaver. 1949. *The mathematical theory of communication*. Urbana, IL: University of Illinois Press.

Simpson, E. 1949. Simpson EH. Measurement of diversity. *Nature* 163: 688.

Tuomisto, H. 2010. A diversity of beta diversities: Straightening up a concept gone awry. 1. Defining beta diversity as a function of alpha and gamma diversity. *Ecography* 33: 2–22.

Washington, H.G. 1984. Diversity, biotic and similarity indices. A review with special relevance to aquatic ecosystems. *Water Research* 18: 653–694.

Whittaker, R.H. 1960. Vegetation of the Siskiyou Mountains, Oregon and California. *Ecological Monographs* 30: 279–338.

Whittaker, R.H. 1967. Gradient analysis of vegetation. *Biological Reviews* 42: 207–264.

Whittaker, R.H. 1969. Evolution of diversity in plant communities. *Brookhaven Symposia in Biology* 22: 178–196.

Whittaker, R.H. 1972. Evolution and measurement of species diversity. *Taxon* 21: 213–251.

Wilson, M.V., and C.L. Mohler. 1983. Measuring compositional change along gradients. *Vegetatio* 54: 129–141.

Chapter 7
Exploratory Analysis of Microbiome Data and Beyond

We can divide methods of microbiome community composition study into two major components: analysis of taxonomic diversities and multivariate analysis of microbiome composition. The multivariate analysis includes various multivariate techniques, such as clustering and (unconstrained and constrained) ordination and hypothesis testing differences among groups. Although the unconstrained ordination involves post hoc hypothesis, it belongs to exploratory analysis per se. The constrained ordination is a hypothesis testing. In this chapter, we will use various graphical techniques to explore taxonomic diversities and use clustering and ordination techniques to explore microbiome compositions. In Chap. 8, we will present comparisons of taxa diversities. Chapter 9 will focus on hypothesis testing of multivariate analysis of compositions.

7.1 Datasets from Mice and Human

7.1.1 Vdr$^{-/-}$ Mice Data Set

We will continue to use $Vdr^{-/-}$ mice data set, which was introduced in Chap. 6. The murine intestinal microbiome data (Jin et al. 2015) were collected from fecal and cecal stool samples. Here, the fecal samples are used.

7.1.2 Cigarette Smokers Data Set

The second data set is from Charlson et al. (2010) and Chen (2012), which includes studies on the effect of smoking on the upper respiratory tract microbiome. The original data set contains samples from both throat and nose microbiomes, and from

© Springer Nature Singapore Pte Ltd. 2018
Y. Xia et al., *Statistical Analysis of Microbiome Data with R*,
ICSA Book Series in Statistics, https://doi.org/10.1007/978-981-13-1534-3_7

both body sides. The data set used in this chapter is from the throat microbiome of left body side. It contains 60 subjects (32 non-smokers and 28 smokers). The data set includes three data: abundance count, tree, and meta-data. It is suitable to illustrate tree plotting and constrained ordination analysis.

7.2 Exploratory Analysis with Graphic Summary

Microbiome data can be explored through various graphs. Here, we illustrate the five commonly used plots: richness, abundance bar, heatmap, network and phylogenetic tree using above two data sets. The plots are generated by the phyloseq package (McMurdie and Holmes 2013). The phyloseq package is a tool to import, store, analyze, and graphically display complex phylogenetic sequencing data. The input data used in this package can be OTUs or abundant count data. This package uses advanced/flexible graphic systems (ggplot2) to easily produce publication-quality graphics of data.

7.2.1 Plot Richness

The estimated alpha diversities can be summarized via a graph using the function plot_richness() in the phyloseq package. Although its name suggests plotting "richness," which usually refers to plot the total number of species/taxa/OTUs in a sample or environment, actually the function not only plots richness, also generates figures of observed and other estimated diversities. First, we need load the phyloseq and ggplot2 packages, and the $Vdr^{-/-}$ mice data set.

```
> library(phyloseq)
> library(ggplot2)
> abund_table=read.csv("VdrFecalGenusCounts.csv",row.names=1,
check.names=FALSE)
> abund_table<-t(abund_table)
```

The critical step when you use the phyloseq package is to build a phyloseq-class object. The following chunk of R codes build a *phyloseq* class object called *physeq* using the constructor phyloseq(). The phyloseq class object is built from its component data: otu table, sample data, taxonomy table and phylo tree. As an experiment-level object, two or more component data objects must be provided. The order of arguments does not matter.

```
> meta_table <-
data.frame(row.names=rownames(abund_table),t(as.data.frame(strsplit
(rownames(abund_table),"_"))))
```

```
> meta_table$Group <- with(meta_table,ifelse(as.factor(X2)%in%
c(11,12,13,14,15),c("Vdr-/-"), c("WT")))

> #Convert the data to phyloseq format
> OTU = otu_table(as.matrix(abund_table), taxa_are_rows = FALSE)
> SAM = sample_data(meta_table)
> physeq<-merge_phyloseq(phyloseq(OTU),SAM)
> physeq
phyloseq-class experiment-level object
otu_table()   OTU Table:          [ 248 taxa and 8 samples ]
sample_data() Sample Data:        [ 8 samples by 4 sample variables ]
```

After build a physeq object, we can use the function plot_richness() through the ggplot2 package to plot the observed and estimated alpha diversities.

```
> plot_richness(physeq, x = "Group", color = "Group")
```

The input data "physeq" is required, which is phyloseq-class, or alternatively, an otu table-class. The optional argument "x" is a variable to map to the horizontal axis; x can be either a character string or a vector. The default value is "samples", which will map each sample's name to a separate horizontal position in the plot. In this case, x = "Group" will map group membership to the x axis. The argument color is also optional. It will specify the sample variable to map to different colors. Like argument x, this can be a single character string or a vector.

In alpha diversity estimation, the noise can be trimmed; however since many richness estimates and even the "observed" richness are highly dependent on the number of singletons. Thus, if you want meaningful results, you must use untrimmed datasets (McMurdie and Holmes 2013).

Figure 7.1 is generated by the above R codes.

You can also choose the alpha-diversity measures that you want to plot. For example, the following R codes plot Chao1 and Shannon diversities only.

```
> plot_richness(physeq, measures = c("Chao1", "Shannon"),
x = "Group", color
= "Group")
```

7.2.2 Plot Abundance Bar

The phyloseq function plot_bar() is powerful and flexible. Its main purpose is to quickly and easily create informative summary graphics of the differences in taxa abundance between samples in an experiment (McMurdie and Holmes 2013). One usage is given below:

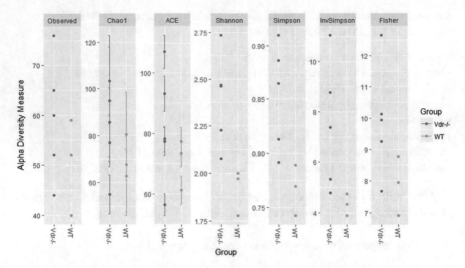

Fig. 7.1 Alpha diversity measure plots with $Vdr^{-/-}$ and WT groups in fecal samples

plot_bar(physeq,   x="Sample",   y="Abundance",   fill=NULL,   title=NULL, facet_grid=NULL)

Both "x" and "y" arguments are optional and character strings. The variables in the data will be mapped to the x-axis, and the y-axis, respectively. Typically "y" argument will be "Abundance" to quantitatively display the abundance values for each OTU/group. Other two sophisticated and customized optional arguments are "fill" and "facet_grid". The "fill" option is a character string to specify which sample variable will be used to map to the fill color of the bars. The "facet_grid" option is a formula object to specify the faceting you want to be displayed in the "ggplot2" graphics.

Let's adjust the default theme first.

```
> theme_set(theme_bw())
```

The default barplot without any parameters being given will plot with every sample individually mapped to the x-axis, and abundance values mapped to the y-axis. The abundance values for each OTU/sample are stacked in the order from greatest to least, separated by a thin horizontal line.

```
> plot_bar(physeq)
```

The following R codes are used to fill different colors for $Vdr^{-/-}$ and WT groups to which each sample belongs.

```
> plot_bar(physeq, fill="Group")
```

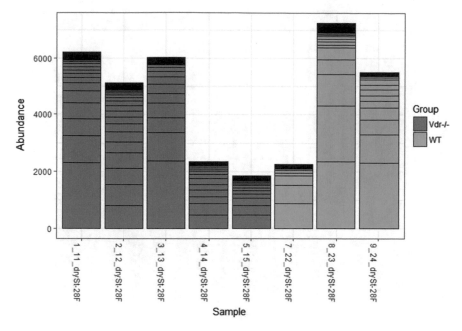

Fig. 7.2 Abundance bar plots with $Vdr^{-/-}$ and WT groups in fecal samples

In Fig. 7.2, all abundance values are plotted, if you just want to know the top five most abundant bacteria, then you can use following R code chunk (Fig. 7.3).

```
> TopNGenus <- names(sort(taxa_sums(physeq), TRUE)[1:5])
> Top5Genus <- prune_taxa(TopNGenus, physeq)

> plot_bar(Top5Genus, fill="Group", facet_grid=~Group)
```

So far, we illustrate "fill" and "facet_grid" options using variable group. Actually, more informative way to visualize sample abundance difference between $Vdr^{-/-}$ and WT groups is to use "Genus" to fill the color here, which need to include taxonomy data in the phyloseq object. However, we do not have taxonomy data for this study. The interested readers can use the below sample codes for their own study.

```
> plot_bar(Top5Genus, fill="Genus", facet_grid=~Group)
```

7.2.3 Plot Heatmap

Rajaram and Oono have shown how to create a heatmap to organize the rows and columns using ordination methods instead of hierarchical cluster analysis (Rajaram

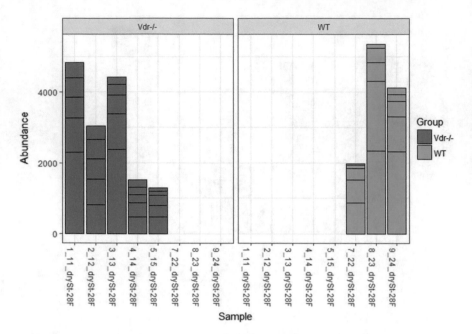

Fig. 7.3 Abundance bar plots of top five most abundant bacteria with $Vdr^{-/-}$ and WT groups in fecal samples

and Oono 2010). The ordination-based ordering is much better than hierarchical-clustering to present microbiome data. There are many useful examples of phyloseq heatmap graphics in the phyloseq online tutorials. The interested readers can reference these sample heatmaps to do their owns. Here, we focus on illustrating the plot_heatmap() function based on the NMDS and PCA ordination methods.

One usage of plot_heatmap() function is given below.

plot_heatmap(physeq, method = "NMDS", distance = "bray", sample.label = NULL, taxa.label = NULL, low = "#000033", high = "#66CCFF", na.value = "black")

The input data argument "physeq" is required. It is a phyloseq-class object (otu_table). Both method and distance augments are optional. The ordination method is to use for organizing the heatmap. The ecological distance method is a character string for using in the ordination. Both "sample.label" and "taxa.label" are character strings and optional to use to label the sample (horizontal) axis and re-label the taxa/species/OTU (vertical) axis, respectively. Both low and high augments are character strings and optional. They are used to choose color options support in R. R understands over 600 colors. You can type colors() in R to check the names.

```
> colors()
```

You can also find a table summary of these colors at the R Cookbook (http://www.cookbook-r.com/Graphs/Colors_(ggplot2)/).

In the heatmap, zero-values are treated as NA, and set to "black", to represent a background color. The low option is used to represent the lowest non-zero value, and the default of low argument is a dark blue color, "#000033"; while the high option is used to represent the highest value and the default is "#66CCFF".

In the *heatmap* plot, too many taxa (in this case, genera) will make the figure be too crowded to be seen clearly. We need to limit the number of taxa to be plotted. The following R codes choose the top five most abundant genera to make a heatmap.

```
> TopNGenus <- names(sort(taxa_sums(physeq), TRUE)[1:5])
> Top5Genus <- prune_taxa(TopNGenus, physeq)
> plot_heatmap(Top5Genus)
```

The following R codes use NMDS ordination method and Bray-Curtis distance method to plot the top five genera.

```
> (p <- plot_heatmap(Top5Genus, "NMDS", "bray"))
```

You can try different colors for heatmap to meet the journal requirements. The following are some examples you can use.

```
> plot_heatmap(Top5Genus, "NMDS", "bray", low="#000033", high="#CCFF66")
> plot_heatmap(Top5Genus, "NMDS", "bray", low="#000033", high="#FF3300")
> plot_heatmap(Top5Genus, "NMDS", "bray", low="#000033", high="#66CCFF")
> plot_heatmap(Top5Genus, "NMDS", "bray", low="#66CCFF", high="#000033",
 na.value="white")
```

You can also try to use different combinations of ecological distances and ordinations. For example, the following heatmap uses PCoA ordination on the default Bray-Curtis distance (Fig. 7.4).

```
> plot_heatmap(Top5Genus, "PCoA", "bray")
```

7.2.4 Plot Network

There are two functions in the phyloseq package to plot microbiome network using "ggplot2": plot_network() and plot_net(). If you use the function plot_network(), then its first argument need to be an igraph object, and the network itself should be

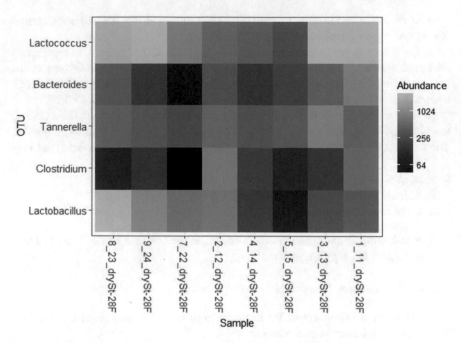

Fig. 7.4 Heatmap of top five most abundant bacteria with $Vdr^{-/-}$ and WT groups in fecal samples

represented using the igraph package. The network object (argument g) can be created using the make_network() function via phyloseq package. The function plot_net() is a performance and interface revision to plot_network(), its first/main argument is a phyloseq-class instance.

The example usages of plot_network() and plot_net() are given below:

plot_network(g, physeq=NULL, type="samples", color="Group", shape= "Group")
plot_net(physeq, distance = "bray", type = "samples", maxdist = 0.7, color = NULL, shape = NULL)

In plot_network(), g is a required igraph-class object created either by the function make_network(), or directly by the igraph-package. The optional argument physeq is a phyloseq-class object on which g is based. Type option indicates whether the network represented in the primary argument, g, is samples or taxa/ OTUs. Default is "samples". Both options color and shape are optional. They are used for color mapping and shape mapping of points.

The required argument physeq in plot_net() function is the phyloseq-class object that you want to represent as a network. The distance option is a distance method or an already-computed dist-class. Default is "bray". The option maxdist means the maximum distance value between two vertices to connect with an edge in the graph. The default value is 0.7.

The following R codes create an igraph-based network based on the default distance method, "Jaccard" and a maximum distance between connected nodes of

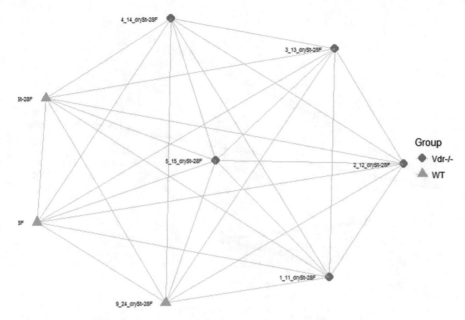

Fig. 7.5 Network plot of $Vdr^{-/-}$ and WT groups in fecal samples by plot_network()

0.8. The "Group" is used to both color and shape mappings to visualize the structure of Vdr$^{-/-}$ and WT mouse samples (Fig. 7.5).

```
> ig <- make_network(physeq, max.dist=0.8)
> plot_network(ig, physeq, color="Group", shape="Group")
```

The above graphic displays some interesting structure, with two subgraphs comprising of the samples from $Vdr^{-/-}$ and WT mice respectively. Also, there seems to be a correlation among samples.

Compared to the function plot_network(), the newer plot_net() function does not require a separate make _network() function call, or a separate igraph object. The following codes create a network based on a maximum distance between connected nodes of 0.5. As we are interested in how the structure of $Vdr^{-/-}$ and WT mouse samples, we use "Group" to color mapping and shape mapping of points (Fig. 7.6).

```
> plot_net(physeq, maxdist = 0.5, color = "Group", shape="Group")
```

7.2.5 Plot Phylogenetic Tree

The function plot_tree() in the phyloseq package is intended to facilitate easy graphical investigation of the phylogenetic tree, as well as sample data. For phylogenetic sequencing of samples with large richness, the tree generated by this

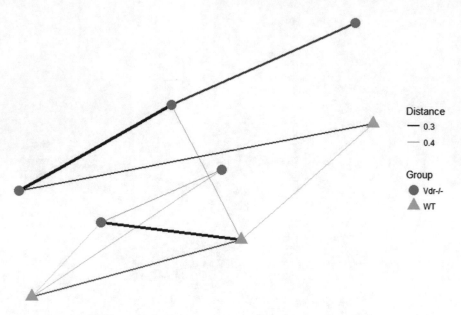

Fig. 7.6 Network plot of $Vdr^{-/-}$ and WT groups in fecal samples by plot_net()

function will be difficult to read and interpretable. A rough "rule of thumb" proposed by the authors of phyloseq package is to use subsets of data with not more than 200 OTUs per plot. One usage of this function is given below:

plot_tree(physeq, method = "sampledodge", color = NULL, shape = NULL, ladderize = FALSE)

The input data "physeq" is required. The data should be the phyloseq-class and contain at minimum a phylogenetic tree component. It is this data that you want to plot and annotate a phylogenetic tree. The "method" option is the name of the annotation method to use. The default "sampledodge" will draw points next to leaves if individuals from that taxon were observed, and a separate point for each sample. Both "color" and "shape" arguments are optional. They provide the names of the variable in physeq to map to point color, and map to point shape, respectively.

The option "ladderize" is used to specify whether or not to ladderize the tree, i.e., reorder nodes according to the depth of their enclosed subtrees prior to plotting. Default is FALSE, no ladderization is applied. When TRUE or "right", "right" ladderization is used. When set to "left", "left" ladderization is applied.

The smokers data set is used to illustrate plotting phylogenetic tree. The data are from GUniFrac package (Charlson et al. 2010; Chen 2012). Let's first load this package and make the data available for use.

```
> library(GUniFrac)
> data(throat.otu.tab)
```

```
> data(throat.tree)
> data(throat.meta)
```

Then, we need to build phyloseq class object through phyloseq package as below.

```
> library(phyloseq)
> #Convert the data to phyloseq format
> OTU = otu_table(as.matrix(throat.otu.tab), taxa_are_rows = FALSE)
> SAM = sample_data(throat.meta)
> TRE <-throat.tree
> physeq<-merge_phyloseq(phyloseq(OTU), SAM, TRE) )
```

Check how many taxa/OTUs in the data set.

```
> ntaxa(physeq)
[1] 856
```

There are 856 OTUs. They are too many to be used for annotation in a phylogenetic tree. The following prune_taxa() function prunes just the first 50 OTUs in the data set. We use these first 50 OTUs to plot and annotate in a phylogenetic tree.

```
> physeq = prune_taxa(taxa_names(physeq)[1:50], physeq)
```

The following R codes map color to smoking status variable (Fig. 7.7).

```
> plot_tree(physeq, ladderize = "left", color = "SmokingStatus")
```

The following R codes map both color and shape to smoking status variable (Fig. 7.8).

```
> plot_tree(physeq, ladderize = "left", color = "SmokingStatus", shape =
"SmokingStatus")
```

Above tree is vertically-oriented tree. It is a Cartesian mapping of the data to a graph. In the literature, a radial tree is frequently used. We can also use the same mapping as in vertically-oriented tree to make a radial tree with ggplot2. The difference is that this time the mapping is with polar coordinates instead (Fig. 7.9).

```
> plot_tree(physeq, color = "SmokingStatus",
shape = "SmokingStatus", ladderize = "left") + coord_polar(theta = "y")
```

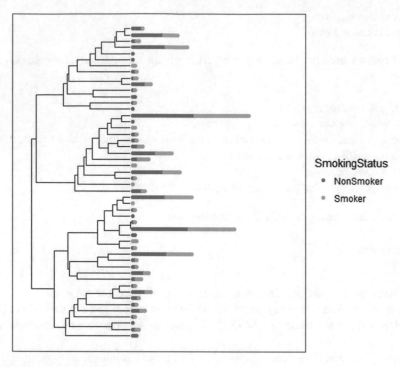

Fig. 7.7 Phylogenetic tree with smoking status (non-smoker and smoker) mapped to the tree using different colors

7.3 Clustering

7.3.1 Introduction to Clustering, Distance and Ordination

Clustering (or classification) and ordination are the two main classes of multivariate methods that microbiome researchers and community ecologists often employ. To certain degree, these two approaches are complementary. The objective of clustering is to put samples into (perhaps hierarchical) classes to reduce complexity (dimensionalities) of data; it may reduce all samples on one dimension (x-axis). However, the data with two or three dimensions are more interpretable than that with one dimension because most community data are continuous. With ordination, community data can be reduced to two or three dimensions. Thus, ordination is usually desired by microbiome researchers and community ecologists. Many multivariate methods have been developed based on ordination in the microbiome and ecology study. When you are doing clustering and ordination, a distance measure need to be provided by a distance method.

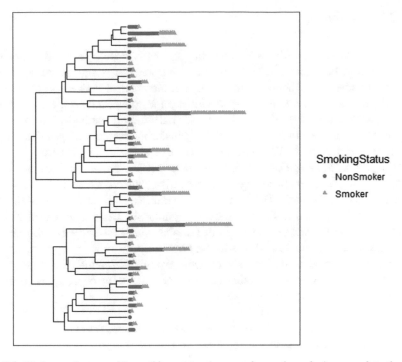

Fig. 7.8 Phylogenetic tree with smoking status (non-smoker and smoker) mapped to the tree using different colors and shapes

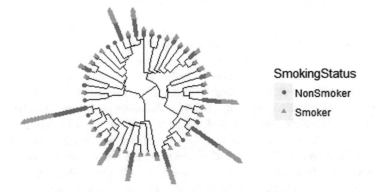

Fig. 7.9 A radial tree with smoking status (non-smoker and smoker) mapped to the tree using different colors and shapes

7.3.2   Clustering

There are several families of clustering methods available in the literature (Legendre and Legendre 2012): sequential or simultaneous algorithms, agglomerative or divisive, monothetic versus polythetic, hierarchical versus non-hierarchical methods, probabilistic versus non-probabilistic methods. Among these categories, Ward's hierarchical clustering and k-means partitioning methods are commonly used in microbiome studies. Hierarchical clustering results are generally represented as dendrograms. We will illustrate several different clustering methods including "single linkage agglomerative clustering", "complete linkage agglomerative clustering", "average linkage agglomerative clustering", and "Ward's minimum variance clustering". The $Vdr^{-/-}$ mouse dataset with fecal samples that you met earlier will be used to illustrate clustering analysis. Here, Bray-Curtis distance is to be used to illustrate classification of samples. Other distances are also applied. If vegan package is not loaded, loading it now.

Let's first normalize the abundance table using the function decostand() and calculate the Bray-Curtis dissimilarities between all pairs of samples using the function vegdist() in vegan package.

```
> abund_table_norm <- decostand(abund_table, "normalize")
> bc_dist<- vegdist(abund_table_norm , method = "bray")
```

Given Bray-Curtis dissimilarities having been calculated, we now apply the hierarchical clustering function hclust() with four different clustering algorithms —"average", "complete", "single" linkage methods, and Ward's clustering method.

7.3.2.1   Single Linkage Agglomerative Clustering

"Agglomerate" means gathered into a cluster; single-linkage agglomerative clustering is also called nearest neighbor sorting. At each step, the clustering combines two samples that contain the shortest pairwise distances (or greatest similarity). The result of the clustering can be visualized as a dendrogram. The drawback of the dendrogram resulting a single linkage clustering often shows chaining of samples. The formed clusters are forced together due to single elements being close to each other, whereas many elements in each cluster maybe very distant to each other. Another relevant drawback of single-linkage clustering is that it could be difficult to interpret in terms of partitions of the data. It is a real disadvantage of single linkage clustering, because we are interested in the data partitions (Fig. 7.10).

```
> cluster_single <- hclust (bc_dist, method = 'single')
> plot(cluster_single)
```

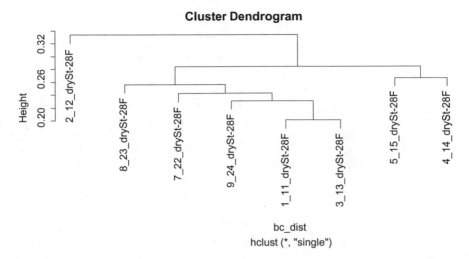

Fig. 7.10 Single linkage agglomerative clustering dendrogram of Bray-Curtis dissimilarity

7.3.2.2 Complete Linkage Agglomerative Clustering

Complete-linkage clustering is also known as farthest neighbor clustering. It allows a sample (or a group) to agglomerate with another sample (or group) only at the distance that is farthest away from each other. Thus, all members of both groups are linked. Complete linkage clustering avoids the drawback of chaining samples by the single linkage method. Complete linkage tends to find many small separate groups (Fig. 7.11).

```
> cluster_complete <- hclust (bc_dist, method = 'complete')
> plot(cluster_complete)
```

7.3.2.3 Average Linkage Agglomerative Clustering

Average linkage clustering allows a sample to be grouped to a cluster at the mean of the distances between this sample and all members of the cluster. The two clusters are joined at the mean of the distances between all members of one cluster and all members of the other. The cluster resulting the dendrogram looks somewhat intermediate between a single and complete linkage clustering (Fig. 7.12).

```
> cluster_average <- hclust (bc_dist, method = 'average')
> plot(cluster_average)
```

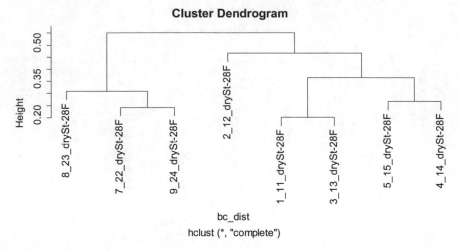

Fig. 7.11 Complete linkage agglomerative clustering dendrogram of Bray-Curtis dissimilarity

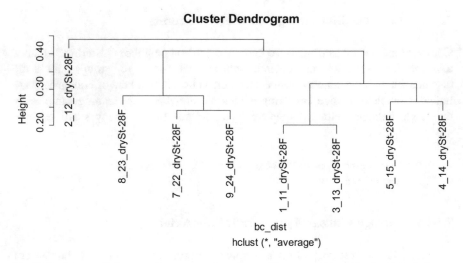

Fig. 7.12 Average linkage agglomerative clustering dendrogram of Bray-Curtis dissimilarity

7.3.2.4 Ward's Minimum Variance Clustering

Ward's minimum variance clustering (a.k.a., Ward's clustering) originally presented by Ward (1963) is based on the linear model criterion of least squares. This method minimizes within-cluster sums of squared (i.e., the squared error of ANOVA) distances between samples. Basically, it looks at cluster analysis as an analysis of variance problem, instead of using distance metrics or measures of association. This method is most appropriate for quantitative variables, and not binary variables. Ward's clustering is implemented through finding the pair of

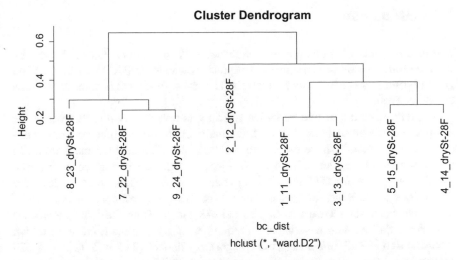

Fig. 7.13 Ward's clustering dendrogram of Bray-Curtis dissimilarity

clusters at each step that leads to minimum increase in total within-cluster variance after merging. This increase is a weighted squared distance between cluster centers. Although the initial cluster distances are defined to be the squared Euclidean distance between points in Ward's clustering, other distance methods can produce meaningful results too (Fig. 7.13).

```
> cluster_ward <- hclust (bc_dist, method = 'ward.D2')
> plot(cluster ward)
```

To draw the results together into one diagram using par (mfrow = c(2,2)) to create one graph with two rows with two panels.

```
> par (mfrow = c(2,2))
> plot(cluster_single)
> plot(cluster_complete)
> plot(cluster_average)
> plot(cluster_ward)
```

Restore the default window panel.

```
> par (mfrow = c(1,1))
```

The comparison among these four dedrograms shows that complete linkage and Ward's clustering generated the same partitioning clusters and have the better performance in terms of partitioning data in the direction of our interest (samples 11, 12, 13, 14, and 15 are from $Vdr^{-/-}$ mice, and 22, 23, and 24 from wild-type mice).

7.4 Ordination

The primary goal of ordination was considered "exploratory" (Gauch 1982a, b), with the introduction of canonical correspondence analysis (CCA), ordination has gone beyond mere "exploratory" analysis (ter Braak 1985) and become hypothesis testing as well.

The data structure of two variables typically is revealed by a scatterplot of the samples. As we presented in Chap. 2, the multivariate microbiome data are multi-dimensional, generally have more than two variables. The microbiome dataset can be viewed as a collection of samples (subjects) positioned in a space where each variable or species (or OTUs/taxa) define one dimension. Thus, there are as many dimensions as variables or species (or OTUs/taxa). For example, in our $Vdr^{-/-}$ mouse fecal data set, there are 8 samples and 248 genera. Thus, the data dimension is 248. For a dataset with n variables, the number of scatterplots need to be drawn would be n (n − 1)/2. In our case, the 248 genera will need (248 × 247)/2 = 30,628 scatterplots. Such large number of scatterplots is not informative to know the data structure; it is also tedious to work on.

Ordination primarily endeavors to represent sample and species (or OTUs/taxa) relationships as faithfully as possible in a low-dimensional space (Gauch 1982a, b). This objective is desirable, because community data are multiple dimensions mixed with noise, low dimensions may ideally and typically represent important and intuitive interpretations of species (or OTUs/taxa)—environment relationships.

For a n × p dataset containing n subjects and p variables, the data structure can be reviewed as n subjects (represented as a cluster of points) in the p-dimensional space. The primary aim of ordination is to represent multiple samples (subjects) in a reduced number of orthogonal (i.e., independent) axes, where the total number of axes is less than or equal to the number of samples (subjects). The importance of ordination axes decreases by order. The first axis of an ordination explains the most variation in the dataset, followed by the second axis, then the third, and so on.

The ordination plots are particularly useful for visualizing the similarity among samples (subjects). For example, in the context of beta diversity, samples that are closer in ordination space have species assemblages that are more similar to one another than samples that are further apart in ordination space.

Ordination methods include constrained and unconstrained ordinations, depending on whether the ordination axes are constrained by environmental factors (variables). As the names suggest, in constrained ordination, ordination axes are constrained by environmental factors: the positions of the samples in the ordination are constrained by the environmental variables. In unconstrained ordination, ordination axes are not constrained by environmental factors. In other words, constrained ordination directly uses environmental variables in the construction of the ordination; whereas in unconstrained ordination, the environmental variables are entered in post hoc analyses.

For the perspective of hypothesis testing, unconstrained ordination analysis per se is primarily descriptive method and not really involves hypotheses testing in multivariate data. Although it involves hypothesis about the explanation of axes using environmental variables, such as using the function envfit() in vegan package, unconstrained ordination is simple. It analyzes one data matrix; its objective is to reveal the major data structure in a graph from a reduced set of orthogonal axes. In contrast, constrained ordination is a "hypothesis driven" ordination: a hypothesis testing method, which directly tests the hypothesis about the influence of environmental factors on species (or OTUs/taxa) composition.

The constrained ordination is related to multivariate linear models as this way: with "dependent" (or the community) variables in left side as responses, "independent" variables (or constraints) in right side as explained factors. Thus, the constrained ordination is non-symmetric.

Here, we cover the most common unconstrained ordinations: principal component analysis (PCA) in Sect. 7.4.1; principal coordinate analysis (PCoA) in Sect. 7.4.2; non-metric multidimensional scaling (NMDS) in Sect. 7.4.3; correspondence analysis (CA) in Sect. 7.4.4; and constrained ordinations: redundancy analysis (RDA) in Sect. 7.4.5; constrained correspondence analysis (CCA) in Sect. 7.4.6; constrained analysis of principal coordinates (CAP) in Sect. 7.4.7.

7.4.1 Principal Component Analysis (PCA)

In term of the vegan package, the environmental variable in our case is genetic conditions ($Vdr^{-/-}$ and WT). We want to know whether the vdr gene deficiency interprets beta diversity in genus composition. We conduct a PCA to explore whether the changes in genus composition of communities (beta diversities) are caused by the genetic factor.

With PCA, the samples are plotted based on abundances of genus A on axis 1, genus B on axis 2, genus C on axis 3, and so on until n samples are plotted in a very high dimensional space. The n samples create $(n − 1)$ number of PCs: PC1 is the first straight line going through the space created by all these samples, PC2 is the second line, perpendicular to PC1, and so the third PC3, until PC$(n − 1)$. The importance of PCs decreases by order. PC1 is the most important PC and explains the most variations among all samples. PC2 explains second most variations, and PC3 explains the third most, and so on the $(n − 1)$ PC explains lest variations of the samples.

Several R functions including prcomp() in preinstalled stats package, rda() in vegan package, pca() in labdsv package can be used to conduct PCA. Here, we use the function rda(). The two extensional functions: evplot() (Borcard et al. 2011) and PCAsignificance() in BiodiversityR package can improve the plots. The evplot() provides visual methods to decide the importance of ordination axes through using Keiser-Guttman criterion and broken stick model. The function PCAsignificance() calculates broken-stick model for PCA axes.

When use the function rda() to conduct PCA, by not specifying the environmental data matrix (i.e., group variable), the function performs unconstrained ordination PCA.

In microbiome data analysis, the absolute abundance counts are not appropriate because the large values will have too high influence in the analysis. Thus, we need to standardize the abundance read data before analysis. Here, we use the function decostand() with total method to standardize read.

```
> stand_abund_table <- decostand(abund_table, method = "total")
> PCA <-rda(stand_abund_table)
> PCA
Call: rda(X = stand_abund_table)

              Inertia Rank
Total          0.0408
Unconstrained  0.0408    7
Inertia is variance

Eigenvalues for unconstrained axes:
    PC1     PC2     PC3     PC4     PC5     PC6     PC7
0.02029 0.01279 0.00371 0.00173 0.00143 0.00077 0.00010
```

In vegan's language, "Inertia" is the general term of "variation" in the data. Total variation of the whole dataset is 0.0408 in this case, and the first axis explains 60.4% of total variation (0.02029/0.0408 = 0.4973). Total variation is a sum of variations of each genus in analyzed matrix. The following R codes check the total variance:

```
> sum (apply (stand_abund_table, 2, var))
[1] 0.04082
```

Then, let's draw the diagrams using the function biplot(). The display option "species" is the vegan package label for OTUs/taxa. Default is "sites" (label for samples) (Fig. 7.14).

```
> biplot(PCA, display = 'species')
```

The above diagrams plotted by biplot() is just drawing arrows for genus, which is not informative. The more informative plot is to use function ordiplot() to draw both genus and sample scores as centroids as below (Fig. 7.15):

```
> ordiplot(PCA, display = "sites", type = "text")
```

In above augments, type="text" or "t" added text labels to figure (default setting adds only points).

As an alternative, we can use function cleanplot.pca() written by François Gillet & Daniel Borcard to intend the drawing PCA results to two diagrams and differing by scaling. This function is to draw two biplots (scaling 1 and scaling 2) from an object of class "rda" in PCA or RDA result from vegan's rda() function. This

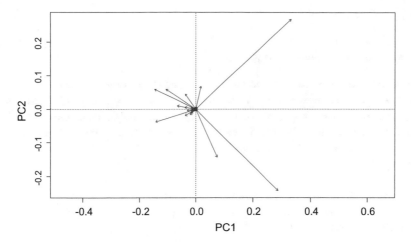

Fig. 7.14 Biplot of two principal components of $Vdr^{-/-}$ mouse fecal data

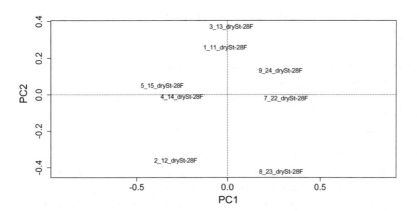

Fig. 7.15 Ordiplot of two principal components of $Vdr^{-/-}$ mouse fecal data with samples labeled

function is provided in Borcard et al's book "Numerical Ecology with R" (Borcard et al. 2011). We run the function cleanplot.pca() first as below.

```
"cleanplot.pca" <- function(res.pca, ax1=1, ax2=2, point=FALSE,
                      ahead=0.07, cex=0.7)
{
  # A function to draw two biplots (scaling 1 and scaling 2) from an object
  # of class "rda" (PCA or RDA result from vegan's rda() function)
  #
  # License: GPL-2
  # Authors: Francois Gillet & Daniel Borcard, 24 August 2012
```

```
require("vegan")

par(mfrow=c(1,2))
p <- length(res.pca$CA$eig)

# Scaling 1: "species" scores scaled to relative eigenvalues
sit.sc1 <- scores(res.pca, display="wa", scaling=1, choices=c(1:p))
spe.sc1 <- scores(res.pca, display="sp", scaling=1, choices=c(1:p))
plot(res.pca, choices=c(ax1, ax2), display=c("wa", "sp"), type="n",
     main="PCA - scaling 1", scaling=1)
if (point)
{
  points(sit.sc1[,ax1], sit.sc1[,ax2], pch=20)
  text(res.pca, display="wa", choices=c(ax1, ax2), cex=cex,
pos=3, scaling=1)
}
else
{
   text(res.pca, display="wa", choices=c(ax1, ax2), cex=cex,
scaling=1)
}
text(res.pca, display="sp", choices=c(ax1, ax2), cex=cex, pos=4,
     col="red", scaling=1)
arrows(0, 0, spe.sc1[,ax1], spe.sc1[,ax2], length=ahead, angle=20,
col="red")
pcacircle(res.pca)

# Scaling 2: site scores scaled to relative eigenvalues
sit.sc2 <- scores(res.pca, display="wa", choices=c(1:p))
spe.sc2 <- scores(res.pca, display="sp", choices=c(1:p))
plot(res.pca, choices=c(ax1,ax2), display=c("wa","sp"), type="n",
     main="PCA - scaling 2")
if (point) {
  points(sit.sc2[,ax1], sit.sc2[,ax2], pch=20)
  text(res.pca, display="wa", choices=c(ax1 ,ax2), cex=cex, pos=3)
}
else
{
   text(res.pca, display="wa", choices=c(ax1, ax2), cex=cex)
}
text(res.pca, display="sp", choices=c(ax1, ax2), cex=cex, pos=4,
col="red")
arrows(0, 0, spe.sc2[,ax1], spe.sc2[,ax2], length=ahead,
angle=20, col="red")
}
```

```
"pcacircle" <- function (pca)
{
   # Draws a circle of equilibrium contribution on a PCA plot
   # generated from a vegan analysis.
   # vegan uses special constants for its outputs, hence
   # the 'const' valuebelow.

   eigenv <- pca$CA$eig
   p <- length(eigenv)
   n <- nrow(pca$CA$u)
   tot <- sum(eigenv)
   const <- ((n - 1) * tot)^0.25
   radius <- (2/p)^0.5
   radius <- radius * const
   symbols(0, 0, circles=radius, inches=FALSE, add=TRUE, fg=2)
}
```

Then call PCA as follows (Fig. 7.16).

```
> cleanplot.pca (PCA)
```

"Scaling" is the way that the ordination results are projected in the reduced space for graphical display (Borcard et al. 2011). The function cleanplot.pca() generates two PCA scalings.

PCA-scaling 1 in the left figure is distance biplot, which focuses on distances among samples. If you're mainly interested to interpret the relationships among samples, choose Scaling 1. The essential features of Scaling 1 are:

The eigenvectors are scaled to unit length and the distances among samples (subjects) in the biplot are approximations of their Euclidean distances in

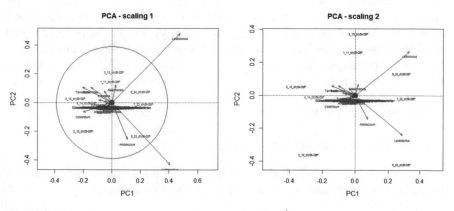

Fig. 7.16 PCA Plots of two principal components of Vdr$^{-/-}$ mouse fecal data using function cleanplot.pca()

multidimensional space. However, the angles among variables (bacteria in this case) vectors are meaningless. The circle is called circle of equilibrium contribution, representing the equilibrium contribution of the variables. For given combination of axes, the variables with vectors longer than the radius of the circle could be interpreted with confidence as most important bacteria, whereas the variables have vectors shorter than the radius of the equilibrium contribution circle contribute little to a given reduced space.

PCA-scaling 2 in the right figure is correlation biplot. It plots the correlation among variables (bacteria in this case). If your main interest focuses on the relationships among variables, choose scaling 2. The essential features of Scaling 2 are:

Each eigenvectors is scaled to the square root of its eigenvalue; the length of vector approximates standard deviation of variables (bacteria); the angles between variables (bacteria in this case) reflect their correlations: the cosine of angle approximates correlation between variables (bacteria); however, the distances among samples (subjects) in the biplot are not approximations of their Euclidean distances in multidimensional space.

7.4.2   Principal Coordinate Analysis (PCoA)

PCoA is also referred to metric multidimensional scaling. PCoA is a flexible ordination technique that allows the user to choose virtually any distance metric (e.g., Jaccard, Bray-Curtis, Euclidean, etc.). As PCA, PCoA uses eigenvalues to measure the importance of a set of returned orthogonal axes. The dimensionality of matrix is reduced by determining each eigenvector and eigenvalue. The principal coordinates are obtained by scaling each eigenvector. PCoA when calculated on Euclidean distances among samples yields the same results as PCA calculated on covariance matrix of the same dataset (if scaling 1 is used).

The R functions, including cmdscale() in vegan package and pcoa() in ape package, can perform PCoA. With vegan, the input data could be calculated by the function vegdist() (default is Bray-Curtis dissimilarity), and the ordination diagram could be drawn with the function ordiplot(). The ordination diagram could be also drawn with the function biplot.pcoa() from ape package. In this case, we use the cmdscale() function and same $Vdr^{-/-}$ mice fecal data to conduct a PCoA. This function needs a resemblance matrix as the input data.

First, let's calculate Bray-Curtis dissimilarity using the function vegdist() and name it as

```
> bc_dist <-vegdist(abund_table, "bray")
```

Then, we are going to explicitly set $k = 2$ (the default values for the number of dimensions to return) and eig = TRUE (which saves the eigenvalues).

```
> PCoA <- cmdscale (bc_dist, eig = TRUE,k = 2)
> PCoA
$points
                       [,1]       [,2]
5_15_drySt-28F   0.35060   0.007035
1_11_drySt-28F  -0.17119   0.137244
2_12_drySt-28F   0.02928   0.115931
3_13_drySt-28F  -0.17013   0.126964
4_14_drySt-28F   0.27190   0.088394
7_22_drySt-28F   0.13943  -0.258936
8_23_drySt-28F  -0.25091  -0.157891
9_24_drySt-28F  -0.19898  -0.058740


$eig
[1]   3.779e-01  1.517e-01  1.170e-01  8.855e-02  2.771e-02
[6]   2.167e-02 -2.515e-17 -4.493e-03

$x
NULL

$ac
[1]  0

$GOF
[1]  0.6713 0.6751
```

The cmdscale() function produces a list of output. The first output *points* contain the coordinates for each sample in each reduced dimension. The second output *eig* contains the eigenvalues. The last three outputs pertain to other options of the analysis that we will not cover here. The following chunk of R codes is used to examine the percent variation in the data set that is explained by the first two axes of the PCoA.

```
> explainedvar1 <- round(PCoA$eig[1] / sum(PCoA$eig), 2) * 100
> explainedvar1
[1] 48
> explainedvar2 <- round(PCoA$eig[2] / sum(PCoA$eig), 2) * 100
> explainedvar2
[1]19

> sum_eig <- sum(explainedvar1, explainedvar2)
> sum_eig
[1] 67
```

First axis explains 48% variations of the data, the second axis 19%. Thus, a large amount of variations of the data (total 67%) has been explained by these two axes.

There are two criteria to assess whether or not the first few PCoA axes capture a disproportionately large amount of the total explained variation: (1) *Kaiser-Guttman criterion* and (2) *broken-stick model*. Kaiser-Guttman criterion states that "the eigenvalues associated with the first few axes should be larger than the average of all the eigenvalues." By the criterion of broken-stick model, the eigenvalues associated with the first few axes are compared to the expectations of the

broken-stick model. The broken stick model assumes that the total sum of eigenvalues decreases sequentially with ordered PCoA axes. We evaluate the performance of PCoA using these two criteria with the following plots:

```
> # Define Plot Parameters
> par(mar = c(5, 5, 1, 2) + 0.1)
> # Plot Eigenvalues
> plot(PCoA$eig, xlab = "PCoA", ylab = "Eigenvalue",
+      las = 1, cex.lab = 1.5, pch = 16)
> # Add Expectation based on Kaiser-Guttman criterion and Broken Stick
Model
> abline(h = mean(PCoA$eig), lty = 2, lwd = 2, col = "blue")
> b_stick <- bstick(8, sum(PCoA$eig))
> lines(1:8, b_stick, type = "l", lty = 4, lwd = 2, col = "red")
> # Add Legend
> legend("topright", legend = c("Avg Eigenvalue", "Broken-Stick"),
+        lty = c(2, 4), bty = "n", col = c("blue", "red"))
```

Figure 7.17 shows that the eigenvalues associated with the first three axes are
larger than the average of all the eigenvalues and are larger than the expectations of
the Broken-Stick model. After evaluating the PCoA output, next we will create an
ordination plot for the two PCoA axes (Fig. 7.18).

```
> # Define Plot Parameters
> par(mar = c(5, 5, 1, 2) + 0.1)
```

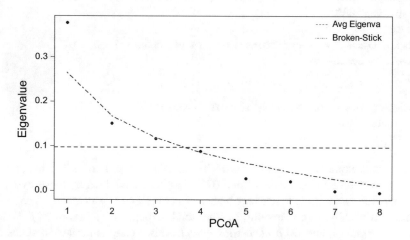

Fig. 7.17 PCoA with Kaiser-Guttman criterion and broken-stick model in *Vdr*$^{-/-}$ mouse fecal
data

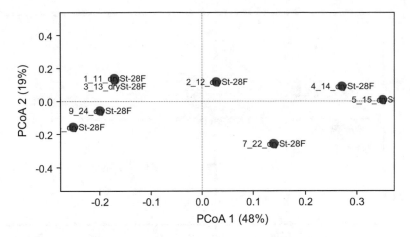

Fig. 7.18 Ordination plot for the two PCoA axes in *Vdr*⁻/⁻ mouse fecal data

```
> # Initiate Plot
> plot(PCoA$points[ ,1], PCoA$points[ ,2], ylim = c(-0.5, 0.5),
+       xlab = paste("PCoA 1 (", explainedvar1, "%)", sep = ""),
+       ylab = paste("PCoA 2 (", explainedvar2, "%)", sep = ""),
+       pch = 5, cex = 1.0, type = "n", cex.lab = 1.0, cex.axis = 1.2,
axes = FALSE)

> # Add Axes
> axis(side = 1, labels = T, lwd.ticks = 2, cex.axis = 1.2, las = 1)
> axis(side = 2, labels = T, lwd.ticks = 2, cex.axis = 1.2, las = 1)
> abline(h = 0, v = 0, lty = 3)
> box(lwd = 2)

> # Add Points & Labels
> points(PCoA$points[ ,1], PCoA$points[ ,2],
+        pch = 19, cex = 3, bg = "blue", col = "blue")
> text(PCoA$points[ ,1], PCoA$points[ ,2],
+      labels = row.names(PCoA$points))
```

Basic ordination plots allow us to see how samples separate from one another. In our example, samples are separating along the PCoA axes owing to variation in the abundance of different mice genera. A logical follow-up question is to ask what genera of the data set are driving the observed divergence among points. Can we identify and visualize these influential genera in PCoA? We can obtain this information using the add.spec.scores() function in the BiodiversityR package. Frist, the relative abundance is calculated as follows:

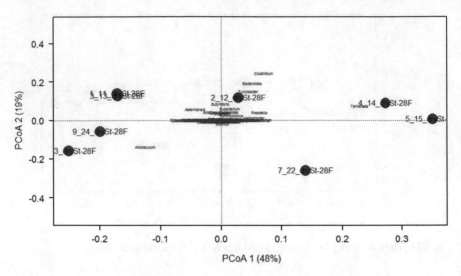

Fig. 7.19 Ordination plot for the two PCoA axes with influential genera in Vdr$^{-/-}$ mouse fecal data

```
> fecalREL <- abund_table
> for(i in 1:nrow(abund_table)){
+   fecalREL[i, ] = abund_table[i, ] / sum(abund_table[i, ])
+ }
```

Then the genera scores are calculated and added to the figure (Fig. 7.19).

```
> require("BiodiversityR")

> PCoA <- add.spec.scores(PCoA,fecalREL,method = "pcoa.scores")
> text(PCoA$cproj[ ,1], PCoA $cproj[ ,2],
+        labels = row.names(PCoA$cproj), col = "black")
```

The add.spec.scores() function can also be used to determine the correlation of each toxon along the PCoA axes. This is a more effectively quantitative approach of identifying influential taxa.

```
> Genus_corr <- add.spec.scores(PCoA, cecalREL, method = "cor.scores")
$cproj
```

To identify and pull out the important taxa, we need to define a correlation-coefficient cutoff value, such as 0.70. Then print out the taxa with the correlation-coefficient greater than 0.70 from either dimension.

```
> corrcut <- 0.7
> genus_corr <- add.spec.scores(PCoA, fecalREL, method = "cor.scores")
$cproj
> import_genus <- genus_corr[abs(genus_corr[, 1]) >= corrcut |
abs(genus_corr[, 2]) >= corrcut, ]
```

The 12 important genera with correlation greater or equal 0.7 along the PCoA axes are printed as below:

```
> import_genus[complete.cases(import_genus),]
                          Dim1      Dim2
Tannerella             0.82046   0.16847
Lactobacillus         -0.30640  -0.86651
Helicobacter           0.74876   0.11758
Paraprevotella         0.74631  -0.08582
Bacillus               0.19803  -0.77265
Pedobacter            -0.24607   0.87028
Limibacter            -0.08244   0.70361
Mycoplasma             0.72268   0.22945
Slackia                0.09773  -0.75775
Fluviicola             0.24247  -0.71075
Caldicellulosiruptor   0.24247  -0.71075
Anaerophaga            0.24247  -0.71075
```

Finally, we use the envfit() function from the vegan package to conduct a permutation test for general abundances across axes on these correlations.

```
> envfit(PCoA, fecalREL, perm = 999)
```

The partial output is given below:

```
                   Dim1    Dim2     r2     Pr(>r)
Tannerella         0.951   0.308   0.70   0.044 *
Lactobacillus     -0.219  -0.976   0.84   0.013 *
Parasutterella    -0.754  -0.657   0.63   0.031 *
Porphyromonas      0.359  -0.933   0.56   0.072 .
Bacillus           0.160  -0.987   0.64   0.056 .
Pedobacter        -0.176   0.984   0.82   0.015 *
Slackia            0.081  -0.997   0.58   0.085 .
---
Signif. codes:  0 '***' 0.001 '**' 0.01 '*' 0.05 '.' 0.1 ' ' 1
Permutation: free
Number of permutations: 999
```

The genera with p-value less than 0.05 are displayed with plot below (Fig. 7.20):

```
> fit <- envfit(PCoA, fecalREL, perm = 999)
> plot(fit, p.max = 0.05, col = "red")
```

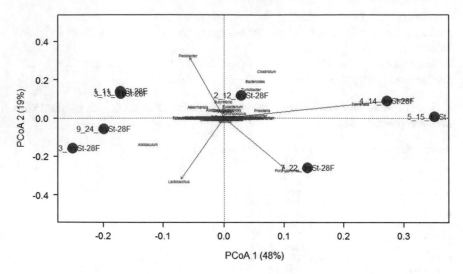

Fig. 7.20 Ordination plot for the two PCoA axes of influential genera with p-value < 0.05 in $Vdr^{-/-}$ mouse fecal data

7.4.3 Non-metric Multidimensional Scaling (NMDS)

NMDS is the non-metric alternative to PCoA analysis. NMDS has been recognized as a good ordination method because it uses ecologically meaningful ways to measure community dissimilarities and any distance (dissimilarities) measure among samples as input. Thus, it is the recommended method in community ordination. The main focus of NMDS analysis is to project the relative position of sample points into low dimensional ordination space (two or three axes).

The function metaMDS() in vegan package performs NMDS analysis. To simplify, the algorithm of NMDS analysis is summarized as below:

First, it uses the function vegdist() to get adequate dissimilarity measures; then it runs NMDS several times with random starting configurations and compares the results via the function procrustes(), and stops after finding twice a similar minimum stress solution. Finally, it scales and rotates the solution, and adds species (or OTUs/taxa) scores to the configuration as weighted averages using the function wascores(). After the algorithm is finished, the final solution is rotated using PCA to ease its interpretation.

In this case, we use vegan package and same $Vdr^{-/-}$ mice fecal data to illustrate NMDS analysis.

First, we use function vegdist() to get the Bray-Curtis dissimilarity measures (the default method) using the default setting of metaMDS() function. It automatically transforms data and checks solution robustness. Wisconsin double standardization and sqrt transformation were combinedly used in the metaMDS() function call. The function call produces stress value of 7.57%.

```
> bc_nmds <- metaMDS(abund_table, dist = "bray")
Square root transformation
Wisconsin double standardization
Run 0 stress 0.07574
Run 1 stress 0.1562
Run 2 stress 0.1284
Run 3 stress 0.1801
Run 4 stress 0.1284
Run 5 stress 0.1562
Run 6 stress 0.1678
Run 7 stress 0.1393
Run 8 stress 0.1562
Run 9 stress 0.1284
Run 10 stress 0.1393
Run 11 stress 0.1192
Run 12 stress 0.1764
Run 13 stress 0.1192
Run 14 stress 0.1551
Run 15 stress 0.1562
Run 16 stress 0.1562
Run 17 stress 0.07574
... Procrustes: rmse 1.314e-06  max resid 2.644e-06
... Similar to previous best
Run 18 stress 0.1284
Run 19 stress 0.1899
Run 20 stress 0.07574
... Procrustes: rmse 1.503e-06  max resid 2.229e-06
... Similar to previous best
*** Solution reached
> bc_nmds

Call:
metaMDS(comm = abund_table, distance = "bray")

global Multidimensional Scaling using monoMDS

Data:      wisconsin(sqrt(abund_table))
Distance:  bray

Dimensions:  2
Stress:        0.07574
Stress type 1, weak ties
Two convergent solutions found after 20 tries
Scaling: centring, PC rotation, halfchange scaling
Species: expanded scores based on 'wisconsin(sqrt(abund_table))'
```

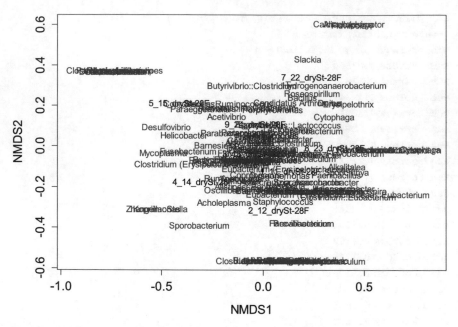

Fig. 7.21 Ordiplot of two NMDS axes with text labels in Vdr$^{-/-}$ mouse fecal data

Second, we use function ordiplot() to draw the results of NMDS. The default setting adds only points to the figure, we use the type = 't' or type = 'text' to add text labels in this figure (Fig. 7.21).

```
> ordiplot (bc_nmds, type = 't')
```

To plot site (sample) scores as text (Fig. 7.22):

```
> ordiplot(bc_nmds, display = "sites", type = "text")
```

Finally, the function stressplot() is used to draw the Shepards stress plot. The function stressplot() generates two figures: one plots ordination distances versus observed dissimilarity (the chosen community dissimilarities), along with a monotone step line to show the fit; another plots goodness of fit to assess goodness of ordination of NMDS2 versus NMDS1 of particular samples. The following R codes are used to divide plotting window into two panels:

```
> par (mfrow = c(1,2))
```

The function plot() draws NMDS ordination diagram with sites (samples):

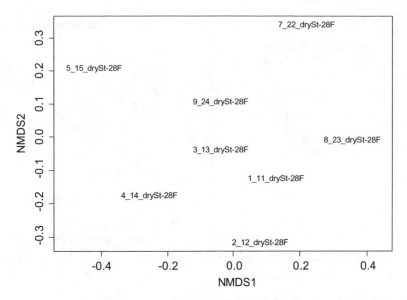

Fig. 7.22 Ordiplot of two NMDS axes with sample labels in $Vdr^{-/-}$ mouse fecal data

```
> stressplot (bc_nmds)
> plot (bc_nmds, display = 'sites', type = 't', main = 'Goodness of fit')
```

The function points() adds the points with size reflecting goodness of fit (bigger = worse fit) (Fig. 7.23).

```
> points (bc_nmds, display = 'sites', cex = goodness (bc_nmds)*300))
```

The stressplot shows the relationship between real distances between samples in resulting m dimensional ordination solution, and their particular compositional dissimilarities expressed by selected Bray-Curtis dissimilarity measure. There are two correlation-like statistics of goodness of fit; the correlation based on stress: $R^2 = 1 - S^2$ (non-metric fit = 0.994) and the correlation between the fitted values and ordination distances, or between the step line and the points: "fit-based R^2" (linear fit = 0.956).

7.4.4 Correspondence Analysis (CA)

CA is another unconstrained ordination method. It uses chi-square distances among samples in the multidimensional space of all ordination axes and gives high weight to rare species (e.g., low occurrence species with many zeros). The same as PCA and PCoA, CA uses eigenvalues to measure the importance of returned orthogonal axes.

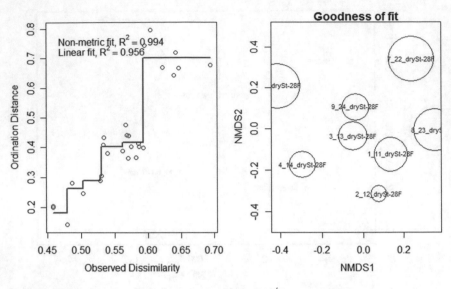

Fig. 7.23 Shepards stress plot and goodness of fit in $Vdr^{-/-}$ mouse fecal data

In PCA ordination diagram, taxa are vectors and samples are points, whereas in CA, taxa and samples are represented by points. Similar to PCA, CA has two types of scalings: Scalings 1 and 2. In the reduced ordination space, the distances among samples (Scaling 1) approximate their chi-square distance. For example, any sample near the point representing a taxon likely contains a high contribution to that taxon.

The distances among taxa (Scaling 2) also approximate their chi-square distances. For example, any taxon close to the point representing a sample more likely has higher frequency in that sample.

The function cca() in vegan package can be used to perform unconstrained correspondence analysis. We use function cca() to conduct CCA and function evplot() to select important ordination axes based on Kaiser-Guttman criterion or broken stick model. The function evplot(), written by Borcard et al. (2011), is used here to plot eigenvalues and percentages of variation of an ordination object.

When the function cca() (cca = canonical compoent analysis) is used to perform unconstrained CA, do not specify the environmental matrix or grouping information.

```
> fecal_genus_cca=cca(abund_table)
> fecal_genus_cca
Call: cca(X = abund_table)

                Inertia Rank
Total            0.502
Unconstrained    0.502     7
Inertia is mean squared contingency coefficient
122 species (variables) deleted due to missingness

Eigenvalues for unconstrained axes:
   CA1    CA2    CA3    CA4    CA5    CA6    CA7
0.2036 0.1256 0.0747 0.0374 0.0322 0.0200 0.0090
```

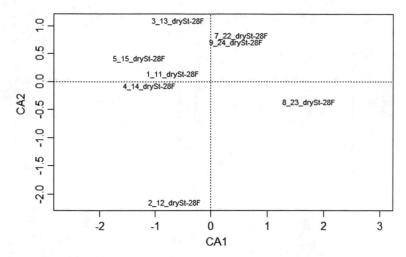

Fig. 7.24 Plotting the ordination and only showing the samples in the figure in *Vdr*$^{-/-}$ mouse fecal data

The total heterogeneity of the data (inertia) is 0.502, and the first axis captures 40.56% of total variation in genus composition (0.2036/0.502 = 0.4056, where 0.2036 is eigenvalue of the first axis CA1, and 0.502 is the total heterogeneity of the data).

The following R codes are used to plot the ordination and display the sample names in the figure (Fig. 7.24):

```
> plot(fecal_genus_cca, display="sites")
```

If you don't want the graph to be overcrowded, use the following R codes to just show points instead of sample names in the figure:

```
> plot(fecal_genus_cca, display="sites", type="p")
```

The following ordination diagram reveals the pattern of samples and genera in ordination diagram (Fig. 7.25):

```
> ordiplot (fecal_genus_cca)
```

The following post CA analysis using the function evplot() is to illustrate how to decide which CA axis should be used for interpretation of results. The syntax of the function evplot() is evplot(ev), where ev is a vector of eigenvalues. First, we run the function.

```
evplot <- function(ev)
{# Broken stick model
```

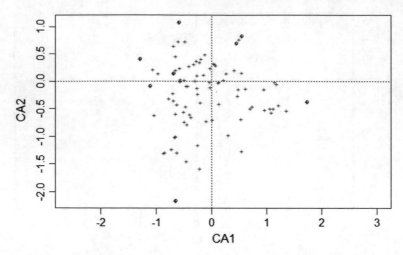

Fig. 7.25 Plotting the ordination and showing the pattern of samples and genera in ordination diagram in $Vdr^{-/-}$ mouse fecal data. The circles represent samples, whereas plus represents genera.

```
n <- length(ev)
bsm <- data.frame(j=seq(1:n), p=0)
bsm$p[1] <- 1/n
for (i in 2:n) bsm$p[i] <- bsm$p[i-1] + (1/(n + 1 - i))
bsm$p <- 100*bsm$p/n
# Plot eigenvalues and % of variation for each axis
op <- par(mfrow=c(2,1))
barplot(ev, main="Eigenvalues", col="bisque", las=2)
abline(h=mean(ev), col="red")
legend("topright", "Average eigenvalue", lwd=1, col=2, bty="n")
barplot(t(cbind(100*ev/sum(ev), bsm$p[n:1])), beside=TRUE,
        main="% variation", col=c("bisque",2), las=2)
legend("topright", c("% eigenvalue", "Broken stick model"),
        pch=15, col=c("bisque",2), bty="n")
par(op)
}

# Plot eigenvalues and % of variance for each axis
ev <- fecal_genus_cca$CA$eig

windows(title="CA eigenvalues")
evplot(ev)
```

As presented in section of PCoA, to assess whether the first few CA axes of the analysis capture a disproportionately large amount of the total explained variation, two additional post-ways using graphics are *Keiser-Guttman criterion* and *broken*

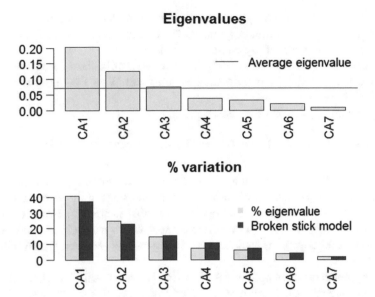

Fig. 7.26 Plotting eigenvalues and percentages of variation with Keiser-Guttman criterion and broken stick model in $Vdr^{-/-}$ mouse fecal data

stick model. Based on *Kaiser-Guttman criterion,* the eigenvalues associated with the first few axes should be larger than the average of all the eigenvalues; with *broken-stick model,* the eigenvalues associated with the first few axes are compared to the expectations. Both Keiser-Guttman criterion and broken stick model show that first three axes are important (Fig, 7.26).

7.4.5   Redundancy Analysis (RDA)

Counterparting to three basic ordination methods, the vegan package has three versions of constrained ordination: redundancy analysis (RDA, related to principal components analysis), constrained analysis of principal coordinates (CAP, related to metric scaling), and constrained correspondence analysis (CCA, related to correspondence analysis).

RDA in the function rda() is based on Euclidean distances and combines multiple regression with PCA. With RDA, each canonical axis is linear combination of all explanatory variables. The number of canonical axes corresponds to the number of explanatory variables, or more precisely to the number of degrees of freedoms (Borcard et al. 2011).

You can use two different syntaxes to calculate an RDA via the function rda ()
from vegan: matrix and formula syntaxes. The matrix syntax is simplest: just list the
names of objects separated by commas as below.

RDA = rda(Y, X, W), where Y is the response matrix (taxa composition), X is
the explanatory matrix (environmental factors) and W is the optional matrix of
co-variables.

The formula syntax is given below:

$$RDA = rda\,(Y \sim var\,1 + factor\,A + var\,2 * var\,3 + condition\,(var\,4), data = XW).$$

The left side of the formula, Y, is the response matrix (taxa composition);
constrainted or explanatory variables are in the right sides of the formula, including
a quantitative variable var 1, a categorical variable factor A, an interaction term
between var 2 and var 3, and co-variable var 4 which can be partialled out. The
explanatory and covariable variables are in object XW data set, which must be a
data frame.

The hypothesis test is not the case in PCA. However, with two data sets Y and
X, in RDA we can test a null hypothesis of absence of linear relationship between
them. We use smoker data set to illustrate the usage of RDA.

First, load data from GUniFrac Package and use the function select() from dplyr
package to create a subset of explanatory variables.

```
> library(GUniFrac)
> data(throat.otu.tab)
> data(throat.meta)

> library(dplyr)
> throat_meta <- select(throat.meta, SmokingStatus, Age, Sex, PackYears)
```

For the purpose of RDA, we transform the taxa data using Hellinger's
transformation:

```
> abund_hell <- decostand (throat.otu.tab, 'hell')
```

The RDA is calculated by the function rda() if matrix of environmental variables
is supplied (if not, PCA will be calculated as we did in Sect. 7.4.1).

```
> rda_hell<- rda(abund_hell ~ ., throat_meta)
> summary (rda_hell)
```

We print the partial output here.

```
Call:
rda(formula = abund_hell ~ SmokingStatus + Age + Sex + PackYears,        data =
throat_meta)

Partitioning of variance:
              Inertia Proportion
Total         0.46271    1.0000
Constrained   0.04823    0.1042
Unconstrained 0.41448    0.8958

Eigenvalues, and their contribution to the variance

Importance of components:
                        RDA1     RDA2     RDA3     RDA4     PC1     PC2     PC3
Eigenvalue           0.02393  0.01330 0.005969 0.005039  0.0683 0.05946 0.03554
Proportion Explained 0.05172  0.02874 0.012900 0.010890  0.1476 0.12849 0.07681
Cumulative Proportion0.05172  0.08045 0.093350 0.104240  0.2518 0.38034 0.45715

Accumulated constrained eigenvalues
Importance of components:
                        RDA1    RDA2     RDA3     RDA4
Eigenvalue           0.02393  0.0133 0.005969 0.005039
Proportion Explained 0.49612  0.2757 0.123740 0.104460
Cumulative Proportion 0.49612 0.7718 0.895540 1.000000

Scaling 2 for species and site scores
* Species are scaled proportional to eigenvalues
* Sites are unscaled: weighted dispersion equal on all dimensions
* General scaling constant of scores:  2.285815

Species scores

          RDA1        RDA2        RDA3        RDA4        PC1         PC2
4695  1.921e-03 -1.129e-02 -7.088e-03 -2.362e-03 -7.858e-04 -5.495e-04
2983  2.385e-03 -1.850e-03 -4.702e-03  4.402e-03  8.961e-04 -3.710e-03
(...)

Site scores (weighted sums of species scores)

                RDA1       RDA2      RDA3      RDA4       PC1        PC2
ESC_1.1_OPL  -0.444360 -0.479468 -0.17464 -0.351952  0.081583 -0.135377
ESC_1.3_OPL   0.601039 -0.226340 -0.10553 -0.275939  0.183698 -0.077295
(...)

Site constraints (linear combinations of constraining variables)

                RDA1       RDA2      RDA3       RDA4       PC1        PC2
ESC_1.1_OPL  -0.30617 -0.220346  0.030881 -0.328152  0.081583 -0.135377
ESC_1.3_OPL   0.32421  0.055762 -0.132139  0.107388  0.183698 -0.077295
(...)
Biplot scores for constraining variables

                        RDA1    RDA2     RDA3    RDA4 PC1 PC2
SmokingStatusSmoker   0.9064 -0.3399 -0.1354 0.21095   0   0
Age                   0.2275 -0.0442  0.7482 0.62172   0   0
SexMale               0.4961  0.8360  0.1026 0.21097   0   0
PackYears             0.6576 -0.1515  0.7376 0.02219   0   0


Centroids for factor constraints

                          RDA1     RDA2     RDA3     RDA4 PC1 PC2
SmokingStatusNonSmoker -0.2502  0.09382  0.03738 -0.05823   0   0
SmokingStatusSmoker     0.2860 -0.10723 -0.04273  0.06655   0   0
SexFemale              -0.1995 -0.33619 -0.04127 -0.08484   0   0
SexMale                 0.1074  0.18103  0.02222  0.04568   0   0
```

The four constrained ordination axes (named RDA1 to RDA4) are related to the 4 environmental variables (SmokingStatus, Age, Sex, PackYears). Unconstrained axes are named as PC axes.

The total variances are partitioned into constrained variance and unconstrained variance. The constrained variance is explained by constrained axes (i.e., environmental variables); whereas the unconstrained variance is explained by unconstrained axes (i.e., variance not explained by environmental factors). The constrained variance is the amount of variance that the Y matrix is explained by the explanatory variables. It is an equivalent to a biased, unadjusted R^2 in the multiple regression. The table for partitioning of variance shows that 4.8% (0.04823) of the proportion of the total variance is explained by all these 4 environmental factors.

The function coef() retrieves the canonical coefficients (the equivalent of regression coefficients) for each explanatory variable on each canonical axis.

```
> coef(rda_hell)
                         RDA1      RDA2      RDA3      RDA4
SmokingStatusSmoker   0.177040 -0.120402 -0.187134   0.15184
Age                  -0.004452 -0.002161  0.002997   0.01757
SexMale               0.092005  0.267873 -0.027579   0.01856
PackYears             0.005257 -0.000520  0.011633  -0.01596
```

We can use the function RsquareAdj() to extract the value of R^2 and adjusted R^2 from results of ordination.

```
> RsquareAdj(rda_hell)
$r.squared
[1] 0.1042

$adj.r.squared
[1] 0.03909
```

The function returns two R^2s: one is ordinary R^2 (r.squared), another is adjusted version R^2_{adj} (adj.r.squared). Note that R^2_{adj} is always lower than R^2, and the difference increases with increasing number of explanatory variables. R^2_{adj} can be negative, which means explanatory variables explaining less variation than the same number of randomly generated variables.

Apply Kaiser-Guttman criterion to residual axes.

```
> rda_hell$CA$eig[rda_hell$CA$eig
> mean(rda_hell$CA$eig)]
     PC1      PC2      PC3      PC4      PC5      PC6      PC7
0.068299 0.059456 0.035542 0.024040 0.017406 0.015601 0.014898
     PC8      PC9     PC10     PC11     PC12     PC13
0.012182 0.010314 0.009654 0.009245 0.008760 0.007745
```

Next, we plot the results of RDA. Based on which ordination of your interest, you can choose to plot type 1 scaling or type 2 scaling. If you are primarily interested in the ordination of samples, scaling 1 is your most appropriate choice. If you are primarily interested in the ordination of taxa, then, scaling 2 is your most appropriate choice.

Type 1 scaling emphasizes the relationships among samples. The essential features (Borcard et al. 2011; Legendre and Legendre 2012) are samples act as the centroids of the response variables (columns) and the distances between sample points indicate their χ^2 distances. The interpretation is based on: (1) sample points that are close each other are likely to be relative similar regarding to their relative frequencies; (2) samples near centroids representing states of categorical or qualitative variables are more likely to possess the state for that species/taxon; and (3) a right-angled projection of an sample point onto a vector representing a quantitative explanatory variable approximates the value of the variable realized for that sample.

Type 2 scaling emphasizes the relationships among response variables. The essential features are response variables (columns) act as the centroids of the samples and the distances between response variable points indicate their χ^2 distances. The interpretation is based on: (1) species/taxon points that close to each other are likely to have similar relative frequencies along the samples; (2) the closer a response variable(a species/taxon) is to the centroid representing a state of a categorical explanatory variable, the more likely that response variable is to have higher values at that state; and (3) a right-angled projection of a point representing a response variable (a species/taxon) onto an arrow representing an explanatory variable indicates the position of the maximum value (the optimum) of the response variable along that explanatory variable.

In constrained ordination, one additional source data is available for plot: explanatory (environmental) variables. Thus, three different data are available for plotting: samples, response variables, and explanatory variables. If you display all data from three sources, you have 'triplot'. If you display two source data, you have 'biplot'. The following R codes generate a type 2 scaling triplot:

```
> plot(rda_hell, display=c("sp", "lc", "cn"),main="Triplot
RDA - scaling 2")
```

In above codes, "sp" stands for species (display = "sp"), and "cn" for constraints or the explanatory variables (display = "cn"). There are two sample scores in vegan package: weighted sums of species/taxa (display = "wa"), and fitted sample scores or "LC scores" (display = "lc"), i.e., linear combinations of explanatory variables. You can choose one of them to display in one plot.

The following R codes are used to add arrows to display species/taxa. The argument of the scores() function "choices=c(1,2)" is the axes to plot. The defaults plot the axes 1 and 2. Therefore, we can omit the codes "choices=c(1,2)" (Fig. 7.27).

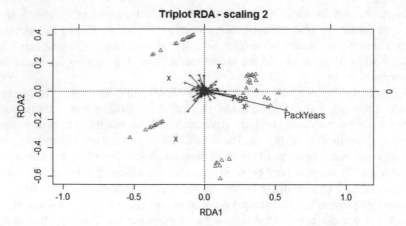

Fig. 7.27 RDA triplot of the smoker throat abundance constrained by SmokingStatus, Age, Sex, PackYear with type 2 Scaling

```
> taxa_scores <- scores(rda_hell, choices=c(1,2), display="sp")
> arrows(0, 0, taxa_scores[,1], taxa_scores[,2], length=0, lty=1,
col="red")
```

In above triplot RDA-scaling 2, green hollow triangles represent samples, blue crosses represent the states of a categorical explanatory variable (e.g., male, femal, or smoker, non-smoker), and blue arrows for quantitative explanatory variables (here, PackYears and Age) with arrowheads indicating their direction of increase, and the species/taxa are shown as red plus.

To test the significance of the variation in the smoker community data explained by explanatory variables, we can conduct a Monte Carlo permutation test via the function anova.cca() in vegan package. This function can test the significances of the global model (default), all axes (by = "axis"), individual explanatory variables (by = "terms"), the first constrained axis (first = TRUE), or variation explained by individual explanatory variables after removing variation of all other variables in the model (by = "margin"). We illustrate its capability by testing the global model, each axis and each explanatory variable, respectively.

To ensure getting same result of permutation test each time you run, set the same seed.

```
> set.seed (123)
```

The following R codes test the significance of the global model. The argument "step" specifies the minimal number of permutations.

```
> anova(rda_hell, step=1000)
Permutation test for rda under reduced model
Permutation: free
Number of permutations: 999
Model: rda(formula = abund_hell ~ SmokingStatus + Age + Sex + PackYears, data
= throat_meta)
          Df Variance    F Pr(>F)
Model      4   0.048  1.6  0.006 **
Residual 55   0.414
---
Signif. codes:  0 '***' 0.001 '**' 0.01 '*' 0.05 '.' 0.1 ' ' 1
```

The global test is statistically significant. Now let's test each axis.

```
> anova(rda_hell, by="axis", step=1000)
Permutation test for rda under reduced model
Marginal tests for axes
Permutation: free
Number of permutations: 999

Model: rda(formula = abund_hell ~ SmokingStatus + Age + Sex + PackYears, data
= throat_meta)
          Df Variance     F Pr(>F)
RDA1       1   0.024  3.18  0.001 ***
RDA2       1   0.013  1.76  0.032 *
RDA3       1   0.006  0.79  0.735
RDA4       1   0.005  0.67  0.886
Residual 55   0.414
---
Signif. codes:  0 '***' 0.001 '**' 0.01 '*' 0.05 '.' 0.1 ' ' 1
```

We can see that the first and second axis are significant.

Now let's test the significance of each explanatory variable.

```
> anova(rda_hell, by="terms", step=1000)
Permutation test for rda under reduced model
Terms added sequentially (first to last)
Permutation: free
Number of permutations: 999

Model: rda(formula = abund_hell ~ SmokingStatus + Age + Sex + PackYears, data
= throat_meta)
              Df Variance     F Pr(>F)
SmokingStatus  1   0.022  2.86  0.001 ***
Age            1   0.006  0.75  0.787
Sex            1   0.014  1.92  0.017 *
PackYears      1   0.007  0.88  0.601
Residual      55   0.414
---
Signif. codes:  0 '***' 0.001 '**' 0.01 '*' 0.05 '.' 0.1 ' ' 1
```

We can see that both SmokingStatus and Sex are significant.

Finally, we use forward selection to reduce the number of explanatory variables entering the analysis, while optimazing the variation explained by them.

Curently, three functions are available in RDA for forward selection: ordistep(), ordiR2step(), and forward.sel().The first two functions are from package vegan. The third is available from package "adespatial". These functions use different criteria for variable selection. The function ordistep() uses the AIC criteria and p-values from Monte Carlo permutation test for the comparison of variable.The function ordiR2step() uses R^2_{adj}. The function forward.sel() uses the preselected significance level of α as the variable selection criterion.

Although the function forward.sel() has different logic for setting arguments, comparing to the other two functions, basically the returned results are same as ordiR2step(). Thus, we only illustrate the first two functions. The procedure ordistep() is applicable with functions rda(), cca() or cmdscale(). The ordiR2step() can be applied only to rda() and capscale(), but not for cca() because cca() doesn't return R^2_{adj}.

The following R codes use the function ordistep() to run forward selection. Options for stepwise and backward selection are also available. This function allows the use of factors.

```
> step_forward <- ordistep(rda(abund_hell ~ 1, data=throat_meta),
+     scope=formula(rda_hell), direction="forward", pstep=1000)

Start: abund_hell ~ 1

                 Df    AIC    F  Pr(>F)
+ SmokingStatus  1  -46.1 2.83  0.005 **
+ Sex            1  -45.3 2.01  0.015 *
+ PackYears      1  -45.1 1.80  0.045 *
+ Age            1  -44.1 0.83  0.720
---
Signif. codes:  0 '***' 0.001 '**' 0.01 '*' 0.05 '.' 0.1 ' ' 1


Step: abund_hell ~ SmokingStatus

             Df    AIC    F  Pr(>F)
+ Sex        1  -46.0 1.87  0.025 *
+ PackYears  1  -45.0 0.87  0.650
+ Age        1  -44.9 0.74  0.820
---
Signif. codes:  0 '***' 0.001 '**' 0.01 '*' 0.05 '.' 0.1 ' ' 1


Step: abund_hell ~ SmokingStatus + Sex

             Df    AIC    F  Pr(>F)
+ PackYears  1  -45.0 0.85  0.66
+ Age        1  -44.9 0.81  0.69
```

This procedure chooses variables SmokingStatus and Sex. The following forward selection uses the function ordiR2step().The default setting for this procedure to include a new variable is based on R^2_{adj} and their comparison with that of the global model (with all variables). The selection will be stopped if the new variable is not significant or the R^2_{adj} of the model including this new variable would exceed the R^2_{adj} of the global model.

```
> step_forward <- ordiR2step(rda(abund_hell ~ 1, data=throat_meta),
+                            scope=formula(rda_hell), direction="forward",
  pstep=1000)
Step: R2.adj= 0
Call: abund_hell ~ 1

                  R2.adjusted
<All variables>      0.039094
+ SmokingStatus     0.030093
+ Sex               0.016765
+ PackYears         0.013326
<none>              0.000000
+ Age              -0.002834


                 Df   AIC    F Pr(>F)
+ SmokingStatus   1 -46.1 2.83  0.002 **
---
Signif. codes:  0 '***' 0.001 '**' 0.01 '*' 0.05 '.' 0.1 ' ' 1

Step: R2.adj= 0.03009
Call: abund_hell ~ SmokingStatus

                  R2.adjusted
+ Sex                0.04449
<All variables>      0.03909
<none>               0.03009
+ PackYears          0.02786
+ Age                0.02574
```

The variable smoking status is selected by the forward selection using the function ordiR2step().

After running forward selection procedure, we fit the final parsimonious RDA model and test with the global model, each axis and each variable:

```
> rda_final<-rda(abund_hell~SmokingStatus+Sex, data=throat_meta)

> anova(rda_final, step=1000)

Permutation test for rda under reduced model
Permutation: free
Number of permutations: 999

Model: rda(formula = abund_hell ~ SmokingStatus + Sex, data = throat_meta)
            Df Variance    F Pr(>F)
Model        2    0.036 2.37  0.001 ***
Residual    57    0.427
---
Signif. codes:  0 '***' 0.001 '**' 0.01 '*' 0.05 '.' 0.1 ' ' 1
```

```
> anova(rda_final, by="axis", step=1000)
Permutation test for rda under reduced model
Marginal tests for axes
Permutation: free
Number of permutations: 999

Model: rda(formula = abund_hell ~ SmokingStatus + Sex, data = throat_meta)
          Df Variance     F Pr(>F)
RDA1       1    0.023  3.01  0.001 ***
RDA2       1    0.013 1.74  0.031 *
Residual 57    0.427
---
Signif. codes:  0 '***' 0.001 '**' 0.01 '*' 0.05 '.' 0.1 ' ' 1

> anova(rda_final, by="terms", step=1000)
Permutation test for rda under reduced model
Terms added sequentially (first to last)
Permutation: free
Number of permutations: 999

Model: rda(formula = abund_hell ~ SmokingStatus + Sex, data = throat_meta)
              Df Variance     F Pr(>F)
SmokingStatus  1    0.022 2.87  0.003 **
Sex            1    0.014 1.87  0.022 *
Residual      57    0.427
---
Signif. codes:  0 '***' 0.001 '**' 0.01 '*' 0.05 '.' 0.1 ' ' 1
```

7.4.6 Constrained Correspondence Analysis (CCA)

CCA is also known as canonical correspondence analysis. Since its introduction in 1986, it has been one of the most popular ordination methods in community ecology and accepted by microbiome researchers (ter Braak 1986). Just like RDA relating to PCA, CAP relates to PCoA, and CCA relates to CA. CCA shares the basic properties of CA and combines them into a constrained ordination. CCA is performed by the function cca(). Its algorithm is based on Legendre and Legendre's (1998): it preserves the χ^2 distance among samples, and taxa are represented as points in the tripplots (Borcard et al. 2011). The calculated χ^2 distance is subjected to weighted linear regression on constraining variables, and the fitted values are passed to correspondence analysis performed via singular value decomposition (svd). Thus, it is a weighted form of RDA.

Like RDA, there are two kinds of syntaxes of CCA. One is simple (default) matrix syntax:

$$cca\,(X, Y, Z)$$

where, X = community data matrix or data frame, it must be given; Y = constraining matrix or data frame, typically of environmental variables (can be omitted); If matrix Y is supplied, it is used to conduct CCA, if not supplied, it calculates CA. Z = conditioning matrix or data frame (also can be omitted). If matrix Z is supplied, then the effect will be partialled out from the community matrix.

Another is formula syntax:

cca(formula, data, na.action = na.fail, subset = NULL)

where, formula is typical model formula: the left side of the formula must be the community data matrix(X); right side defines the constraining model: the constraining variables can contain ordered or unordered factors, interactions among variables and functions of variables; and conditioning variables can be given within a special function condition for conditioning variables (covariables) partialled out before analysis. So the following commands are equivalent: cca(X, Y, Z), cca (X ~ Y + condition(Z)), where Y and Z refer to constraints and conditions matrices respectively. The data is a data frame containing the variables on the right hand side of the model formula. The na.action() is used to handle the missing values in constraints or conditions. The default (na.fail) is to stop with missing value; na. omit is to remove all rows with missing values; na.exclude is to keep all observations but give NA for results that cannot be calculated. However, missing values are never allowed in dependent community data. The subset is used to subset of data rows.

In this section, we will use smoker data to conduct CCA through the function cca () from vegan package. We mentioned earlier, to conduct CCA, the matrix of environmental variables must be supplied, and otherwise the function cca() calculates CA. As recall, smoker data have two data sets: throat.otu.tab (community abundance data frame) and throat.meta(meta data including two binary variables SmokingStatus and Sex, and two continuous variables Age and PackYears). To run a CCA, load vegan library now and do not transform the community abundance data by Hellinger method as we did in RDA. Otherwise, the χ^2 distance cannot be calculated and the results cannot be interpreted.

In the following CCA, smoker abundance data are constrained by four environmental variables in the throat.meta data including SmokingStatus, Age, Sex, and PackYears.

```
> smoker_cca <- cca(throat.otu.tab ~ ., throat_meta)
> smoker_cca
Call: cca(formula = throat.otu.tab ~ SmokingStatus + Age
+ Sex + PackYears, data = throat_meta)

              Inertia Proportion Rank
Total          4.9330     1.0000
Constrained    0.3782     0.0767    4
Unconstrained  4.5548     0.9233   55
Inertia is mean squared contingency coefficient

Eigenvalues for constrained axes:
   CCA1    CCA2    CCA3    CCA4
 0.1517  0.0912  0.0781  0.0572

Eigenvalues for unconstrained axes:
   CA1    CA2    CA3    CA4    CA5    CA6    CA7    CA8
 0.457  0.358  0.325  0.299  0.237  0.187  0.165  0.160
(Showed only 8 of all 55 unconstrained eigenvalues)
```

The first section after the "Call:" give the "mean squared contingency coefficients" of the analysis. They play the same role in CCA that total variance plays in RDA. Since the community matrix is converted to χ^2 distance, the entries are contingency coefficients. The total variation before the matrix is subjected to weighted regression is 4.9330; this is the variation that could be explained. The variation in the community matrix that explained after weighted regression is 0.3782; this is the variation that will be explained by the axes in the CCA. The variance of the residuals of the regression is 4.5548; this is the variation that will not be explained by the axes in the CCA, which can be subjected to CA.

Here, we notice that the CCA is not very successful because only 0.3782/4.9330 or 0.0767 (see the column Proportion and row Constrained) of the total variation of data was captured in the CCA by all four variables. The variance explained by particular axes could be found by summary() function:

```
> summary(smoker_cca)
Call:
cca(formula = throat.otu.tab ~ SmokingStatus + Age + Sex + PackYears, data =
throat_meta)

Partitioning of mean squared contingency coefficient:
                Inertia Proportion
Total            4.933     1.0000
Constrained      0.378     0.0767
Unconstrained    4.555     0.9233

Eigenvalues,and their contribution to the mean squared contingency
coefficient

Importance of components:
                        CCA1    CCA2    CCA3    CCA4     CA1     CA2
Eigenvalue            0.1517  0.0912  0.0781  0.0572  0.4567  0.3581
Proportion Explained  0.0307  0.0185  0.0158  0.0116  0.0926  0.0726
Cumulative Proportion 0.0307  0.0492  0.0651  0.0767  0.1692  0.2418
(...)

Accumulated constrained eigenvalues
Importance of components:
                        CCA1    CCA2    CCA3    CCA4
Eigenvalue            0.152   0.0912  0.0781  0.0572
Proportion Explained  0.401   0.2411  0.2066  0.1512
Cumulative Proportion 0.401   0.6422  0.8488  1.0000
(...)


Biplot scores for constraining variables
                       CCA1    CCA2     CCA3    CCA4 CA1 CA2
SmokingStatusSmoker   0.831   0.452   0.0597 0.3181   0   0
Age                   0.202  -0.179  -0.7738 0.5729   0   0
SexMale               0.683  -0.730   0.0444 0.0112   0   0
PackYears             0.615   0.163  -0.7704 0.0303   0   0
Centroids for factor constraints
                          CCA1    CCA2     CCA3     CCA4 CA1 CA2
SmokingStatusNonSmoker  -0.746  -0.406  -0.0531 -0.28569   0   0
SmokingStatusSmoker      0.926   0.503   0.0660  0.35459   0   0
SexFemale               -0.922   0.985  -0.0599 -0.01516   0   0
SexMale                  0.505  -0.540   0.0328  0.00831   0   0
```

The variance explained by first four constrained axes (CCA1, CCA2, CCA3, CCA4): 3.07, 1.85 1.58, and 1.16%, respectively. The variance explained by first unconstrained axis (CA1) is 9.26%.

The section of "Accumulated constrained eigenvalues" provides the eigenvalues associated with the projection. Because we have four variables in our environmental dataframe, there are four constrained eigenvalues. As shown here, the first axis accounts for approximately 40% of the constrained variation, with the second axis at 24%, the third at 21%, and the fourth at 15%.

Next, we plot the results of CCA for type 1 scaling using the plot() function. In the plot, we want to display linear constraints or "LC scores" (display = "lc") and centroids of levels of factor variables (display = "cn").

```
plot(smoker_cca,scaling=1,display = c("lc","cn"),main="Biplot
CCA-scaling 1")
```

The type 1 scaling shows four groups of samples, with smoker group linked to PackYears. In this analysis, the first axis is associated with increasing PackYears while the second is associated with decreasing Age (Fig. 7.28).

Similar as in RDA, let's conduct a permutation test for the global model, each axis and each explanatory variable. To ensure getting the same result of permutation test, each time you run, set the same seed.

```
> set.seed (123)
```

The following R codes test the significance of the global model.

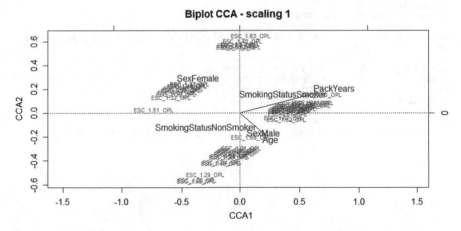

Fig. 7.28 CCA biplot of the smoker throat abundance constrained by SmokingStatus, Age, Sex, PackYear with type 1 Scaling

```
> anova(smoker_cca, step=1000)
Permutation test for cca under reduced model
Permutation: free
Number of permutations: 999

Model: cca(formula = throat.otu.tab ~ SmokingStatus + Age + Sex + PackYears,
data = throat_meta)
         Df ChiSquare    F Pr(>F)
Model     4     0.38 1.14    0.2
Residual 55     4.55
```

The result is not statistically significant.

Then test the significance of each axis.

```
> anova (smoker_cca, by = 'axis',step=1000)
Permutation test for cca under reduced model
Marginal tests for axes
Permutation: free
Number of permutations: 999

Model: cca(formula = throat.otu.tab ~ SmokingStatus + Age + Sex + PackYears,
data = throat_meta)
         Df ChiSquare    F Pr(>F)
CCA1      1     0.15 1.83  0.004 **
CCA2      1     0.09 1.10  0.350
CCA3      1     0.08 0.94  0.611
CCA4      1     0.06 0.69  0.959
Residual 55     4.55
---
Signif. codes:  0 '***' 0.001 '**' 0.01 '*' 0.05 '.' 0.1 ' ' 1
```

We can see that the first axis is significant.

Now let's test the significance of each explanatory variable.

```
> anova (smoker_cca, by = 'terms')
Permutation test for cca under reduced model
Terms added sequentially (first to last)
Permutation: free
Number of permutations: 999

Model: cca(formula = throat.otu.tab ~ SmokingStatus + Age + Sex + PackYears,
data = throat_meta)
                Df ChiSquare    F Pr(>F)
SmokingStatus    1      0.13 1.56  0.009 **
Age              1      0.07 0.89  0.751
Sex              1      0.10 1.27  0.104
PackYears        1      0.07 0.85  0.768
Residual        55      4.55
---
Signif. codes:  0 '***' 0.001 '**' 0.01 '*' 0.05 '.' 0.1 ' ' 1
```

We can see that SmokingStatus is significant with p-value of 0.009.

Finally, let's do forward selection using the function ordistep() in vegan package. As we stated in RDA, the function ordistep() is applicable with functions rda(), cca() or cmdscale().

Comparing variables is based on AIC criteria and p-values from Monte Carlo permutation test.

```
> ordistep(cca(throat.otu.tab ~ 1
  ,data=throat_meta),scope=formula(smoker_cca), direction="forward",
pstep=1000)

Start: throat.otu.tab ~ 1

                  Df    AIC      F Pr(>F)
+ SmokingStatus  1 539.05 1.5638   0.015 *
+ Sex            1 539.17 1.4378   0.025 *
+ PackYears      1 539.34 1.2775   0.225
+ Age            1 539.73 0.8914   0.795
---
Signif. codes:  0 '***' 0.001 '**' 0.01 '*' 0.05 '.' 0.1 ' ' 1

Step: throat.otu.tab ~ SmokingStatus

              Df    AIC      F Pr(>F)
+ Sex        1 539.71 1.2838   0.075 .
+ PackYears  1 540.04 0.9688   0.555
+ Age        1 540.12 0.8877   0.760
---
Signif. codes:  0 '***' 0.001 '**' 0.01 '*' 0.05 '.' 0.1 ' ' 1

Call: cca(formula = throat.otu.tab ~ SmokingStatus, data = throat_meta)

                Inertia Proportion Rank
Total           4.93301    1.00000
Constrained     0.12951    0.02625    1
Unconstrained   4.80350    0.97375   58
Inertia is mean squared contingency coefficient

Eigenvalues for constrained axes:
   CCA1
0.12951
```

```
Eigenvalues for unconstrained axes:
   CA1    CA2    CA3    CA4    CA5    CA6    CA7    CA8
0.4840 0.3834 0.3322 0.3025 0.2486 0.1884 0.1774 0.1614
(Showed only 8 of all 58 unconstrained eigenvalues)

> ordistep(cca(throat.otu.tab ~ 1, data=throat_meta),
scope=formula(smoker_cca), direction="forward", pstep=1000)

Start: throat.otu.tab ~ 1

                Df AIC     F Pr(>F)
+ SmokingStatus  1 539 1.56  0.005 **
+ Sex            1 539 1.44  0.045 *
+ PackYears      1 539 1.28  0.190
+ Age            1 540 0.89  0.710
---
Signif. codes:  0 '***' 0.001 '**' 0.01 '*' 0.05 '.' 0.1 ' ' 1


Step: throat.otu.tab ~ SmokingStatus

            Df AIC      F Pr(>F)
+ Sex        1 540 1.28   0.08 .
+ PackYears  1 540 0.97   0.54
+ Age        1 540 0.89   0.78
---
Signif. codes:  0 '***' 0.001 '**' 0.01 '*' 0.05 '.' 0.1 ' ' 1

Call: cca(formula = throat.otu.tab ~ SmokingStatus, data = throat_meta)

              Inertia Proportion Rank
Total          4.9330     1.0000
Constrained    0.1295     0.0263    1
Unconstrained  4.8035     0.9737   58
Inertia is mean squared contingency coefficient

Eigenvalues for constrained axes:
  CCA1
0.1295

Eigenvalues for unconstrained axes:
  CA1   CA2   CA3   CA4   CA5   CA6   CA7   CA8
0.484 0.383 0.332 0.302 0.249 0.188 0.177 0.161
(Showed only 8 of all 58 unconstrained eigenvalues)
```

The selected variable is SmokingStatus. The final model is fitted below.

```
> (smoker_cca_final <- cca(throat.otu.tab ~ SmokingStatus, data=throat_meta))
> anova.cca(smoker_cca_final, step=1000)
Call: cca(formula = throat.otu.tab ~ SmokingStatus, data = throat_meta)

                Inertia Proportion Rank
Total            4.9330    1.0000
Constrained      0.1295    0.0263     1
Unconstrained    4.8035    0.9737    58
Inertia is mean squared contingency coefficient
Eigenvalues for constrained axes:
  CCA1
0.1295

Eigenvalues for unconstrained axes:
   CA1   CA2   CA3   CA4   CA5   CA6   CA7   CA8
 0.484 0.383 0.332 0.302 0.249 0.188 0.177 0.161
(Showed only 8 of all 58 unconstrained eigenvalues)

> anova.cca(smoker_cca_final, step=1000)
Permutation test for cca under reduced model
Permutation: free
Number of permutations: 999

Model: cca(formula = throat.otu.tab ~ SmokingStatus, data = throat_meta)
          Df ChiSquare    F Pr(>F)
Model      1      0.13 1.56  0.007 **
Residual 58      4.80
---
Signif. codes:  0 '***' 0.001 '**' 0.01 '*' 0.05 '.' 0.1 ' ' 1
```

Smoking Status reaches the same level of significance with p-value of 0.007. However, the parsimony model has paid off with larger residual.

7.4.7   Constrained Analysis of Principal Coordinates (CAP)

CAP (also called constrained analysis of proximities in vegan package), is an ordination method similar to RDA. It is simply a redundancy analysis of results of principal coordinates analysis (or metric multidimensional scaling) (Anderson and Willis 2003). CAP allows non-Euclidean dissimilarity indices, such as Manhattan or Bray-Curtis distance. If Euclidean distance is specified as the ordination method, the results will be identical to RDA.

The function capscale() from vegan package is used to implement CAP. It needs a dissimilarity matrix as input data set, which can be calculated using functions vegdist(), dist(), or any other method producing similar matrices. Two steps are needed: first, it uses the function cmdscale () to ordinate the dissimilarity matrix, then uses RDA to analyze these results. Unlike RDA, in which both matrix and formula syntaxes can be used, the function capscale() can be called only with the formula syntax. One usage of the function capscale() is listed below.

$$\text{capscale(formula, data, distance} = ''\text{bray}'', \text{dfun} = \text{vegdist)}$$

where, formula is a typical model formula as defined in rda() and cca(). The left side of the formula must be either a community data matrix (frame) or a dissimilarity matrix, which can be estimated from the function vegdist() or dist(). If the left side of the formula is a data matrix (frame) instead of dissimilarity matrix, then a dissimilarity (or distance) index must be provided as input of distance. The right side of the formula defines the constraints. The constraining variables can be continuous variables, factors, interaction terms or a special term condition used as defining variables to be partialled out. The data are a data frame containing the variables on the right hand side of the model formula. The dfun is the distance or dissimilarity function used.

The basic CAP can be done with following codes. The constraining variables include two binary variables (SmokingStatus and Sex), and two continuous variables (PackYears and Age). The special term condition (Age) is used to be partialled out age effect.

```
> throat_cap <- capscale(throat.otu.tab ~ SmokingStatus + Sex + PackYears +
Condition(Age), throat_meta, dist="bray")
> throat_cap
Call: capscale(formula = throat.otu.tab ~ SmokingStatus + Sex + PackYears +
Condition(Age), data = throat_meta, distance = "bray")

              Inertia Proportion Eigenvals Rank
Total         14.0932     1.0000   14.5356
Conditional    0.2020     0.0143    0.2084    1
Constrained    1.2438     0.0883    1.2623    3
Unconstrained 12.6473     0.8974   13.0648   46
Imaginary                          -0.4425   13
Inertia is squared Bray distance

Eigenvalues for constrained axes:
 CAP1  CAP2  CAP3
0.731 0.376 0.155

Eigenvalues for unconstrained axes:
 MDS1  MDS2  MDS3  MDS4  MDS5  MDS6  MDS7  MDS8
2.278 1.994 1.144 0.925 0.749 0.615 0.534 0.473
(Showed only 8 of all 46 unconstrained eigenvalues)
```

The first three axes are called "CAP1", "CAP2", and "CAP3", and then followed by original MDS. We can see that the three constrained variables (SmokingStatus, Sex and PackYears) explain 8.83% of the total variation of whole data set.

```
> anova(throat_cap)
Permutation test for capscale under reduced model
Permutation: free
Number of permutations: 999

Model: capscale(formula = throat.otu.tab ~ SmokingStatus + Sex + PackYears +
Condition(Age), data = throat_meta, distance = "bray")
         Df SumOfSqs    F Pr(>F)
Model     3     1.24  1.8  0.004 **
Residual 55    12.65
---
Signif. codes:  0 '***' 0.001 '**' 0.01 '*' 0.05 '.' 0.1 ' ' 1
```

The model is statistically significant with p-value of 0.004.

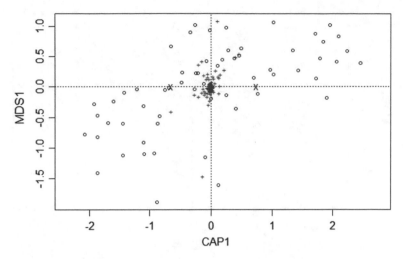

Fig. 7.29 Basic plot of CAP in smoker throat data

The default plot() function generates the following figure, it is not informative (Fig. 7.29).

```
> plot(throat_cap)
```

As we are interested in the different dissimilarities between smokers vs. non-smokers, let's extract the group information here.

```
> groups <- throat.meta$SmokingStatus
> groups
 [1] NonSmoker Smoker    Smoker    Smoker    Smoker    Smoker
 [7] NonSmoker NonSmoker NonSmoker NonSmoker Smoker    NonSmoker
[13] NonSmoker Smoker    NonSmoker Smoker    Smoker    NonSmoker
[19] NonSmoker NonSmoker NonSmoker NonSmoker NonSmoker NonSmoker
[25] NonSmoker NonSmoker NonSmoker NonSmoker NonSmoker NonSmoker
[31] NonSmoker NonSmoker NonSmoker Smoker    NonSmoker NonSmoker
[37] NonSmoker NonSmoker NonSmoker Smoker    NonSmoker Smoker
[43] NonSmoker Smoker    Smoker    Smoker    Smoker    Smoker
[49] Smoker    Smoker    Smoker    Smoker    Smoker    Smoker
[55] Smoker    Smoker    Smoker    NonSmoker Smoker    Smoker
Levels: NonSmoker Smoker
```

In the following bunch of R codes, the function plot() generates an empty CAP ordination diagram; the function points() adds points to the ordination diagram (low-level plotting function) created by the plot. The function ordispider() creates spiderplot by connecting individual members of the group with the group centroid. The function ordiellipse() encircles the clouds of points within the group by ellipse like the envelopes (Fig. 7.30).

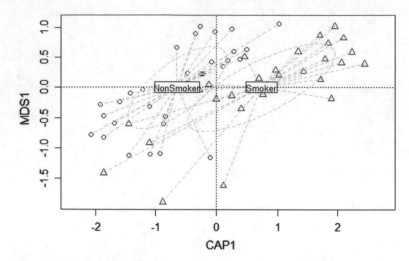

Fig. 7.30 Ordispider and ordiellipse plots of CAP in smoker throat data

```
> plot(throat_cap, type="n")
> points(throat_cap, col=as.numeric(as.factor(groups)),
+        pch=as.numeric(as.factor(groups)))
> ordispider(throat_cap, groups, lty=2, col="grey", label=T)
> ordiellipse(throat_cap, groups, lty=2, col="grey", label=F)
```

Similar as in RDA and CCA, let's conduct a permutation test for the global model, each axis and each explanatory variable.

To ensure getting same result of permutation test each time you run, set the same seed.

```
> set.seed(123)
```

The following codes test the significance of the global model.

```
> anova(throat_cap, step=1000)
Permutation test for capscale under reduced model
Permutation: free
Number of permutations: 999

Model: capscale(formula = throat.otu.tab ~ SmokingStatus + Sex + PackYears +
Condition(Age), data = throat_meta, distance = "bray")
         Df SumOfSqs    F Pr(>F)
Model     3    1.24   1.8  0.003 **
Residual 55   12.65
---
Signif. codes:  0 '***' 0.001 '**' 0.01 '*' 0.05 '.' 0.1 ' ' 1
```

The result is statistically significant with *p*-value of 0.003.

Then test the significance of each axis.

```
> anova(throat_cap, by="axis", step=1000)
Permutation test for capscale under reduced model
Marginal tests for axes
Permutation: free
Number of permutations: 999

Model: capscale(formula = throat.otu.tab ~ SmokingStatus + Sex + PackYears +
Condition(Age), data = throat_meta, distance = "bray")
          Df SumOfSqs    F  Pr(>F)
CAP1       1    0.73  3.08  0.001 ***
CAP2       1    0.38  1.58  0.073 .
CAP3       1    0.16  0.65  0.869
Residual  55   13.06
---
Signif. codes:   0 '***' 0.001 '**' 0.01 '*' 0.05 '.' 0.1 ' ' 1
```

We can see that the first axis is significant with *p*-value of 0.001 and second axis is marginally significant with *p*-value of 0.073.

Now let's test the significance of each explanatory variable.

```
> anova(throat_cap, by="terms", step=1000)
Permutation test for capscale under reduced model
Terms added sequentially (first to last)
Permutation: free
Number of permutations: 999

Model: capscale(formula = throat.otu.tab ~ SmokingStatus + Sex + PackYears +
Condition(Age), data = throat_meta, distance = "bray")
               Df SumOfSqs    F  Pr(>F)
SmokingStatus   1    0.63  2.72  0.003 **
Sex             1    0.44  1.89  0.035 *
PackYears       1    0.18  0.79  0.682
Residual       55   12.65
---
Signif. codes:   0 '***' 0.001 '**' 0.01 '*' 0.05 '.' 0.1 ' ' 1
```

We can see that both SmokingStatus and Sex are significant with *p*-values = 0.003, and 0.035, respectively.

Now, let's do forward selection using the function ordistep() in vegan package. As we stated in RDA and CCA, the function compares variables based on AIC criteria and *p*-values from Monte Carlo permutation test.

```
> step_forward <- ordistep(capscale(throat.otu.tab ~ 1, data=throat_meta),
+                 scope=formula(throat_cap), direction="forward", pstep=1000)

Start: throat.otu.tab ~ 1


                 Df AIC     F  Pr(>F)
+ SmokingStatus  1 712 2.05  0.035 *
+ Sex            1 712 1.68  0.090 .
+ PackYears      1 712 1.27  0.215
+ Condition(Age) 1 713 0.00
---
Signif. codes:  0 '***' 0.001 '**' 0.01 '*' 0.05 '.' 0.1 ' ' 1

Step: throat.otu.tab ~ SmokingStatus

                 Df AIC     F  Pr(>F)
+ Sex            1 712 1.53  0.14
+ PackYears      1 713 0.58  0.78
+ Condition(Age) 1 713 0.00
```

The selected variable is Smoking Status. The final model is fitted below.

```
> cap_final<- capscale(throat.otu.tab ~ SmokingStatus, throat_meta,
dist="bray")
> anova(cap_final, step=1000)
Permutation test for capscale under reduced model
Permutation: free
Number of permutations: 999

Model: capscale(formula = throat.otu.tab ~ SmokingStatus, data = throat_meta,
distance = "bray")
           Df SumOfSqs   F  Pr(>F)
Model       1    0.65 2.8  0.004 **
Residual 58     13.44
---
Signif. codes:  0 '***' 0.001 '**' 0.01 '*' 0.05 '.' 0.1 ' ' 1
```

Smoking Status reaches the significance with p-value of 0.004, but the parsimony model has paid off with larger residual.

7.5 Summary and Discussion

In this chapter, we used mouse and human data sets to illustrate exploratory analysis of microbiome data. We first used the phyloseq package to illustrate the five plots, including richness, abundance bar, heatmap, network and phylogenetic tree. Then, we introduced several families of clustering methods available in the ecology and microbiome studies, and focused on illustrating four clustering methods (single linkage agglomerative, complete linkage agglomerative, average linkage agglomerative, and Ward's minimum variance). We also briefly described the relationship of clustering, ordination and distance measure. Finally, we illustrated the most common unconstrained and constrained ordinations: PCA, PCoA, NMDS, CA, RDA, CCA, and CAP.

The characteristics of unconstrained ordinations are considered 'exploratory'. However, the capabilities of constrained ordinations are beyond merely exploratory data analysis, and become hypothesis testing as well. We introduced the different characteristics of unconstrained and constrained ordinations. Reader can further understand these ordinations through the real examples.

We illustrated exploratory analysis and hypothesis testing (in terms of constrained ordinations) of microbiome data through using the specifically developed package for analyzing microbiome census data "phyloseq" and the packages that commonly used in ecology such as vegan package. The extending functions, i.e., cleanplot.pca() and evplot() are attractive and two criteria to evaluate the performance of ordinations (Kaiser-Guttman criterion and broken-stick model) are helpful for evaluating the ordination analyses.

References

Anderson, M.J., and T.J. Willis. 2003. Canonical analysis of principal coordinates: A useful method of constrained ordination for ecology. *Ecology* 84: 511–525.

Borcard, D., F. Gillet, et al. 2011. *Numerical ecology with R*. New York: Springer.

Charlson, E.S., J. Chen, et al. 2010. Disordered microbial communities in the upper respiratory tract of cigarette smokers. *PLoS ONE* 5 (12): 0015216.

Chen, J. 2012. GUniFrac: Generalized UniFrac distances. R package version 1.0. https://CRAN.R-project.org/package=GUniFrac.

Gauch Jr., H.G. 1982a. Noise reduction by eigenvalue ordinations. *Ecology* 63: 1643–1649.

Gauch Jr., H.G. 1982b. *Multivariate analysis and community structure*. Cambridge: Cambridge University Press.

Jin, D., S. Wu, et al. 2015. Lack of vitamin D receptor causes dysbiosis and changes the functions of the murine intestinal microbiome. *Clinical Therapeutics* 37(5): 996–1009.

Legendre, P., and L. Legendre. 1998. *Numerical ecology*. Amsterdam: Elsevier.

Legendre, P., and L. Legendre. 2012. *Numerical ecology*. Amsterdam: Elsevier.

McMurdie, P.J., and S. Holmes. 2013. phyloseq: An R package for reproducible interactive analysis and graphics of microbiome census data. *PLoS ONE* 8 (4): e61217.

Rajaram, S., and Y. Oono. 2010. Neatmap—Non-clustering heat map alternatives in R. *BMC Bioinformatics* 11 (1): 45.

ter Braak, C.J.F. 1985. *CANOCO—A FORTRAN program for canonical correspondence analysis and detrended correspondence analysis*. The Netherlands: Wageningen.

ter Braak, C.J.F. 1986. Canonical correspondence analysis: A new eigenvector technique for multivariate direct gradient analysis. *Ecology* 67: 1167–1179.

Ward Jr., J.H. 1963. Hierarchical grouping to optimize an objective function. *Journal of the American Statistical Association* 58: 236–244.

Chapter 8
Univariate Community Analysis

We divide microbiome community composition study into two major components: (1) hypothesis testing of taxonomic diversities, OTUs and taxa and (2) analysis of dissimilarities among groups. The first component primarily belongs to univariate community analysis. The second component can be further divided into various multivariate techniques, such as clustering and ordinations, and hypothesis testing of multivariate analysis of dissimilarities. In Chap. 7, we covered these multivariate techniques. We will focus on comparisons of diversities, OTUs and taxa in this chapter. Hypothesis testing of multivariate analysis of dissimilarities among groups will be presented in Chap. 9.

8.1 Comparisons of Diversities Between Two Groups

In our $Vdr^{-/-}$ mouse study, one of the purposes is to test the difference of diversities between two groups ($Vdr^{-/-}$ and wild type mices) in fecal and cecal sites. In Chap. 6, we calculated the Shannon diversity using the fecal samples. Here, to illustrate univariate community analysis, we shall compare the calculated Shannon diversity using various testing statistics.

8.1.1 Two-Sample Welch's t-Test

The t-statistic was introduced in 1908 by William Sealy Gosset. A two-sample *t*-test is used to test the means of two populations are equal. It is most commonly applied when the test statistic would follow a normal distribution. If the two groups have the same variance, the t statistic can be calculated as follows:

© Springer Nature Singapore Pte Ltd. 2018   251
Y. Xia et al., *Statistical Analysis of Microbiome Data with R*,
ICSA Book Series in Statistics, https://doi.org/10.1007/978-981-13-1534-3_8

$$t = \frac{\bar{X}_1 - \bar{X}_2}{s_p \sqrt{\frac{1}{n_1} + \frac{1}{n_2}}}, \tag{8.1}$$

where, $s_p = \sqrt{\frac{(n-1)s_1^2 + (n_2-1)s_2^2}{n_1 + n_2 - 2}}$ is an estimator of the pooled standard deviation of the two samples. Welch's t-test or unequal variances t-test is adapted from t-test (Welch 1947). The Welch's t-test statistic is given:

$$t = \frac{\bar{X}_1 - \bar{X}_2}{s_{\bar{\Delta}}}, \tag{8.2}$$

where, $s_{\bar{\Delta}} = \sqrt{\frac{s_1^2}{n_1} + \frac{s_2^2}{n_2}}$; s_1^2 and s_2^2 are the unbiased estimator of the variance of samples 1 and 2, respectively. When the two samples have unequal variances and unequal sample sizes, Welch's t-test is considered as more reliable (Ruxton 2006). Thus, here we use Welch's t-test to our $Vdr^{-/-}$ mouse data.

First, load and transpose the data set as previously in Chaps. 6 and 7.

```
> abund_table=read.csv("VdrGenusCounts.csv",row.names=1,
check.names=FALSE)
> abund_table<-t(abund_table)
```

In order to incorporate group information from data set directly to the comparison, we need to do data management. In the data set, sample id and group information are in a character striple. We first extract them from there.

```
> grouping<-data.frame(row.names=rownames(abund_table),t(as.data.frame
(strsplit(rownames(abund_table),"_"))))

> grouping$Location <- with(grouping, ifelse(X3%in%"dryst-28F", "Fecal",
"Cecal"))
> grouping$Group <- with(grouping,ifelse(as.factor(X2)%in% c(11,12,13,14,15),
c("Vdr-/-"), c("WT")))
> grouping <- grouping[,c(4,5)]
> grouping
                  Location  Group
5_15_dryst-28F      Fecal  Vdr-/-
20_12_Cest-28F      Cecal  Vdr-/-
1_11_dryst-28F      Fecal  Vdr-/-
2_12_dryst-28F      Fecal  Vdr-/-
3_13_dryst-28F      Fecal  Vdr-/-
4_14_dryst-28F      Fecal  Vdr-/-
7_22_dryst-28F      Fecal     WT
8_23_dryst-28F      Fecal     WT
9_24_dryst-28F      Fecal     WT
19_11_Cest-28F      Cecal  Vdr-/-
21_13_Cest-28F      Cecal  Vdr-/-
22_14_Cest-28F      Cecal  Vdr-/-
23_15_Cest-28F      Cecal  Vdr-/-
25_22_Cest-28F      Cecal     WT
26_23_Cest-28F      Cecal     WT
27_24_Cest-28F      Cecal     WT
```

The Shannon diversity was calculated in Chap. 6, we repeat here for the convenience.

```
> library(vegan)
> H<-diversity(abund_table, "shannon")
```

We make a dataframe of Shannon diversity.

```
> df_H<-data.frame(sample=names(H),value=H,measure=rep("Shannon",
length(H)))
```

Then we combine diversity and grouping data frames to make a new data frame.

```
> df_G <-cbind(df_H, grouping)
> rownames(df_G)<-NULL
> df_G
            sample value measure Location  Group
1   5_15_dryST-28F 2.461 Shannon    Fecal Vdr-/-
2  20_12_CeST-28F 2.340 Shannon    Cecal Vdr-/-
3   1_11_dryST-28F 2.228 Shannon    Fecal Vdr-/-
4   2_12_dryST-28F 2.734 Shannon    Fecal Vdr-/-
5   3_13_dryST-28F 2.077 Shannon    Fecal Vdr-/-
6   4_14_dryST-28F 2.467 Shannon    Fecal Vdr-/-
7   7_22_dryST-28F 1.777 Shannon    Fecal     WT
8   8_23_dryST-28F 2.000 Shannon    Fecal     WT
9   9_24_dryST-28F 1.972 Shannon    Fecal     WT
10 19_11_CeST-28F 1.345 Shannon    Cecal Vdr-/-
11 21_13_CeST-28F 2.016 Shannon    Cecal Vdr-/-
12 22_14_CeST-28F 1.955 Shannon    Cecal Vdr-/-
13 23_15_CeST-28F 1.614 Shannon    Cecal Vdr-/-
14 25_22_CeST-28F 1.959 Shannon    Cecal     WT
15 26_23_CeST-28F 2.271 Shannon    Cecal     WT
16 27_24_CeST-28F 2.002 Shannon    Cecal     WT
```

Next, we subset fecal data from the new data frame.

```
> Fecal_G<- subset(df_G, Location=="Fecal")
> Fecal_G
           sample value measure Location  Group
1 5_15_dryST-28F 2.461 Shannon    Fecal Vdr-/-
3 1_11_dryST-28F 2.228 Shannon    Fecal Vdr-/-
4 2_12_dryST-28F 2.734 Shannon    Fecal Vdr-/-
5 3_13_dryST-28F 2.077 Shannon    Fecal Vdr-/-
6 4_14_dryST-28F 2.467 Shannon    Fecal Vdr-/-
7 7_22_dryST-28F 1.777 Shannon    Fecal     WT
8 8_23_dryST-28F 2.000 Shannon    Fecal     WT
9 9_24_dryST-28F 1.972 Shannon    Fecal     WT
```

Now the data is ready for statistical analysis. Before conducting hypothesis testing, let's explore the distribution of the Shannon diversity values using the function ggplot() from the ggplot2 package and the function ddply() in plyr package.

```
> library(ggplot2)
```

We split the plot into two panels using facet_grid.

```
> p<-ggplot(Fecal_G, aes(x=value))+
+    geom_histogram(color="black", fill="black")+
+    facet_grid(Group ~ .)
```

The package plyr is used to calculate the average Shannon diversity values of each group.

```
> library(plyr)
> mu <- ddply(Fecal_G, "Group", summarise, grp.mean=mean(value))
> head(mu)
    Group grp.mean
1 Vdr-/-    2.393
2    WT     1.916
```

Add the mean lines to the plot.

```
> p+geom_vline(data=mu, aes(xintercept=grp.mean, color="red"),
+                     linetype="dashed")
```

The distribution (Fig. 8.1) shows that *Vdr* knockout results in higher diversity because the histogram for this group is shifted to the right (higher diversity values) relative to the WT group. To test the null hypothesis of no difference in Shannon diversity, a Welch's *t*-test was used resulting in *p*-value = 0.01 (t = 3.6, df = 5.9). Thus, we reject the null hypothesis of no difference in favor of the alternative that the Shannon diversities are different in the two groups.

```
> fit_t <- t.test(value ~ Group, data=Fecal_G)
> fit_t
        Welch Two Sample t-test

data:  value by Group
t = 3.6, df = 5.9, p-value = 0.01
alternative hypothesis: true difference in means is not equal to 0
95 percent confidence interval:
 0.1518 0.8026
sample estimates:
mean in group Vdr-/-    mean in group WT
               2.393                  1.916
```

8.1.2   Wilcoxon Rank Sum Test

Wilcoxon rank sum test is equivalent to the Mann-Whitney *U* test developed by Mann and Whitney (1947). It is a nonparametric alternative to the two sample *t*-test that uses ranks of two independent sample data to test the null hypothesis: the two independent samples come from populations with the same distribution (that is, the two populations are identical). Unlike the *t*-test, Wilcoxon rank sum test does not require the assumption of normal distributions, and is nearly as efficient as the *t*-test. Therefore, it is widely used in microbiome study. It takes three main steps to conduct the Wilcoxon rank sum test for finding the value of the test statistic:

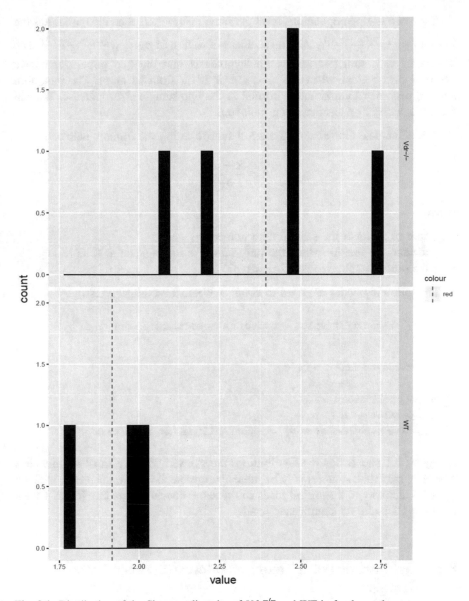

Fig. 8.1 Distribution of the Shannon diversity of $Vdr^{-/-}$ and WT in fecal samples

Step 1. Assign ranks to all the observations, the smallest value gets a rank of 1. Where values are tied, assign the mean of the ranks involved in the tie.

Step 2. Sum the ranks for either one of the two samples. The sum of ranks in another sample can be determinated since the sum of all the ranks equals N $(N + 1)/2$, where N is the total number of observations.

If the two testing populations have the same distribution, then the rank R has the mean of $\mu_R = \frac{n_1(n_1+n_2+1)}{2}$, and the standard deviation of $\sigma_R = \sqrt{\frac{n_1 n_2(n_1+n_2+1)}{12}}$. The Wilcoxon rank sum test rejects the hypothesis that the two populations have identical distributions when the rank sum R is far from its mean. The rank sum statistic becomes approximately normal as the two sample sizes increase. We can form the statistic by standardizing rank sum.

Step 3. Calculate the value of the z test statistic using the formula below:

$$z = \frac{R - \mu_R}{\sigma_R},$$

(8.3)

where

R sum of ranks of the sample with number n_1
n_1 the sample size for which the rank sum R is found (such as sample 1)
n_2 the other sample size (such as sample 2).

The following codes are used to conduct Wilcoxon rank-sum test.

```
> fit_w <- wilcox.test(value ~ Group, data=Fecal_G)
> fit_w

        Wilcoxon rank sum test

data:  value by Group
W = 15, p-value = 0.04
alternative hypothesis: true location shift is not equal to 0
```

Figure 8.1 shows that the distributions are skewed with the small sample size. The Wilcoxon rank sum test may be more appropriate; however, the p = 0.04 given by the Wilcoxon rank sum test leads to the same conclusion as the Welch's t-test with p = 0.01 at 0.05 significance level.

8.2   Comparisons of a Taxon of Interest Between Two Groups

8.2.1   Comparison of Relative Abundance Using Wilcoxon Rank Sum Test

When we analyze microbiome abundance data, it is inappropriate to draw inferences regarding the total abundance in the ecosystem from the abundance of OTUs or abundance of taxa in the samples. Instead, we can use the relative abundance in the sample to inference its relative abundance of a taxon in the ecosystem. The reason underling it is that it exists a compositional constraint: all microbial relative abundances within a sample sum to one, which results in compositional data residing in a simplex (Aitchison 1982, 1986) rather than the Euclidean space. Thus, it is often to standardize the data to a common scale to facilitate the comparison of the abundance of the taxon across groups. The way is to divide the taxon count by the total number of reads time 100 to convert the abundance to the percentage of reads in the sample, scale the data to "the number of taxon per 100 reads".

When we select a specific single taxon to test across groups, it is important to make sure the specified taxon is based on hypothesis or theory to reduce the chance to inflate the false positive rate (i.e., rejects the null hypothesis when it should not be rejected).

Vdr in mice substantially affects beta diversity and consistently influences individual bacterial taxa, such as *Parabacteroides* (Wang et al. 2016). In this section, we illustrate Wilcoxon rank sum test to compare bacterial *Bacteroides* in the *Vdr* mouse data set using fecal samples.

First, check total abundance in each sample.

```
> apply(abund_table,1, sum)
 5_15_dryst-28F 20_12_Cest-28F  1_11_dryst-28F  2_12_dryst-28F  3_13_dryst-28F
           1853            3239            6211            5115            6016
 4_14_dryst-28F  7_22_dryst-28F  8_23_dryst-28F  9_24_dryst-28F 19_11_Cest-28F
           2343            2262            7255            5502            5067
21_13_Cest-28F 22_14_Cest-28F 23_15_Cest-28F 25_22_Cest-28F 26_23_Cest-28F
           2397            3788            9264            2072            6903
27_24_Cest-28F
           6327
```

Then, calculate relative abundance by dividing each value by sample total abundance.

```
> relative_abund_table<-decostand(abund_table, method = "total")
```

Check the total abundance in each sample to make the above calculations are correct.

```
> apply(relative_abund_table, 1, sum)
 5_15_dryst-28F 20_12_Cest-28F  1_11_dryst-28F  2_12_dryst-28F  3_13_dryst-28F
              1              1              1              1              1
 4_14_dryst-28F  7_22_dryst-28F  8_23_dryst-28F  9_24_dryst-28F 19_11_Cest-28F
              1              1              1              1              1
21_13_Cest-28F 22_14_Cest-28F 23_15_Cest-28F 25_22_Cest-28F 26_23_Cest-28F
              1              1              1              1              1
27_24_Cest-28F
              1
```

Take a look at the transformed data.

```
> relative_abund_table[1:16,1:8]
                Tannerella Lactococcus Lactobacillus Lactobacillus::Lactococcus
5_15_dryST-28F   0.256881    0.17593      0.05073                    0.0005397
20_12_CeST-28F   0.020685    0.22754      0.18432                    0.0037048
1_11_dryST-28F   0.088392    0.36983      0.06988                    0.0040251
2_12_dryST-28F   0.113001    0.10714      0.14057                    0.0009775
3_13_dryST-28F   0.165559    0.39528      0.05352                    0.0028258
4_14_dryST-28F   0.172429    0.20102      0.08749                    0.0004268
7_22_dryST-28F   0.141026    0.38992      0.28470                    0.0057471
8_23_dryST-28F   0.072502    0.27195      0.32254                    0.0020675
9_24_dryST-28F   0.077063    0.41948      0.18175                    0.0025445
19_11_CeST-28F   0.000000    0.08328      0.06513                    0.0013815
21_13_CeST-28F   0.002503    0.07217      0.26658                    0.0000000
22_14_CeST-28F   0.005280    0.15312      0.16711                    0.0007920
23_15_CeST-28F   0.003994    0.52537      0.19635                    0.0026986
25_22_CeST-28F   0.018340    0.34122      0.30164                    0.0043436
26_23_CeST-28F   0.011734    0.20339      0.19716                    0.0014486
27_24_CeST-28F   0.037142    0.30235      0.05769                    0.0020547
                Parasutterella Helicobacter Prevotella Bacteroides
5_15_dryST-28F      0.0005397     0.048030   0.0652995    0.147329
20_12_CeST-28F      0.0000000     0.000000   0.0021612    0.010497
1_11_dryST-28F      0.0001610     0.000000   0.0465303    0.154242
2_12_dryST-28F      0.0007820     0.002542   0.0193548    0.073705
3_13_dryST-28F      0.0003324     0.003989   0.0556848    0.087434
4_14_dryST-28F      0.0000000     0.013658   0.0610329    0.085361
7_22_dryST-28F      0.0000000     0.001326   0.0490716    0.038019
8_23_dryST-28F      0.0016540     0.000000   0.0122674    0.058442
9_24_dryST-28F      0.0001818     0.000000   0.0152672    0.036714
19_11_CeST-28F      0.0000000     0.000000   0.0000000    0.000000
21_13_CeST-28F      0.0000000     0.000000   0.0004172    0.002086
22_14_CeST-28F      0.0000000     0.000000   0.0007920    0.005280
23_15_CeST-28F      0.0002159     0.000000   0.0010794    0.003346
25_22_CeST-28F      0.0000000     0.000000   0.0033784    0.009170
26_23_CeST-28F      0.0002897     0.000000   0.0007243    0.006664
27_24_CeST-28F      0.0000000     0.000000   0.0039513    0.019282
```

Our interested bacterial *Bacteroides* is in column 8. Let's subset this bacterial.

```
> (Bacteroides <-relative_abund_table[,8])
5_15_dryST-28F 20_12_CeST-28F 1_11_dryST-28F 2_12_dryST-28F 3_13_dryST-28F
      0.147329       0.010497       0.154242       0.073705       0.087434
4_14_dryST-28F 7_22_dryST-28F 8_23_dryST-28F 9_24_dryST-28F 19_11_CeST-28F
      0.085361       0.038019       0.058442       0.036714       0.000000
21_13_CeST-28F 22_14_CeST-28F 23_15_CeST-28F 25_22_CeST-28F 26_23_CeST-28F
      0.002086       0.005280       0.003346       0.009170       0.006664
27_24_CeST-28F
      0.019282
```

Now, combine *Bacteroides* and grouping data frames and subset fecal sanmples for later use.

```
  Bacteroides Location  Group
1  0.14732866    Fecal  Vdr-/-
3  0.15424247    Fecal  Vdr-/-
4  0.07370479    Fecal  Vdr-/-
5  0.08743351    Fecal  Vdr-/-
6  0.08536065    Fecal  Vdr-/-
7  0.03801945    Fecal     WT
8  0.05844245    Fecal     WT
9  0.03671392    Fecal     WT
```

The boxplot() function is used to generate a simple boxplot of Bacteroides with group (Fig. 8.2).

```
  Bacteroides Location  Group
1     0.14733     Fecal Vdr-/-
3     0.15424     Fecal Vdr-/-
4     0.07370     Fecal Vdr-/-
5     0.08743     Fecal Vdr-/-
6     0.08536     Fecal Vdr-/-
7     0.03802     Fecal    WT
8     0.05844     Fecal    WT
9     0.03671     Fecal    WT
```

```
> boxplot(Bacteroides ~ Group,data=Fecal_Bacteroides_G, col=rainbow
(2),main="Bacteroides in Vdr WT/KO mice")
```

The following codes are used to generate boxplot using function ggplot() (Fig. 8.3).

```
> ggplot(Fecal_Bacteroides_G, aes(x=Group, y=Bacteroides,col=factor
(Group)))+ geom_boxplot(notch=FALSE)
> ggplot(Fecal_Bacteroides_G, aes(x=Group, y=Bacteroides)) +
geom_boxplot(outlier.colour="red", outlier.shape=8, outlier.size=4) +
layer(stat_params = list(binwidth = 2))
```

The boxplots display taxa (*Bacteriodes*) in wild type (WT, n = 3) and *Vdr* knockout mice (KO, n = 5).

```
> fit_w_b=wilcox.test(Bacteroides~Group,data=Fecal_Bacteroides_G)
> fit_w_b

        Wilcoxon rank sum test

data: Bacteroides by Group
W = 15, p-value = 0.04
```

Fig. 8.2 Boxplot of bacterial *Bacteroides* with $Vdr^{-/-}$ and WT groups in fecal samples

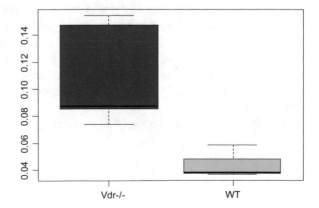

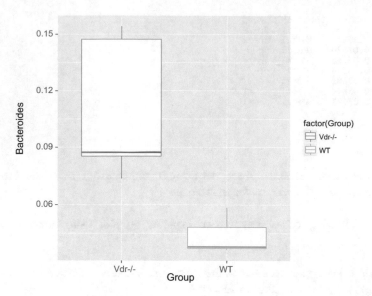

Fig. 8.3 Boxplot of bacterial *Bacteroides* with $Vdr^{-/-}$ and WT groups in fecal samples generated using ggplot

```
alternative hypothesis: true location shift is not equal to 0
```

The above Wolcoxon test indicates that a statistical significance of a relative abundance of *Bacteriodes* exisits between $Vdr^{-/-}$ and WT mice. We can conclude that *Vdr* knockout enriches *Bacteriodes*.

8.2.2   Comparison of Present or Absent Taxon Using Chi-Square Test

A chi-square test, also written as χ^2 test, often used as short for Pearson's chi-square test, was proposed and first investigated its properties by Karl Pearson in 1900 (Pearson 1900). χ^2 test is applied to sets of categorical data to test whether an observed frequency distribution differs from a claimed or theoretical distribution (tests of goodness of fit) and to investigate whether the row variable and the column variable in a contingency table are independent of each other (tests of independence).

The test statistic of goodness of fit is given by:

$$\chi^2 = \sum_{i=1}^{n} \frac{(O_i - E_i)^2}{E_i} = N \sum_{i=1}^{n} \frac{(O_i/N - p_i)^2}{p_i}, \tag{8.4}$$

where

χ^2	Pearson's test statistic, which asymptotically approaches a χ^2 distribution
O_i	number of observations of category i
N	total number of observations
$E_i = Np_i$	expected (theoretical) frequency of category i under the null hypothesis
p_i	probability of category i in the population
n	number of cells in the table.

The test statistic of independence is given below:

$$\chi^2 = \sum_{i=1}^{r} \sum_{j=1}^{c} \frac{(O_{i,j} - E_{i,j})^2}{E_{i,j}} = N \sum_{i,j} p_{i.} p_{.j} \left(\frac{(O_{i,j}/N) - p_{i.} p_{.j}}{p_{i.} p_{.j}} \right)^2, \tag{8.5}$$

where

N	total sample size (the sum of all cells in the table)
$E_{ij} = Np_{i.} p_{.j}$	expected (theoretical) frequency under the null hypothesis of independence
$p_{i.} = \frac{O_{i.}}{N} = \sum_{j=1}^{c} \frac{O_{i,j}}{N}$	probability of observations of category i ignoring the column attribute (probability of row totals)
$p_{.j} = \frac{O_{.j}}{N} = \sum_{i=1}^{r} \frac{O_{i,j}}{N}$	probability of observations of category j ignoring the row attribute (probability of column totals).

As a rule of thumb, it requires that all expected cell counts equal or exceed 5 to provide an adequate approximation to the distribution of Chi-square distribution (Wackerly et al. 2002), although Cochran (1952) noted that this value could be as low as 1 for some situations.

In this section, we illustrate χ^2 test to compare bacterial *Parabacteroides* in the *Vdr* mouse data set using cecal samples. To illustrate the χ^2 test, we transform the abundance count data of *Parabacteroides* into a binary variable. The count data in the abundance table for the taxon *Parabacteroides* would be transformed to 0 if the taxon is absent in the sample or to 1 if the taxon is present in the sample. The transformed data are summarized in Table 8.1.

First, look at the abundance data to identify bacterial *Parabacteroides* and subset this bacterial.

Table 8.1 Distribution of the *Parabacteroides* rate across *Vdr*$^{-/-}$ and WT cecal samples obtained from the *Vdr* mouse data set

Group	Presence	Absence	Total
Vdr$^{-/-}$	3 (60%)	2 (40%)	5
WT	3 (100%)	0 (0%)	3

```
> abund_table[1:16,1:27]
> (Parabacteroides <- abund_table[,27])
```

Then, combine the subsetted data with grouping data frame.

```
> Parabacteroides_G <-cbind(Parabacteroides, grouping)
> rownames(Parabacteroides_G)<-NULL
```

Since the combined dataframe includes both fecal and cecal samples, let's subset cecal data from this dataframe.

```
> Cecal_Parabacteroides_G <- subset(Parabacteroides_G, Location=="Cecal")
> Cecal_Parabacteroides_G
   Parabacteroides Location  Group
2                0    Cecal Vdr-/-
10               0    Cecal Vdr-/-
11               1    Cecal Vdr-/-
12               4    Cecal Vdr-/-
13              15    Cecal Vdr-/-
14               5    Cecal    WT
15               4    Cecal    WT
16               6    Cecal    WT
```

Recode a binary variable "Present" for Chi-square test.

```
> Cecal_Parabacteroides_G$Present <- ifelse((Cecal_Parabacteroides_G$Parabact
eroides > 0), "Present","Absent")
> Cecal_Parabacteroides_G
   Parabacteroides Location  Group Present
2                0    Cecal Vdr-/-  Absent
10               0    Cecal Vdr-/-  Absent
11               1    Cecal Vdr-/- Present
12               4    Cecal Vdr-/- Present
13              15    Cecal Vdr-/- Present
14               5    Cecal    WT Present
15               4    Cecal    WT Present
16               6    Cecal    WT Present
```

The following codes are used to conduct Chi-square test.

```
> library(MASS)
> tbl = table(Cecal_Parabacteroides_G$Group, Cecal_Parabacteroides_G$Present)
> tbl

          Absent Present
  Vdr-/-      2      3
  WT          0      3
> chisq.test(tbl)

        Pearson's Chi-squared test with Yates' continuity correction

data:  tbl
X-squared = 0.18, df = 1, p-value = 0.7

Warning message:
In chisq.test(tbl) : Chi-squared approximation may be incorrect
```

Table 8.1 shows the distribution of these rates—3 (60%) out of 5 $Vdr^{-/-}$ cecal samples had *Parabacteroides*, while 3 (100%) out of 3 wild type samples did. To test the null hypothesis that of no difference in the rates of occurrence between the two groups a chi-square test gave a *P*-value 0.7 (X-squared = 0.18, df = 1), so we can not reject the null hypothesis of no difference between the two groups, and conclude that they do not have different rates of occurrence. Note that because the small sample size, there is a warning message in the output. Typically if the cell values are small (such as <5) in the contingency table, Chi-square test may be incorrect, a Fisher's exact test is applied.

```
> fisher.test(tbl)

        Fisher's Exact Test for Count Data

data: tbl
p-value = 0.5
alternative hypothesis: true odds ratio is not equal to 1
95 percent confidence interval:
 0.109    Inf
sample estimates:
odds ratio
       Inf
```

The result of Fisher's exact test is not significant either with *p*-value of 0.5, which is consistent with that of Chi-square test. However, the test is hard to conclude with the infinite confidence interval.

8.3   Comparisons Among More than Two Groups Using ANOVA

8.3.1   One-Way ANOVA

Analysis of variance (ANOVA) was proposed by Ronald Fisher in 1918 (Fisher 1918) and became well known after Fisher's book "*Statistical Methods for Research Workers*" was published in 1925. ANOVA generalizes the two-sample *t*-test to more than two groups. The null hypothesis of ANOVA is: all the means of compared groups are equal. The analysis using ANOVA relies on an assumption of normality of the underlying data. However, most of microbiome community composition data, especially multivariate data, are not normally distributed, thus, ANOVA is only used for comparing univariate analysis of alpha diversity measures in this book. For multivariate community composition data, either a non-parametric version of ANOVA or other suitable statistical methods are applied.

The formation of testing statistic is through using traditional partitioning of the sum of squares (portioning of variation). The definitional equation of sample variance is

$$s^2 = \frac{1}{n-1} \sum_{i=1}^{n} (y_i - \bar{y})^2, \tag{8.6}$$

where s^2 = sample variance. The sample variance is calculated by the sum of squares (SS) divided by n − 1 (called degrees of freedom, DF). The result is called the mean square (MS) and the squared terms are deviations from the sample mean.

The fundamental technique of ANOVA partitions the total sum of squares (SS) of deviations into two components: sum of squares related to treatment and sum of squares related to error:

$$SS_{Total} = SS_{Treatments} + SS_{Error}$$

The number of degrees of freedom, $DF,$ can be partitioned in a similar way:

$$DF_{Total} = DF_{Treatments} + DF_{Error}$$

The *F*-test is used for comparing the factors of the total deviation. The *F*-value is obtained by dividing the variance between treatments by the variance within treatments. The F test statistic in one-way ANOVA is given below:

$$F = \frac{MS_{Treatments}}{MS_{Error}} = \frac{SS_{Treatments}/(K-1)}{SS_{Error}/(N-1)} \tag{8.7}$$

where MS = mean square, K = number of treatments and N = total number of samples.

To illustrate ANOVA in microbiome community composition study, we use our $Vdr^{-/-}$ mouse data. One hypothsis of this study is that Vdr status and intestinal location have no effects on the bacterial community in the gut. We analyze Chao 1 alpha diversity measures using ANOVA to address this hypothsis.

For your convenience, we copy the codes used in Chap. 6 to calculate Chao 1 richness measures below. The results were wrapped up a data frame. The group information is merged for the ANOVA test.

The following codes make a dataframe of Chao1 richness and add group information into this dataframe.

```
> CH=estimateR(abund_table)[2,]
> df_CH <-data.frame(sample=names(CH),value=CH,measure=rep("Chao1",length(CH)
))
> df_CH_G <-cbind(df_CH, grouping)
> rownames(df_G)<-NULL
> df_CH_G
                         sample  value measure Location  Group
5_15_dryST-28F 5_15_dryST-28F   94.75   Chao1    Fecal  Vdr-/-
20_12_CeST-28F 20_12_CeST-28F   59.80   Chao1    Cecal  Vdr-/-
1_11_dryST-28F 1_11_dryST-28F   77.00   Chao1    Fecal  Vdr-/-
2_12_dryST-28F 2_12_dryST-28F  103.27   Chao1    Fecal  Vdr-/-
3_13_dryST-28F 3_13_dryST-28F   85.67   Chao1    Fecal  Vdr-/-
4_14_dryST-28F 4_14_dryST-28F   55.14   Chao1    Fecal  Vdr-/-
7_22_dryST-28F 7_22_dryST-28F   62.75   Chao1    Fecal      WT
8_23_dryST-28F 8_23_dryST-28F   67.67   Chao1    Fecal      WT
9_24_dryST-28F 9_24_dryST-28F   80.50   Chao1    Fecal      WT
19_11_CeST-28F 19_11_CeST-28F   52.17   Chao1    Cecal  Vdr-/-
21_13_CeST-28F 21_13_CeST-28F   55.00   Chao1    Cecal  Vdr-/-
22_14_CeST-28F 22_14_CeST-28F   59.00   Chao1    Cecal  Vdr-/-
23_15_CeST-28F 23_15_CeST-28F   60.88   Chao1    Cecal  Vdr-/-
25_22_CeST-28F 25_22_CeST-28F   51.00   Chao1    Cecal      WT
26_23_CeST-28F 26_23_CeST-28F  112.86   Chao1    Cecal      WT
27_24_CeST-28F 27_24_CeST-28F   78.06   Chao1    Cecal      WT
```

The new four levels of group are generated using interaction of Location and Group.

```
> df_CH_G$Group4<- with(df_CH_G, interaction(Location,Group))
> df_CH_G
                         sample  value measure Location  Group       Group4
5_15_dryST-28F 5_15_dryST-28F   94.75   Chao1    Fecal  Vdr-/-  Fecal.Vdr-/-
20_12_CeST-28F 20_12_CeST-28F   59.80   Chao1    Cecal  Vdr-/-  Cecal.Vdr-/-
1_11_dryST-28F 1_11_dryST-28F   77.00   Chao1    Fecal  Vdr-/-  Fecal.Vdr-/-
2_12_dryST-28F 2_12_dryST-28F  103.27   Chao1    Fecal  Vdr-/-  Fecal.Vdr-/-
3_13_dryST-28F 3_13_dryST-28F   85.67   Chao1    Fecal  Vdr-/-  Fecal.Vdr-/-
4_14_dryST-28F 4_14_dryST-28F   55.14   Chao1    Fecal  Vdr-/-  Fecal.Vdr-/-
7_22_dryST-28F 7_22_dryST-28F   62.75   Chao1    Fecal      WT     Fecal.WT
8_23_dryST-28F 8_23_dryST-28F   67.67   Chao1    Fecal      WT     Fecal.WT
9_24_dryST-28F 9_24_dryST-28F   80.50   Chao1    Fecal      WT     Fecal.WT
19_11_CeST-28F 19_11_CeST-28F   52.17   Chao1    Cecal  Vdr-/-  Cecal.Vdr-/-
21_13_CeST-28F 21_13_CeST-28F   55.00   Chao1    Cecal  Vdr-/-  Cecal.Vdr-/-
22_14_CeST-28F 22_14_CeST-28F   59.00   Chao1    Cecal  Vdr-/-  Cecal.Vdr-/-
23_15_CeST-28F 23_15_CeST-28F   60.88   Chao1    Cecal  Vdr-/-  Cecal.Vdr-/-
25_22_CeST-28F 25_22_CeST-28F   51.00   Chao1    Cecal      WT     Cecal.WT
26_23_CeST-28F 26_23_CeST-28F  112.86   Chao1    Cecal      WT     Cecal.WT
27_24_CeST-28F 27_24_CeST-28F   78.06   Chao1    Cecal      WT     Cecal.WT
```

We explore the Chao 1 index using boxplot() (Fig. 8.4).

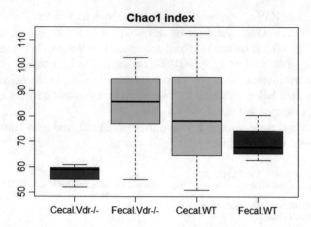

Fig. 8.4 Boxplot of Chao 1 index with four groups generated using function boxplot()

```
> boxplot(value~Group4, data=df_CH_G, col=rainbow
(4), main="Chao1 index")
```

The following ggplot() generates high quality boxplot for publication use (Fig. 8.5).

```
> p <- ggplot(df_CH_G, aes(x=Group4, y=value),col=rainbow
(4), main="Chao1 index") + geom_boxplot()
```

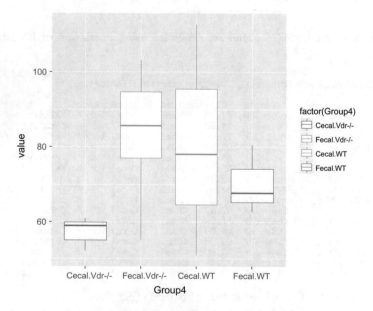

Fig. 8.5 Boxplot of Chao 1 index with four groups generated using ggplot()

```
> p + coord_flip()
> ggplot(df_CH_G, aes(x=Group4, y=value,col=factor(Group4))) +
+    geom_boxplot(notch=FALSE)
```

Except visual inspection of normality of the underlying data, homogeneity of variance can be tested. Sokal and Rohlf (2011) describe three such tests: the Bartlett's test for homogeneity, Hartley's F_{max} test and the log-anova, or Scheffé-Box test. To proceed with the verification of using ANOVA, we must first test for homogeneity of variances. The software R provides two tests: the Bartlett's test, and the Fligner-Killeen test.

To illustrate the test for homogeneity of variances, we use the Chao 1 richness measures of $Vdr^{-/-}$ and WT mouse data from both fecal and cecal locations. The null hypothesis (H_0) is that all variances in four groups are the same.

We begin with the Bartlett's test. For convenience of processing the Bartlett's test, we use the function select() from dplyr package to select the relevant group and Chao 1 value columns.

```
> library(dplyr)

> df_CH_G4 <- select(df_CH_G, Group4,value)
> df_CH_G4
                        Group4  value
5_15_drySt-28F Fecal.Vdr-/-  94.75
20_12_CeSt-28F Cecal.Vdr-/-  59.80
1_11_drySt-28F Fecal.Vdr-/-  77.00
2_12_drySt-28F Fecal.Vdr-/- 103.27
3_13_drySt-28F Fecal.Vdr-/-  85.67
4_14_drySt-28F Fecal.Vdr-/-  55.14
7_22_drySt-28F      Fecal.WT  62.75
8_23_drySt-28F      Fecal.WT  67.67
9_24_drySt-28F      Fecal.WT  80.50
19_11_CeSt-28F Cecal.Vdr-/-  52.17
21_13_CeSt-28F Cecal.Vdr-/-  55.00
22_14_CeSt-28F Cecal.Vdr-/-  59.00
23_15_CeSt-28F Cecal.Vdr-/-  60.88
25_22_CeSt-28F      Cecal.WT  51.00
26_23_CeSt-28F      Cecal.WT 112.86
27_24_CeSt-28F      Cecal.WT  78.06
```

The R codes below conduct the Bartlett's test of homegeneity of variances:

```
> bartlett.test(df_CH_G4, Group4)

        Bartlett test of homogeneity of variances

data: df_CH_G4
Bartlett's K-squared = 62, df = 1, p-value = 3e-15
```

The function gives us the K squared value of the statistical tests, and the p-value. It shows that the null hypothesis can be rejected at the 5% level. Alternatively, we can compare the Bartlett's K-squared with the value of chi-square tables, using the same level of alpha and degrees of freedom at the qchisq() function. If Chi-squared > Bartlett's K-squared, we accept the null hypothesis H_0 (homogeneity of variances), elsewise reject the null hypothesis.

```
> qchisq(0.95, 1)
[1] 3.841
```

Because Chi-squared is less than Bartlett's K-squared, we reject the null hypothesis H_0 and conclude that the variances are not same.

We now use Fligner-Killeen test to check the homoscedasticity. The syntax as below is quite similar.

```
> fligner.test(df_CH_G4, Group4)


    Fligner-Killeen test of homogeneity of variances

data: df_CH_G4
Fligner-Killeen:med chi-squared = 21, df = 1, p-value = 6e-06
```

The conclusions are similar as the test of Bartlett: the variances are not the same. However, for the purpose of illustration, we proceed to analyze the data by ANOVA regardless of the test results of homegeneity of variances.

The following R codes fit the model:

```
> fit = lm(formula = value~Group4,data=df_CH_G)
```

Then we analyze the ANOVA model:

```
> anova (fit)
Analysis of Variance Table

Response: value
          Df Sum Sq Mean Sq F value Pr(>F)
Group4     3   1926     642    2.19   0.14
Residuals 12   3513     293
```

Or just use the following concise R codes: aov() function nested within summary () function.

```
> summary(aov(value~Group4, data=df_CH_G))
          Df Sum Sq Mean Sq F value Pr(>F)
Group4     3   1926     642    2.19   0.14
Residuals 12   3513     293
```

You may also want print out the intercept by using below R codes.

```
> aov_fit <- aov(value~Group4,data=df_CH_G)
> summary(aov_fit, intercept=T)
```

The output of the function is a classical ANOVA table.

```
            Df Sum Sq Mean Sq F value Pr(>F)
(Intercept) 1  83450   83450  285.08 1e-09 ***
Group4      3   1926     642    2.19  0.14
Residuals  12   3513     293
---
Signif. codes:  0 '***' 0.001 '**' 0.01 '*' 0.05 '.' 0.1 ' ' 1
```

As p-value > 0.05, we accept the null hypothesis H_0: the four means are not different. You can also compare the computed F-value with the tabulated F-value:

```
> qf(0.95, 12, 3)
[1] 8.745
```

Because the tabulated F-value is larger than the computed F-value, we accept the null hyptohesis.

The outputs from ANOVA are some kind of messy. You can use broom package to obtain the tidy and more informative tables.

```
> library(broom)
> tidy(aov_fit)
       term df sumsq meansq statistic p.value
1    Group4  3  1926  641.9     2.193  0.1418
2 Residuals 12  3513  292.7        NA      NA
> augment(aov_fit)
        .rownames  value       Group4 .fitted .se.fit   .resid   .hat .sigma   .cooksd
1  5_15_dryST-28F  94.75 Fecal.Vdr-/-   83.17   7.651   11.584 0.2000  17.44 0.0358109
2  20_12_CeST-28F  59.80 Cecal.Vdr-/-   57.37   7.651    2.432 0.2000  17.85 0.0015781
3  1_11_dryST-28F  77.00 Fecal.Vdr-/-   83.17   7.651   -6.166 0.2000  17.75 0.0101485
4  2_12_dryST-28F 103.27 Fecal.Vdr-/-   83.17   7.651   20.106 0.2000  16.53 0.1078934
5  3_13_dryST-28F  85.67 Fecal.Vdr-/-   83.17   7.651    2.500 0.2000  17.85 0.0016683
6  4_14_dryST-28F  55.14 Fecal.Vdr-/-   83.17   7.651  -28.024 0.2000  15.17 0.2095941
7  7_22_dryST-28F  62.75    Fecal.WT   70.31   9.878   -7.556 0.3333  17.65 0.0365658
8  8_23_dryST-28F  67.67    Fecal.WT   70.31   9.878   -2.639 0.3333  17.84 0.0044605
9  9_24_dryST-28F  80.50    Fecal.WT   70.31   9.878   10.194 0.3333  17.47 0.0665687
10 19_11_CeST-28F  52.17 Cecal.Vdr-/-   57.37   7.651   -5.202 0.2000  17.78 0.0072213
11 21_13_CeST-28F  55.00 Cecal.Vdr-/-   57.37   7.651   -2.368 0.2000  17.85 0.0014970
12 22_14_CeST-28F  59.00 Cecal.Vdr-/-   57.37   7.651    1.632 0.2000  17.86 0.0007105
13 23_15_CeST-28F  60.88 Cecal.Vdr-/-   57.37   7.651    3.507 0.2000  17.83 0.0032819
14 25_22_CeST-28F  51.00    Cecal.WT   80.64   9.878  -29.639 0.3333  14.13 0.5626776
15 26_23_CeST-28F 112.86    Cecal.WT   80.64   9.878   32.218 0.3333  13.33 0.6648948
16 27_24_CeST-28F  78.06    Cecal.WT   80.64   9.878   -2.580 0.3333  17.84 0.0042631
   .std.resid
1      0.7570
2      0.1589
3     -0.4030
4      1.3139
5      0.1634
6     -1.8313
7     -0.5409
8     -0.1889
9      0.7298
10    -0.3399
11    -0.1548
12     0.1066
13     0.2292
14    -2.1217
15     2.3063
16    -0.1847
> glance(aov_fit)
  r.squared adj.r.squared sigma statistic p.value df logLik   AIC   BIC deviance
1    0.3541        0.1926 17.11     2.193  0.1418  4 -65.84 141.7 145.5     3513
  df.residual
1          12
```

8.3.2   Pairwise and Tukey Multiple Comparisons

The ANOVA results give the overall test of group difference (in this case, 4 groups with fecal, cecal, $Vdr^{-/-}$, and WT combination). Our purpose is to also test each pair difference associated with Chao 1 richness. The following steps are to illustrate the capabilities of pairwise t-test and Tukey's ad hoc multiple comparisons in R.

Let's run unadjusted pairwise t-test for all the four groups. The default setting in R for this test is to adjust p-values as a post hoc using the Holm method, so to get un-adjusted p-values, you need to specify p.adjust = "none". R's default is to assume homogeneity of variance, therefore, it is unnecessary to specify pool. sd = T. If your data have unequal variance, you need to use pool.sd = F.

```
> #Pairwise tests of mean differences
> pairwise.t.test(df_CH_G$value, df_CH_G$Group4,p.adjust="none",pool.sd=T)

        Pairwise comparisons using t tests with pooled SD

data:   df_CH_G$value and df_CH_G$Group4

             Cecal.Vdr-/- Fecal.Vdr-/- Cecal.WT
Fecal.Vdr-/- 0.03         -            -
Cecal.WT     0.09         0.84         -
Fecal.WT     0.32         0.32         0.47

P value adjustment method: none
```

If we don't make any adjustments to our p-values, there are statistically differences between fecal $Vdr^{-/-}$, cecal $Vdr^{-/-}$, and marginally statistically differences between cecal WT and cecal $Vdr^{-/-}$. These differences are visualized in above boxplot.

As we notice, the *p.adjust()* function is nested within the *pairwise.t.test()* function. This is a basic and very useful R function. It can be used to control the family-wise Type I error. The p.adjust() function can be nested in other function, or be independently called. In an independent call, the syntax is given below:

$$p.adjust(p, method = p.adjust.methods, n = length(p))$$

where, p = numeric vector of p-values, method = correction method, n = number of comparisons, must be at least length(p). The adjustment methods include c ("bonferroni", "holm", "hochberg", "hommel", "BH", "BY", "fdr", "none"). Where "bonferroni" is the Bonferroni correction in which the p-values are multiplied by the number of comparisons; "holm", "hochberg", "hommel", "BH", "BY", "fdr", are refered to Holm (1979), Hochberg (1988), Hommel (1988), Benjamini and Hochberg (1995) and Benjamini and Yekutieli (2001), and "fdr" is alias of "BH". They are less conservative corrections.

```
> #conservative Bonferroni adjustment
> pairwise.t.test(df_CH_G$value, df_CH_G$Group4, p.adjust="bonferroni", pool.
sd = T)

        Pairwise comparisons using t tests with pooled SD

data:   df_CH_G$value and df_CH_G$Group4

             Cecal.Vdr-/- Fecal.Vdr-/- Cecal.WT
Fecal.Vdr-/- 0.2          –            –
Cecal.WT     0.5          1.0          –
Fecal.WT     1.0          1.0          1.0

P value adjustment method: bonferroni
```

```
> #Holm method
> pairwise.t.test(df_CH_G$value, df_CH_G$Group4, p.adjust="holm",pool.sd = T)

        Pairwise comparisons using t tests with pooled SD

data:   df_CH_G$value and df_CH_G$Group4

             Cecal.Vdr-/- Fecal.Vdr-/- Cecal.WT
Fecal.Vdr-/- 0.2          –            –
Cecal.WT     0.4          1.0          –
Fecal.WT     1.0          1.0          1.0

P value adjustment method: holm
```

```
> #Benjamini & Hochberg(BH)
> pairwise.t.test(df_CH_G$value, df_CH_G$Group4, p.adjust="BH", pool.sd = T)

        Pairwise comparisons using t tests with pooled SD

data:   df_CH_G$value and df_CH_G$Group4

             Cecal.Vdr-/- Fecal.Vdr-/- Cecal.WT
Fecal.Vdr-/- 0.2          –            –
Cecal.WT     0.3          0.8          –
Fecal.WT     0.5          0.5          0.6

P value adjustment method: BH
```

```
> #Benjamini & Yekutieli
> pairwise.t.test(df_CH_G$value, df_CH_G$Group4, p.adjust="BY", pool.sd = T)

        Pairwise comparisons using t tests with pooled SD

data:   df_CH_G$value and df_CH_G$Group4

             Cecal.Vdr-/- Fecal.Vdr-/- Cecal.WT
Fecal.Vdr-/- 0.5          –            –
Cecal.WT     0.6          1.0          –
Fecal.WT     1.0          1.0          1.0

P value adjustment method: BY
```

All four adjustments above give no significant differences of pairwise comparisons. The conservative Bonferroni and Benjamini & Yekutieli adjustments have

Fig. 8.6 Plot of Tukey
multiple comparisons of
means and their confidence
intervals in $Vdr^{-/-}$ mouse data

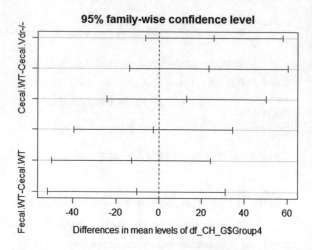

largest *p*-values. With the Benjamini & Hochberg method none of the comparisons
are significant either, but their adjusted *p*-values are smaller. The Benjamini &
Hochberg method is more powerful in this case.

Both Benjamini & Hochberg (BH) and Benjamini & Yekutieli (BY) methods are
for adjusting for the "False Discovery Rate". Actually it is not a true control of
family-wise error. The False Discovery Rate methods find the same results: all
pairwise comparisons are not significant differences.

Next, let's show using the TukeyHSD () function to do Tukey multiple comparisons of means and obtain their confidence intervals. The way to call this
function is similar to the summary() function. It takes the variable from the original
ANOVA calculation as one of its arguments (Fig. 8.6).

```
> #Tukey multiple comparisons of means
> TukeyHSD(aov_fit, conf.level=.95)
  Tukey multiple comparisons of means
    95% family-wise confidence level

Fit: aov(formula = value ~ Group4, data = df_CH_G)

$Group4
                              diff     lwr   upr  p adj
Fecal.Vdr-/--Cecal.Vdr-/-   25.798  -6.328 57.92 0.1334
Cecal.WT-Cecal.Vdr-/-       23.270 -13.825 60.37 0.2935
Fecal.WT-Cecal.Vdr-/-       12.937 -24.159 50.03 0.7328
Cecal.WT-Fecal.Vdr-/-       -2.528 -39.624 34.57 0.9969
Fecal.WT-Fecal.Vdr-/-      -12.861 -49.957 24.23 0.7362
Fecal.WT-Cecal.WT          -10.333 -51.807 31.14 0.8792


> plot(TukeyHSD(aov(df_CH_G$value~df_CH_G$Group4), conf.level=.95))
```

This plot represents all possible pairwise tests and the p-values, and 95% confidence intervals. The default 95% confidence level can be changed based on your choice. Because all confidence lines cross 0, for this example, there are no significantly different terms after adjustment using Tukey multiple comparisons.

8.4 Comparisons Among More than Two Groups Using Kruskal-Wallis Test

8.4.1 Kruskal-Wallis Test

The Kruskal-Wallis test or One-way ANOVA on ranks, named after William Kruskal and W.Allen Wallis, is a non-parametric method for testing whether samples are originated from the same distribution (Kruskal and Wallis 1952; Daniel 1990). The parametric equivalent of the Kruskal-Wallis test is the one-way ANOVA. It extends the Mann-Whitney U test to more than two groups. The null hypothesis of the Kruskal-Wallis test is that the mean ranks of the groups are the same. Unlike the analogous one-way ANOVA, the non-parametric Kruskal-Wallis test does not assume a normal distribution of the underlying data. It has been widely used in microbiome research. For example, the post-sequencing microbiome data are not normally distributed and contain some strong outliers. Therefore, it is appropriate to use ranks rather than actual values to avoid the testing being affected by the presence of outliers or by non-normal distribution. The test statistic takes four main steps:

Step 1. Rank all data from all groups together in a single series in ascending order, i.e., rank the data from 1 to N ignoring group membership.
Step 2. Assign any tied values by averaging their rank position.
Step 3. Sum up the different ranks, e.g., R_1 R_2 R_3... for each of the different groups.
Step 4. Calculate the test statistic by applying the following formula:

$$H = \frac{12}{n(n+1)} \sum_{i=1}^{k} \frac{R_i^2}{n_i} - 3(n+1), \tag{8.8}$$

where

H Kruskal-Wallis test statistic
n   total number of measurements in all samples
n_i number of measurements in sample from population i
k   number of populations
R_i rank sum for sample i.

The Kruskal-Wallis test statistic is approximately a chi-square distribution, with $k - 1$ degrees of freedom if n_i values are 'large.' The approximation is generally accepted to be adequate when each of the n_i values is greater than or equal 5.

8.4.2   Compare Diversities Among Groups

Kruskal-Wallis test or Kruskal-Wallis one-way ANOVA is performed to compare multiple groups that data do not follow a normal distribution. This test is similar to the Wilcoxon rank sum test for two samples. We first use our $Vdr^{-/-}$ mouse data to illustrate this test.

```
> library(dplyr)
> Data <- mutate(df_CH_G, Group = factor(df_CH_G$Group4, levels=unique
(df_CH_G$Group4)))
```

Obtain Descriptive Statistics

```
> library(FSA)
> Summarize(value ~ Group4, data = df_CH_G)
         Group4 n  mean     sd   min    Q1 median     Q3     max
1 Cecal.Vdr-/- 5 57.37  3.659 52.17 55.00  59.00 59.80   60.88
2 Fecal.Vdr-/- 5 83.17 18.494 55.14 77.00  85.67 94.75  103.27
3     Cecal.WT 3 80.64 31.009 51.00 64.53  78.06 95.46  112.86
4     Fecal.WT 3 70.31  9.165 62.75 65.21  67.67 74.08   80.50
```

Generate Histograms by Group (Fig. 8.7).

```
> #Individual plots in panel of 2 columns and 2 rows
> library(lattice)
> histogram(~ value|Group4, data=df_CH_G, layout=c(2,2))
```

The histogram shows that the distributions of values among groups are different in this case. We now conduct Kruskal-Wallis test to compare the differences of medians using the kruskal.test() function.

```
> #kruskal wallis test of Chao 1 richness
> kruskal.test(value ~ Group4, data = df_CH_G)

        Kruskal-Wallis rank sum test
```

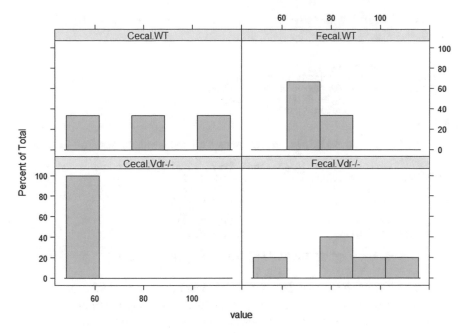

Fig. 8.7 Histograms of four groups in *Vdr* mouse fecal and cecal data

```
data:  value by Group4
Kruskal-Wallis chi-squared = 5.2, df = 3, p-value = 0.2
```

The value of the test statistic is 5.2 with *p*-value greater than 0.05 and it is also lower than the chi-square-tabulation:

```
> qchisq(0.950, 3)
[1] 7.815
```

Thus we accept the null hypothesis H_0: the medians of the 4 groups are statistically equal at 5% significant level.

Generally, a post hoc analysis is further conducted to find which levels of the groups are different from each other if the Kruskal-Wallis test is significant. In this case, the Kruskal-Wallis test is not significant. For the purpose of illustration, we conduct two post hoc tests: Nemenyi test and Dunn test. Similar to ANOVA, we can choose a method to adjust the *p*-values to control the familywise error rate or to control the false discovery rate. When you enter *?p.adjust* in R or RStudio, it appears a link to the document "Adjust *P*-values for Multiple Comparisons". You can check the details of adjustment methods from this link.

Nemenyi Test for Multiple Comparisons
Nemenyi test is performed via the NemenyiTest() function in DescTools package. We first load the DescTools package and call the function NemenyiTest(). The

method for adjusting the *p*-values should be one of "tukey", "chisq". We here choose the Tukey method.

```
> library(DescTools)
> #Tukey method for adjusting p-values
> Test_N = NemenyiTest(x = df_CH_G$value,
+                      g = df_CH_G$Group4,
+                      dist="tukey")
> Test_N

 Nemenyi's test of multiple comparisons for independent samples (tukey)

                             mean.rank.diff    pval
Fecal.Vdr-/--Cecal.Vdr-/-          6.6000  0.1254
Cecal.WT-Cecal.Vdr-/-             4.7333  0.5237
Fecal.WT-Cecal.Vdr-/-             5.0667  0.4636
Cecal.WT-Fecal.Vdr-/-            -1.8667  0.9501
Fecal.WT-Fecal.Vdr-/-            -1.5333  0.9713
Fecal.WT-Cecal.WT                 0.3333  0.9998
---
Signif. codes:  0 '***' 0.001 '**' 0.01 '*' 0.05 '.' 0.1 ' ' 1
```

Nemenyi's test shows that there is no significant mean rank differences of Chao 1 diversity among locations and genotypes in fecal and cecal vdr knockout samples using Tukey adjustment method. However, when the groups have unequal numbers of observations, Nemenyi test is inappropriate, and the Dunn test is appropriate (Zar 2010). We run the Dunn test as below.

Dunn Test for Multiple Comparisons

The most popular post hoc Kruskal-Wallis test is the Dunn test. We can perform the Dunn test using the dunnTest() function from FSA package. In following, we call the function dunnTest() and use Benjamini and Hochberg method to adjust the *p*-values.

```
> library(FSA)
> # "bh" suggests Benjamini and Hochberg  method for adjusting p-values
> Test_N = dunnTest(df_CH_G$value ~ df_CH_G$Group4,data=df_CH_G, method="bh")
> Test_N
Dunn (1964) Kruskal-Wallis multiple comparison
  p-values adjusted with the Benjamini-Hochberg method.

                     Comparison       Z P.unadj  P.adj
1      Cecal.Vdr-/- - Cecal.WT -1.36136 0.17340 0.3468
2 Cecal.Vdr-/- - Fecal.Vdr-/- -2.19190 0.02839 0.1703
3      Cecal.WT - Fecal.Vdr-/- -0.53688 0.59135 0.8870
4      Cecal.Vdr-/- - Fecal.WT -1.45723 0.14505 0.4352
5          Cecal.WT - Fecal.WT -0.08575 0.93167 0.9317
6      Fecal.Vdr-/- - Fecal.WT  0.44100 0.65921 0.7911
```

Dunn test shows that there is a statistical significant difference of Chao 1 diversity between cecal and fecal $Vdr^{-/-}$ samples. However, after the multiple comparison *p*-values are adjusted with the Benjamini-Hochberg method, there are no statistical significant terms among the locations and genotypes in the samples.

8.4.3 Find Significant Taxa Among Groups

In this section, we use Kruskal-Wallis test to illustrate how to find significant taxa among groups. Suppose we want to know if there exist any significant taxa among samples of $Vdr^{-/-}$ and WT mice from fecal and cecal locations. We use the Kruskal-Wallis test to each one of the 248 taxa (bacteria) in the data set.

First, normalize the abundance data and make the data to a data frame. One normalization method is to use log transformation.

```
> data<-log((abund_table+1)/(rowSums(abund_table)+dim(abund_table)
[2])))
> df<-as.data.frame(data)
```

Another normalization method is to convert the adundance count into relative abundance.

```
> df <- as.data.frame(abund_table/rowSums(abund_table))
```

Then, use the kruskal.test() function and an iterative R function to perform 248 tests (each for one bacterium). The kruskal.test() function have several key components:

- The test is looping for all taxa (columns) with the codes "for (i in 1:dim(df)[2])".
- For each loop, run Kruskal-Wallis test with codes "KW_test <- kruskal.test(df[,i], g=Group4)".
- The results are stored in a dataframe with one row per sample, and one column per each *p*-value of the KW test.
- Report the number of tests with cat function "cat(paste("Kruskal-Wallis test for ",names(df)[i]," ", i, "/", dim(df)[2], "; *p*-value=", KW_test$p.value,"\n", sep=""))".

```
> KW_table <- data.frame()
> for (i in 1:dim(df)[2]) {
+    #run KW test for each bacterium
+    KW_test <- kruskal.test(df[,i], g=df_CH_G$Group4)
+    # Store the result in the data frame
+    KW_table <- rbind(KW_table,
+                      data.frame(id=names(df)[i],
+                      p.value=KW_test$p.value
+                      ))
+    # Report number of bacteria tested
```

```
+   cat(paste("Kruskal-Wallis test for ",names(df)[i]," ", i, "/",
+        dim(df)[2], "; p-value=", KW_test$p.value,"\n", sep=""))
+ }
```

Check the dataframe table to make sure the function works:

```
> #Check the data frame table
> head(kw_table)
                       id  p.value
1              Tannerella 0.005289
2            Lactococcus 0.407302
3          Lactobacillus 0.058626
4 Lactobacillus::Lactococcus 0.476355
5          Parasutterella 0.120519
6            Helicobacter 0.140053
```

8.4.4   Multiple Testing and E-value, FWER and FDR

Several different types of multiple testing corrections exist in the literature. Among them the Bonferroni correction is more conservative. The correction is simply to divide the alpha by the number of tests. We have illustrated p-value adjustment using Bonferroni, Holm, Tukey methods and two versions of method adjusting for the "False Discovery Rate" in pairwise comparisons and tests using ANOVA in Sect. 8.3.2, and post hoc of Kruskal-Wallis test in Sect. 8.4.2. In this section, we present general multiple testing corrections: E-value, Family-Wise Error Rate (FWER), and FDR.

8.4.4.1   E-value

The E-value is the expected number of false positives by chance when you make multiple tests. You can simply multiply the p-value with the number of taxa on which the test is performed to get it: E-value = p-value × the number of tests. Please note that on the E-value, the base correction is to use the original alpha, the p-value from testing rather than the nominal p-value.

```
> #E-value
> KW_table$E.value <-KW_table$p.value * dim(KW_table)[1]
> KW_table$E.value
```

Since the E-value is just multiplying the p-value by the number of tests, it can be larger than 1. If there are many taxa in the dataframe for testing, this correction method is not easy to find the significant taxa. Significant taxa are those for which the E-value is much smaller than 1. The following codes are used to check whether or not the E-values are added to the result data frame:

```
> #check E-value in result data frame
> head(kW_table)
                          id p.value E.value
1                  Tannerella 0.005289   1.312
2                 Lactococcus 0.407302 101.011
3                Lactobacillus 0.058626  14.539
4 Lactobacillus::Lactococcus 0.476355 118.136
5               Parasutterella 0.120519  29.889
6                 Helicobacter 0.140053  34.733
```

8.4.4.2 FWER

FWER is the probability that you make at least one false positive (type I error). In other words, it is the probability that you did not reject the null hypothesis H_0: there are no differences among groups while making multiple tests. The formula is given by:

$$FWER = 1 - (1 - p - value)^T, \qquad (8.9)$$

where, T = the number of tests. In order to avoid rounding errors caused by direct calculation using above formula, in R it is better to compute FWER with a right-tail binomial distribution test. The R codes are given as below.

```
> #FWER
> KW_table$FWER <- pbinom(q=0, p=KW_table$p.value,size=dim(KW_table)[1],
lower.tail=FALSE)
```

Check the dataframe to see if FWER are added to the result data frame:

```
> #check the dataframetable
> head(kW_table)
                          id p.value E.value    FWER
1                  Tannerella 0.005289   1.312 0.7316
2                 Lactococcus 0.407302 101.011 1.0000
3                Lactobacillus 0.058626  14.539 1.0000
4 Lactobacillus::Lactococcus 0.476355 118.136 1.0000
5               Parasutterella 0.120519  29.889 1.0000
6                 Helicobacter 0.140053  34.733 1.0000
```

8.4.4.3 FDR

Last but not least important is the FDR. Benjamini and Hochberg (1995) defined the false discovery rate as follows:

FDR = expected proportion of erroneous rejections among all rejections.

In this case, FDR is the proportion of false positives among those taxa accepted as positive when you make multiple tests. The Benjamini-Hochberg correction consists in following steps.

First, order p-values from smallest to largest and make a rank (1, 2, 3,..., k,..., T); the codes are given below:

```
> #FDR
> #order p-values from smallest to largest
> kw_table <- kw_table[order(kw_table$p.value, decreasing=FALSE), ]
> head(kw_table)
               id  p.value E.value    FWER
8      Bacteroides 0.003976   0.986 0.6277
19       Alistipes 0.004637   1.150 0.6842
7       Prevotella 0.005174   1.283 0.7238
39 Butyricimonas 0.005174   1.283 0.7238
1       Tannerella 0.005289   1.312 0.7316
10    Odoribacter 0.008189   2.031 0.8699
```

Next, calculate the q-value using following equation and codes:

$$\text{q-value} = p - value * \text{T/k}, \tag{8.10}$$

```
> #calculate q-value
> kw_table$q.value.factor <- dim(kw_table)[1] / 1:dim(kw_table)[1]
> head(kw_table$q.value.factor)
[1] 248.00 124.00  82.67  62.00  49.60  41.33
```

```
> kw_table$q.value <- kw_table$p.value * kw_table$q.value.factor
> head(kw_table$q.value)
[1] 0.9860 0.5749 0.4277 0.3208 0.2623 0.3385
```

```
> #check to see if q-value added to the result data frame
> head(kw_table)
               id  p.value E.value    FWER q.value.factor q.value
8      Bacteroides 0.003976   0.986 0.6277         248.00  0.9860
19       Alistipes 0.004637   1.150 0.6842         124.00  0.5749
7       Prevotella 0.005174   1.283 0.7238          82.67  0.4277
39 Butyricimonas 0.005174   1.283 0.7238          62.00  0.3208
1       Tannerella 0.005289   1.312 0.7316          49.60  0.2623
10    Odoribacter 0.008189   2.031 0.8699          41.33  0.3385
```

Then, specify the target FDR and identify the last item of the ranked list having a q-value equal or less that the specified alpha by using the below codes:

```
> #set up alpha value
> KW_alpha=0.05
> #identify the last item of the ranked list with a q-value =< alpha
> last.significant.item <- max(which(KW_table$q.value <= KW_alpha))
Warning message:
In max(which(KW_table$q.value <= KW_alpha)) :
  no non-missing arguments to max; returning -Inf
> last.significant.item
[1] -Inf
```

In our case, there are no q-value less than or equal to the specified alpha, so the program returns negative infinite.

Finally, display the result frame table and chosen taxa:

```
> #display the chosen results
> selected <- 1:5
> #selected <- 1:last.significant.item
> print(kw_table[selected,])
                id  p.value E.value    FWER q.value.factor q.value
8      Bacteroides 0.003976   0.986 0.6277         248.00  0.9860
19       Alistipes 0.004637   1.150 0.6842         124.00  0.5749
7       Prevotella 0.005174   1.283 0.7238          82.67  0.4277
39   Butyricimonas 0.005174   1.283 0.7238          62.00  0.3208
1       Tannerella 0.005289   1.312 0.7316          49.60  0.2623

> diff.taxa.factor <- kw_table$id[selected]
> diff.taxa <- as.vector(diff.taxa.factor)
> diff.taxa
[1] "Bacteroides"   "Alistipes"     "Prevotella"
[4] "Butyricimonas" "Tannerella"
```

Because there are no q-value less or equal the specified alpha = 0.05 in this case, the above displayed 5 taxa are not based on FDR. They are the chosen taxa with smallest *p*-values. The Benjamini-Hochberg correction is less stringent than the other multiple testing corrections presented above and thus has a higher sensitivity. FDR is widely used in microbiome (Le Chatelier et al. 2013; Ballou et al. 2016) and other study fields (Jungquist et al. 2010) and many R functions.

8.5 Summary

In this chapter, we presented a variety of common and classic methods in all research fields. Some of them are widely applied in microbiome studies. We illustrated these methods for analyzing microbiome data with step-by-step implementation in the R system. The data sets are from our own publications (Jin et al. 2015; Wang et al. 2016). Readers may use the R codes and explanations provided in this chapter to analyze their own microbiome data. We focused on hypothesis testing for univariate community microbiome data in this chapter. In the coming Chap. 9, we will emphasize on hypothesis testing multivariate community microbiome data.

References

Aitchison, J. 1982. The statistical analysis of compositional data. *Journal of the Royal Statistical Society. Series B (Methodological)* 44 (2): 139–177.

Aitchison, J. 1986. *The statistical analysis of compositional data.* Chapman & Hall; reprinted in 2003, with additional material, by The Blackburn Press.

Ballou, A.L., R.A. Ali, et al. 2016. Development of the Chick microbiome: How early exposure influences future microbial diversity. *Frontiers in Veterinary Science* 3: 2.

Benjamini, Y. and Y. Hochberg 1995. Controlling the false discovery rate: A practical and powerful approach to multiple testing. *Journal of the Royal Statistical Society Series B* (57): 289–300.

Benjamini, Y., and D. Yekutieli. 2001. The control of the false discovery rate in multiple testing under dependency. *The Annals of Statistics* 29 (4): 1165–1188.

Cochran, W.G. 1952. The $\chi 2$ test of goodness of fit. *Annals of Mathematical Statistics* 25: 315–345.

Daniel, W. W. 1990. Kruskal–Wallis one-way analysis of variance by ranks. *Applied nonparametric statistics* (2nd ed.), 226–234. Boston, PWS-Kent.

Fisher, R.A. 1918. The correlation between relatives on the supposition of mendelian inheritance. *Philosophical Transactions of the Royal Society of Edinburgh* 52: 399–433.

Hochberg, Y. 1988. A sharper Bonferroni procedure for multiple tests of significance. *Biometrika* 75 (4): 800–802.

Holm, S. 1979. A simple sequentially rejective multiple test procedure. *Scandinavian Journal of Statistics* 6: 65–70.

Hommel, G. 1988. A stagewise rejective multiple test procedure based on a modified Bonferroni test.

Jin, D., S. Wu, et al. 2015. Lack of vitamin D receptor causes dysbiosis and changes the functions of the murine intestinal microbiome. *Clinical Therapeutics* 37 (5): 996–1009. e1007.

Jungquist, C.R., C. O'Brien, et al. 2010. The efficacy of cognitive-behavioral therapy for insomnia in patients with chronic pain. *Sleep Medicine* 11 (3): 302–309.

Kruskal, W.II., and W.A. Wallis. 1952. Use of ranks in one-criterion variance analysis. *Journal of the American Statistical Association* 47 (260): 583–621.

Le Chatelier, E., T. Nielsen, et al. 2013. Richness of human gut microbiome correlates with metabolic markers. *Nature* 500 (7464): 541–546.

Mann, H.B., and D.R. Whitney. 1947. On a test of whether one of two random variables is stochastically larger than the other. *Annals of Mathematical Statistics* 18 (1): 50–60.

Pearson, K. 1900. On the criterion that a given system of deviations from the probable in the case of a correlated system of variables is such that it can be reasonably supposed to have arisen from random sampling. *Philosophical Magazine Series* 5.50 (302): 157–175.

Ruxton, G.D. 2006. The unequal variance t-test is an underused alternative to student's t-test and the Mann-Whitney U test. *Behavioral Ecology* 17 (4): 688–690.

Sokal, R. R. and F. J. Rohlf, 2011. Biometry: The principles and practice of statistics in biological research, Freeman, W. H. & Company.

Wackerly, D. D., W. Mendenhall, et al. 2002. Mathematical statistics with applications. Duxbury Press.

Wang, J., L.B. Thingholm, et al. 2016. Genome-wide association analysis identifies variation in vitamin D receptor and other host factors influencing the gut microbiota. *Nature Genetics* 48 (11): 1396–1406.

Welch, B.L. 1947. The generalization of "Student's" problem when several different population variances are involved. *Biometrika* 34 (1–2): 28–35.

Zar, J.H. 2010. Biostatistical analysis. Upper Saddle River, NJ: Pearson Prentice Hall.

Chapter 9
Multivariate Community Analysis

The main goal of microbiome community studies is to compare the composition of different communities (beta diversity). In Chap. 6, we introduced beta diversities and illustrated how to calculate beta diversity indices. After we obtain beta diversity indices, we can conduct statistical analysis on them. The beta diversity analyses in studies of microbiome fall into two categories: exploratory techniques and statistical tests of significance. We illustrated clustering and ordination in Chap. 7. In this chapter, we focus on statistical tests of significance on beta diversity. Several methods or models have been developed to test for differences in microbiome community composition. We will introduce statistical tests of beta diversity using permutational multivariate analysis of variance (PERMANOVA), Mantel test, analysis of similarity (ANOSIM) , multi-response permutation procedures (MRPP) and generalized UniFrac distance via PERMANOVA.

9.1 Hypothesis Testing Among Groups Using Permutational Multivariate Analysis of Variance (PERMANOVA)

9.1.1 Introduction of PERMANOVA

The traditional multivariate analysis of variance (MANOVA) is simply an ANOVA with several dependent variables. ANOVA is used to test the null hypothesis: there are no differences in means between two or more groups; in contract, MANOVA could be used to test the null hypothesis: there are no differences in two or more vectors of means. Thus, it is particularly powerful for analysis of multivariate data. However, the traditional MANOVA assumes the dependent variable should be normally distributed within groups (normal distribution), the linear relationships among all pairs of dependent variables, all pairs of covariates, and all dependent

© Springer Nature Singapore Pte Ltd. 2018
Y. Xia et al., *Statistical Analysis of Microbiome Data with R*,
ICSA Book Series in Statistics, https://doi.org/10.1007/978-981-13-1534-3_9

variable-covariate pairs in each cell (linearity), the dependent variables exhibit equal levels of variance across the range of predictor variables (homogeneity of variances) and homogeneity of variances and covariances. Due to these stringent assumptions, the traditional MANOVA is not appropriate for most microbiome multivariate data sets. For example, it is not suitable to analyze the relationships between microbiome composition and environment factors (i.e., different treatment groups or conditions).

In 2001, Anderson (2001) proposed a nonparametric procedure for testing the hypothesis of no difference between two or more groups of samples based on the analysis and partitioning sums of square distances. It is called permutational MANOVA (formerly "nonparametric MANOVA", abbreviated as NP-MANOVA). Anderson's permutational MANOVA is formulated by the dissimilarity matrix. Let's consider a matrix of distances between every pair of observations and let $N = an$, the total number of observations (points), and d_{ij} be the distance between observation $i = 1,...,N$, and observation $j = 1,...,N$, then the total sum of squares is given below:

$$SS_T = \frac{1}{N} \sum_{i=1}^{N-1} \sum_{j=i+1}^{N} d_{ij}^2 \qquad (9.1)$$

The sum adds up the squares of all of the distances in the half sub-diagonal (or upper-diagonal) of the distance matrix (but not including the diagonal) and divide by N. SS_T is used to calculate average distance among all samples. Similarly, the within-group or residual sum of squares is

$$SS_W = \frac{1}{n} \sum_{i=1}^{N-1} \sum_{j=i+1}^{N} d_{ij}^2 \varepsilon_{ij} \qquad (9.2)$$

Where ε_{ij} is an indicator and takes the value 1 if observation i and observation j are in the same group, otherwise it takes the value of zero. That is, add up the squares of all of the distances between observations that occur in the same group and divide by n, the number of observations per group. With this formulation, SS_W is used to calculate average distance among samples within groups.

The sum of squares used to calculate average distance among groups can be obtained through subtract SS_T by SS_W. That is, $SS_A = SS_T - SS_W$. A pseudo F-ratio to test the multivariate hypothesis is given:

$$F = \frac{SS_A/(a-1)}{SS_W/(N-1)} \qquad (9.3)$$

The rationale for this test statistics lies in the fact if the points from different groups have different central locations (centroids in the case of Euclidean distances) in multivariate space, then the among-group distances will be relatively large compared to the within-group distances, and the resulting pseudo F-ratio will be relatively large.

From formula (9.3) as the F test statistic, we can see that the bigger the ratio between $SS_A/(a-1)$ to $SS_W/(N-1)$ (called the signal to noise ratio), the larger the F value, and thus results in a smaller p-value. The question is: how we can obtain a p-value? The individual variables in microbiome and ecology are typically not normally distributed and we do not expect that the Euclidean distance will necessarily be used for the analysis. As Anderson (2001) noticed, even if each of the variables were normally distributed and the Euclidean distance used, the mean squares calculated for the multivariate data would not each consist of sums of independent χ^2 variables, because, although individual observations are expected to be independent, individual species (OTUs or taxa) variables are not independent of one another. Thus, traditional tabled p-values cannot be used.

Anderson proposed to randomly shuffled (permuted) the variables within the dataset to generate empirical distribution. The algorithm underlying this is that under the null hypothesis, the groups are not really different, and then the multivariate observations (rows) would be exchangeable among the different groups. The random shuffling can be repeated for all possible re-orderings of the rows, such as 1000 times, and then 1000 distributions specific to the type of data are generated. The p-value, which indicates the significance between groups, will be obtained from the empirical F distribution.

Now, let us explain how we can obtain p-value from permutation testing. As presented above, permutations mean randomly assigning sample observations to groups. The p-value is calculated by comparing the permuted F-ratio to the observed F-ratio. The significance test is simply the fraction of permuted F-ratio that are greater than the observed F-ratio. Briefly, we take one-way test as an example to explain what permutations actually do. In a one-way test, our interest is to see whether a statistic is either less than or greater than what can be expected by chance. The p-value is calculated from the proportion of permuted pseudo F-statistics which are greater than or equal to the observed F-statistic. In another words, we want to know whether the permuted data sets following the PERMANOVA yield a better resolution of groups relative to the actual data set. If more than 5% of the permuted F-statistics has values greater than that of the observed F statistic, the p-value is greater than 0.05. Then, we can conclude that any difference among groups is not statistically significant.

PERMANOVA has at least two advantages over the traditional MANOVA. First, it does not require any assumptions about distributions. Second, it can use the distance matrix calculated by any distance metric. Obviously, non-distribution assumption is an advantage, but the later feature is also important, because the Euclidean distances-based analysis is to calculate average distance among samples within groups. In other words, it is to measure the central location for the group in Euclidean space, called a centroid. However, for many distance measures, it is difficult to calculate the central location. For example, in ecological and micro-biome studies, there exist many situations when the semi-metric Bray-Curtis measure is more appropriate; however, we cannot easily calculate the central location directly from the sample data in multivariate Bray-Curtis space.

9.1.2 Implementing PERMANOVA Using Vegan Package

PERMANOVA is implemented through the function adonis() in the vegan package. The function adonis() is used to analyze and partition sums of squares using semi-metric and metric distance matrices (Oksanen et al. 2016). Typical uses of adonis() include analysis of ecological and microbiome community data (samples by species (taxa) matrices) or genetic data with a limited number of samples of individuals and thousands or millions of columns of gene expression. The function adonis() allows ANOVA-like tests of the variance in beta diversity explained by continuous and/or categorical predictors. ADONIS is a recommended method in the vegan package. Other methods in vegan include MRPP and ANOSIM. However, both MRPP and ANOSIM handle only categorical predictors, and they are less robust than ADONIS (Oksanen et al. 2016).

To implement of PERMANOVA, you need to choose a distance measure. For regular measurements, usually the "euclidean" distance is the choice, but for community microbiome data, "bray" (the Bray-Curtis distance) is more appropriate. In the literature, four beta-diversity measures including Bray-Curtis distance, Jaccard distance, weighted and unweighted UniFrac distances typically have been reported (Linnenbrink et al. 2013).

One example of usages is given below:

adonis(formula, data, permutations = 1000, method = "bray", contr.unordered = "contr.sum", contr.ordered = "contr.poly")

In above syntax, formula = model formula, such as $Y \sim A + B + C * D$, where, Y can be a dissimilarity object (inheriting from class "dist"), a data frame or a matrix; A, B, C, and D may be factors or continuous variables.

data	the data frame.
permutations	number of replicate permutations used for the hypothesis tests (F tests).
method	name of any method used in the function vegdist () to calculate pairwise distances if the left hand side of the formula was a data frame or a matrix.
contr.unordered	contrasts used for the design matrix; in general, R default uses dummy or treatment contrasts for unordered factors. However, the default contrasts in vegan package are different; they use "sum" or "ANOVA" contrasts.
contr.ordered	contrasts used for the design matrix for ordered factors.

In Chap. 6, we calculate several beta-diversity measures including Bray-Curtis index using Vdr mouse sample data. After obtaining these beta-diversity indices, we can conduct multivariate community analysis to test how the composition of microbiome communities varies across different samples. In this case, first we want to test whether the composition of microbiome communities varies in fecal and cecal sites and differentiates between groups ($Vdr^{-/-}$ and WT mice). We also want to test within same site, such as fecal samples, whether genetic deficient group ($Vdr^{-/-}$ mice) has different microbiome composition, compared to the WT group.

Prepare Implementation of PERMANOVA Using Vegan Package

Since the location and group information is not directly given in our data set, we need additional programming to extract them from the sample ids, as we did in Chaps. 6, 7 and 8. The following codes are used to split string sample ids as three components as X1, X2, and X3.

```
> grouping<-data.frame(row.names=rownames(abund_table),t(as.data.frame(strsplit(rownames
(abund_table),"_"))))
> grouping<-data.frame(row.names=rownames(abund_table),t(as.data.frame
(strsplit(rownames(abund_table),"_"))))
> grouping
                    X1 X2         X3
5_15_dryST-28F     5 15 dryST-28F
20_12_CeST-28F    20 12  CeST-28F
1_11_dryST-28F     1 11 dryST-28F
2_12_dryST-28F     2 12 dryST-28F
3_13_dryST-28F     3 13 dryST-28F
4_14_dryST-28F     4 14 dryST-28F
7_22_dryST-28F     7 22 dryST-28F
8_23_dryST-28F     8 23 dryST-28F
9_24_dryST-28F     9 24 dryST-28F
19_11_CeST-28F    19 11  CeST-28F
21_13_CeST-28F    21 13  CeST-28F
22_14_CeST-28F    22 14  CeST-28F
23_15_CeST-28F    23 15  CeST-28F
25_22_CeST-28F    25 22  CeST-28F
26_23_CeST-28F    26 23  CeST-28F
27_24_CeST-28F    27 24  CeST-28F
```

In the data set, "dryST" indicates that the samples come from fecal, "CeST" indicates that the samples come from cecal. Thus, we create a location variable to group the samples from fecal and cecal sites.

```
> grouping$Location <- with(grouping, ifelse(X3%in%"dryST-28F",
"Fecal", "Cecal"))
```

We further separate $Vdr^{-/-}$ samples from WT samples within fecal and cecal sites as below:

```
> grouping$Group <- with(grouping,ifelse(as.factor(X2)%in% c
(11,12,13,14,15),c("Vdr-/-"), c("WT")))
```

Check variable names and remove X1, X2, and X3 from the data set.

```
> names(grouping)
> grouping <- grouping[,c(4,5)]
> grouping
                  Location  Group
5_15_dryST-28F     Fecal  Vdr-/-
20_12_CeST-28F     Cecal  Vdr-/-
1_11_dryST-28F     Fecal  Vdr-/-
2_12_dryST-28F     Fecal  Vdr-/-
3_13_dryST-28F     Fecal  Vdr-/-
4_14_dryST-28F     Fecal  Vdr-/-
7_22_dryST-28F     Fecal     WT
8_23_dryST-28F     Fecal     WT
9_24_dryST-28F     Fecal     WT
19_11_CeST-28F     Cecal  Vdr-/-
21_13_CeST-28F     Cecal  Vdr-/-
22_14_CeST-28F     Cecal  Vdr-/-
23_15_CeST-28F     Cecal  Vdr-/-
25_22_CeST-28F     Cecal     WT
26_23_CeST-28F     Cecal     WT
27_24_CeST-28F     Cecal     WT
```

After creating location and group variables, now we can call function adonis() to conduct PERMANOVA. The input data of the function adonis () can either be dissimilarities or data frame; in the latter case, adonis() uses vegdist() to find the dissimilarities. To illustrate, we choose the Bray-Curtis, Jaccard, and Sørensen beta-diversity measures. They were calculated in Chap. 6, so we can directly use them here.

Test Difference of the Bray-Curtis Dissimilarity Between Genotypes
The simplest R codes to implement PERMANOVA to test difference of the Bray-Curtis dissimilarity between $Vdr^{-/-}$ and wild type samples in vegan is as below.

```
> set.seed(123)
> # adonis="analysis of dissimilarity"
> adonis(bray ~ Group,data=grouping,permutations = 1000)

Call:
adonis(formula = bray ~ Group, data = grouping, permutations = 1000)

Permutation: free
Number of permutations: 1000

Terms added sequentially (first to last)

          Df SumsOfSqs MeanSqs F.Model    R2 Pr(>F)
Group      1     0.23    0.230     1.5 0.097   0.18
Residuals 14     2.14    0.153         0.903
Total     15     2.37                  1.000
```

If the Bray-Curtis dissimilarity measure is not given, the following codes give the same results.

```
> adonis(abund_table ~ Group,data=grouping,permutations = 1000, method =
"bray")

Call:
adonis(formula = abund_table ~ Group, data = grouping, permutations = 1000,
method = "bray")

Permutation: free
Number of permutations: 1000

Terms added sequentially (first to last)

          Df SumsOfSqs MeanSqs F.Model    R2 Pr(>F)
Group      1     0.23   0.230     1.5 0.097   0.19
Residuals 14     2.14   0.153         0.903
Total     15     2.37                 1.000
```

Except the difference of p-value due to round up, all statistics are same in these two outputs. The p-value was obtained by permutation test. The R^2 for group is 0.097, which means that 9.7% of total variance can be explained by group. Performing 1000 randomizations of the rows and columns of Bray-Curtis distance matrix generate the R^2 under the null hypothesis. Out of these 1000 values, 180 was larger than the observed value of 0.097, so that the chance of obtaining a value as large as the observed is smaller than 180/1000, indicating a p-value of 0.18. Thus, we conclude that the Bray-Curtis distance differences between $Vdr^{-/-}$ and wild type samples tend to be by chance.

Test Difference of the Jaccard Dissimilarity Between Genotypes

Similarly, we can implement PERMANOVA to test difference of the Jaccard dissimilarity between $Vdr^{-/-}$ and wild type samples.

```
> adonis(jaccard ~ Group,data=grouping,permutations = 1000)

Call:
adonis(formula = jaccard ~ Group, data = grouping, permutations = 1000)

Permutation: free
Number of permutations: 1000

Terms added sequentially (first to last)

          Df SumsOfSqs MeanSqs F.Model    R2 Pr(>F)
Group      1     0.33   0.334    1.37 0.089   0.17
Residuals 14     3.40   0.243         0.911
Total     15     3.74                 1.000
```

Test Difference of the Sørensen Dissimilarity Between Genotypes

```
> adonis(Sørensen ~ Group,data=grouping,permutations = 1000)

Call:
adonis(formula = Sørensen ~ Group, data = grouping, permutations = 1000)

Permutation: free
Number of permutations: 1000

Terms added sequentially (first to last)

          Df SumsOfSqs MeanSqs F.Model   R2 Pr(>F)
Group      1    0.119  0.1191     1.3 0.085   0.21
Residuals 14    1.282  0.0916         0.915
Total     15    1.401                 1.000
```

The PERMANOVA were performed using analysis of dissimilarity ("adonis") applied to Bray-Curtis, Jaccard and Sørensen beta-diversity measures. The $Vdr^{-/-}$ and WT mice samples displayed non-significant separation according to Bray-Curtis distance (adonis, $R^2 = 0.097$, $P = 0.18$), Jaccard distance ($R^2 = 0.089$, $P = 0.17$), and Sørensen distance ($R^2 = 0.085$, $P = 0.21$). We can conclude that given small sample size, with combined fecal and cecal samples, these three dissimilarities have no difference between $Vdr^{-/-}$ and WT mice at the 0.05 of statistical significance level.

Test Difference of the Bray-Curtis Dissimilarity Between Locations

The following R codes are used to test if the Bray-Curtis dissimilarities are different between fecal and cecal samples.

```
> adonis(bray ~ Location,data=grouping,permutations = 1000)

Call:
adonis(formula = bray ~ Location, data = grouping, permutations = 1000)

Permutation: free
Number of permutations: 1000

Terms added sequentially (first to last)

          Df SumsOfSqs MeanSqs F.Model   R2 Pr(>F)
Location   1    0.533   0.533    4.06 0.225  0.001 ***
Residuals 14    1.840   0.131         0.775
Total     15    2.374                 1.000
---
Signif. codes:  0 '***' 0.001 '**' 0.01 '*' 0.05 '.' 0.1 ' ' 1
```

The R^2 is 0.225, which suggests that 22.5% of total variance can be explained by location. Performing 1000 randomizations of the rows and columns of Bray-Curtis distance matrix generate the R^2 under the null hypothesis. Out of these 1000 values, one was larger than the observed value of 0.225, so that the chance of obtaining a value as large as the observed is smaller than 1/1000, indicating a p-value of 0.001.

Thus, we can conclude that the Bray-Curtis distance differences between fecal and cecal samples not tend to be by chance.

Test Difference of the Jaccard Dissimilarity Between Locations

The following R codes are used to test if the Jaccard dissimilarities are different between fecal and cecal samples:

```
> adonis(jaccard ~ Location,data=grouping,permutations = 1000)

Call:
adonis(formula = jaccard ~ Location, data = grouping, permutations = 1000)

Permutation: free
Number of permutations: 1000

Terms added sequentially (first to last)

          Df SumsOfSqs MeanSqs F.Model    R2 Pr(>F)
Location   1    0.64    0.645   2.92 0.173  0.006 **
Residuals 14    3.09    0.221        0.827
Total     15    3.74                 1.000
---
Signif. codes:  0 '***' 0.001 '**' 0.01 '*' 0.05 '.' 0.1 ' ' 1
```

Test Difference of the Sørensen Dissimilarity Between Locations

The following R codes are used to test if the Sørensen dissimilarities are different between fecal and cecal samples:

```
> adonis(Sørensen ~ Location,data=grouping,permutations = 1000)

Call:
adonis(formula = Sørensen ~ Location, data = grouping, permutations = 1000)

Permutation: free
Number of permutations: 1000

Terms added sequentially (first to last)

          Df SumsOfSqs MeanSqs F.Model    R2 Pr(>F)
Location   1    0.352   0.352   4.71 0.252  0.001 ***
Residuals 14    1.049   0.075        0.748
Total     15    1.401                1.000
---
Signif. codes:  0 '***' 0.001 '**' 0.01 '*' 0.05 '.' 0.1 ' ' 1
```

The fecal and cecal mice samples displayed significant separation according to Bray-Curtis distance (adonis, $R^2 = 0.225$, $P = 0.001$), Jaccard distance (adonis, $R^2 = 0.173$, $P = 0.006$), and Sørensen (adonis, $R^2 = 0.252$, $P = 0.001$). We can conclude that the differences between the two sites are statistically significant and that around 22.5%, 17.3% and 25.2% of the "variance" is accounted for by site differences according to Bray-Curtis distance, Jaccard distance and Sørensen distance, respectively.

Sequential Test the Bray-Curtis Dissimilarity Ordering by Group to Location

In testing of group, the $Vdr^{-/-}$ and WT samples are not differentiated from fecal or cecal location. In testing of location, the fecal and cecal samples are not differentiated from $Vdr^{-/-}$ or WT group. Actually, given two variables group and location, we can conduct a sequential test of permutation ANOVA. To illustrate, we use the Bray-Curtis dissimilarity to conduct the sequential test. The interested readers can try their own tests using Jaccard and Sørensen distance measures.

```
> adonis(bray ~ Group*Location,data=grouping,permutations = 1000)

Call:
adonis(formula = bray ~ Group * Location, data = grouping, permutations
= 1000)

Permutation: free
Number of permutations: 1000

Terms added sequentially (first to last)
```

	Df	SumsOfSqs	MeanSqs	F.Model	R2	Pr(>F)	
Group	1	0.230	0.230	1.77	0.097	0.123	
Location	1	0.533	0.533	4.10	0.225	0.001	***
Group:Location	1	0.051	0.051	0.39	0.021	0.928	
Residuals	12	1.559	0.130		0.657		
Total	15	2.374			1.000		

```
---
Signif. codes:  0 '***' 0.001 '**' 0.01 '*' 0.05 '.' 0.1 ' ' 1
```

Sequential Test the Bray-Curtis Dissimilarity Ordering Location by Group

```
> adonis(bray ~ Location*Group,data=grouping,permutations = 1000)

Call:
adonis(formula = bray ~ Location * Group, data = grouping, permutations
= 1000)

Permutation: free
Number of permutations: 1000

Terms added sequentially (first to last)
```

	Df	SumsOfSqs	MeanSqs	F.Model	R2	Pr(>F)	
Location	1	0.533	0.533	4.10	0.225	0.002	**
Group	1	0.230	0.230	1.77	0.097	0.095	.
Location:Group	1	0.051	0.051	0.39	0.021	0.909	
Residuals	12	1.559	0.130		0.657		
Total	15	2.374			1.000		

```
---
Signif. codes:  0 '***' 0.001 '**' 0.01 '*' 0.05 '.' 0.1 ' ' 1
```

Notice that the order of variables matters. However, either the group test first or location first, location is statistically significant with $p < 0.05$.

Test Difference of the Bray-Curtis Dissimilarity Among Four Levels of Group

Actually, we can implement PERMANOVA to test dissimilarity among four levels of group combining two genotypes and two locations. The following R codes create a group variable with 4 levels combining genotype variable and location variable. The default separator is '.'.

```
> grouping$Group4<- with(grouping, interaction(Location,Group))
> grouping
              Location  Group      Group4
5_15_drySt-28F    Fecal  Vdr-/- Fecal.Vdr-/-
20_12_CeSt-28F    Cecal  Vdr-/- Cecal.Vdr-/-
1_11_drySt-28F    Fecal  Vdr-/- Fecal.Vdr-/-
2_12_drySt-28F    Fecal  Vdr-/- Fecal.Vdr-/-
3_13_drySt-28F    Fecal  Vdr-/- Fecal.Vdr-/-
4_14_drySt-28F    Fecal  Vdr-/- Fecal.Vdr-/-
7_22_drySt-28F    Fecal      WT    Fecal.WT
8_23_drySt-28F    Fecal      WT    Fecal.WT
9_24_drySt-28F    Fecal      WT    Fecal.WT
19_11_CeSt-28F    Cecal  Vdr-/- Cecal.Vdr-/-
21_13_CeSt-28F    Cecal  Vdr-/- Cecal.Vdr-/-
22_14_CeSt-28F    Cecal  Vdr-/- Cecal.Vdr-/-
23_15_CeSt-28F    Cecal  Vdr-/- Cecal.Vdr-/-
25_22_CeSt-28F    Cecal      WT    Cecal.WT
26_23_CeSt-28F    Cecal      WT    Cecal.WT
27_24_CeSt-28F    Cecal      WT    Cecal.WT
```

A PERMANOVA is implemented to test dissimilarity among four levels of group.

```
> adonis(bray ~ Group4,data=grouping,permutations = 1000)
Call:
adonis(formula = bray ~ Group4, data = grouping, permutations = 1000)

Permutation: free
Number of permutations: 1000

Terms added sequentially (first to last)

          Df SumsOfSqs MeanSqs F.Model    R2 Pr(>F)
Group4     3    0.814   0.271    2.09 0.343  0.018 *
Residuals 12    1.559   0.130         0.657
Total     15    2.374                 1.000
---
Signif. codes:  0 '***' 0.001 '**' 0.01 '*' 0.05 '.' 0.1 ' ' 1
```

The samples displayed significant separation according to Bray-Curtis distance (adonis, $R^2 = 0.343$, $P = 0.018$). We can conclude that the differences among the four levels of group are statistically significant; based on Bray-Curtis dissimilarity, around 34.3% of the "variance" is accounted for by group differences.

Change the Default Dummy Contrasts in R to the Default "Sum" Contrasts in Vegan Package

For unordered factors in the design matrix, R default uses dummy or treatment contrasts. The vegan package default uses "sum" or ANOVA contrasts. The "sum" contrasts for unordered factors are used to change the default contrasts in R.

```
> adonis(bray ~ Group4,data=grouping,permutations = 1000,contr.unordered =
"contr.sum")

Call:
adonis(formula = bray ~ Group4, data = grouping, permutations = 1000,
contr.unordered = "contr.sum")

Permutation: free
Number of permutations: 1000

Terms added sequentially (first to last)

          Df SumsOfSqs MeanSqs F.Model   R2 Pr(>F)
Group4     3    0.814   0.271   2.09 0.343  0.009 **
Residuals 12    1.559   0.130        0.657
Total     15    2.374                1.000
---
Signif. codes:  0 '***' 0.001 '**' 0.01 '*' 0.05 '.' 0.1 ' ' 1
```

Add the Contrasts for Ordered Factors

The following R codes add a "poly" contrasts for ordered factors to the test.

```
> adonis(bray ~ Group4,data=grouping,permutations = 1000,contr.unordered =
"contr.sum",contr.ordered = "contr.poly")

Call:
adonis(formula = bray ~ Group4, data = grouping, permutations = 1000,
contr.unordered = "contr.sum", contr.ordered = "contr.poly")

Permutation: free
Number of permutations: 1000

Terms added sequentially (first to last)

          Df SumsOfSqs MeanSqs F.Model   R2 Pr(>F)
Group4     3    0.814   0.271   2.09 0.343  0.011 *
Residuals 12    1.559   0.130        0.657
Total     15    2.374                1.000
---
Signif. codes:  0 '***' 0.001 '**' 0.01 '*' 0.05 '.' 0.1 ' ' 1
```

Test the Global Differences Among Groups

We can conduct a permutational MANOVA to test the global differences among these four levels of group using one of following two sample calls. Both calls give same output.

```
> adonis(bray ~ grouping$Group4,permutations = 1000)

Call:
adonis(formula = bray ~ grouping$Group4, permutations = 1000)

Permutation: free
Number of permutations: 1000

Terms added sequentially (first to last)

                Df SumsOfSqs MeanSqs F.Model     R2 Pr(>F)
grouping$Group4  3     0.814   0.271    2.09 0.343  0.017 *
Residuals       12     1.559   0.130         0.657
Total           15     2.374                 1.000
---
Signif. codes:  0 '***' 0.001 '**' 0.01 '*' 0.05 '.' 0.1 ' ' 1


> adonis(abund_table ~ Group4,data=grouping,permutations = 1000, method =
"bray")

Call:
adonis(formula = abund_table ~ Group4, data = grouping, permutations =
1000,method = "bray")

Permutation: free
Number of permutations: 1000

Terms added sequentially (first to last)

          Df SumsOfSqs MeanSqs F.Model     R2 Pr(>F)
Group4     3     0.814   0.271    2.09 0.343   0.01 **
Residuals 12     1.559   0.130         0.657
Total     15     2.374                 1.000
---
Signif. codes:  0 '***' 0.001 '**' 0.01 '*' 0.05 '.' 0.1 ' ' 1
```

9.1.3 Implementing Pairwise Permutational MANOVA Using RVAideMemoire Package

In ANOVA, a significant testing result in permutational MANOVA indicates that there is a significant difference among the defined groups; however, there is no way to know which groups are separated significantly. After the PERMANOVA is conducted using the vegan, a pairwise permutational MANOVA can be performed by using the function pairwise.perm.manova() from the RVAideMemoire package (Hommel 1988) to do pairwise comparisons of each group level with corrections for multiple testing.

One example call of this function is as below.

pairwise.perm.manova(resp, fact, test = c("Pillai", "Wilks","Hotelling-Lawley", "Roy", "Spherical"), nperm = 1000, progress = TRUE, p.method = "fdr") where, resp = response, either a typical matrix (one column per variable), or a distance matrix, or a data frame; fact = grouping factor; test = choice of test statistic when response is a matrix; nperm = number of permutations to obtain the *p*-value; progress = logical indicating if the progress bar should be displayed; and p.method = method for *p*-values correction.

As in multiple comparisons using ANOVA in Sect. 8.3.2, Kruskal-Wallis Test in Sect. 8.4.2, several *p*-value adjustment methods are available in pairwise permutational MANOVA including:

"bonferroni" (Bonferroni 1936), "holm" (Holm 1979), "hochberg" and "hommel" (Hochberg 1988),

"BH" or its alias "fdr" (Benjamini and Hochberg 1995), "BY" (Benjamini and Yekutieli 2001).

Tukey method is not available in this package. Type? p.adjust() to check the options and references in R. If you do not want to adjust the p-value, use the pass-through option ("none").

To perform a pairwise permutational MANOVA, we first need to install and load the RVAideMemoire package.

```
> install.packages("RVAideMemoire")
> library(RVAideMemoire)
```

We then can use either one of following three sample calls to conduct a pairwise permutational MANOVA.

```
> set.seed(0)
> pairwise.perm.manova(bray,grouping$Group4,nperm=1000)

> # or
> pairwise.perm.manova(vegdist(abund_table,"bray"),grouping$Group4,
nperm=1000)
> # or
> pairwise.perm.manova(bray, grouping$Group4, test = c("Pillai",
"Wilks","Hotelling-Lawley", "Roy", "Spherical"),
nperm = 1000,
+                       progress = TRUE, p.method = "fdr")
```

Adjust the P-Values Using "none" Method
The *p*-value is not adjusted when using p.method = "none".

```
> pairwise.perm.manova(bray, grouping$Group4, test = c("Pillai", "Wilks",
"Hotelling-Lawley", "Roy", "Spherical"), nperm = 1000,
+                         progress = TRUE, p.method = "none")
        Pairwise comparisons using permutation MANOVAs on a distance matrix

data:  bray by grouping$Group4
1000 permutations

            Cecal.Vdr-/- Fecal.Vdr-/- Cecal.WT
Fecal.Vdr-/- 0.02          -            -
Cecal.WT     0.64          0.07         -
Fecal.WT     0.08          0.16         0.50

P value adjustment method: none
```

Adjust the P-Values Using "bonferroni" Method

```
> pairwise.perm.manova(bray, grouping$Group4, test = c("Pillai", "Wilks",
"Hotelling-Lawley", "Roy", "Spherical"), nperm = 1000,
+                         progress = TRUE, p.method = "bonferroni")
        Pairwise comparisons using permutation MANOVAs on a distance matrix

data:  bray by grouping$Group4
1000 permutations

            Cecal.Vdr-/- Fecal.Vdr-/- Cecal.WT
Fecal.Vdr-/- 0.1          -            -
Cecal.WT     1.0          0.3          -
Fecal.WT     0.4          1.0          1.0

P value adjustment method: bonferroni
```

Adjust the P-Values Using "holm" Method

```
> pairwise.perm.manova(bray, grouping$Group4, test = c("Pillai", "Wilks",
"Hotelling-Lawley", "Roy", "Spherical"), nperm = 1000,
+                         progress = TRUE, p.method = "holm")
        Pairwise comparisons using permutation MANOVAs on a distance matrix

data:  bray by grouping$Group4
1000 permutations

            Cecal.Vdr-/- Fecal.Vdr-/- Cecal.WT
Fecal.Vdr-/- 0.09          -            -
Cecal.WT     1.00          0.24         -
Fecal.WT     0.27          0.52         1.00

P value adjustment method: holm
```

Adjust the P-Values Using "hochberg" Method

```
> pairwise.perm.manova(bray, grouping$Group4, test = c("Pillai", "Wilks",
"Hotelling-Lawley", "Roy", "Spherical"), nperm = 1000,
+                        progress = TRUE, p.method = "hochberg")
        Pairwise comparisons using permutation MANOVAs on a distance matrix

data:  bray by grouping$Group4
1000 permutations
```

	Cecal.Vdr-/-	Fecal.Vdr-/-	Cecal.WT
Fecal.Vdr-/-	0.06	–	–
Cecal.WT	0.65	0.23	–
Fecal.WT	0.26	0.45	0.65

```
P value adjustment method: hochberg
```

Adjust the P-Values Using "hommel" Method

```
> pairwise.perm.manova(bray, grouping$Group4, test = c("Pillai", "Wilks",
"Hotelling-Lawley", "Roy", "Spherical"), nperm = 1000,
+                        progress = TRUE, p.method = "hommel")
        Pairwise comparisons using permutation MANOVAs on a distance matrix

data:  bray by grouping$Group4
1000 permutations
```

	Cecal.Vdr-/-	Fecal.Vdr-/-	Cecal.WT
Fecal.Vdr-/-	0.07	–	–
Cecal.WT	0.64	0.20	–
Fecal.WT	0.30	0.53	0.64

```
P value adjustment method: hommel
```

Adjust the P-Values Using "BH" Method

```
> pairwise.perm.manova(bray, grouping$Group4, test = c("Pillai", "Wilks",
"Hotelling-Lawley", "Roy", "Spherical"), nperm = 1000,
+                        progress = TRUE, p.method = "BH")
        Pairwise comparisons using permutation MANOVAs on a distance matrix

data:  bray by grouping$Group4
1000 permutations
```

	Cecal.Vdr-/-	Fecal.Vdr-/-	Cecal.WT
Fecal.Vdr-/-	0.1	–	–
Cecal.WT	0.7	0.2	–
Fecal.WT	0.2	0.2	0.6

```
P value adjustment method: BH
```

Adjust the P-Values Using "fdr" Method

```
> pairwise.perm.manova(bray, grouping$Group4, test = c("Pillai", "Wilks",
"Hotelling-Lawley", "Roy", "Spherical"), nperm = 1000,
+                      progress = TRUE, p.method = "fdr")
        Pairwise comparisons using permutation MANOVAs on a distance matrix

data:  bray by grouping$Group4
1000 permutations

             Cecal.Vdr-/- Fecal.Vdr-/- Cecal.WT
Fecal.Vdr-/- 0.1          –            –
Cecal.WT     0.6          0.1          –
Fecal.WT     0.1          0.3          0.6

P value adjustment method: fdr
```

Adjust the P-Values Using "BY" Method

```
> pairwise.perm.manova(bray, grouping$Group4, test = c("Pillai", "Wilks",
"Hotelling-Lawley", "Roy", "Spherical"), nperm = 1000,
+                      progress = TRUE, p.method = "BY")
        Pairwise comparisons using permutation MANOVAs on a distance matrix

data:  bray by grouping$Group4
1000 permutations

             Cecal.Vdr-/- Fecal.Vdr-/- Cecal.WT
Fecal.Vdr-/- 0.3          –            –
Cecal.WT     1.0          0.3          –
Fecal.WT     0.3          0.6          1.0

P value adjustment method: BY


             Cecal.Vdr-/- Fecal.Vdr-/- Cecal.WT
Fecal.Vdr-/- 0.02         –            –
Cecal.WT     0.64         0.07         –
Fecal.WT     0.08         0.16         0.50

P value adjustment method: none
```

Without adjusting, fecal $Vdr^{-/-}$ and cecal $Vdr^{-/-}$ samples are significantly separated with p-value of 0.02. However, after adjustment using either method, none pairwise items have significant at the 0.05 significance level.

9.1.4   Test Group Homogeneities Using the Function betadisper()

After testing the group mean differences using the function adonis(), we can test the differences in group homogeneities by the function betadisper(). The adonis() is analogous to multivariate analysis of variance, and the betadisper() is analogous to Levene's test of the equality of variances.

```
> homo <-with(grouping,betadisper(bray, Group4))
> homo

          Homogeneity of multivariate dispersions

Call: betadisper(d = bray, group = Group4)

No. of Positive Eigenvalues: 11
No. of Negative Eigenvalues: 4

Average distance to median:
Cecal.Vdr-/- Fecal.Vdr-/-    Cecal.WT    Fecal.WT
     0.342        0.285       0.309        0.239

Eigenvalues for PCoA axes:
PCoA1 PCoA2 PCoA3 PCoA4 PCoA5 PCoA6 PCoA7 PCoA8
0.775 0.628 0.358 0.174 0.161 0.116 0.100 0.045
```

The function has plot and boxplot methods for graphical display. The following R code produces the plot of PCoA in Fig. 9.1.

```
> plot(homo)
```

The following R code produces the boxplot for four groups of distance to centroid in Fig. 9.2.

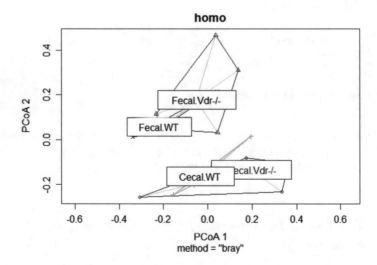

Fig. 9.1 Plot of PCoA for inspecting the homogeneity of multivariate dispersions

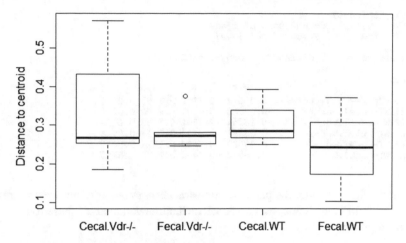

Fig. 9.2 Boxplot for four groups of distance to centroid

```
> boxplot(homo)
```

We can use either standard parametric ANOVA or permutation tests (permutest) to analyze the significance of the fitted model.

```
> anova(homo)
Analysis of Variance Table

Response: Distances
          Df Sum Sq Mean Sq F value Pr(>F)
Groups     3  0.021 0.00701    0.54   0.67
Residuals 12  0.157 0.01305
```

```
> permutest(homo)

Permutation test for homogeneity of multivariate dispersions
Permutation: free
Number of permutations: 999

Response: Distances
          Df Sum Sq Mean Sq      F N.Perm Pr(>F)
Groups     3  0.021 0.00701 0.54      999   0.67
Residuals 12  0.157 0.01305
```

Both parametric and permutation tests show that multivariate dispersions are not statistically different at 0.05 significance level.

Furthermore, the pairwise differences between groups can be analyzed using parametric Tukey's HSD test as follows:

```
> TukeyHSD(homo)
  Tukey multiple comparisons of means
    95% family-wise confidence level

Fit: aov(formula = distances ~ group, data = df)

$group
                              diff     lwr    upr  p adj
Fecal.Vdr-/--Cecal.Vdr-/- -0.05622 -0.2707 0.1583 0.8629
Cecal.WT-Cecal.Vdr-/-     -0.03273 -0.2804 0.2150 0.9786
Fecal.WT-Cecal.Vdr-/-     -0.10244 -0.3501 0.1453 0.6221
Cecal.WT-Fecal.Vdr-/-      0.02349 -0.2242 0.2712 0.9918
Fecal.WT-Fecal.Vdr-/-     -0.04623 -0.2939 0.2015 0.9437
Fecal.WT-Cecal.WT         -0.06972 -0.3466 0.2072 0.8760
```

The results show that the pairwise comparisons among these four groups are not statistically different. Thus, we can conclude that the variances of these four groups are homogeneous.

9.2   Hypothesis Tests Among Group-Differences Using Mantel Test (MANTEL)

9.2.1   Introduction of Mantel and Partial Mantel Tests for Dissimilarity Matrices

Mantel initiated a permutational testing procedure (Mantel 1967) to test the correlation between two distance matrices and further developed in Mantel and Valand (Mantel and Valand 1970). Because of this initiation, the procedure has known as the Mantel test in the biological and environmental sciences, and it is also referred to as Mantel and Valand's nonparametric MANOVA in the statistical literature.

Typically, correlation analysis is used to quantify the association between two continuous variables either between an independent and a dependent variable or between two independent variables. Mantel's test has the advantage: it can be applied to different types of variables including categorical, rank, or interval-scale data because it uses a distance (dissimilarity) matrix as its input data. The setting of Mantel's test is a regression analysis in which the variables themselves are distance or dissimilarity matrices summarizing pairwise similarities among sample locations. With this setting, the dependent variable is not the "abundance of taxon X on sample i", instead it might be "similarity of the average amount of taxon X on samples i and j"; similarly, the predictor variable is not the "condition" for a single sample, it might be "similarity of condition" between samples.

In summary, Mantel's test is a correlation analysis because it analyzes the association between two variables or distance matrices. It is merely a regression on distance matrices. Actually, the power and versatility of Mantel's test lie in it handling the distance matrices and framing the regression analysis. The capabilities of including categorical variables in correlation analysis, and converting these variables to distance (dissimilarity) metrics make the metrics better for hypothesis testing, which is especially useful for ecologists and microbiome researchers. Thus, Mantel's test is recognized as overcoming some of the problems inherent in explaining species-environment relationships (Legendre and Fortin 1989) or in general taxa-environment relationships.

Generally, the null hypothesis in Mantel's test is constructed like this: the distances among samples in a matrix of response variables are not linearly correlated with another matrix of explanatory variables. The operative questions we can ask are something like these: "do samples that are similar in terms of the predictor (environmental) variables also tend to be similar in terms of the dependent (taxon) variable?" Or "are samples that are close together also compositionally similar?" Or put another way, "are samples that are in different groups or environmentally dissimilar from each other also different in terms of compositions of taxa or compositionally dissimilar?" The test statistic is given as follows:

$$z = \sum_{i=1}^{n-1} \sum_{j=i+1}^{n} x_{ij} y_{ij} \tag{9.4}$$

where, z = test statistic, is Hadamard product (matrices), was named after French mathematician Jacques Hadamard. In the product, the two matrices with the same dimensions produce another matrix where each element ij is the product of elements ij of the original two matrices; Y_{ij} is the dependent distance matrix or condensed vectors; X_{ij} is the predictor matrix or contrast matrix for groups taking 0 if the sample in sample groups, taking 1 if the sample in different groups. The appropriate distance metric can be univariate (e.g., "similarity in *Bacteroides* abundance") or multivariate (e.g., Bray-Curtis', Jaccard's, Sørenson's index of similarity); n is the number of samples.

We can divide the process of Mantel's test into following four main steps:

Step 1: calculate dissimilarity matrices.
Step 2: calculate test statistic Z.
Step 3: test the significance.

Mantel test compares two sets of dissimilarities by judging whether similarity (or closeness) in one set of variables is related to similarity (or closeness) in another set of variables. Basically, it is the correlation between dissimilarity entries. Because the elements of a distance matrix are not independent and there are too many dissimilarities among N samples (N(N − 1)/2), normal significance tests are not applicable. Mantel developed asymptotic test statistics, but in vegan package, the function mantel() uses permutation tests. As in PERMANOVA test, the p-value of test statistic z is obtained through randomly rearranging of the rows and columns of one of the input distance matrices (the first dissimilarity matrix). The significance test is simply the fraction of permuted Z's that are greater than the observed Z. It is the probability of a Z given this large or larger. If randomizations frequently produce a correlation greater or equal to the observed data little evidence that correlation differs from zero. If these two distances are rank transformed, Mantel's test is the same as ANOSIM and similar to rank-transformed MRPP.

Step 4: calculate the correlation r of the two matrices to determine the strength of the relationship between them. The standardized Mantel statistic r is given below:

$$r = \frac{\sum_i \sum_j \left[\frac{(x_{ij}-\bar{x})}{s_x}\right]\left[\frac{(y_{ij}-\bar{y})}{s_y}\right]}{n-1}$$

(9.5)

The standardized Mantel statistic r is interpreted like a correlation coefficient which is a measure of "effect size" as other type of correlation coefficient such as Pearson's coefficient r. The value of r falls in the range of -1 to $+1$, where being close to -1 indicates strong negative correlation and $+1$ indicates strong positive correlation. If the average within-group distance between samples is less than the average overall distance between samples, then $r > 0$; the larger the r, the more correlated the groups.

While the Mantel test is used to compare between two distance (dissimilarity) matrices, such as A and B, the partial Mantel test is used to estimate the correlation between these two matrices, while controlling for the effect of a control matrix C. The goal is to remove spurious correlations. In ecological literature, one typical example of the partial Mantel test is used to compare a community distance matrix with another distance matrix derived from an environmental parameter, while using geographic distance as the third "control" distance matrix. In microbiome study, the third matrix C could be either an environmental matrix or an experimental design matrix created from an environmental matrix or another variable such as treatment membership or conditions. But remember, both the environmental and the design matrices derived from an environmental parameter need to be numeric/continuous in nature; and also need to be distance (dissimilarity) matrices. If the created matrix is not a distance (dissimilarity) matrix, you should use a distance function to convert it to distance (dissimilarity) matrix before you use it as a control matrix in the partial Mantel test.

The partial Mantel test is constructed through two steps: First, to conduct the regression between **A** and **C** to construct a matrix of residuals, **A'**, and the regression between **B** and **C** to construct a matrix of residuals, **B'**; then compare the two residual matrices, **A'** and **B'** by a standard Mantel test.

9.2.2 Illustrating Mantel Test Using Vegan Package

9.2.2.1 Test the Correlation of Two Community Distance Matrices

With high-depth sampling was conducted, Bray-Curtis, Jaccard and Sørensen dissimilarity indices usually have higher correlation. We can conduct a mantel test for these matrices. Mantel test can be performed by vegan, ape and ade4 packages. Here, we use the vegan package for this test. One syntax is given as below:

mantel(xdis, ydis, method = "pearson", permutations = 1000)

where, xdis, ydis are dissimilarity matrices or a distance objects; method is correlation method, is a character string, accepted as "pearson", "spearman" or "kendall"; permutations are the number of permutations need to be specified in assessing significance.

In Chap. 7, we used the smoker data set from the GUniFrac package to plot tree and illustrate ordination techniques. In this section, we use it again to illustrate Mantel test. The following R codes load the package, access and subset the data.

```
> library(GUniFrac)
> data(throat.otu.tab)
> otu_table <-throat.otu.tab
> data(throat.meta)
> data(throat.tree)
> library(dplyr)
> throat_meta <- select(throat.meta, SmokingStatus, Age, Sex, PackYears)
```

Test Pearson's Product-Moment Correlation of Bray-Curtis and Jaccard Dissimilarities
The correlation of Bray-Curtis and Jaccard dissimilarity indices is estimated as below.

```
> library(vegan)
> mantel(bray, jaccard,"pearson",permutations=1000)

Mantel statistic based on Pearson's product-moment correlation

Call:
mantel(xdis = bray, ydis = jaccard, method = "pearson", permutations = 1000)

Mantel statistic r: 0.993
      Significance: 0.001

Upper quantiles of permutations (null model):
  90%    95% 97.5%    99%
0.154 0.201 0.233 0.266
Permutation: free
Number of permutations: 1000
```

The Mantel test can be interpreted this way:

We specified permutations = 1000 to perform 1000 randomizations of the rows and columns of Bray-Curtis distance matrix that generate the distribution of correlations under the null hypothesis: the distances among samples in Bray-Curtis matrix are not linearly correlated with Jaccard matrix. The results show that, in this case, out of these 1000 values, none was larger than the observed value of 0.993 (that is, number of permutations < observed = 1000; number of permutations > observed = 0; number of permutations = observed = 1), so that the chance of obtaining a value as large as the observed is smaller than 1/1000, indicating a p-value of 0.001. Because a large correlation generated by chance is so small, we can conclude that Bray-Curtis

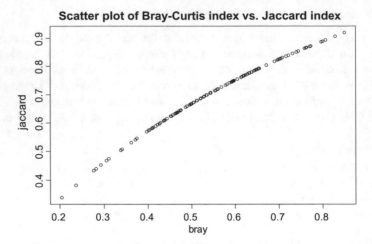

Fig. 9.3 Scatterplot of Pearson correlation between Bray-Curtis and Jaccard matrices

distance differences increase linearly with Jaccard distances; in other words, these two dissimilarity indices are highly positively correlated.

We can plot Pearson correlation of Bray-Curtis and Jaccard matrices as below:

```
> plot(bray, jaccard, main="Scatter plot of Bray-Curtis index vs. Jaccard
index")
```

The Pearson's coefficient r is 0.993 with a *p*-value of 0.001. The scatterplot of elements in Bray-Curtis and Jaccard matrices suggests a linear relationship between these two distances/dissimilarities as shown in Fig. 9.3.

Test Spearman's Rank Correlation of Bray-Curtis and Sørensen Dissimilarities
We calculate the correlation of Bray-Curtis and Sørensen dissimilarity indices using Spearman methods as bellow:

```
> mantel(bray, Sørensen,"spearman",permutations=1000)

Mantel statistic based on Spearman's rank correlation rho

call:
mantel(xdis = bray, ydis = Sørensen, method = "spearman", permutations
= 1000)

Mantel statistic r: 0.514
      Significance: 0.001

Upper quantiles of permutations (null model):
   90%   95% 97.5%   99%
0.132 0.178 0.206 0.241
Permutation: free
Number of permutations: 1000
```

Test Kendall's Rank Correlation of Jaccard and Sørensen Dissimilarities
Below we calculate the correlation of Jaccard and Sørensen dissimilarity indices
using Kendall method.

```
> mantel(jaccard,Sørensen,"kendall",permutations=1000)

Mantel statistic based on Kendall's rank correlation tau

Call:
mantel(xdis = jaccard, ydis = Sørensen, method = "kendall", permutations
= 1000)

Mantel statistic r: 0.358
      Significance: 0.001

Upper quantiles of permutations (null model):
   90%    95% 97.5%    99%
0.0961 0.1285 0.1521 0.1849
Permutation: free
Number of permutations: 1000
```

9.2.2.2 Test the Correlation of a Community Matrix and a Design Matrix

In Sect. 9.2.2.1, the Mantel tests were conducted between two community
matrices. Here we illustrate the test by choosing the Bray-Curtis matrix as the
dependent distance matrix, the smoking status from meta-data as the design
matrix. We will test whether the Bray-Curtis dissimilarities are different between
samples from smokers and non-smokers. The variable SmokingStatus is in throat.
meta data set.

The following R codes extract this variable and convert it to a distance matrix.

```
> library(dplyr)
> group <-select(throat.meta, SmokingStatus)
> group$Status <- with(group, ifelse(SmokingStatus%in%"Smoker", 1, 0))
> group <- group[,-1]
> group_dist <- vegdist(scale(group), "euclid")
```

The following R codes conduct the Mantel test of the Pearson's product-moment
correlation of the Bray-Curtis matrix (the dependent distance matrix) and the
smoking status (the predictor matrix).

```
> mantel(group_dist,bray,"pearson",permutations = 1000)

Mantel statistic based on Pearson's product-moment correlation

Call:
mantel(xdis = group_dist, ydis = bray, method = "pearson", permutations
= 1000)

Mantel statistic r: 0.0728
      Significance: 0.003

Upper quantiles of permutations (null model):
   90%     95%  97.5%     99%
0.0245 0.0336 0.0436 0.0581
Permutation: free
Number of permutations: 1000
```

The Mantel statistic r of 0.0728 with p-value of 0.003 indicates that the results are statistically significant at an α of 0.05. Hence, we conclude that smoking status really predicts the Bray-Curtis dissimilarities although there is relatively weak positive correlation between these two matrices. The *p*-value is obtained by specifying 1000 permutations.

9.2.2.3   Partial Mantel Test the Correlation of Two Distance Matrices Controlling the Third Matrix

The Mantel partial test is used to conduct correlation analysis of a community distance matrix and a design distance matrix while controlling an environmental distance matrix (Smouse et al. 1986). For example, the Mantel partial test can be used to determine if there is significant correlation of the Bray-Curtis distance (dissimilarity) matrix and the smoking status distance matrix when control the matrix with age, gender, and pack per year.

Suppose we would like to know "How much of the variability in Bray-Curtis dissimilarity (the dependent matrix) is explained by the smoking status (the design matrix) while controlling the environmental matrix (the predictor matrix: with age, gender, and pack per year)?" Then, the test statistic is calculated by constructing a matrix of residuals, **A'**, of the regression between the smoking status and the predictor matrix with age, gender, and pack per year, and a matrix of residuals, **B'**, of the regression between Bray-Curtis dissimilarity and the predictor matrix with age, gender, and pack per year. The two residual matrices, **A'** and **B'**, are then compared by a standard Mantel test.

The following R codes subset an environmental data set from throat meta data set.

```
> meta <- select(throat.meta, Age,Sex,PackYears)
```

In the original data set, sex is a character variable labeled as "Male" and "Female". In order to convert this data set into a numerical distance matrix, we need to recode it as a numerical value. The following R codes create a numerical variable Gender.

```
> meta$Gender <- with(meta,ifelse(Sex%in%"Male", 1, 0))
> env <-select(meta, Age,Gender,PackYears)
```

The following R codes convert this data set into a distance matrix using the function vegdist() in vegan package.

```
> env_dist <- vegdist(scale(env), "euclid")
```

Mantel partial test is conducted using Pearson method as below.

```
> mantel.partial(group_dist,bray,env_dist, method = "pearson", permutations
=1000)
Partial Mantel statistic based on Pearson's product

Call:
mantel.partial(xdis = group_dist, ydis = bray, zdis = env_dist,      method
="pearson", permutations = 1000)

Mantel statistic r: 0.068
      Significance: 0.008

Upper quantiles of permutations (null model):
   90%     95%  97.5%     99%
0.0215 0.0321 0.0438 0.0641
Permutation: free
Number of permutations: 1000
```

The Mantel r statistic of 0.068 indicates that there is relatively not strong positive correlation between the smoking status and Bray-Curtis distance (dissimilarity) matrices while controlling for differences in environmental matrix with age, gender and pack per year. However, the p-value of 0.008 indicates that the results are statistically significant at $\alpha = 0.05$.

9.3   Hypothesis Tests Among-Group Differences Using ANOSIM

9.3.1   Introduction of Analysis of Similarity (ANOSIM)

ANOSIM is simply a modified version of the Mantel Test based on a standardized rank correlation between two distance matrices.

ANOSIM test was developed by Clarke (1993), a distribution-free method of multivariate data analysis frequently used by community ecologists and micro-biome researchers. It is a nonparametric procedure for testing the hypothesis of no difference between two or more groups of samples based on permutation test of among-and within-group similarities (Clarke 1993). It compares the variation in species (or any other taxa) abundance and composition among sampling units (e.g., beta diversity) in terms of the grouping factor or experimental treatment levels. Similarly as in ANOVA analysis, ANOSIM treats group membership or treatment levels as factors and model them as the explanatory variable. Analysis of similarity is based on the simple idea: if the tested groups are meaningful, then samples within the groups should be more similar in composition than samples from different groups. The null hypothesis is therefore: there are no differences between the members of the testing groups or treatment conditions. Bray-Curtis measure of similarity method is used in this test.

The anosim test statistic is based on the difference of mean ranks between groups and within groups. It is given below:

$$R = \frac{\bar{r}_B - \bar{r}_W}{M/2} \tag{9.6}$$

where,

R   test statistic, is an index of relative within-group dissimilarity.
$M = N(N-1)/2$ number of sample pairs.
N   is the total number of samples (subjects).
$\bar{r}_B$ is the mean of the ranked similarity between groups.
$\bar{r}_W$ is the mean of the ranked similarity within groups.

There are five main steps to conduct ANOSIM:

Step 1: calculate dissimilarity matrix.
Step 2: calculate rank dissimilarities and assign a rank of 1 to the smallest dissimilarity.
Step 3: calculate the mean among-and within-group rank dissimilarities.
Step 4: calculate test statistic R using the above formula $R = \frac{\bar{r}_B - \bar{r}_W}{M/2}$.

R is interpreted like a correlation coefficient which is a measure of "effect size" as other types of correlation coefficient such as Pearson's coefficient. The test statistic is to test there is no difference among groups under the null hypothesis. If the null hypothesis is correct, then $R = 0$, which suggests that among-and within-group dissimilarities are the same on average. It occurs when the high and low similarities are perfectly mixed and bear no relationship to the group. If the null hypothesis is rejected, then $R \neq 0$, which suggests that all pairs of samples within groups are more similar than to any pair of samples from different groups. For example, in the case, all the most similar samples are within the sample groups, then $R = 1$. Theoretically, it is also possible that $R < 0$, but practically such case is unlikely in ecological and microbiome studies. The extreme case, R = −1, which indicates that the most similar samples are all not in the groups.

Step 5: test for significance.

As in PERMANOVA test, the *p*-value of test statistic R is obtained by permutation: randomly assigning sample observations to groups. Then, the ranked similarity within and between groups is compared with the similarity that would be generated by random chance. The significance test is simply the fraction of permuted R's that are greater than the observed value of R. It is the probability of an R given this large or larger. The algorithm behind the hypothesis testing is same as PERMANOVA: if two groups of sampling units are really different in their species (or other taxa) composition, then compositional dissimilarities between the groups ought to be greater than those within the groups.

9.3.2   Illustrating Analysis of Similarity (ANOSIM) Using Vegan Package

Analysis of similarities (ANOSIM) provides a way to statistically test whether there is a significant difference between two or more groups of sampling units. The analysis of similarity is implemented via the function anosim() in the vegan package. The function assumes that all ranked dissimilarities within groups have about equal median and range. The input data is a dissimilarity matrix, which can be produced by the function dist() or vegdist(). The function also has summary and plot methods to perform the post modeling analysis. The following is one example of syntax.

anosim (data, grouping, permutations = 1000, distance = "bray")

where, data = data matrix or data frame in which rows are samples and columns are response variable(s), or a dissimilarity object or a symmetric square matrix of dissimilarities; grouping = grouping variable (a factor); permutations = number of permutation to assess the significance of the ANOSIM statistic; distance = distance or dissimilarity measure. If the input data does not have the dissimilarity structure or is a symmetric square matrix, then the distance needs to be specified.

The *Vdr* mouse fecal data are used here to illustrate ANOSIM test. First, we need to load data and the vegan package if they have not been loaded yet. The grouping information is obtained as previously described.

```
> abund_table=read.csv("VdrFecalGenusCounts.csv",row.names=1,
check.names=FALSE)
> abund_table<-t(abund_table)
> grouping<-data.frame(row.names=rownames(abund_table),t(as.data.frame
(strsplit(rownames(abund_table),"_"))))
```

```
> grouping$Group <- with(grouping,ifelse(as.factor(X2)%in% c
(11,12,13,14,15),c("Vdr-/-"), c("WT")))
> grouping<- grouping[,c(4)]
```

Fit ANOSIM using the Bray-Curtis Dissimilarity

The following R codes run ANOSIM using Bray-Curtis dissimilarity matrix as input data.

```
> library(vegan)
> bray<-vegdist(abund_table, "bray")
> anosim(bray, grouping,permutations = 1000)

Call:
anosim(dat = bray, grouping = grouping, permutations = 1000)
Dissimilarity: bray

ANOSIM statistic R: 0.19
      Significance: 0.2

Permutation: free
Number of permutations: 1000
```

It can be seen from the output in the function anosim() that it includes the modeling formula along with the dissimilarity method used from the function call, the value of ANOSIM statistic R, the significance from permutation and the number of permutation values of R. The p-value of 0.2 is greater than 0.05, which indicates that within-group similarity is not greater than between-group similarity at 0.05 significant level. We can conclude that there is no evidence that the within-group samples are more similar than would be expected by random chance.

The following R codes run ANOSIM using abundance data frame as input data.

```
> anosim(abund_table, grouping, permutations = 1000, distance = "bray")

Call:
anosim(dat = abund_table, grouping = grouping, permutations = 1000,
distance = "bray")
Dissimilarity: bray

ANOSIM statistic R: 0.19
      Significance: 0.19

Permutation: free
Number of permutations: 1000
```

The ANOSIM fit results can be summarized by the function summary().

```
> fit <- anosim(bray, grouping,permutations = 1000)
> summary(fit)

Call:
anosim(dat = bray, grouping = grouping, permutations = 1000)
Dissimilarity: bray

ANOSIM statistic R: 0.19
      Significance: 0.18

Permutation: free
Number of permutations: 1000

Upper quantiles of permutations (null model):
  90%   95% 97.5%   99%
0.282 0.323 0.538 0.846

Dissimilarity ranks between and within classes:
         0% 25% 50%    75% 100%  N
Between   2 9.5  17 21.50   28 15
Vdr-/-    1 6.5  14 19.75   25 10
WT        5 8.0  11 16.50   22  3
```

Finally, we can plot the results (Fig. 9.4):

```
> plot(fit)
```

Fit ANOSIM Using the Jaccard Dissimilarity
The following R codes fit ANOSIM using the Jaccard method.

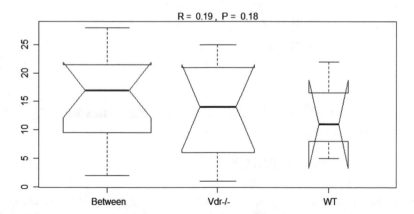

Fig. 9.4 Boxplot of the fitted between and within Bray-Curtis dissimilarities in the WT and $Vdr^{-/-}$ mouse data

```
> anosim(abund_table, grouping, permutations = 1000, distance = "jaccard")

Call:
anosim(dat = abund_table, grouping = grouping, permutations = 1000,
distance= "jaccard")
Dissimilarity: jaccard

ANOSIM statistic R: 0.19
      Significance: 0.2

Permutation: free
Number of permutations: 1000
```

Fit ANOSIM Using the Sørensen Dissimilarity

The following R codes fit ANOSIM using Sørensen method.

```
> fit_S <- anosim(abund_table, grouping, permutations = 1000,distance =
"Sørensen")
> summary(fit_S)

Call:
anosim(dat = abund_table, grouping = grouping, permutations = 1000)
Dissimilarity: bray

ANOSIM statistic R: 0.19
      Significance: 0.19

Permutation: free
Number of permutations: 1000

Upper quantiles of permutations (null model):
   90%    95% 97.5%    99%
 0.282 0.344 0.546 0.846

Dissimilarity ranks between and within classes:
         0% 25% 50%    75% 100%  N
Between   2 9.5  17 21.50   28  15
Vdr-/-    1 6.5  14 19.75   25  10
WT        5 8.0  11 16.50   22   3
```

9.4   Hypothesis Tests of Multi-response Permutation Procedures (MRPP)

9.4.1   Introduction of MRPP

Multi-response permutation procedures (MRPP) is a nonparametric procedure for testing the hypothesis of no difference between two or more groups of samples based on permutation test of among-and within-group dissimilarities (Mielke 1984, 1991). The testing difference may be differences in mean (location) or differences in within-group distance (spread) (Warton et al. 2012).

Similar as PERMANOVA, in both concept and method, MRPP is allied with ANOVA: it compares dissimilarities within and among groups. The underlying idea is also same. The MRPP test statistic is based on the difference of weighted mean between-and within-group dissimilarities. It is given below:

$$delta = \delta = \sum_{i=1}^{g} C_i \overline{d}_i \tag{9.7}$$

where, δ = MRPP test statistic, is the overall weighted mean of within-group means of the pairwise dissimilarities among sampling units; $C_i = n_i/N$; N = total number of items; and n_i = number of items in group i.

There are five main steps to conduct MRPP:

Step 1: calculate distance matrix using Euclidean distance for general cases, proportional city-block measures for community data.

Step 2: calculate average distance in each group $\overline{d}_i$.

Step 3: calculate delta for g groups.

Step 4: determine the effect size. The statistic A, which is a measure of effect size, is interpreted like R in ANOISIM; it is obtained as a comparison of within-group homogeneity to the random expectation.

$$A = 1 - \frac{\delta}{\mu_\delta} = 1 - \frac{observed\ \delta}{expected\ \delta} \tag{9.8}$$

The test statistic is to test there is no difference among groups under the null hypothesis. If within-group heterogeneity equals expectation by chance, then A = 0; when all items are identical within groups, then A = 1. $A < 0.1$ is common in ecology; $A > 0.3$ is fairly high in ecology. However, based on our knowledge, there is no reporting criterion of effect size in microbiome literature.

Step 5: test for significance. As in PERMANOVA and ANOSIM tests, the p-value of test statistic δ is obtained through Monte Carlo permutations. The significance test is simply the fraction of permuted deltas that are less than the observed delta, with a small sample correction. It is the probability of a delta given this small or smaller.

9.4.2   Illustrating MRPP Using Vegan Package

MRPP provides a way to statistically test whether there is a significant difference between two or more groups of sampling units. The MRPP is implemented via the function mrpp() in vegan package. If the input data is dissimilarity, it can be directly used. If it is a matrix with observations by responses data structure, then the dissimilarity needs to be calculated by the function vegdist() before use. The default distance is Euclidean method, but other dissimilarities in vegdist() also are applied. The function has summary and plot methods to perform post modeling analysis.

The following is one sample syntax:

mrpp(data, grouping, permutations = 1000, distance = "bray")

where, data = data matrix or data frame in which rows are observations and columns are responses, or a dissimilarity object or a symmetric square matrix of dissimilarities. The response(s) may be univariate or multivariate; grouping = grouping variable (a factor); permutations = number of permutation to assess the significance of the MRPP statistic; distance = distance or dissimilarity measure. If the input data does not have the dissimilarity structure or is a symmetric square matrix, then the distance needs to be specified.

As in ANOSIM test, we need to access the data and load the vegan package.

Fit MRPP Using the Bray-Curtis Dissimilarity
The following R codes run MRPP using Bray-Curtis dissimilarity matrix as input data.

```
> mrpp(bray, grouping,permutations = 1000)

Call:
mrpp(dat = bray, grouping = grouping, permutations = 1000)

Dissimilarity index: bray
Weights for groups:  n

Class means and counts:

      Vdr-/-  WT
delta 0.44    0.427
n     5       3

Chance corrected within-group agreement A: 0.0502
Based on observed delta 0.4353 and expected delta 0.4583

Significance of delta: 0.17
Permutation: free
Number of permutations: 1000
```

The observed and expected deltas are 0.4353 and 0.4583, respectively. The significance of delta is 0.13 with the chance corrected within-group agreement A of 0.0502. Given the small sample size, we conclude that there is no statistically significant difference of the two genus clusters at the 0.05 of significance level.

The following codes run MRPP using abundance data frame as input data:

```
> mrpp(abund_table, grouping, permutations = 1000, distance = "bray")

Call:
mrpp(dat = abund_table, grouping = grouping, permutations = 1000,
distance= "bray")

Dissimilarity index: bray
Weights for groups:  n

Class means and counts:

       Vdr-/- WT
delta 0.44   0.427
n     5      3

Chance corrected within-group agreement A: 0.0502
Based on observed delta 0.4353 and expected delta 0.4583

Significance of delta: 0.15
Permutation: free
Number of permutations: 1000
```

Obtain Mean Distance Matrix Using meandist()

The function meandist() calculates a matrix of mean within-cluster (block) dis-similarities (diagonal) and between-cluster (block) dissimilarities (off-diagonal elements), and an attribute n of grouping counts.

```
> meandist(bray, grouping,permutations = 1000)
        Vdr-/-     WT
Vdr-/- 0.4401 0.4766
WT     0.4766 0.4273
attr(,"class")
[1] "meandist" "matrix"
attr(,"n")
grouping
Vdr-/-    WT
    5     3
```

Obtain Mean Distances and Summary Statistics Using meandist() and summary()

We can use the function summary() to the function meandist() object to find the within-class, between-class and overall means of these dissimilarities, and the MRPP statistics with all weight.type options and the classification strength.

```
> bray_mrpp <- meandist(bray, grouping,permutations = 1000,distance =
"bray",weight.type = 1)
> summary(bray_mrpp)

Mean distances:
                Average
within groups   0.4372
between groups  0.4766
overall         0.4583

Summary statistics:
                        Statistic
MRPP A weights n         0.05016
MRPP A weights n-1       0.04900
MRPP A weights n(n-1)    0.04612
Classification strength  0.04131
```

9.5   Compare Microbiome Communities Using the GUniFrac Package

9.5.1   Introduction to UniFrac, Weighted UniFrac and Generalized UniFrac Distance Metrics

In multivariate microbiome composition analysis, the measures of unweighted and weighted UniFrac distances are most widely used to measure two microbiome communities.

The UniFrac distance, also known as unweighted UniFrac distance, was introduced by Lozupone et al. in 2005 (Lozupone and Knight 2005). It is a measure to estimate the difference between microbiome samples that based on phylogenetic distance. The goal of the UniFrac distance metric was to enable objective comparison between microbiome samples from different conditions. The unweighted UniFrac is defined as follows:

$$d^U = \sum_{i=1}^{n} \frac{b_i \left| I\left(p_i^A > 0\right) - I\left(p_i^B > 0\right) \right|}{\sum_{i=1}^{n} b_i} \tag{9.9}$$

where, d^U = unweighted UniFrac distance; A, B = microbiome community A and B, respectively; n = rooted phylogenetic tree's branches; b_i =length of the branch i. p_iA and p_iB= taxa proportions descending from the branch i for community A and B, respectively. $I(.)$ is the indicator function to indicate if species presence/absence in branch i. In above formula, both taxa proportions descending from the branch i for community A and B are defined as >0 with $I\left(p_i^A > 0\right)$ and $I\left(p_i^B > 0\right)$.

As defined this way, the UniFrac measure is calculated by dividing the branch lengths that are not shared between the two samples by the branch lengths covered by either sample, but not both (Lozupone and Knight 2005). A distance of 0 indicates that the two samples are identical, and a distance of 1 indicates that the two samples share no taxa in common. As a binary test of absence, the unweighted UniFrac distance considers only taxa presence and absence information; it is most efficient in detecting abundance change in rare lineages. However, such definition of distance measure completely ignores the taxa abundance information (Chen et al. 2012).

In 2007, Lozupone et al. added a proportional weighting to the original unweighted method (Lozupone et al. 2007), hence called this new UniFrac measure as weighted UniFrac. Weighted UniFrac distance uses taxa abundance information and weights the branch length with abundance difference; in a weighted UniFrac distance measure, each branch length of the phylogenetic tree is weighted by the difference in proportional abundance of the taxa between the two samples, instead of looking only at the presence or absence of taxa. The weighted UniFrac distance (Lozupone et al. 2007) is defined as

$$d^W = \frac{\sum_{i=1}^{n} b_i \left| p_i^A - p_i^B \right|}{\sum_{i=1}^{n} b_i (p_i^A + p_i^B)} \tag{9.10}$$

where, d^W = (normalized) weighted UniFrac distance; A, B = microbiome community A and B, respectively; n = rooted phylogenetic tree's branches; b_i =length of the branch i.

There are several features with formulation of this definition: (1) it weights the branch length with abundance difference; (2) d^W can not be reduced to d^U even if we convert abundance data into presence/absence data; and (3) d^W uses the absolute proportion difference, which results in the value of d^W is determined mainly by branches with large proportions and is less sensitive to the abundance changes on the branches with small proportions (Chen et al. 2012). By adding a proportional weighting to UniFrac distance, weighted UniFrac distance reduces the problem of low abundance taxa being represented as a 0 or by a low count depending on sampling depth. In weighted UniFrac, low abundance taxa have a much lower weight and so will have a lower impact on the total distance reported by the metric (Wong et al. 2016). Thus, weighted UniFrac can detect both changes in how many sequences from each lineage are present, as well as in which taxa are present (Lozupone et al. 2007); it is most sensitive to detect change in abundant lineages (Chen et al. 2012). However, either unweighted or weighted UniFrac distances may not be very powerful in detecting change in moderately abundant lineages (Chen et al. 2012) bacause they assign too much weight either to rare lineages or to most abundant lineages. Thus, Chen et al. proposed the following generalized UniFrac distances to unify weighted UniFrac and unweighted UniFrac distances.

$$d^{(\alpha)} = \frac{\sum_{i=1}^{n} b_i (p_i^A + p_i^B)^\alpha \left| \frac{p_i^A - p_i^B}{p_i^A + p_i^B} \right|}{\sum_{i=1}^{n} b_i (p_i^A + p_i^B)^\alpha} \tag{9.11}$$

where, $d^{(\alpha)}$ = generalized UniFrac distances; $\alpha \in [0, 1]$ is used to controls the contribution from high-abundance branches; A, B = microbiome community A and B, respectively; n = rooted phylogenetic tree's branches; b_i =length of the branch i; $\sum_{i=1}^{n} b_i (p_i^A + p_i^B)^\alpha$ = normalizing factor to ensure $d^{(\alpha)}$ value in [0,1]. Generalized UniFrac distance contains an extra parameter α controlling the weight on abundant lineages so the distance is not dominated by highly abundant lineages. $\alpha = 0.5$ has overall the best power.

The unified formulation of UniFrac distances has several features: (1) the weight on branches with large proportions is attenuated through using the relative difference $\left| p_i^A - p_i^B \right| / (p_i^A + p_i^B)$. The weight value is in [0,1]; (2) with this formulation, now d^W can be reduced to d^U if we convert abundance data into presence/absence data; when we put $\alpha = 1$ in above (9.11), $d^{(\alpha)}$ is reduced to d^W.

$$d^{(1)} = \frac{\sum_{i=1}^{n} b_i (p_i^A + p_i^B)^1 \left| \frac{p_i^A - p_i^B}{p_i^A + p_i^B} \right|}{\sum_{i=1}^{n} b_i (p_i^A + p_i^B)^1} = \frac{\sum_{i=1}^{n} b_i |p_i^A - p_i^B|}{\sum_{i=1}^{n} b_i (p_i^A + p_i^B)} = d^W \qquad (9.12)$$

When $\alpha = 0$, we get

$$d^{(0)} = \frac{\sum_{i=1}^{n} b_i (p_i^A + p_i^B)^0 \left| \frac{p_i^A - p_i^B}{p_i^A + p_i^B} \right|}{\sum_{i=1}^{n} b_i (p_i^A + p_i^B)^0} = \frac{\sum_{i=1}^{n} b_i \left| \frac{p_i^A - p_i^B}{p_i^A + p_i^B} \right|}{\sum_{i=1}^{n} b_i} \qquad (9.13)$$

The pseudo-F statistic based on UniFrac distances is defined as

$$F = \frac{tr(HGH)/(m-1)}{tr[(I-H)G(I-H)]/(n-m)}, \qquad (9.14)$$

where tr(.) is the trace function of a matrix, $H = X(X^T X)^{-1} X^T$ is the hat (projection) matrix of the design matrix $\mathbf{X}$, G is Gower's centered matrix, and n and m is the number of samples and the number of predictors, respectively. Let d_{ij} be the generalized UniFrac distance between community i and j and denote $A = (a_{ij}) = \left(-\frac{1}{2} d_{ij}^2 \right)$. The Gower's matrix is defined as $G = \left(I - \frac{11'}{n} \right) A \left(I - \frac{11'}{n} \right)$. For details of the test statistic and unified formulation of unweighted, weighted UniFrac distances and generalized UniFrac distances, readers can reference the authors' original paper (Chen et al. 2012).

9.5.2   Breast Milk Data Set

The breast milk data set comes from two recently published studies (Urbaniak et al. 2016; Wong et al. 2016). It collects 58 microbiome samples taken from lactating Caucasian Canadian women. Human milk is an important source of bacteria for the developing infant and influences the bacterial composition of the newborn infant, which in turn can affect disease risk later in life. In the first publication, the authors used this data set to compare bacterial profiles between preterm and term births, C section (elective and non-elective) and vaginal deliveries, and male and female infants. In the second publication, the same data set was used to illustrate the authors' own developed tools including unweighted UniFrac, weighted UniFrac, information UniFrac and ratio UniFrac. Here we use this data set to compare microbiome communities using the GUniFrac package.

9.5.3 Comparing Microbiome Communities Using the GUniFrac Package

The package GUniFrac (Chen 2012) was developed to implement the generalized uniFrac distance to compare microbiome communities (Chen et al. 2012). As the PERMANOVA procedure, in GUniFrac package the significance of the pseudo-F statistics is assessed based on permutations. If the fraction of the tree unique to one environment is greater than would be expected by chance, then the two communities are considered different. In this package, the unweighted and weighted UniFrac, and variance adjusted weighted UniFrac distances can also be implemented. The UniFrac distances can be calculated and used to compare microbiome communities in the GUniFrac package including d^W, $d^{(0.5)}$, $d^{(0)}$, d^U and variance adjusted weighted UniFrac distance d^{VAW}. In above section, we present the formulas of $d^W, d^{(0)}$, and d^U. The $d^{(0.5)}$ represents the distance in middle of the distance series; it is given by: $d^{(0.5)} = \dfrac{\sum_{i=1}^{n} b_i \sqrt{p_i^A + p_i^B} \left| \frac{p_i^A - p_i^B}{p_i^A + p_i^B} \right|}{\sum_{i=1}^{n} b_i \sqrt{p_i^A + p_i^B}}$. It can be derived by plugging 0.5 to α in formula (9.11).

The variance-adjusted weighted UniFrac distance d^{VAW} is given by $d^{VAW} = \dfrac{\sum_{i=1}^{n} b_i \frac{|p_i^A - p_i^B|}{m_i(m - m_i)}}{\sum_{i=1}^{n} b_i \frac{p_i^A - p_i^B}{m_i(m - m_i)}}$, where m_i is the total number of individuals/reads from both communities on the ith branch and m is total number of individuals/reads. It was developed to account for the fact that weighted UniFrac distance does not consider the variation of the weights under random sampling resulting in less power detecting the differences between communities (Chang et al. 2011). The GUniFrac package is dependent on vegan and ape packages and the author also suggests using package ade4. One usage is given as below.

GUniFrac(otu.tab, tree, alpha = c(0, 0.5, 1))

where, out.tab = OTU count table with row (=sample) and column (=OTU); tree = rooted phylogenetic tree of R class "phylo"; alpha = parameter controlling weight on abundant lineages.

UniFrac measure calculations require two pieces of information: a table of counts and a phylogenetic tree. Thus, two data sets are needed to run GUniFrac package: a table of counts such as OTU table and a phylogenetic tree.

In the following, we step-by-step illustrate how to use the GUniFrac package to comparing microbiome communities.

Step 1: Load and Read OTU Table with Appropriate Formats
Set the directory the same way as we did in previous chapters. The
"td_OTU_tag_mapped_lineage.txt" data set includes two pieces of information:
OTU count table and taxonomy in the last column. The partial R codes from the
original dataset's authors are useful. We modify them here, and explain and
comment on what the codes are doing for.

```
> setwd("E:/Home/MicrobiomeStatUsingR/Analysis/")
> otu_tab <- read.table("td_OTU_tag_mapped_lineage.
txt", header=T, sep="\t", row.names=1, comment.
char="", check.names=FALSE)
```

In the arguments, row.names = 1 argument specifies the column 1 of the table
which contains the row names; comment.char = "" is used to turn off the interpretation of comments altogether. It is very faster than the default read.table(). The
first 6 rows of the dataset "td_OTU_tag_mapped_lineage.txt" are given below:

```
> head(otu_tab)
    S31     S1    S42 S13_T2   S30   S50   S43   S20   S29 S47U   S26 S13_T3   S33  S8L
0    38     36     30     14    13    18    27    38    49    7  5251     12    17   35
1  2866  15069  42985   3292  1223  1056  3959  3021  7023 1856  7993   2571 13306 1101
2   437   9831   4628   4231  4473   718  3843   441  4311 2496  5672   4940  4112 4830
3  3356   7407   5355     62   121    14  3616  6184   334  108    31     30    13   56
4    12    478     16    342    23     8    18    97   390  126     4    271    53    7
5   145    238    234      3    56     1   109   156   374   28     0     45     0    1
......
                                                                           taxonomy
0
Bacteria;Proteobacteria;Gammaproteobacteria;Pasteurellales;Pasteurellaceae;Pasteurella;|93
1
Bacteria;Firmicutes;Bacilli;Bacillales;Staphylococcaceae;Staphylococcus;|77
2
Bacteria;Proteobacteria;Gammaproteobacteria;Pseudomonadales;Pseudomonadaceae;Pseudomonas;|92
3 Bacteria;Proteobacteria;Gammaproteobacteria;Enterobacteriales;Enterobacteriaceae;Escherichia-
Shigella;|98
4
Bacteria;Proteobacteria;Gammaproteobacteria;Enterobacteriales;Enterobacteriaceae;Klebsiella;|75
5
Bacteria;Actinobacteria;Actinobacteria;Corynebacteriales;Corynebacteriaceae;Corynebacterium;|88
```

However, for correctly using GUniFrac package, the OTU table should be a
numeric matrix. The following R codes are used to remove taxonomy column from
the original dataset.

```
> taxonomy <- otu_tab$taxonomy
> otu_tab <- otu_tab[-length(colnames(otu_tab))]
```

The otu table needs to be transposed into a sample by otu matrix.

```
> otu_tab <- t(as.matrix(otu_tab))
> head(otu_tab)
         0     1    2    3    4   5     6  7   8    9 10  11  12  13    14   15  16  17
S31     38  2866  437 3356  12 145    43  0  20   19 33  27  16  21    79   40  30  12
S1      36 15069 9831 7407 478 238  1368 25 306 2821 91 169 323 475  1290 3795 532 186
S42     30 42985 4628 5355  16 234 14491  2 357  153 48 109 136 520   781  617 727 867
S13_T2  14  3292 4231   62 342   3   282  1 188   51 64 168 161 574   557   33 408   7
S30     13  1223 4473  121  23  56     3  0 123    3 13   3 279 207   703  123 617   5
S50     18  1056  718   14   8   1     3  1  20    5  0   1  35  49   119   28  83   5
......
```

Step 2: Use Rarefaction to Normalize the Sample OTU Counts to a Standard Sequencing Depth

The rarefied data is recommended to be used by the authors of UniFrac (Carcer et al. 2011) and was used to calculate the unweighted UniFrac distance matrix, while the non-rarefied data was used for weighted, information, and ratio UniFrac using their custom UniFrac script (Wong et al. 2016). However, in GUniFrac package manual, the rarefied data were used for all UniFrac distance calculations. Because GUniFrac is sensitive to different sequencing depth, to compare microbiomes on an equal basis, rarefaction might be used (Chen 2012). Thus, we follow the package manual; rarefy the samples before performing unweighted, weighted UniFrac, and variance-adjusted weighted UniFrac distances. The rarefaction can be done using either function rrarefy() or rarefy() from vegan package.

```
> library(vegan)
> otu_tab_rarefy <- rrarefy(otu_tab, min(apply(otu_tab,1,sum)))
```

Step 3: Read Phylogenetic Tree

The GUniFrac package requires a rooted tree as input data. We can use the function midpoint() from the phangorn package to obtain the rooted tree.

```
> library(phangorn)
> otu_tree <- midpoint(otu_tree)
> otu_tree

Phylogenetic tree with 115 tips and 114 internal nodes.

Tip labels:
        1, 11, 6686, 18, 230, 82, ...
Node labels:
        NA, 71.9, 79.1, 86.9, 87.1, 52.4, ...

Rooted; includes branch lengths.
```

Step 4: Calculate the UniFracs

Now, the UniFracs can be calculated using the GUniFrac package.

```
> library(GUniFrac)
> #Calculate the UniFracs
> unifracs <- GUniFrac(otu_tab_rarefy, otu_tree, alpha=c(0, 0.5, 1))
$unifracs
```

```
> dw <- unifracs[,, "d_1"] # Weighted UniFrac
> du <- unifracs[,, "d_UW"] # Unweighted UniFrac
> dv <- unifracs[,, "d_VAW"]# Variance adjusted weighted UniFrac
> d0 <- unifracs[,, "d_0"] # GUniFrac with alpha 0
> d5 <- unifracs[,, "d_0.5"]# GUniFrac with alpha 0.5
```

Step 5: Conduct PERMANOVA to Compare One UniFrac Measure
In order to test hypothesis on these UniFrac measures, the group information is
needed to be extracted from the meta data. We use the function read.table() to read
the metadata as follows:

```
> meta_tab<- read.table("metadata.txt", header=T, sep="\t",
row.names=1, comment.char="", check.names=FALSE)
```

The OTU table and metadata are matched to keep the samples that only appear in
both datasets.

```
> otu_meta_matched <- match(rownames(meta_tab),rownames(otu_tab))
> otu_meta_matched <- otu_meta_matched[!is.na(otu_meta_matched)]
> otu_tab <- otu_tab[otu_meta_matched,]
> meta_tab_Ordered <- meta_tab[match(rownames(otu_tab),rownames
(meta_tab)),]
```

The following R codes use the function adonis() in vegan package to conduct
PERMANOVA to compare the distance in middle of the distance series of gestation. The interested readers can try other UniFrac distance metrics.

```
> set.seed(123)
> adonis(as.dist(d5) ~ meta_tab$Gestation)

Call:
adonis(formula = as.dist(d5) ~ meta_tab$Gestation)

Permutation: free
Number of permutations: 999

Terms added sequentially (first to last)

                   Df SumsOfSqs  MeanSqs F.Model      R2 Pr(>F)
meta_tab$Gestation  4    0.4336 0.108391  1.2001 0.08305   0.22
Residuals          53    4.7869 0.090319         0.91695
Total              57    5.2205                  1.00000
```

Similarly, gender and milktype effects can be tested as below.

```
> adonis(as.dist(d5) ~ meta_tab$Gender)

Call:
adonis(formula = as.dist(d5) ~ meta_tab$Gender)

Permutation: free
Number of permutations: 999

Terms added sequentially (first to last)

                 Df SumsOfSqs  MeanSqs F.Model     R2 Pr(>F)
meta_tab$Gender   2    0.1864 0.093197  1.0182 0.0357  0.381
Residuals        55    5.0341 0.091529         0.9643
Total            57    5.2205                  1.0000


> adonis(as.dist(d5) ~ meta_tab$milktype)

Call:
adonis(formula = as.dist(d5) ~ meta_tab$milktype)

Permutation: free
Number of permutations: 999

Terms added sequentially (first to last)

                   Df SumsOfSqs  MeanSqs F.Model      R2 Pr(>F)
meta_tab$milktype   3    0.4019 0.133976  1.5014 0.07699  0.06 .
Residuals          54    4.8186 0.089233         0.92301
Total              57    5.2205                  1.00000
---
Signif. codes:  0 '***' 0.001 '**' 0.01 '*' 0.05 '.' 0.1 ' ' 1
```

Step 6: Conduct PERMANOVA to Compare Multiple UniFrac Measures Using the Function PermanovaG()

Combining multiple distance matrices can add power for hypothesis testing. The following R codes use d(0), d(0.5), d(1) and the function PermanovaG() to conduct the permutational multivariate analysis of variance.

```
> PermanovaG(unifracs[, , c("d_0", "d_0.5", "d_1")] ~ meta_tab$Gestation)
$aov.tab
                      F.Model p.value
meta_tab$Gestation 1.262764   0.263
```

9.6 Summary and Discussion

In this chapter, we presented hypothesis testing on multivariate community microbiome data and their step-by-step implementations in the R system. The data we used to illustrate are from our own studies (Jin et al. 2015; Wang et al. 2016) or are publicly availble. Readers may use the R codes and explanations provided in this chapter to analyze their own microbiome data.

About multivariate community analysis of beta diversity, two approaches exist in the ecological literature: "raw-data approach" and "distance (Mantel) approach" (Legendre et al. 2005; Tuomisto and Ruokolainen 2006; Laliberte 2008). PERMANOVA, redundancy analysis (RDA), distance-based RDA (db-RDA), and canonical analysis of principal coordinates are belong to raw data based approaches, while Mantel test is typical distance based approach. ANOSIM is simply a modified version of the Mantel test based on a standardized rank correlation between two distance matrices. Thus, it also belongs to distance based approach. The domain of application of the Mantel test is also applied to the analysis of similarity (ANOSIM) as well (Legendre et al. 2005).

The question is which approach is more appropriate for analyzing multivariate community microbiome data? In ecological literature, there are many discussions about this topic (McArdle and Anderson 2001; Legendre et al. 2005; Legendre 2007; Laliberte 2008; Legendre et al. 2008; Pélissier et al. 2008; Tuomisto and Ruokolainen 2008; Anderson et al. 2011; Legendre and Legendre 2012).

The distance-based methods have the problems: (1) they do not correctly partition the variation in the data and do not provide the correct Type-I error rates, therefore are not appropriate for analyzing beta diversity; (2) as point out by Anderson et al., what is even more problematic is the use of partitioning methods to make direct inferences regarding the relative importance of underlying processes driving patterns in beta diversity (Anderson et al. 2011). For example, ANOSIM and Mantel tests have been shown that they are inappropriate for testing hypotheses concerning variation of the raw data (Legendre et al. 2005). Thus, they are suggested to restrict to analyzing the variation of beta diversity, but not beta diversity. The alternative raw data based approaches have been thought to offer a more appropriate and more powerful tools for analysis of beta diversity. However, the distance-based methods do have some advantages. For example, the Mantel test was thought as a valid approach to relate two distance matrices (Anderson et al. 2011) and offered more flexibility, allowing the use of other types of distance functions such as Jaccard or Steinhaus/Bray-Curtis (Legendre et al. 2005), and it may be appropriate for hypotheses concerning the variation in beta diversity among groups of sites (samples) (Legendre et al. 2005).

Compared to the simple Mantel test, ecological studies have also pointed out that the partial Mantel approach for some time to be problematic for interpretation (e.g., Legendre et al. 2005; Anderson et al. 2011).

About the uses of functions in vegan package, the authors of this package recommend adonis() over mrpp() and anosim(). The reasons lie on that the function adonis() allows ANOVA-like tests of the variance in beta diversity explained by continuous and/or categorical predictors. However, both mrpp() and anosim() only handle categorical predictors, and they are less robust than adonis() (Oksanen et al. 2016).

So far, most discussions about multivariate community analysis are limited in ecological and other relevant study fields, but not in microbiome area. However, microbiome studies have adopted these methods and approaches, the advantages and limitations of these methods are also applicable to microbiome research.

References

Anderson, M.J. 2001. A new method for non-parametric multivariate analysis of variance. *Austral Ecology* 26: 32–46.

Anderson, M.J., T.O. Crist, et al. 2011. Navigating the multiple meanings of beta diversity: A roadmap for the practicing ecologist. *Ecology Letters* 14 (1): 19–28.

Benjamini, Y., and Y. Hochberg. 1995. Controlling the false discovery rate: A practical and powerful approach to multiple testing. *Journal of the Royal Statistical Society Series B* 57: 289–300.

Benjamini, Y., and D. Yekutieli. 2001. The control of the false discovery rate in multiple testing under dependency. *Annals of Statistics* 29: 1165–1188.

Bonferroni, C.E. 1936. Teoria statistica delle classi e calcolo delle probabilitàby. *Pubblicazioni del R Istituto Superiore di Scienze Economiche e Commerciali di Firenze* 8: 3–62 Key: citeulike:1778138.

Carcer, D.A., S.E. Denman, et al. 2011. Evaluation of subsampling-based normalization strategies for tagged high-throughput sequencing data sets from gut microbiomes. *Applied and Environment Microbiology* 77 (24): 8795–8798.

Chang, Q., Y. Luan, et al. 2011. Variance adjusted weighted UniFrac: A powerful beta diversity measure for comparing communities based on phylogeny. *BMC Bioinformatics* 12 (1): 118.

Chen, J. 2012. GUniFrac: Generalized UniFrac distances. R package version 1.0. https://CRAN.R-project.org/package=GUniFrac.

Chen, J., K. Bittinger, et al. 2012. Associating microbiome composition with environmental covariates using generalized UniFrac distances. *Bioinformatics* 28 (16): 2106–2113.

Clarke, K.R. 1993. Non-parametric multivariate analysis of changes in community structure. *Australian Journal of Ecology* 18: 117–143.

Hochberg, Y. 1988. A sharper Bonferroni procedure for multiple tests of significance. *Biometrika* 75: 800–803.

Holm, S. 1979. A simple sequentially rejective multiple test procedure. *Scandinavian Journal of Statistics* 6: 65–70.

Hommel, G. 1988. A stagewise rejective multiple test procedure based on a modified Bonferroni test. *Biometrika* 75: 383–386.

Jin, D., S. Wu, et al. 2015. Lack of Vitamin D receptor causes dysbiosis and changes the functions of the murine intestinal microbiome. *Clinical Therapeutics* 37 (5): 996–1009, e1007.

Laliberte, E. 2008. Analyzing or explaining beta diversity? comment. *Ecology* 89 (11): 3232–3237.

Legendre, P. 2007. Studying beta diversity: Ecological variation partitioning by multiple regression and canonical analysis. *Journal of Plant Ecology* 1 (1): 3–8.

Legendre, P., and L. Legendre. 2012. *Numerical ecology*. Amsterdam: Elsevier Science BV.

Legendre, P., and M.J. Fortin. 1989. Spatial pattern and ecological analysis. *Vegetatio* 80 (2): 107–138.

Legendre, P., D. Borcard, et al. 2005. Analyzing beta diversity: Partitioning the spatial variation of community composition data. *Ecological Monographs* 75 (4): 435–450.

Legendre, P., D. Borcard, et al. 2008. Analyzing or explaining beta diversity? comment. *Ecology* 89 (11): 3238–3244.

Linnenbrink, M., J. Wang, et al. 2013. The role of biogeography in shaping diversity of the intestinal microbiota in house mice. *Molecular Ecology* 22 (7): 1904–1916.

Lozupone, C., and R. Knight. 2005. UniFrac: A new phylogenetic method for comparing microbial communities. *Applied and Environmental Microbiology* 71 (12): 8228–8235.

Lozupone, C.A., M. Hamady, et al. 2007. Quantitative and qualitative beta diversity measures lead to different insights into factors that structure microbial communities. *Applied and Environment Microbiology* 73 (5): 1576–1585.

Mantel, N. 1967. The detection of disease clustering and a generalized regression approach. *Cancer Research* 27: 209–220.

Mantel, N., and R.S. Valand. 1970. A technique of nonparametric multivariate analysis. *Biometrics* 26 (3): 547–558.

McArdle, B.H., and M.J. Anderson. 2001. Fitting multivariate models to community data: A comment on distance-based redundancy analysis. *Ecology* 82 (1): 290–297.

Mielke, P.W. 1984. Meteorological applications of permutation techniques based on distance functions. In *Handbook of statistics*, vol. 4, ed. P.R. Krishnaiah and P.K. Sen, 813–830. Amsterdam, North-Holland: Elsevier Science Publishers.

Mielke Jr., P.W. 1991. The application of multivariate permutation methods based on distance functions in the earth sciences. *Earth-Science Reviews* 31: 55–71.

Oksanen, J., F. Guillaume Blanchet, et al. 2016. Vegan: Community ecology package. R package version 2.4-1. http://CRAN.R-project.org/package=vegan.

Pélissier, R., P. Couteron, et al. 2008. Analyzing or explaining beta diversity? comment. *Ecology* 89 (11): 3227–3232.

Smouse, P.E., J.C. Long, et al. 1986. Multiple regression and correlation extensions of the mantel test of matrix correspondence. *Systematic Zoology* 35 (4): 627–632.

Tuomisto, H., and K. Ruokolainen. 2006. Analyzing or explaining beta diversity? Understanding the targets of different methods of analysis. *Ecology* 87: 2697–2708.

Tuomisto, H., and K. Ruokolainen. 2008. Analyzing or explaining beta diversity: Reply. *Ecology* 89: 3244–3256.

Urbaniak, C., M. Angelini, et al. 2016. Human milk microbiota profiles in relation to birthing method, gestation and infant gender. *Microbiome* 4 (1): 1.

Wang, J., L.B. Thingholm, et al. 2016. Genome-wide association analysis identifies variation in vitamin D receptor and other host factors influencing the gut microbiota. *Nature Genetics* 48 (11): 1396–1406.

Warton, D.I., S.T. Wright, et al. 2012. Distance-based multivariate analyses confound location and dispersion effects. *Methods in Ecology and Evolution* 3 (1): 89–101.

Wong, R.G., J.R. Wu, et al. 2016. Expanding the UniFrac toolbox. *PLoS ONE* 11 (9): e0161196.

Chapter 10
Compositional Analysis of Microbiome Data

This chapter focuses on compositional analysis of microbiome data. In Sect. 10.1, we introduce the concepts, principles, statistical methods and tools of compositional data analysis. Section 10.2 introduce the reasons that microbiome dataset can be treated as compositional. In Sect. 10.3, we illustrate some graphics of exploratory compositional data analysis. Section 10.4 is covered by the ALDEx2 package for hypothesis testing between the groups. In Sect. 10.5, we introduce the concept of proportionality for correlation analysis for relative data and illustrate its use. In Sect. 10.6, we summarize this chapter and discuss the limitations of compositional data analysis.

10.1 Introduction to Compositional Analysis

10.1.1 What Are Compositional Data?

According to Webster's II New College Dictionary, composition is "the act of putting together parts or elements to form a whole", or it is "the way in which such parts are combined or related: constitution". Compositional data quantitatively describe the parts of whole and provide only relative information between their components (Hron et al. 2010; Egozcue and Pawlowsky-Glahn 2011; Pawlowsky-Glahn et al. 2015). Thus, compositional data exist as the proportions, or fractions, of a whole or portions of a total (van den Boogaart and Tolosana-Delgado 2013), conveying exclusively relative information, and have the properties: the elements of the composition are non-negative and sum to unity (Bacon-Shone 2011).

From a practical point of view, if researchers are really only interested in relative frequencies, not the absolute amount of data, then the data are compositional. Therefore, compositional data frequently arise in different fields of science:

© Springer Nature Singapore Pte Ltd. 2018
Y. Xia et al., *Statistical Analysis of Microbiome Data with R*,
ICSA Book Series in Statistics, https://doi.org/10.1007/978-981-13-1534-3_10

genomics, population genetics, demography, ecology, biology, chemistry, geology, petrology, sedimentology, geochemistry, planetology, psychology, marketing, survey analysis, economics, probability, and statistics.

10.1.2 Aitchison Simplex

Mathematically, a data is defined as compositional, if it contains D multiple parts of nonnegative numbers whose sum is 1 (Aitchison 1986, p. 25) or any constant-sum constraint (Pawlowsky-Glahn et al. 2015, p. 10). It can be formally stated as:

$$S^D = \left\{ X = [x_1, x_2, \ldots, x_D] | x_i > 0,\, i = 1, 2, \ldots, D;\, \sum_{i=1}^{D} x_i = \kappa \right\} \qquad (10.1)$$

The formula states that compositional data can be represented by constant sum real vectors with positive components. This defines the sample space of compositional data as a hyperplane, called the simplex (Aitchison 1986, p. 27; Mateu-Figueras et al. 2011; van den Boogaart and Tolosana-Delgado 2013, p. 37; Pawlowsky-Glahn et al. 2015, p. 10).

Note that κ is arbitrary. Depending on the units of measurement or rescaling, frequent values are 1 (per unit, proportions), 100 (percent, %), 10^6 (ppm, parts per million), and 10^9 (ppb, parts per billion).

10.1.3 Problems with Standard Statistical Methods

Standard data analysis techniques, such as correlation analysis, rely on the assumption of the Euclidean geometry in real space (Eaton 1983). Applying them to compositional data may yield misleading results because the compositional data represent the special properties of the sample space, the simplex.

In Chap. 3 of "The Statistical Analysis of Compositional Data" (Aitchison 1986), John Aitchison reviewed and discussed some challenging problems in compositional data analysis. We summarize the key points and give further explanations here.

First, there is a spurious correlation, which results in being difficult to interpret the correlations between proportions in any meaningful way, mainly because uncorrelated proportions are not necessarily independent. Earlier in 1897, Pearson first observed the problem of "spurious correlation" between ratios of variables. i.e., while statistically independent variables X, Y, and Z are not correlated, their ratios X/Z and Y/Z must be, because of their common divisor (Pearson 1897; Lovell et al. 2015). For example, in microbiome study, relative abundance data can make statistically independent components appear correlated (Lovell et al. 2011). Thus, correlation of relative abundances is thought as just wrong and correlation analysis of relative abundances is considered to tell us absolutely nothing (Lovell et al. 2015).

Second, the difficulties of high dimensionality arise in compositional data analysis, which results in graphical distortions of the multivariate pattern of variability. When the analysis is restricted to a selection of subcompositions rather than the compositions as a whole, then it projects a partial analysis and loses a picture of the multivariate pattern of variability. Due to unit-sum constraint confines compositional vectors to a simplex, graphical distortions happened: graphical pattern seen is no guarantee as the same in familiar space such as R^2.

Third, constant-sum problem (also called negative bias problem) makes it difficult to interpret the correlation and covariance in their usual ways. Using the traditional way, the interdependence of the compositions of a D-part composition vector is expressed through product-moment covariances. However, the covariance structure is not interpretable.

The difficulties have been expressed in a variety of ways: negative bias difficulty, subcomposition difficulty, basis difficulty, and null correlation difficulty.

Subject to unit-sum or constant-sum constraint, there must be at least one negative element in each row of the (raw) covariance matrix. In other words, at least D of its entries must be negative. For example, in each sample if the amount of one kind of taxa in the ecosystem increases, the amounts of one or more other kinds of taxa must decrease. Hence subject to the non-negative definiteness of the covariance or correlation matrix, the values of correlations are not in the usual interval $(-1, 1)$ (Aitchison 1986, 1999). This is called negative bias difficulty.

Similarly, the unit-sum constraint precludes relationship between the raw covariance matrix of a subcomposition and that of the full composition. Moreover, the raw correlations may change substantially when we move from full composition to its subcompositions and variances may display different and unrelatable rank orderings as we form subcompositions. Aitchison called this as subcomposition difficulty.

When we construct a composition from a basis vector, the correlations between the elements of constructed vector are different from their basis vector, which results in difficulty in relating the raw covariance matrix of the composition to the covariance matrix of its basis: basis difficulty.

Furthermore, due to negative bias, it is difficult to use the value zero to present no association or independence of random variables. Actually, uncorrelated components of the bases yields null correlations, but not necessarily zero. The concept of null correlation here is analogous to Pearson's spurious correlation. This is null correlation difficulty. Thus, compositional constraints are notorious for their impacts on the covariance and correlation structures of data (Aitchison 1986) (Sect. 3.3).

Finally, it is difficult to use parametric distributions into the simplex sample space to model compositional data (difficulty of parametric modeling). Regression and multivariate analysis rely on the assumption of multivariate normality and are conducted in the real sample space. A unit sum constraint places a much more fundamental restriction on the freedom of the components of composition than the non-negative restriction. Because of analyzing the parts from the whole or subject to non-negative restriction and a unit sum constraint, components cannot be normally distributed, due to the bounded range of values. Therefore, the multinormal and its transformed multivariate lognormal parametric class of distributions are not appropriate statistical tools to analyze compositional data (Aitchison 1986).

In standard factorial experimental design and associated ANOVA and linear models, the independence of factors allows us to test their additive effect on the response or specific interaction terms exist (Cameron and Trivedi 1998). However, in simplex space, because of the unit-sum constraint, the factors (D parts of a composition) are not independent; actually they are the mixture. If we change one component, we had to change at least one other component, and not linear (especially at the boundaries). Thus, it is difficult to formulate meaningful hypotheses about the nature of the effect of the mixture on the response. Aitchison called it as the mixture variation difficulty.

The main properties of Dirichlet distribution shown by Aitchison are: the correlation structure of a Dirichlet composition is completely negative, which makes it inappropriate to analyze data patterns for which some such correlations are definitely positive. Every Drichlet composition has a very strong implied independence structure, unlikely being used to describe compositions with even weak forms of dependence (Aitchison 1986). Thus, even the Dirichlet classes turn out to be totally inadequate for the description of the variability of compositional data.

In summary, composition data violate the assumptions of all standard statistical tests; i.e., differences between parts are linear or additive. It makes most standard statistical methods and tests invalid: (1) spurious correlations preclude correlation analysis; (2) graphical distortions make the visualizing tools (e.g., scatter plot, QQ plot, et al.) impossible; (3) lack of multivariate normality of compositions preclude multivariate parametric modeling of compositional data; and (4) dependence of the mixture makes ANOVA and linear regression meaningless to be used to test hypotheses on the response.

10.1.4   Statistical Analysis of Compositional Data

10.1.4.1   Fundamental Principles

Aitchison proposed three fundamental principles for the analysis of compositional data, and suggested that we should adhere to these principles when analyzing compositional data (Aitchison 1982, 1986). They have been reformulated several times (Barceló-Vidal et al. 2001; Martín-Fernández et al. 2003; Aitchison and Egozcue 2005; Egozcue 2009; Egozcue and Pawlowsky-Glahn 2011) according to new theoretical developments. The principles are all rooted in the definition of compositional data: only ratios of components carry information.

(i) **Scaling invariance.**
   It states that analyses must treat vectors with proportional positive components as representing the same composition (Lovell et al. 2015). In other words, statistical inferences about compositional data should not depend on the scale used. Thus, the vector of per-units and the vector of percentages convey exactly the same information (Egozcue and Pawlowsky-Glahn 2011). We should obtain exactly the same results from analyzing proportions and percentages. For example, the vectors $a = [11, 2, 5]$, $b = [110, 20, 50]$, and $c = [1100, 200, 500]$ represent all the same composition because the relative importance (the *ratios*) between their components is the same (van den Boogaart and Tolosana-Delgado 2013).

(ii) **Subcompositional coherence.**
   It states that analyses should depend only on data about components (or parts) within that subset, not depend on other non-involved components (or parts) (Egozcue and Pawlowsky-Glahn 2011); and statistical inferences about subcompositions (a particular subset of components) should be consistent, regardless of whether the inference is based on the subcomposition or the full composition (Lovell et al. 2015).

(iii) **Permutation invariance.**
   It states that the conclusions of a compositional analysis should not depend on the order (the sequence) of the components (the parts) (Egozcue and Pawlowsky-Glahn 2011; van den Boogaart and Tolosana-Delgado 2013; Lovell et al. 2015). In compositional analysis, the information from the order of the different components plays no role. For example, it does not matter that we choose which component to be the "first", which component to be the "second" and so on, which one to be the "last".

10.1.4.2 A Family of Log-Ratio Transformations

The major problem with compositional data is that the data points do not map to Euclidean space, but instead to the Aitchison simplex (Aitchison 1986). The question is: how to analyze compositional data? Should we move or stay with the simplex? Because standard statistical methods cannot solve the compositional data problems in simplex, the critical step towards compositional data analysis is to provide an approach for a one-to-one mapping onto a real space.

Log and Log-Ratio Transformations
The approach of solving the compositional data problems in simplex is expected to be completed through several steps: first transform compositions into real space using a log-ratio transformation, then to apply standard statistical methods to the

transformed data, finally, return to the simplex by using the inverse log-ratio transformation (Mateu-Figueras et al. 2011). The log-ratio transformation of compositional data is thought to legally restore much usage of traditional statistical analysis tools in situations such as relative abundance.

Although using a log-ratio transformation is considered as a critical approach to release compositional constraint, it has taken a long time to reach the currently suitable versions.

To remove the non-negative constraint from compositional data, the first and maybe the easy way is to use log-normal distributions. Over a hundred years, from Galton-McAlister's introduction (Galton 1879; McAlister 1879) to the text book of Aitchison and Brown for the log-normal distribution (Aitchison and Brown 1969), the log transform techniques are readily available. By taking a log transform of the data, the non-negative constraint is removed, and then assuming a normal distribution. The approach is analogous to using logistic link function to model binary data with generalized linear model framework (McCullagh and Nelder 1989). However, the log transformation approach only addresses the non-negative constraint of compositional data and does not address the unit sum constraint (Bacon-Shone 2011). It is until Aitchison in the 1980s developed methodology based on a variety of log-ratio transformation (Aitchison and Egozcue 2005), the unit sum constraint problem began to solve. Aitchison in the 1980s realized that compositions only provide the information about relative, not absolute values of parts or components. Thus, he used the ratios of components to present every statement about a composition (Aitchison 1981, 1982, 1983, 1984). Because mathematically log-ratios are easier to handle than ratios, and a log-ratios transformation provides a one-to-one mapping onto a real space, it opens a path for researchers to develop methodology based on a variety of log-ratio transformation (Aitchison and Egozcue 2005). The algorithm behind the log-ratio transformation principle is based on the fact that there is a one-to-one correspondence between compositional vectors and associated log-ratio vectors, so that any statement about compositions can be reformed in terms of log-ratios, and vice versa (Pawlowsky-Glahn et al. 2015).

With log-ratio transformations, the problem of a constrained sample space, the simplex, is removed, and data are projected into multivariate real space. Therefore, open up all available standard multivariate techniques (Pawlowsky-Glahn et al. 2015). The log-ratio transformation methodology was accepted by statisticians and researchers in geology, ecology and other fields (Aitchison 1982; Pawlowsky-Glahn and Buccianti 2011; van den Boogaart and Tolosana-Delgado 2013; Pawlowsky-Glahn et al. 2015).

In a seminal work (1986) (Aitchison 1986), in order to transform the simplex to the real space, Aitchison developed an axiomatic approach to compositional data analysis with a set of fundamental principles. Based on these fundamental principles, a variety of methods, operations, and tools, including additive log-ratio (alr), centered log-ratio (clr) and isometric log-ratio (ilr) transformations, have been developed by Aitchison and others. We briefly describe these three log-ratio transformations appropriate for compositional data as below:

Additive Log-Ratio (alr) Transformation
The original approach proposed in Aitchison (1986) for the compositional data analysis was based on the additive log-ratio (alr) transformation. It is defined as:

$$\text{alr}(x) = \left[\ln\left(\frac{x_1}{x_D}\right), \ldots, \ln\left(\frac{x_i}{x_D}\right), \ldots, \ln\left(\frac{x_{D-1}}{x_D}\right) \right]. \tag{10.2}$$

The distinguishing feature of this formula is to map a composition in the D-part Aitchison simplex none isometrically to a D-1 dimensional Euclidean vector. Thus, the log-ratio transformation transforms raw compositional data from simplex to real/Euclidean space. The log-ratio transformed data can then be analyzed by all standard statistical methods, which are not relied on a distance. Its inverse transforms from real/Euclidean space back to the simplex (Aitchison 2003).

The additive log-ratio (alr) transformation is the simplest one which chooses one component as a reference. It is still in wide use. For example, in studying the association of obesity and microbiome, the ratio of *Bacteroidetes* to *Firmicutes* has been reported in many publications (Ley et al. 2005, 2006; Turnbaugh et al. 2006, 2009; Arumugam et al. 2011; Knights et al. 2011; The Human Microbiome Project 2012; Sweeney and Morton 2013; Finucane et al. 2014; Walters et al. 2014; Sze and Schloss 2016).

Centered Log-Ratio (clr) Transformation
Centered log-ratio (clr) transformation maps a composition in the D-part Aitchison simplex isometrically to a D-1 dimensional Euclidean vector. The clr representation of composition $x = (x_1, \ldots, x_i, \ldots, x_D)$ is defined as the logarithm of the components after dividing by the geometric mean of x:

$$\text{clr}(x) = \left[\ln\left(\frac{x_1}{g_m(x)}\right), \ldots, \ln\left(\frac{x_i}{g_m(x)}\right), \ldots, \ln\left(\frac{x_D}{g_m(x)}\right) \right], \tag{10.3}$$

with $g_m(x) = \sqrt[D]{x_1 \cdot x_2 \cdots x_D}$ ensuring that the sum of the elements of clr(x) is zero. The clr transforms the composition to the Euclidean sample space, and hence providing the possibility of using standard unconstrained statistical methods for analyzing compositional data (Aitchison. 2003). Dividing all components in a composition by the geometric mean $g_m(x)$ or any constant does not alter the ratios of components. Just like the alr, the inverse of clr also exists.

For example, the clr-approach transforms each taxon within a sample by taking the log-ratio of the counts for that taxon divided by the geometric mean of the counts of all taxa, instead of using one reference taxon. This algorithm has been adopted by some software developments (Fernandes et al. 2013; van den Boogaart and Tolosana-Delgado 2013) for microbiome research and argued that this transformation could be used to successfully analyze microbiome data, as well as RNA-seq data and next-generation sequence data set (Fernandes et al. 2014).

Isometric Log-Ratio (ilr) transformation
The isometric log-ratio (ilr) transformation was defined by Egozcue et al. (2003) as below:

$$y = \mathrm{ilr}(x) = (y_i, \ldots, y_{D-1}) \in R^{D-1}. \tag{10.4}$$

where, $y_i = \dfrac{1}{\sqrt{i(i+1)}} \ln \left[\dfrac{\prod_{j=1}^{i} x_j}{(x_i+1)i} \right]$.

Like the clr, the ilr transformation maps a composition in the D-part Aitchison simplex isometrically to a D-1 dimensional Euclidian vector. Like alr and clr, the isometric log-ratio (ilr) can transform the data from simplex to real space according to isometric log-ratio transformation. It also has inverse. All standard statistical methods can be applied into analysis of the ilr-transformed data.

The ilr transformation is the product of the clr and the transpose of a matrix which consists of elements. The elements are clr-transformed components of an orthonormal basis. This ilr transformation is an orthonormal isometry. It addresses certain difficulties of alr and clr, but its interpretability is subject to the selection of its basis, which has somewhat limited its adoption (Egozcue et al. 2003).

Which Transformation We Should Choose?
The difference among these three log-ratio transformations is to choose the divisor. In other words, is to choose which value to be used to normalize all the values in a sample. Each transformation has its own weaknesses or advantages.

Theoretically, one shortcoming of alr transformation is that the transformation by definition, is asymmetric in the parts of the composition (Egozcue et al. 2003), thus, the distances between points in the transformed space are not the same for different divisors (Bacon-Shone 2011). Therefore, it means alr transformed data should not be analyzed by standard statistical methods, such as ANOVA and t-test, although as shown in Aitchison (1986) and further developed in Aitchison et al. (2000), this weakness is a conceptual rather than practical problem (Aitchison et al. 2000). The main drawback of alr transformation is: it is not an isometric transformation from the simplex, with the Aitchison metric, onto the real alr-space, with the ordinary Euclidean metric. Although using an appropriate metric with oblique coordinates in real additive log-ratio (alr)-space could solve this weakness. However, it is not a standard practice (Aitchison and Egozcue 2005).

In practice, the alr transformation or choosing reference taxa is relatively simple to interpret the results, because the relation to the original D-1 first parts is preserved. It is the advantage of alr. However, there may not always be an obvious reference to choose, the choice of reference taxon is somewhat arbitrary (Li 2015) and results may vary substantially dependent on the choice of reference (Tsilimigras and Fodor 2016). It may be one of the reasons that the alr transformation was not used for analysis of compositional data in "Analyzing Compositional Data with R" (van den Boogaart and Tolosana-Delgado 2013), although there was a choice for the alr function.

By avoiding alr transformation problem of choosing a divisor (e.g., using one reference taxon), the clr transformation is to divide by the geometric mean. The advantage of the clr is that it is an isometric transformation of the simplex with the Aitchison metric, onto a subspace of real space with the ordinary Euclidean metric (Egozcue et al. 2003). However, the disadvantage is that the clr covariance matrix is singular, making it difficult to use in some standard statistical procedures without adaption (Bacon-Shone 2011). Additionally, the orthogonal references in its subspace are not obtained in a straightforward manner (Egozcue et al. 2003), which is thought as its prominent weakness.

The ilr avoids the arbitrariness of alr and the singularity of clr. It has significant conceptual advantages (Bacon-Shone 2011); however there is no one-to-one relation between the original components and the transformed variables, it is difficult to interpret the results. Thus, in practice, ilr has limited adoption in use.

10.1.4.3   How to Deal Zeros in Compositional Data Analysis

One critical progress in compositional data analysis since the 1980s was to use the log-ratio methods. However, the log-ratio methods did not solve zero problems, instead, highlighted the importance of dealing zeros. Because the logarithm of zero is not defined, log and log-ratio transformations require non-zero elements in the data matrix; as a consequence, compositional data analysis must be preceded by a treatment of the zeros.

The three log-ratio transformations have difficulties to meet the central challenges arisen from the complexity of sequencing data sets, especially to solve zero problems. We have reviewed the topic of zero in Chap. 2, and will further cover this topic in zero-inflated models in Chap. 12. Here we review how the compositional data analysts deal with different kinds of zeros.

The zeros are caused by many complicated reasons and currently, no simple general treatment strategy exists (Martín-Fernández et al. 2011). Compositional data analysts try to find the underlying reason and determine the appropriate approach to be applied. Since Aitchison proposed his initial approaches to zeros by replacement and using a model (Aitchison 1986), several treatment approaches have been developed in compositional data analysis.

Deal with Rounded Zeros
For rounds zeros, most approaches treat them as a particular NMAR (Not Missing At Random) case, and deal with them by using both nonparametric *multiplicative replacement* (Martín-Fernández et al. 2003) and more sophisticated model-based replacements parametric methods: to replace them with a small, nonzero value (Martín-Fernández et al. 2012, 2015).

Technically, the non-parametric methods for rounded zeros essentially are to replace a small quantity for each zero by imputation (Martín-Fernández et al. 2003, 2011); while several strategies for rounded compositional zeros have been proposed in the literature. One of the parametric methods for rounded zeros uses a modification of the common expectation-maximization (EM) algorithm in combination with the alr transformation to generate suitable estimates for the values below the detection limit (Palarea-Albaladejo et al. 2007; Mateu-Figueras and Pawlowsky-Glahn 2008; Palarea-Albaladejo and Martín-Fernández 2008; Martín-Fernández et al. 2011).

The aim of imputation of zero is to avoid taking logarithms of zero using the log-ratio transformations. However, in real study, it is difficult to replace zeros with the particular imputed small non-zero values and while do not distort statistical estimates, especially if the degree of sparsity changes dramatically and outlier occurs (Filzmoser et al. 2012; Martín-Fernández et al. 2012; Palarea-Albaladejo and Martín-Fernández 2015; Palarea-Albaladejo and Martín-Fernández 2015).

Deal with Sampling Zeros

Sampling zeros are assumed to be a consequence of the sampling process, not genuine zeros, and specialized methods are required (Martín-Fernández 2015). To address the sampling zero problem, a Bayesian-multiplicative (BM) treatment combining with the Dirichlet distribution has been proposed (Martín-Fernández et al. 2011, 2015). The Bayesian replacement techniques are considered as the most popular way to deal with count zeros (Martín-Fernández et al. 2015).

A new version of Bayesian-multiplicative method for compositional data analysis was proposed by Martín-Fernández et al. (2015). It involves *Bayesian* inference on the zero values and a *multiplicative* modification of the non-zero values in the vector of counts. A zero value is replaced by its posterior Bayesian estimate. The non-zero parts are modified in a *multiplicative* way. This modification preserves the original ratios between parts, as well as the total sum representation of the vector (Martín-Fernández et al. 2015) and has a minor distortion of the association between the parts (Martín-Fernández et al. 2003, 2015).

Based on the valuable information: the average of a compositional vector is equal to its geometric mean (Aitchison 1986), the Geometric BM (GBM) prior and the GBM replacement (Martín-Fernández et al. 2015) are developed to replace zero. However, although the GBM replacements result in the best behavior among the Bayesian replacement techniques, none of the Bayesian methods, neither the GBM replacement, do fully account for the scale invariance. Because it is not fully compatible with the principle of scale invariance of compositional data analysis (Egozcue 2009), researchers cast further doubts on the Bayesian replacement (Martín-Fernández et al. 2015) and back to directly use a model-based replacement procedure to impute the values below the detection limit and developed R software to implement it. For example, a version of this procedure is currently implemented in the function impRZilr() in the library "robCompositions" (Bacon-Shone 2003).

Deal with Structural Zeros

There are various attempts to address the structural zero problem. Relevant contributions specifically focused on the treatment of this kind of zero are by Aitchison and Kay (2003) and Bacon-Shone (2003, 2008). Although currently there is no general method for dealing with the structural zero, it is clear that strategies for replacing it by a small value are not appropriate (Martín-Fernández et al. 2011, 2015).

Under the framework of compositional data analysis, most early researches take the responsibility of the decision on whether a zero is structural or not. They thought that structural zeros can be present in data sets where the components are continuous variables or percentages (Aitchison and Kay 2003) or appear in discrete compositions of count data (Bacon-Shone 2008) and modeled them based on a binomial conditional logistic normal model (Aitchison and Kay 2003) and based on the Poisson-log normal distribution (Bacon-Shone 2008), respectively. Although these two approaches have modeled structural zeros with some success, however, structural zero issue is by far the most complicated problem; it needs the specific models to consider combining zero and non-zero components (Martín-Fernández et al. 2011).

In summary, the approaches of differentiating zero sources and modeling them based on distinct categories: rounded, sampling, or structural zeros under the framework of compositional data analysis, have difficulties, troubles, and challenges, especially in the field of omics researches. In omics, the zero issues are more complicated since it is not easy to separate sampling zeros from structural zeros. Microbiome read counts are generated through two high-throughput sequencing-based approaches: either by sequencing the 16S rRNA marker gene or the shotgun sequencing, which sequences all the microbial genomes presented in the sample. After the sequencing reads are obtained, the data are quantified by aligning to some known reference sequences, and normalized to the relative abundances to make the compositional data comparable (Chen and Li 2016). Generally, we can say that lots of zeros occur due to the process of data generating. However, the presence of zero values in a compositional data set can be due to multiple and different reasons. The zero measurements exist, either because a component was not present, or because it was present but not sampled, or because some measurement error occurred (Lovell et al. 2011).

10.1.4.4 Statistical Tools for Compositional Data Analysis

Statistical Software Under the Classic Framework of Aitchison's CODA
In 2001, compositional data researchers noticed that the original set of routines programmed by John Aitchison (1986) under the name of CODA (with Basic as the language) and NEWCODA (with Matlab 5) were difficult to use for scientists and other users with no programming skills (Aitchison and Greenacre 2002). Since then many R packages have been developed by compositional data researchers and are available for use. We can divide these tools into two categories: exploratory analysis and statistical modeling.

CoDaPack 3D

CoDaPack 3D belongs to the first category. It is publicly available as freeware at http://ima.udg.edu/CoDaPack. Compositional data analysis, following Aitchison's approach, is mainly based on the study and interpretation of log-ratios. CoDaPack 3D provides a user-friendly freeware environment that performs most of the techniques of this approach (Aitchison and Greenacre 2002; Gotelli 2008). CoDaPack 3D is implemented as a set of menus from an ExcelR datasheet and returns numerical results either on the same sheet or as graphical results in an independent window. Compositional data techniques do not permit zero values because of the use of logarithms. In order to replace the zeros, CoDaPack 3D has a routine on the operation menu.

Compositions

Three frequently used R packages for compositional data analysis with Aitchison's approach are compositions (van den Boogaart et al. 2014), robCompositions (Templ et al. 2011), and zCompositions (Palarea-Albaladejo and Martin-Fernandez 2015).

The "compositions" is a unified R package to analyze compositional data (Greenacre 1993). The package provides functions for the consistent analysis of compositional data. Especially, it offers methods for the statistical analysis of four different scales of amount data: (1) acomp: compositional data with relative geometry (Aitchison Simplex); (2) rcomp: compositional data in absolute geometry (Classical Simplex); (3) aplus: positive data with relative geometry (Log-scale analysis); and (4) rplus: positive data with absolute geometry $(R + {}^\wedge d)$. It provides:

- descriptive statistics (e.g., variation matrix, Aitchison mean)
- basic plotting (e.g., ternary diagrams, log-geometry boxplots)
- advanced plotting (e.g., confidence ellipsoids, Aitchison lines)
- multivariate analysis (e.g., compositional principle components)
- all operations in all four geometries (e.g., perturbation, norm)
- standard transforms (e.g., ilr, clr)
- complexity reduction (e.g., marginal compositions, grouping)
- examples.

All data sets from Aitchison (1986) on compositional data are available in the package compositions.

robCompositions

While the compositions package is devoted in particular to classical statistical procedures, the robCompositions package provides tools of exploratory compositional data analysis (Templ et al. 2011): a robust statistical analysis of compositional data together with corresponding graphical tools (Barnett 1981). The robCompositions package provides for the alr, clr and ilr transformations. However, their implementations of transformations are different from the compositions package; in the robCompositions package, variable names and absolute values are preserved. It also provides a comprehensive tool for robust statistical analysis of compositional data, including principal component analysis, factor analysis, discriminant analysis, missing values imputation, multivariate outlier detection, and the accordingly graphic tools (e.g., compositional biplot), etc.

zCompositions

A common left-censoring problem in data sets susceptible to a compositional analysis is the presence of rounded zeros. The zCompositions package implements methods for imputing zeros in compositional count data sets (Palarea-Albaladejo and Martin-Fernandez 2015). It performs imputation of multivariate data with left-censored values under a compositional approach (Palarea-Albaladejo and Martin-Fernandez 2015). The novelty of zCompositions package is to consider both the multivariate structure of the data and methods for left-censored data compatible with a compositional approach to data analysis. Thus, it was adopted by other packages (e.g., ALDEx2).

Statistical Methods and Packages for Correlation and Graphical Network
CCREPE

The CCREPE (Compositionality Corrected by REnormalizaion and PErmutation) package (Egozcue and Pawlowsky-Glahn 2005; Gevers et al. 2014; Weiss et al. 2015) was designed to assess the significance of general similarity measures in compositional datasets, by using permutation-based methods, which implemented through two functions: ccrepe()ccrepe() and nc.score()nc.score(). The first function calculates similarity measures, *p*-values and q-values for relative abundances, using bootstrap and permutation matrices of the data, while the second function calculates species-level co-variation and co-exclusion patterns based on an extension of the checkerboard score to ordinal data. The package takes the sum to one constraint into account when assigning *p*-values to similarity measures between the taxa.

SparCC

A common goal of genomic surveys is to identify correlations between taxa within ecological communities. As an alternative to CCREPE, SparCC (Sparse Correlations for Compositional data) (Friedman and Alm 2012a, b) was specifically designed to estimate the linear Pearson correlations between the log-transformed components from compositional data.

SpiecEasi

SPIEC-EASI (SParse InversE Covariance Estimation for Ecological Association Inference) (Kurtz et al. 2015) is a statistical method for the inference of microbial ecological networks from amplicon sequencing that addresses the two issues: (1) the microbial abundances are compositional, and therefore are not independent; and (2) the much larger number of taxa (OTUs) when compared with the number of samples. The SPIEC-EASI and package SpiecEasi addresses these issues by taking advantage of the proportionality invariance of relative abundance data and making assumptions about the underlying network structure when the number of taxa in the dataset is larger than the number of sampled communities (Kurtz et al. 2015).

The software including CCREPE, SPARCC, SPIEC-EASI, addresses different difficulties arising from the compositional nature of microbiome analyses (Tsilimigras and Fodor 2016). It adopts all the algorithms that have been developed to appropriately analyze compositional data. However, the proposed approaches have the fundamental limitations: they are all built on the assumptions about the underlying data, and no "gold standard" to validate the assumptions and general features of such data sets (Kurtz et al. 2015), although there are no guiding assumptions.

For example, CCREPE's permutation approach has been argued that will fail to adequately control for compositional effects and lead to "false confidence" in the observed correlations (Friedman and Alm 2012a, b; Tsilimigras and Fodor 2016). There are two arguable issues of SparCC model. First, it assumes that there are a sufficiently large number of taxa, and that these taxa on average are uncorrelated with each other leading to a sparse network, which potentially has overestimated the underlying association networks. Second, it eliminates zero fractions by adding small pseudocounts (Friedman and Alm 2012a, b), which obviously simplifies the complication of zero problem.

In SPIEC-EASI, the problem of producing less consistent and sparser interaction networks by SparCC and CCREPE has been investigated. Actually, SPIEC-EASI constructed more highly reproducible association networks, compared to SparCC and CCREPE. Although these two methods are designed to account for these compositional biases and represent the state of the art in the field, it is not clear that correlation is the proper measure of association (Kurtz et al. 2015).

Statistical Tools for Examining Differences in Taxon Abundance Using the CoDa

ANCOM

ANCOM (Analysis of Composition of Microbiomes) (Mandal et al. 2015) was developed to account for the compositional constraints to reduce false discoveries in detecting differences in microbial mean taxa abundance at an ecosystem level. It is based on the compositional log-ratios. ANCOM allows researchers to compare microbial taxa abundance in two or more populations, including detecting trends over time in longitudinal or cross sectional studies, while adjusting for covariates if necessary. The method is implemented via ANCOM package. The method of ANCOM is one of two currently available tools for statistical analysis and hypothesis testing of differences in taxon (OTU) abundance that use the CoDa analysis approach. The other is ALDEx2.

ALDEx2

As reviewed in Chap. 3, to our knowledge, most existing tools for compositional data analysis have been used in the other fields, such as geology and ecology, but not in microbiome studies. These existing tools can be readily adapted and is a valid approach to analyze microbiome high-throughput sequencing data (Gloor and Reid 2016). The R packages called ALDEx and ALDEx2 were developed to analyze

ANOVA-like differential express (Fernandes et al. 2013; Gloor et al. 2016) and to unify the analysis of high-throughput sequencing datasets including RNA sequencing (RNA-seq), chromatin immunoprecipitation sequencing (ChIP-seq), sequencing of 16S rRNA gene fragments, metagenomic analysis and selective growth experiments (Fernandes et al. 2014).

ALDEx and ALDEx2 are compositional data analysis tools that use Bayesian methods to infer technical and statistical error. It incorporates a Bayesian estimate of the posterior probability of taxon abundance into a compositional framework: using a Dirichlet distribution to transform the observed data, then estimates the distribution of taxon abundance by random sampling instances of the transformed data. ALDEx and ALDEx2 are robust statistical methods developed in a traditional ANOVA-like framework that decompose sample-to-sample variation into four parts: within-condition variation, between-condition variation, sampling variation, and general (unexplained) error. They evaluate the taxon (OTU) abundance in microbiome datasets using both statistical testing of significance and measuring the effect size based on CoDa approach.

As a CoDa analysis approach, ALDEx is not interested in the total number of reads, but the proportions from counts. Let n_i present the number of counts observed in taxon i, and assume that each taxon's read count was sampled from a Poisson process with rate μ_i, i.e., $n_i \sim Poisson(\mu_i)$ with $n = \sum_i n_i$. The equivalency between Poisson and multinomial processes can then be used to assert that the set of joint counts with given total has a multinomial distribution, i.e., $\{[n_1, n_2, \ldots] | n\} \sim$ Multinomial $(p_1, p_2, \ldots | n)$ where each $p_i = \mu_i / \sum_k \mu_k$.

Based on the fact of equivalence between Poisson and multinomial processes, traditional methods use n_i to estimate μ_i and then use the set of μ_i to estimate p_i. The methods ignore that most datasets of this type contain large numbers of taxa with zero or small read counts, thus the maximum-likelihood estimate of p_i this way is often exponentially inaccurate. Therefore, ALDEx estimates the set of proportions p_i directly from the set of counts n_i.

ALDEx uses standard Bayesian techniques to infer the posterior distribution of $[p_1, p_2, \ldots]$ as the product of the multinomial likelihood with a Dirichlet $(\frac{1}{2}, \frac{1}{2}, \ldots)$ prior. Considering the large variance and extreme non-normality of the marginal distributions p_i when the associated n_i are small, ALDEx does not summarize the posterior of p_i using point-estimates. Instead, it performs all inferences using the full posterior distribution of probabilities drawn from the Dirichlet distribution such that $[p_1, p_2, \ldots] \sim$ Dirichlet $([n_1, n_2, \ldots] + \frac{1}{2})$.

Adding 0.5 to the Dirichlet distribution, the multivariate distribution avoids the zero problem for the inferred proportions even if the associated count is zero, and conserves the probability, i.e., $\sum_k p_k = 1$. After obtaining the multivariate Dirichlet proportional distributions, to make a meaningful comparison between-sample values from proportional distributions, ALDEx uses the procedures developed by Aitchison, Egozcue, and others (Egozcue et al. 2003; Aitchison and Egozcue 2005; Egozcue and Pawlowsky-Glahn 2005) to transform component proportions into linearly independent components.

ALDEx takes the component-wise logarithms and subtracts the constant $\frac{1}{m}\sum_k \log(p_k)$ from each log-proportion component for a set of m proportions $[p_1, p_2, \ldots, p_m]$, because mathematically log-proportions are easily manipulated. This results in the values of the relative abundances $q_i = \log(p_i) - \frac{1}{m}\sum_{k=1}^m \log(p_i)$ where $\sum_k q_k$ is always zero. Most important, it projects q onto a $m-1$ dimensional Euclidean vector space with linearly independent components. Thus, a traditional ANOVA-like framework can be formed to analyze the q values $[q_1, q_2, \ldots, q_m]$.

The software estimates the distribution of q from multiple Monte Carlo realizations of p given $[n_1, n_2, \ldots, n_m]$, because it is cumbersome to directly compute q distribution.

The distribution of $p \sim$ Dirichlet (α) has the following properties:

$$E\{\log(p_i)\} = \psi(\alpha_i) - \psi\left(\sum \alpha_k\right), \tag{10.5}$$

and

$$\mathrm{cov}\{\log(p_i), \log(p_j)\} = \psi'(\alpha_i)\delta_{ij} - \psi'\left(\sum \alpha_k\right) \tag{10.6}$$

where ψ, ψ', and δ represent the digamma, trigamma, and Kronecker-delta functions, respectively.

Let $i = \{1, 2, \ldots, I\}$ index genes (taxa), $j = \{1, 2, \ldots, J\}$ index the conditions, and $k = \{1, 2, \ldots, K_j\}$ index the replicate of a given condition, using the framework of random-effect ANOVA models, the proposed ALDEx is given by:

$$q_{ijk} = \mu_{ij} + \nu_{ijk} + \tau_{ijk} + \varepsilon_{ijk}, \tag{10.7}$$

where,

q_{ijk} adjusted log-expression (abundance)
μ_{ij} expected expression (abundance) of gene (taxon) i within each condition j
ν_{ijk} sample-specific expression (abundance) change for replicate k
τ_{ijk} sampling variation from inferring expression (abundance) from read counts
ε_{ijk} remaining nonspecific error.

As the usual ANOVA assumptions, ν_{ijk} is assumed to be approximately normal. The distribution of the sampling error τ_{ijk} is given by the adjusted log-marginal distributions of the Dirichlet posterior and is very Gaussian-like.

ALDEx does not assume that within condition sample-to-sample variation is small and essentially negligible, which is more appropriate for the analysis of high-throughput sequencing datasets.

Under the ANOVA framework, we can test the hypotheses:

$$H_0 : \mu_{ij} = \mu_{ij'}$$

The authors of the model emphasize the statistical significance by this hypothesis test does not imply that the conditions j and j' are meaningfully different. Instead, such meaning can be inferred through an estimated effect-size that compares predicted between condition differences to within-condition differences.

Given the set of random variables p_{ijk} and q_{ijk}, the within-condition distribution is:

$$W(i,j) = \sum_{k=1}^{K_j} q_{ijk}, \qquad (10.8)$$

the absolute fold difference between-condition distribution is:

$$\Delta_A(i,j,j') = W(i,j) - W(i,j'), \qquad (10.9)$$

the between sample, within-condition difference:

$$\Delta_W(i,j) = \max_{k \neq k'} |q_{ijk} - q_{ijk'}|, \qquad (10.10)$$

and the relative effect-size:

$$\Delta_R(i,j,j') = \Delta_A(i,j,j')/\max\{\Delta_W(i,j), \Delta_W(i,j')\}. \qquad (10.11)$$

The distributions are estimated from multiple independent Monte Carlo realizations of their underlying Dirichlet-distributed proportions for all genes i simultaneously.

10.2   Why Microbiome Dataset Can Be Treated as Compositional?

There are several reasons that microbiome dataset can be treated as compositional.

The Structure of Microbiome Data Set is Compositional.
In his 1986 seminar work (Aitchison 1986), Aitchison summarized that a compositional data set has four characteristic features: (1) each row of the data array corresponds to a replicate, a single experimental or observational unit; (2) each column corresponds to a specific ingredient or part of each composition; (3) each entry is non-negative; and (4) the sum of the entries in each row is 1, or equivalently 100%. The relative abundance table of microbiome data meets the characteristic features of a compositional data set.

Relative Values of Microbiome Data May be the Interest of Microbiome Study.

In some circumstances the genuinely interest of microbiome study is to compare relative amounts, or the relative abundance of different components. That is, researchers are really interested in the truly relative feature of different components (Lovell et al. 2011). For example, in the obesity microbiome study, one of the research interests is the ratio of the relative abundance of *Bacteroidetes* to that of *Firmicutes* (Ley et al. 2005; Sze and Schloss 2016). Under this situation, the total number of reads for a particular sample is not itself informative or not itself important.

The Source of Microbiome Data May Make the Total Values of the Data Meaningless.

From the sequencing perspective, datasets generated from high throughput sequencing are predefined or constrained to some constants. The omics datasets including RNA sequencing (RNA-seq), sequencing of 16S rRNA gene fragments (Illumina HiSeq or 454 pyrosequencing), chromatin immunoprecipitation sequencing (ChIP-seq), metagenomic analysis and selective growth experiments are composed of counts of sequencing reads mapped to a large number of features (e.g., OTUs, genes, species, or any taxonomic levels) in each sample. The capacity of the machine (the sequencing platform used) and the number of samples that are multiplexed in the run determine the observed number of reads (sequencing depth) (Fernandes et al. 2014). Thus, although the total of reads reported from the high-throughput sequencing methods are large but finite.

Sample Preparation Limits Microbiome Data Carry Only Relative Information.

Sample preparation and DNA/RNA extraction process have made the measurements of omics in ways that ensure that data carry only relative information (Lovell et al. 2011). For example, RNA sequencing starts with a fixed weight or volume tissue sample, a fixed weight or volume of DNA/RNA are extracted, and a finite number of sequence fragment reads are obtained from a fixed volumes of total RNA.

In summary, essentially, the common feature of microbiome data is compositional (Lovell et al. 2011, 2015; Friedman and Alm 2012a, b; Fernandes et al. 2013, 2014) based on the criteria defined by Aitchison (1986). Thus the approaches of compositional data analysis can be applied to microbiome data.

Practical Rules of Choosing Compositional Approach to Analyze Microbiome Data.

In practice, how do we judge whether a compositional approach is appropriate? Generally, when we are interested in the ratios between their components, rather than the total sum of the vectors, then a compositional approach is appropriate (Martín-Fernández et al. 2015). Specially, the appropriateness of a data transformation for compositional data can be addressed by answering two questions (van den Boogaart and Tolosana-Delgado 2008; Fernandes et al. 2014). First, is the total sum of the counts of the data useful? And second, is the absolute difference between observations important? When we answer yes to both questions, then it means that the data belongs to Euclidean space, and the traditional statistical methods are valid. If we answer no to both questions, it means that the data belongs to the Aitchison simplex, and it must be transformed prior to analysis. Most RNA-seq analysis tools, for example, the major tools used for 16S rRNA gene analysis (qiime, mothur and vegan) and tools to analyze ChIP-seq, assume that the values in the dataset are Euclidean and the absolute differences are important. The interested readers can reference the papers of Fernandes et al. (2014) on how to unify the analysis of high-throughput sequencing datasets by compositional data analysis.

10.3 Exploratory Compositional Data Analysis

10.3.1 Compositional Biplot

The compositional biplot is one of the most widely used tools for exploring multivariate compositional data. The compositional biplot is considered as the first exploratory data analysis tool that should be used whenever exploring a microbiome dataset. The plot shows whether or not the samples separate into different groups; what taxa are driving this separation and what taxa are irrelevant to the analysis.

In Chap. 7, the biplot was used when we introduced principal component analysis (PCA), but without details. Here, we further introduce its concept and use. The biplot, proposed by Gabriel (1971, 1981), displays the observations (objects or samples) and variables in the same plot, in a way that depicts their joint relationships. The prefix "bi" in the name biplot refers to the simultaneous display of both rows (observations or samples) and columns (variables) of the data matrix, not to a two-dimensionality of the plot. The biplot is usually used to graphic display of matrices with application to PCA (called principal component biplot). As displays of more than two dimensions are generally difficult to make and even more difficult to interpret, most biplots show only the two dimensions which account for the maximum amount of variation in the data matrix (Kroonenberg 2008).

Biplots were used in biomedical research (Gabriel and Odoroff 1990), compositional data analysis (Aitchison and Greenacre 2002) and currently in microbiome studies (Gloor and Reid 2016) in the form of compositional biplot. In microbiome study, the compositional biplot displays both samples and taxa (OTUs) of a data matrix graphically in the form of scores and loadings of a principal component analysis. Usually, samples are displayed as points while taxa are displayed either as vectors or rays. Biplots essentially are a projection of the multidimensional data onto two dimensions by displaying the two principle components from PCA. Thus, ideally, the first two principle components can explain all the variation of the data.

The most basic property of a biplot is that the inner product of the samples vector and the taxa vector in the plot is the best approximation to the corresponding value in the data matrix. Under a perfect fit condition (two dimensions), then the inner products are identical to the values in the data matrix. Several interpretational rules have been formed from this basic property. Generally, samples are preferably displayed as points and taxa as vectors or arrows. If the angle between two sample vectors is small, they have similar response patterns over taxa. If the angle between two taxon vectors is small, they are strongly associated. Specifically, several rules of interpretation in terms of compositional biplot have been summarized (Gloor and Reid 2016):

(1) rays show the variance exhibited by each taxon, with longer rays indicate more variation across all samples; (2) the locations of sample names show the variable relationship related to other samples; (3) samples that are highly variable and in the same direction as a long ray for a taxon suggest those samples contain that taxon in high abundance; (4) two taxa with co-incident rays and the same length indicate that the ratio of these two taxa is nearly identical across all samples; (5) taxa with orthogonal rays are uncorrelated; (6) taxa having very far distant tips of the rays indicate highly variable ratios across the samples; (7) three or more taxa lying on a common link suggest that they are positively or negatively correlated; (8) the cosine of the angle between links is proportional the correlation between the pairs of ratios, or groups of ratios.

We illustrate the compositional biplot using our *Vdr* mouse dataset. There are 8 samples including 5 $Vdr^{-/-}$ and 3 wild type mice. We use the compositional biplot to examine the relationship between samples and taxa. Two critical procedures need to be performed by applying biplot to compositional data. One is to convert the microbiome data to the centered log-ratio because the compositional biplot based on clr-transformed compositions is easily interpreted. Another is to use a statistical method to replace zero values. We illustrate the compositional biplot step-by-step as below:

Step 1: Load the Data and Convert the Data to the Appropriate Format.
For the plot, the data format needs to be samples being rows, taxa being columns. We load the "VdrFecalGenusCounts" mouse data as previously, and convert the data to the appropriate format.

```
> abund_table=read.csv("VdrFecalGenusCounts.csv",row.names=1,check.names=
FALSE)
> abund_table_t<-t(abund_table)
> head(abund_table_t)
               Tannerella Lactococcus Lactobacillus
5_15_dryst-28F        476         326            94
1_11_dryst-28F        549        2297           434
2_12_dryst-28F        578         548           719
3_13_dryst-28F        996        2378           322
               Lactobacillus::Lactococcus Parasutterella Helicobacter
5_15_dryst-28F                          1              1           89
1_11_dryst-28F                         25              1            0
2_12_dryst-28F                          5              4           13
3_13_dryst-28F                         17              2           24
```

Step 2: Replace 0 Values Using the zCompositions Package.

The following R codes use the function cmultRepl() from the zCompositions package to replace 0 values with the count zero multiplicative method and output counts. This function expects the samples to be in rows and taxa (or OTUs) to be in columns. Because the abund_table_t dataset already have the appropriate data format, we directly use here. But in order to convert the count data to proportion, we use the t() function to transpose the data back to taxa by samples format.

```
> library (zCompositions)
> abund_table_r <- t(cmultRepl((abund_table_t), method="CZM", output="counts"
))
No. corrected values: 54
```

No. Corrected values: 54

```
> head(abund_table_r)
                            5_15_dryst-28F 1_11_dryst-28F 2_12_dryst-28F
Tannerella                             476       549.0000            578
Lactococcus                            326      2297.0000            548
Lactobacillus                           94       434.0000            719
Lactobacillus::Lactococcus               1        25.0000              5
Parasutterella                           1         1.0000              4
Helicobacter                            89         0.3281             13
                            3_13_dryst-28F 4_14_dryst-28F 7_22_dryst-28F
Tannerella                             996       404.0000       319.0000
Lactococcus                           2378       471.0000       882.0000
Lactobacillus                          322       205.0000       644.0000
Lactobacillus::Lactococcus              17         1.0000        13.0000
Parasutterella                           2         0.3343         0.3348
Helicobacter                            24        32.0000         3.0000
                            8_23_dryst-28F 9_24_dryst-28F
Tannerella                        526.0000       424.0000
Lactococcus                      1973.0000      2308.0000
Lactobacillus                    2340.0000      1000.0000
Lactobacillus::Lactococcus         15.0000        14.0000
Parasutterella                     12.0000         1.0000
Helicobacter                        0.3278         0.3288
```

Step 3: Convert the Data to Proportions.

After replace the zero counts, we convert the data to proportions using the function apply() by samples (columns).

```
> abund_table_prop <- apply(abund_table_r, 2, function(x){x/sum(x)})
> head(abund_table_prop)
                              5_15_dryst-28F 1_11_dryst-28F 2_12_dryst-28F
Tannerella                         0.2487268       8.755e-02      0.1117660
Lactococcus                        0.1703465       3.663e-01      0.1059650
Lactobacillus                      0.0491183       6.921e-02      0.1390308
Lactobacillus::Lactococcus         0.0005225       3.987e-03      0.0009668
Parasutterella                     0.0005225       1.595e-04      0.0007735
Helicobacter                       0.0465056       5.233e-05      0.0025138
                              3_13_dryst-28F 4_14_dryst-28F 7_22_dryst-28F
Tannerella                         0.1638771      0.1676255      0.1368797
Lactococcus                        0.3912647      0.1954248      0.3784574
Lactobacillus                      0.0529803      0.0850575      0.2763340
Lactobacillus::Lactococcus         0.0027971      0.0004149      0.0055782
Parasutterella                     0.0003291      0.0001387      0.0001437
Helicobacter                       0.0039488      0.0132773      0.0012873
                              8_23_dryst-28F 9_24_dryst-28F
Tannerella                         0.0718879       7.617e-02
Lactococcus                        0.2696479       4.146e-01
Lactobacillus                      0.3198054       1.796e-01
Lactobacillus::Lactococcus         0.0020500       2.515e-03
Parasutterella                     0.0016400       1.796e-04
Helicobacter                       0.0000448       5.907e-05
```

Step 4: Perform Abundance and Sample Filtering and Deal Sparsity.

We filter the data to remove all taxa that are less than 0.1% abundance in any sample using the function apply() again.

```
> abund_table_prop_f <- abund_table_r[apply(abund_table_prop, 1, min) > 0.001
,]
> head(abund_table_prop_f)
                 5_15_dryst-28F 1_11_dryst-28F 2_12_dryst-28F 3_13_dryst-28F
Tannerella                  476            549            578            996
Lactococcus                 326           2297            548           2378
Lactobacillus                94            434            719            322
Prevotella                  121            289             99            335
Bacteroides                 273            958            377            526
Eubacterium                  52            144            238            129
                 4_14_dryst-28F 7_22_dryst-28F 8_23_dryst-28F 9_24_dryst-28F
Tannerella                  404            319            526            424
Lactococcus                 471            882           1973           2308
Lactobacillus               205            644           2340           1000
Prevotella                  143            111             89             84
Bacteroides                 200             86            424            202
Eubacterium                  90             20             88            192
```

Step 5: Perform the clr Data Transform.

After filter the data, we want to make a reduced dataset before convert the data to the centered log-ratio. First, we add the names again and sort by abundance to check which taxa are most top in samples. Then obtain the taxa in the reduced dataset by name. Finally, make the compositional dataset and transpose it to samples by taxa format.

```
> names_add <- rownames(abund_table_prop_f)[
+   order(apply(abund_table_prop_unord, 1, sum), decreasing=T) ]
> abund_table_prop_reduced <- abund_table_prop_f[names_add,]
> head(abund_table_prop_reduced)
                     5_15_drySt-28F 1_11_drySt-28F 2_12_dryST-28F 3
_13_dryST-28F
Lactococcus                326           2297           548        2378
Lactobacillus               94            434           719         322
Tannerella                 476            549           578         996
Bacteroides                273            958           377         526
Clostridium                130            597           815         203
Akkermansia                 48            102            85         519
                 4_14_dryST-28F 7_22_dryST-28F 8_23_dryST-28F 9_24_dryST-28F
Lactococcus             471            882           1973         2308
Lactobacillus           205            644           2340         1000
Tannerella              404            319            526          424
Bacteroides             200             86            424          202
Clostridium             232             43            114          184
Akkermansia             113             27            111          513
```

```
> abund_clr <- t(apply(abund_table_prop_reduced, 2, function(x){log(x) - mean
(log(x))}))
> head(abund_clr)
               Lactococcus Lactobacillus Tannerella Bacteroides Clostridium
5_15_dryST-28F    1.4104       0.1668      1.7889      1.2329      0.4910
1_11_dryST-28F    2.1759       0.5096      0.7447      1.3014      0.8285
2_12_dryST-28F    0.9113       1.1829      0.9646      0.5373      1.3083
3_13_dryST-28F    2.2679       0.2684      1.3976      0.7592     -0.1929
4_14_dryST-28F    1.4623       0.6305      1.3089      0.6058      0.7542
7_22_dryST-28F    2.4995       2.1850      1.4825      0.1717     -0.5215
               Akkermansia Prevotella Eubacterium Alistipes Butyricimonas
5_15_dryST-28F   -0.50532     0.4193    -0.42528    -1.8116      -2.767
1_11_dryST-28F   -0.93845     0.1030    -0.59361    -1.1326      -2.998
2_12_dryST-28F   -0.95228    -0.7998     0.07734    -0.3198      -2.910
3_13_dryST-28F    0.74576     0.3080    -0.64633    -2.1739      -2.734
4_14_dryST-28F    0.03486     0.2703    -0.19271    -2.1276      -2.747
7_22_dryST-28F   -0.98685     0.4268    -1.28695    -1.8848      -2.085
```

Step 6: Perform the Singular Value Decomposition Using the Function prcomp().

The following R codes do principal component analysis on the compositional dataset using the function prcomp().

```
> abund_PCX <- prcomp(abund_clr)
> abund_PCX$x
                   PC1      PC2      PC3      PC4      PC5      PC6      PC7
5_15_dryST-28F  1.0242  -0.6032  0.80957  -0.32768  0.22770  -0.15661  -0.214411
1_11_dryST-28F  1.0227   0.2804  0.44953   0.96400  0.09902   0.16335  -0.001434
2_12_dryST-28F  1.6109   1.5102  -0.69053  -0.25939  -0.15748  -0.18697  0.072141
3_13_dryST-28F  -0.1694  -1.5474  0.06475   0.13418  -0.08307  -0.28778  0.175535
4_14_dryST-28F  0.6115  -0.6322  -0.01712  -0.52362  0.01342   0.43329  0.089260
7_22_dryST-28F  -1.5161   0.6660  1.03864  -0.07416  -0.60975  0.02074  -0.025307
8_23_dryST-28F  -1.7195   0.8018  0.01231  -0.08533  0.68585  -0.02853  0.048112
9_24_dryST-28F  -0.8642  -0.4756  -1.66715  0.17200  -0.17568  0.04252  -0.143895
                    PC8
5_15_dryST-28F  1.388e-17
1_11_dryST-28F  2.359e-16
2_12_dryST-28F  -1.943e-16
3_13_dryST-28F  -3.504e-16
4_14_dryST-28F  1.041e-17
7_22_dryST-28F  8.327e-17
8_23_dryST-28F  0.000e+00
9_24_dryST-28F  8.327e-17
```

Step 7: Display the Results of Principal Component Analysis by Using Either the biplot() or the coloredBiplot().

In Chap. 7, we used the basic biplot() function, here we illustrate the coloredBiplot () function from the compositions package to generate a simple biplot and allow to color the samples individually. One syntax is given by:

coloredBiplot(x, y, choices = 1:2, var.axes = T, col, cex = rep(par("cex"), 2), xlabs = the names to write for the points of the first set, ylabs = the names to write for the points of the second set, expand = 1, arrow.len = 0.1, main = main title, sub = subtitle, xlab = horizontal axis title, ylab = vertical axis title, xlabs.col = the color(s) to draw the points of the first set, xlabs.pc = the plotting character(s) for the first set, scale = 1)

where:

- x = the co-information to be plotted, given by a result of the prcomp() function or the first set of coordinates to be plotted;
- y = optional, the second set of coordinates to be potted;
- var.axes = T or TRUE, the second set of points have arrows representing them as (unscaled) axes; col = used to specify one color (to be used for the y set) or a vector of two colors (to be used for x and y sets respectively, if xlabs.col is NULL);
- cex = the usual cex parameter for plotting, can be a length-2 vector to format differently x and y labels/symbols;
- expand = an expansion factor to apply when plotting the second set of points relative to the first. This can be used to tweak the scaling of the two sets to a physically comparable scale.
- arrow.len = the length of the arrow heads on the axes plotted in'var.axes' is true. The arrow head can be suppressed by 'arrow.len = 0'.
- choices = the components to be plotted.

- Scale = the way to distribute the singular values on the right or left singular vectors for princomp and prcomp objects. Scale = 0 is to scale the plot based on the samples. Scale = 1 is to scale based on taxa.

```
> library(compositions)
#Sum the total variances
> sum(abund_PCX$sdev[1:2]^2)/mvar(abund_clr)
[1] 0.6894
```

We calculate the total variance explained by the first two principal components by calling the compositions package. The results show that 68.94% of total variances are explained by the first two components.

There are 5 $Vdr^{-/-}$ and 3 wild type samples. In order to have a differentiated visualization of two conditions, we use different colors to label them.

```
> samples <- c(rep(1, 5,rownames(abund_PCX$x)),
+       rep(2, 3,rownames(abund_PCX$x)))
> palette=palette(c(rgb(1,0,0,0.6), rgb(0,0,1,0.6), rgb(.3,0,.3,0.6)))
> palette
[1] "black"      "red"       "green3"    "blue"      "cyan"      "magenta"
"yellow"
[8] "gray"
```

The following R Codes call the function coloredBiplot() from the compositions package to make a covariance biplot of the compositional data (Fig. 10.1).

```
> library(compositions)
> coloredBiplot(abund_PCX, col="black", cex=c(0.6, 0.5),xlabs.col=
samples,
+                     arrow.len=0.05,
+                     xlab=paste("PC1 ", round (sum(abund_PCX$sdev[1]
^2)/mvar(abund_clr),3), sep=""),
+                     ylab=paste("PC2 ", round (sum(abund_PCX$sdev[2]
^2)/mvar(abund_clr),3), sep=""),
+                     expand=0.8,var.axes=T, scale=1, main="Biplot")
```

The plot shows that:

- The first two principle components explain about 69% of the variance in the dataset. Generally, the greater the variance explained by these two components, the greater the distinction from taxa or OTUs (in this case, genera) and samples.
- The samples partition into two groups: 3 wild types (in blue) on the left and 5 $Vdr^{-/-}$ (in red) on the right. They are separated on PC1, which indicates the effects on the split between samples.

Fig. 10.1 The compositional
biplot of the
abundance-filtered Vdr mouse
data. The $Vdr^{-/-}$ and WT
samples are separated very
well. The first two
components explained 69%
total variance (42.7% for
component 1, 26.3% for
component 2) in the dataset

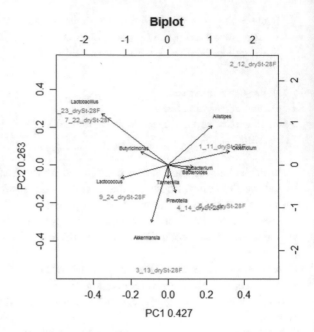

- The length and direction of the arrows (taxa location) is proportional to the standard deviation of the taxon in the dataset. *Lactobacillus* is highly variable genus along the same direction as samples 22 and 23, which indicates that this bacterial is more abundant in WT samples than in $Vdr^{-/-}$ samples.
- *Bacteroides* and *Eubacterium* are very close together. They have a short link. The length of a link is proportional to the variance in their ratios. So the variance of the ratios of these two bacteria is fairly constant.

10.3.2 Compositional Scree Plot

After creating a compositional dataset, we can use a scree plot to display the proportion of the total variation in the dataset that is explained by each of the components in a principle component analysis. This helps us to identify how many of the components are needed to summarize the data. To create a scree plot of the components, we use the screeplot() function. It is the plot method for classes "princomp" and "prcomp". Its default plots the variances against the number of the principal component (Fig. 10.2).

```
> layout(matrix(c(1,2),1,2, byrow=T), widths=c(6,4), heights=c(6,4))
> par(mgp=c(2,0.5,0))
> screeplot(abund_PCX, type = "lines", main="Scree plot")
> screeplot(abund_PCX, type = "barplot", main="Scree plot")
```

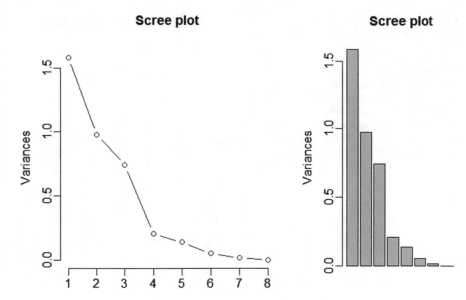

Fig. 10.2 The scree plot of the abundance-filtered *Vdr* mouse data. It shows that the majority of the variability is on components 1 and 2

10.3.3   Compositional Cluster Dendrogram

The biplot suggested that two groups could be defined with our Vdr mouse data. It appears that the samples were separated between the WT samples containing taxa of *Lactobacillus*, *Butyricimonas*, *Lactococcus*, and the $Vdr^{-/-}$ samples containing taxa of *Alistipes*, *Clostridium*, *Eubacterium*, *Bacteroides*, *Tannerella*, *Prevotella*, *Akkermansia*. We can use a compositional cluster analysis (compositional cluster dendrogram) and a compositional barplot to confirm the relationship between the sample clusters and taxa abundance.

   In Chap. 7, we introduced cluster analysis based on Bray-Curtis distance using the same data as use here. Usually in the traditional microbiome analysis, clustering is based on one metric: either the weighted or unweighted unifrac distances, or the Bray-Curtis dissimilarity. However, the Aitchison distance used in compositional data analysis is considered as more robust to the community data. Thus, according to the compositional approach, we here illustrate how to conduct a cluster analysis or plot cluster dendrogram on the log-ratio-transformed data. Euclidian distance can be used because the Aitchison transformed data are linearly related, but all distances should be calculated from the ratios (Fig. 10.3).

```
> # generate the distance matrix
> dist <- dist(abund_clr, method="euclidian")
```

Fig. 10.3 Cluster dendrogram generated by compositional cluster analysis. The figure shows that the samples were separated with WT samples (9_22_drySt-28F, and 9_23_drySt-28F) on the left, and 5 *Vdr*$^{-/-}$ samples on the right, except one WT sample (9_24_drySt-28F)

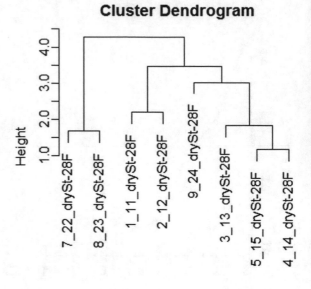

Cluster Dendrogram

dist
hclust (*, "ward.D2")

```
> # cluster the data
> hc <- hclust(dist, method="ward.D2")
> hc
```

Call:
hclust(d = dist, method = "ward.D2")

Cluster method   : ward.D2
Distance   : euclidean
Number of objects: 8

```
> # plot the dendrogram
> plot(hc, cex=1.0)
```

10.3.4 Compositional Barplot

In Sect. 7.2.2 of Chap. 7, we used barplot to display the taxa abundance distribution via the function plot_bar() from the phyloseq package. Here, we conduct the sample bar plot, but on the compositionally transformed data. The following R codes are used to reorder the samples to match the sample orders as cluster dendrogram. We can stack the cluster dendrogram on the top of barplot later.

```
> re_order <- abund_table_prop_reduced[,hc$order]
> re_order
              7_22_dryST-28F 8_23_dryST-28F 1_11_dryST-28F 2_12_dryST-28F
Lactococcus              882           1973           2297            548
Lactobacillus           644           2340            434            719
Tannerella              319            526            549            578
Bacteroides              86            424            958            377
Clostridium              43            114            597            815
Akkermansia              27            111            102             85
Prevotella              111             89            289             99
Eubacterium              20             88            144            238
Alistipes                11             19             84            160
Butyricimonas             9             26             13             12
              9_24_dryST-28F 3_13_dryST-28F 5_15_dryST-28F 4_14_dryST-28F
Lactococcus             2308           2378            326            471
Lactobacillus          1000            322             94            205
Tannerella              424            996            476            404
Bacteroides             202            526            273            200
Clostridium             184            203            130            232
Akkermansia             513            519             48            113
Prevotella               84            335            121            143
Eubacterium             192            129             52             90
Alistipes                27             28             13             13
Butyricimonas             8             16              5              7
```

Now we call the acomp() and barplot() functions to generate the compositional barplot (Fig. 10.4).

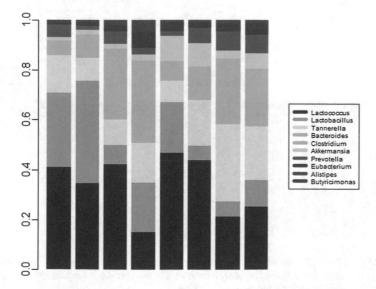

Fig. 10.4 Compositional barplot. The figure shows taxa abundance distribution with the same sample order as that of cluster dendrogram

```
> library(compositions)
> re_order_acomp <- acomp(t(re_order))
> par(mfrow=c(1,2))
> colors <- rainbow(10)
> # plot the barplot below
> barplot(re_order_acomp, legend.text=F, col=colors, axisnames=F,
border=NA, xpd=T)
> # and the legend
> plot(1,2, pch = 1, lty = 1, ylim=c(-10,10),
type = "n", axes = FALSE, ann = FALSE)
> legend(x="center", legend=names_add, col=colors, lwd=5,
cex=.6, border=NULL)
```

Cluster dendrogram visualized the sample separation, but did not provide the information on taxa abundance; bar plot visualized the distribution of taxa abundance, but did not present clear sample information. We can stack the cluster dendrogram on the top of the bar plot to have a better visualization of both sample separation and taxa abundance as Gloor and Reid did in their paper (Gloor and Reid 2016) (Fig. 10.5).

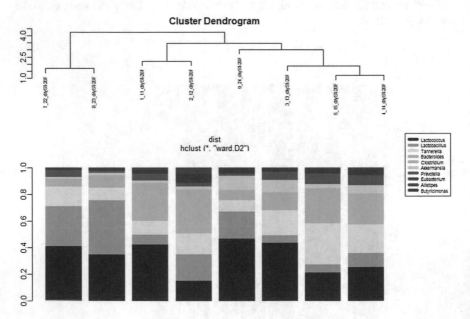

Fig. 10.5 Cluster dendrogram and compositional barplot. With the sample order of cluster dendrogram matched with that of barplot, we can clearly see that taxon *Lactobacillus* enrich in the WT samples, which confirms the results of the biplot

```
> layout(matrix(c(1,3,2,3),2,2, byrow=T), widths=c(5,2), height=c(3,4))
> par(mar=c(3,1,1,1)+0.8)
> # plot the dendrogram
> plot(hc, cex=0.6)
> # plot the barplot below
> barplot(re_order_acomp, legend.text=F, col=colors, axisnames=F,
border=NA, xpd=T)
> # and the legend
> plot(1,2, pch = 1, lty = 1, ylim=c(-10,10),
type = "n", axes = FALSE, ann = FALSE)
> legend(x="center", legend=names_add, col=colors, lwd=5, cex=.6,
border=NULL)
```

10.4 Comparison Between the Groups Using ALDEx2 Package

10.4.1 Vdr Data Set of Fecal and Cecal Sites

The "VdrSitesGenusCounts" data set comes from a part of our microbiome study comparing the effect of Vdr deficiency, which we used in this chapter and previous chapters. Here we focus on comparing the effects of Vdr deficiency and location on microbiome. The data set contains samples of 5 Vdr deficient mice from both fecal and cecal sites (total 10 samples). Here we use this data set to run compositional data analysis using ALDEx2 package.

10.4.2 Compositional Data Analysis Using ALDEx2

There are two essential procedures in ALDEx2: first takes the original input data, and generates a distribution of posterior probabilities of observing each taxon; then uses the centred log-ratio transformation to transform this distribution. After centred log-ratio transforming the distribution, the univariate statistical tests can be conducted by a parametric or nonparametric t-test or ANOVA, and return the p-values and Benjamini-Hochberg adjusted p-values.

In this section, we illustrate the capabilities of ALDEx2 by analyzing data on our Vdr fecal and cecal locations. We first load the abundance table and assign the group variable.

```
> abund_table=read.csv("VdrSitesGenusCounts.csv",row.names=1,
check.names=FALSE)
```

```
> abund_table_t<-t(abund_table)
> ncol(abund_table_t)  # check the number of genera
[1] 248
> nrow(abund_table_t)  # check the number of samples
[1] 10
```

Then extract group information from the abundance table and assign a group variable:

```
> meta_table <- data.frame(row.names=rownames(abund_table_t),t(as.data.
frame(strsplit(rownames(abund_table_t),"_"))))
> meta_table
                 X1 X2      X3
5_15_drySt-28F  5 15 drySt-28F
20_12_CeSt-28F 20 12 CeSt-28F
1_11_drySt-28F  1 11 drySt-28F
2_12_drySt-28F  2 12 drySt-28F
3_13_drySt-28F  3 13 drySt-28F
4_14_drySt-28F  4 14 drySt-28F
19_11_CeSt-28F 19 11 CeSt-28F
21_13_CeSt-28F 21 13 CeSt-28F
22_14_CeSt-28F 22 14 CeSt-28F
23_15_CeSt-28F 23 15 CeSt-28F
> groups <- with(meta_table,ifelse(as.factor(X3)%in% c("drySt-28F"),
c("VdrFecal"), c("VdrCecal")))
> groups
 [1] "VdrFecal" "VdrCecal" "VdrFecal" "VdrFecal" "VdrFecal"
 [6] "VdrFecal" "VdrCecal" "VdrCecal" "VdrCecal" "VdrCecal"
```

ALDEx2 needs the input data with taxa by samples format (row being per-taxon counts, column being each sample). We check to make sure the data format is correct.

```
> abund_table[1:3,1:3]
              5_15_drySt-28F 20_12_CeSt-28F 1_11_drySt-28F
Tannerella               476             67            549
Lactococcus              326            737           2297
Lactobacillus             94            597            434
```

To use the aldex() function to implement compositional data analysis, we need to install package ALDEx2 and call the ALDEx2 library. To install this package, start R and enter:

```
> source("https://bioconductor.org/biocLite.R")
> biocLite("ALDEx2")
```

ALDEx2 can be run using aldex modular or wrapper. To illustrate the capabilities of ALDEx2, we implement both approaches.

Run the ALDEX Modular Step-by-Step.
The aldex modular offers the user the ability to build a data analysis pipeline for her/his experimental designs and tests. Readers can check the manual of ALDEX software for more details. To simplify, the procedure of this approach is just to call aldex.clr(), aldex.ttest(), and aldex.effect() functions in turn and then merge the data into one object.

Step 1: Generate Instances of the Centred Log-Ratio Transformed Values Using the Function aldex.clr().
The function has three inputs: counts table, number of Monte-Carlo instances, and level of verbosity (TRUE or FALSE). The software authors recommend 128 or more mc.samples for the *t*-test, 1000 for a rigorous effect size calculation, and at least 16 for ANOVA.

```
> library(ALDEx2)
> #this operation is fast.
> vdr <- aldex.clr(abund_table, groups, mc.samples=128, verbose=TRUE)
```

Step 2: Perform the Welch's t and Wilcoxon Rank Sum Test Using aldex.ttest().
As in other statistical testing for two conditions, the Welch's *t*-test and Wilcoxon rank sum test can both be used. The function aldex.ttest() has three inputs: the aldex object from aldex.clr(), the vector of conditions, and whether or not a paired test should be conducted (TRUE or FALSE). The aldex.ttest() function returns the values of we.ep (expected *p*-value of Welch's *t* test), we.eBH (expected Benjamini-Hochberg corrected *p*-value of Welch's *t* test), wi.ep (expected *p*-value of Wilcoxon rank sum test), and wi.eBH (expected Benjamini-Hochberg corrected *p*-value of Wilcoxon rank sum test).

```
> vdr_t <- aldex.ttest(vdr, groups, paired.test=FALSE)
> head(vdr_t)
                              we.ep  we.eBH     wi.ep wi.eBH
Tannerella                 0.023164 0.2194  0.007937 0.1030
Lactococcus                0.809151 0.9260  0.850632 0.9448
Lactobacillus              0.005553 0.1275  0.008557 0.1059
Lactobacillus::Lactococcus 0.699612 0.8774  0.712302 0.8796
Parasutterella             0.398490 0.6859  0.428075 0.6801
Helicobacter               0.079861 0.3355  0.077071 0.3308
```

As an alternative to step 2, we can perform the glm and Kruskal-Wallis tests for one-way ANOVA using the function aldex.glm(); however, this is slow. The aldex. glm() function returns the values of kw.ep (expected *p*-value of Kruskal-Wallis test), kw.eBH (expected Benjamini-Hochberg corrected *p*-value of Kruskal-Wallis test), glm.ep (expected *p*-value of glm test), and glm.eBH (expected Benjamini-Hochberg corrected *p*-value of glm test).

```
> # based on the documentation this is slow and not evaluated
> vdr_glm <- aldex.glm(vdr, groups)
```

Step 3: Estimate Effect Size Using the Function aldex.effect().
The aldex.effect() function estimates effect size and the within and between condition values in the case of two conditions. It has four inputs: the aldex object from aldex.clr(), the vector of conditions, a flag indicating whether or not to include values for all samples are used as the denominator, and the level of verbosity.

```
> vdr_effect <- aldex.effect(vdr, groups, include.
sample.summary=FALSE, verbose=FALSE)
```

The aldex.effect() function returns all the values including:

rab.all (median clr value for all samples in the feature)
rab.win.VdrFecal (median clr value for the VdrFecal group of samples)
rab.win. VdrCecal (median clr value for the VdrCecal group of samples)
dif.btw (median difference in clr values between VdrFecal and VdrCecal groups)
dif.win (median of the largest difference in clr values within VdrFecal and VdrCecal groups)
effect (median effect size: diff.btw /max(diff.win) for all instances
overlap (proportion of effect size that overlaps 0 (i.e., no effect): it is overlap between the Bayesian distribution of groups VdrFecal and VdrCecal.

Step 4: Merge all Data into One Object and Make a Data Frame for Result Viewing and Downstream Analysis.

```
> vdr_all <- data.frame(vdr_t, vdr_glm, vdr_effect)
```

The following head() function examines the first few lines of data:

```
> head(vdr_all)
                               we.ep  we.eBH    wi.ep wi.eBH
Tannerella                  0.023164 0.2194 0.007937 0.1030
Lactococcus                 0.809151 0.9260 0.850632 0.9448
Lactobacillus               0.005553 0.1275 0.008557 0.1059
Lactobacillus::Lactococcus  0.699612 0.8774 0.712302 0.8796
Parasutterella              0.398490 0.6859 0.428075 0.6801
Helicobacter                0.079861 0.3355 0.077071 0.3308
                               kw.ep  kw.eBH   glm.ep glm.eBH
Tannerella                  0.009023 0.1171 0.004246 0.03923
Lactococcus                 0.764270 0.8477 0.781273 0.89270
Lactobacillus               0.009571 0.1191 0.001292 0.02153
Lactobacillus::Lactococcus  0.630767 0.7727 0.659656 0.81794
Parasutterella              0.368972 0.5766 0.341531 0.54294
Helicobacter                0.062197 0.2737 0.048052 0.15739
                             rab.all rab.win.VdrCecal
Tannerella                    7.8986           5.2093
Lactococcus                  10.1128          10.1775
Lactobacillus                 9.4856          10.2528
Lactobacillus::Lactococcus    3.5202           3.9320
Parasutterella                0.4034          -0.3646
Helicobacter                  0.6931          -1.1552
                             rab.win.VdrFecal diff.btw diff.win
Tannerella                              9.523   4.5454   1.8002
Lactococcus                             9.837  -0.2911   2.1394
Lactobacillus                           8.773  -1.6159   0.9453
Lactobacillus::Lactococcus              2.434  -0.5853   3.2089
Parasutterella                          1.018   1.2547   3.3765
Helicobacter                            5.099   5.9691   4.3374
                             effect    overlap
Tannerella                   2.4660 0.0002193
Lactococcus                 -0.1482 0.4454829
Lactobacillus               -1.7516 0.0062660
Lactobacillus::Lactococcus  -0.1572 0.4112150
Parasutterella               0.2863 0.3312502
Helicobacter                 1.2005 0.1214960
```

Here, the results actually present ratios between values, rather than abundances. The abundances are determined as the ratio of the abundance of a taxon to all taxa in the sample. Except p-value, all values are on a $\log_2$ scale and should be interpreted as $\log_2$ scale. In addition, because the aldex.clr() function uses Monte Carlo method to sample the data, all the reported values are the mean values over the number of Dirichlet instances as given by the mc.samples variable in the aldex.clr() function (Gloor and Reid 2016).

We check how many significant taxa between fecal versus cecal sites detected in both Welch's t-test and Wilcoxon rank sum tests, and how many remain significant when the p-values are adjusted for multiple testing corrections using the Benjamini-Hochberg's method. Then, we summarize these detected significant taxa with a table.

```
> sig_by_both <- which(vdr_all$we.ep < 0.05 & vdr_all$wi.ep < 0.05)
> sig_by_both
 [1]  1  3  7  8 10 19 22 36 39 57 58
```

```
> sig_by_both_fdr <- which(vdr_all$we.eBH < 0.05 & vdr_all$wi.eBH < 0.05)
> sig_by_both_fdr
integer(0)
```

Eleven taxa are identified as significant by both Welch's *t*-test and GLM, but none of these reach significance when the *p*-values are adjusted for multiple testing corrections using the Benjamini-Hochberg's method.

The following R codes use the xtable() function from xtable package to make a result table. The xtable package is used to create export tables, with converting an R object to an xtable object, which can then be printed as a LaTeX or HTML table. Here, the print.xtable() function is used to export to HTML file. If you want to export the LaTeX file, then use type="latex", file="Vdr_Table.tex" instead.

```
> library(xtable)
> table <-xtable(
+       vdr_all[sig_by_both,c
(12:15,1,3,2,4)], caption="Table of significant taxa", digits=3,
label="sig.table", align=c("l",rep("r",8) )
+ )
> print.xtable(table, type="html", file="Vdr_Table.html")
```

Where, vdr_all[sig_by_both,c(12:15,1,3,2,4)] is a R object; the element of the object "sig_by_both" is the row of output matrix, the element of the object "c(12:15,1,3,2,4)]" is the column of output matrix with the order of columns you want to be in export table. Caption is used to specify the table's caption or title. The label argument is used to specify the LaTeX label or HTML anchor. The align argument indicates the alignment of the corresponding columns, is character vector with the length equal to the number of columns of the resulting table; the resulting table has 8 columns, so the number is 8. If the R object is a data.frame, the length of align is specified to be $1 + \text{ncol}(x)$ because the row names are printed in the first column. The left, right, and center alignment of each column are denoted by "l", "r", and "c", respectively. In this table, align=c("l",rep("r",8) indicates that first column is aligned left, the remaining 8 columns are aligned right. The digits argument is used to specify the number of digits to display in the corresponding columns.

Only those significant taxa detected in both Welch's *t*-test and Wilcoxon rank sum test are printed in Table 10.1. We can interpret the table this way, as the example of *Lactobacillus*, the absolute difference between $Vdr^{-/-}$ fecal and $Vdr^{-/-}$ cecal groups can be up to -1.616, implying that the absolute fold change in the ratio between *Lactobacillus* and all other taxa between $Vdr^{-/-}$ fecal and $Vdr^{-/-}$ cecal groups for this organism is on average $(1/2)^{-1.616} = 3.065$ fold across samples. The difference within the groups of 0.945 is roughly equivalent to the standard deviation, giving an effect size of -1.752.

Table 10.1 Table of significant taxa detected by ALDEx2

	diff. btw	diff. win	effect	overlap	we. ep	wi.ep	we. eBH	wi. eBH
Tannerella	4.545	1.800	2.466	0.000	0.023	0.008	0.219	0.103
Lactobacillus	−1.616	0.945	−1.752	0.006	0.006	0.009	0.127	0.106
Prevotella	5.360	2.021	2.713	0.000	0.007	0.008	0.112	0.103
Bacteroides	4.242	1.802	2.421	0.000	0.020	0.008	0.201	0.103
Odoribacter	4.027	3.284	1.094	0.069	0.045	0.047	0.283	0.227
Alistipes	5.020	2.256	2.184	0.000	0.007	0.008	0.112	0.103
Paraprevotella	4.249	2.808	1.438	0.047	0.028	0.020	0.235	0.153
Butyricimonas	4.972	2.639	1.912	0.003	0.014	0.010	0.163	0.112
Alistipes:: Bacteroides	4.811	2.856	1.510	0.019	0.014	0.013	0.164	0.130
Paraeggerthella	−4.391	3.275	−1.227	0.047	0.033	0.037	0.237	0.194
TM7 (genus)	−3.598	3.176	−1.151	0.075	0.045	0.043	0.268	0.208

Run the ALDEX Wrapper

Currently, the aldex wrapper is limited to two sample tests and one-way ANOVA design. When you run the aldex wrapper, it will link the modular elements together to emulate ALDEx2 prior to the modular approach.

```
> vdr_w <- aldex(abund_table, groups, mc.samples=128, test="t", effect=TRUE,
+               include.sample.summary=FALSE, denom="iqlr", verbose=FALSE)
> head(vdr_w)
                           rab.all rab.win.VdrCecal rab.win.VdrFecal diff.btw diff.win    effect
Tannerella                  7.9905           5.1624           9.7038  4.60318    2.275  2.067398
Lactococcus                10.1374          10.1395          10.1319 -0.01517    1.576 -0.006149
Lactobacillus               9.7087          10.2840           8.4371 -1.75076    1.213 -1.322765
Lactobacillus::Lactococcus  3.4425           3.7795           3.0984 -0.51921    2.870 -0.169915
Parasutterella              0.2524          -0.5844           0.7755  1.70280    3.660  0.344842
Helicobacter                0.7640          -1.0509           4.6825  6.03731    4.118  1.285585
                            overlap  we.ep we.eBH    wi.ep wi.eBH
Tannerella                0.0002193 0.02569 0.2721 0.007937 0.1231
Lactococcus               0.4968750 0.81617 0.9321 0.862661 0.9552
Lactobacillus             0.0968759 0.02981 0.2916 0.050409 0.3025
Lactobacillus::Lactococcus 0.3925235 0.73171 0.8995 0.703497 0.8901
Parasutterella            0.3177572 0.37140 0.6962 0.441468 0.7210
Helicobacter              0.1281257 0.06767 0.3583 0.075707 0.3687
```

Because there are two test groups, this is a two-sample t-test. We specify test="t", and then the effect should be set to TRUE. The "t" option evaluates the data as a two-factor experiment using both the Welch's t-test and the Wilcoxon rank sum test. If the test is "glm", then effect should be specified as FALSE. The "glm" option evaluates the data as a one-way ANOVA using the glm and Kruskal-Wallis test. All tests include a Benjamini-Hochberg correction of the raw p-values.

10.4.3   Difference Plot, Effect Size and Effect Plot

As downstream analyses, we use the merged data graphically present the differences and effect sizes.

Bland-Altman Plot
A Bland-Altman plot, named after J. Martin Bland and Douglas G.Altman, is also
known as difference plot or Tukey mean-difference plot. It analyzes the agreement
between two different measures (Altman and Bland 1983; Martin Bland and
Altman 1986; Bland and Altman 1999). The point underlying the method is that
any two methods designing to measure the same property or parameter should have
agreed sufficiently closely, but not merely highly correlated. ALDEx2 provides a
Bland-Altman (MA) style plot to graphically compare the degree of agreement of
measures between median $\log_2$ between-condition difference and median $\log_2$ relative abundance. We use the aldex.plot() function to generate MA plot.

```
> aldex.plot(vdr_all, type="MA", test="welch", cutoff=0.15, all.
cex=0.7, called.cex=1.1,rare.col="grey", called.col="red")
```

where, type = MA specifies the type of plot to be produced; test="welch" indicates
using Welch's t test to calculate significane; cutoff = 0.15 specifies to use 0.15 for
the Benjamini-Hochberg FDR cutoff, default is 0.1; all.cex = 0.7 specifies the
symbol size; called.cex = is used to specify the character expansion of points with
FDR, $q \leq 0.1$; rare.col = "grey" specifies grey for rare taxa, default black;
called.col = "red" specifies red points to present those taxa that have a mean
Benjamini-Hochberg adjusted Wilcoxon rank sum test's p-value (FDR) of 0.15 or
less (Fig. 10.6).

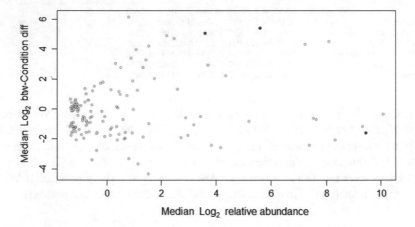

Fig. 10.6 Bland-Altman plot produced by the aldex.plot() function

Effect Size and Effect Size Plot

In ALDEx2, the effect size is defined as a measure of the mean ratio of the difference between groups (diff.btw) and the maximum difference within groups (diff.win or variance). The effect size can be obtained by the aldex.effect() function when you run the aldex modular, or by specifying effect = TRUE argument when you run the aldex wrapper (see Table 10.1).

We can use the aldex.plot() function to plot median between-group difference versus median within-group difference to visualize differential abundance of the sample data. The plots are refer as to "effect size" plots in ALDEx2.

```
> par(mfrow=c(1,2))
> aldex.plot(vdr_all, type="MW", test="welch",cutoff=0.15, all.cex=0.7,
called.cex=1.1, rare.col="black", called.col="red")
> aldex.plot(vdr_all, type="MW",test="wilcox", cutoff=0.15, all.
cex=0.7, called.cex=1.1, rare.col="black", called.col="red")
```

where, type = "MW" specifies the type of plot be MW: a difference between to a variance within. The Welch's t-test or the Wilcoxon rank sum test is used for calculating significance (Fig. 10.7).

The plots show the maximum variance within the $Vdr^{-/-}$ fecal or cecal group versus between group differences. The left and right panel of this figure uses the Welch's t-test, and the Wilcoxon rank sum test, respectively. In both plots, red points represent the differentially abundant taxa with a mean Benjamini-Hochberg adjusted Welch's t-test or Wilcoxon rank sum test's p-value of 0.15 or less ($q < 0.15$). If no red points displayed indicates no significance detected by this test. The grey points represent the abundant taxa, but non-significant. The grey lines

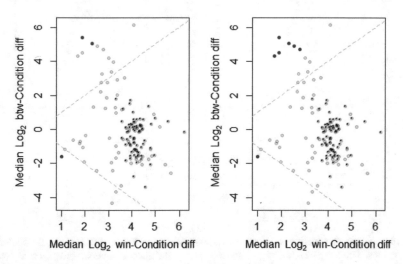

Fig. 10.7 A plot of differential abundance using either the Welch's t-test or the Wilcoxon rank sum test by the aldex.plot() function to exanimate the univariate differences between $Vdr^{-/-}$ fecal and cecal groups

represent the line of equivalence for the within and between group values. Black points are taxa that are less abundant than the mean taxon abundance and non-significant too. Generally, these taxa are difficult to be precisely estimated.

In general, *p*-value is less robust than effect size. Thus, researchers prefer to report effect size more often than the *p*-value. If sample size is sufficiently large, an effect size of 0.5 or greater is considered more likely corresponding to biological relevance. In ALDEx2, an effect size cutoff of 1.5–2 and an overlap cutoff of 0.01 is considered as more appropriate to identify differential taxa of interest (Fernandes et al. 2013). Here, we illustrate two more plots about effect size: (1) plot the effect size versus the *p*-value, and (2) a volcano plot shows the difference between groups versus the *p*-value (Fig. 10.8).

```
> par(mfrow=c(1,2))
> plot(vdr_all$effect, vdr_all$wi.ep, log="y", pch=19, main="Effect",
+          cex=0.5, xlab="Effect size", ylab="Expected P value of
Wilcoxon rank test")
> abline(h=0.05, lty=2,lwd=3, col ='red')
> plot(vdr_all$diff.btw, vdr_all$wi.ep, log="y", pch=19,
main="Volcano",
+          cex=0.5, xlab="Difference", ylab="Expected P value of
Wilcoxon rank test")
> abline(h=0.05, lty=2,lwd=3, col='red')
```

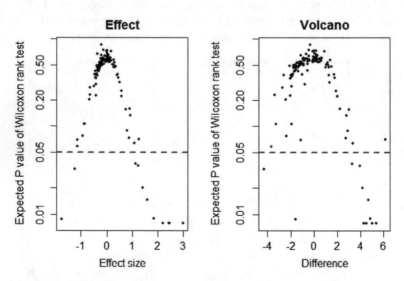

Fig. 10.8 Effect plot exanimating the univariate differences between $Vdr^{-/-}$ fecal and $Vdr^{-/-}$ cecal groups. The left plot of this figure shows a plot of the effect size versus the expected *p*-value of Wilcoxon rank sum test. The right plot of this figure shows a volcano plot where the difference between groups is plotted versus the expected *p*-value of Wilcoxon rank sum test

10.5 Proportionality: Correlation Analysis for Relative Data

10.5.1 Correlation Analysis Is Not Appropriate for Compositional Data

Correlation is a bivariate analysis that measures the strengths of association between two variables and the direction of the relationship. The correlation coefficient has a value between +1 and −1. As the value is near 0, the relationship between the two variables is weaker; while the direction of the relationship is indicated by ±: the + sign indicates a positive relationship between the variables, and the − sign indicates a negative relationship between them.

Usually, there are four types of correlations: Pearson correlation, Spearman correlation, Kendall rank correlation, and the Point-Biserial correlation. Of them, Pearson and Spearman correlations are most frequently used.

Pearson r Correlation
Pearson r correlation is the most widely used correlation statistic to measure the linear correlation between two variables X and Y. The following formula is used to calculate the Pearson r correlation:

$$r = \frac{N \sum XY - (\sum X)(\sum Y)}{\sqrt{N(\sum X^2) - (\sum X)^2}\sqrt{N(\sum Y^2) - (\sum Y)^2}} \tag{10.12}$$

where,

r Pearson r correlation coefficient.
N number of value in each data set.
$\sum XY$ sum of the products of paired values: each X-value should first be multiplied by its corresponding Y-value. After obtaining all such products, find their sum.
$\sum X$ sum of X-values.
$\sum Y$ sum of Y-values.
$\sum X^2$ sum of squared X-values.
$\sum Y^2$ sum of squared Y-values.

The assumptions for appropriate use of the Pearson r correlation include: normality (both variables should be normally distributed), random sampling (the sample of paired (X, Y) data is a random sample of quantitative data), linearity (a straight line relationship between each of the variables), and homoscedasticity (the data is normally distributed about the regression line).

Spearman's Rank Correlation
Spearman r_s correlation is a nonparametric measure of the strength and direction of association between two ranked variables X and Y. It is equal to the Pearson correlation between the rank values of those two variables. The difference is that

Pearson's correlation assesses linear relationships, whereas Spearman's correlation assesses monotonic relationships. A monotonic relationship occurs when the value of X variable increases, the value of the Y variable either increases or decreases (whether linear or not). If there are no repeated data values, a perfect Spearman correlation of +1 or −1 occurs when each of the variables is a perfect monotone function of the other.

Spearman r_s correlation also assumes the sample of paired (X, Y) data has been randomly selected; however, unlike the Pearson r correlation, it does not require that both variables should be normally distributed.

Inappropriateness of Correlation Analysis of Compositional Data

Unfortunately, Pearson and Spearman correlations are inappropriate measures of association in compositional data. The underlying reasons for the failure are: (1) the constraint that all components sum to a constant makes each pair of components of compositional data dependence on each other; while either linear or rank correlation assumes that the sample of paired data is randomly selected (independent), and (2) The relationship between two components of compositional data is not linear or monotonic. Consequently, correlation analysis of compositional data results in meaningless conclusions, because:

(1) Its value depends on which components are analyzed (Aitchison 1986); thus it is not subcompositionally coherent (Aitchison 2003).
(2) Relative abundance data can also make statistically independent components appear correlated (Lovell et al. 2011). For example, although statistically independent variables X, Y, and Z are not correlated, their ratios X/Z and Y/Z must be, because of their common divisor. This was observed by Pearson (Pearson 1897) as "spurious correlation."
(3) In the absence of any other information or assumptions, correlations, including rank correlations or other measures of statistical association between relative abundances, tell us absolutely nothing about the relationship between the absolute abundances that gave rise to them. Lovell et al. show this problem with the plot of pairs of relative abundances (Lovell et al. 2015) and absolute and relative gene expression data (2015).

Therefore, we should caution about correlation and other statistical methods that assume measurements come from real coordinate space. It is suggested that correlation analysis should not be applied to relative abundance data (Lovell et al. 2015). Some researchers pointed out that the available methods, including gene coexpression networks (López-Kleine et al. 2013), weighted gene co-expression network analysis (Zhang and Horvath 2005), and heatmap visualization (Eisen et al. 1998), are potentially misleading if applied to relative data. Lovell et al. extended their concern to the methods based on mutual information (e.g., relevance networks) (Butte and Kohane 2000) and advocated caution to gene co-expression databases that provide correlation coefficients for the relative expression levels of different genes (Obayashi and Kinoshita 2011).

In summary, we should not conduct correlation analysis on the data that carry only relative information.

10.5.2 Introduction to Proportionality

Compositional data analysis is a valid alternative approach for relative data (Shu et al. 2013). To analyze relative data, such as relative abundances in microbiome study, we must obey three principles: scaling invariance, subcompositional coherence, and permutation invariance. Lovell et al. proposed the proportionality measure for analyzing relative data and think that proportionality obeys all three principles (Lovell et al. 2015). The proposed proportionality measure is statistic ϕ, which is used to describe the strength of proportionality between two variables: to assess the extent to which a pair of random variables (x, y) are proportional. Erb and Notredame proposed a symmetric proportionality coefficient, called ρ, partial proportionality, a definition adopted from partial correlations (Erb and Notredame 2016). They think ρ has some advantages over ϕ statistic in that it is symmetric, has a limited range, can also detect reciprocality and allows for the definition of a partial coefficient.

Consider a matrix of D taxon count values measured across N samples subjected to condition, treatment status or time. The condition could be a binary or continuous event. Then the functions phit() and perb() are defined below:

$$\phi(A_i, A_j) = \frac{\text{var}(A_i - A_j)}{\text{var}(A_i)} \tag{10.13}$$

$$\rho(A_i, A_j) = 1 - \frac{\text{var}(A_i - A_j)}{\text{var}(A_i) + \text{var}(A_j)} \tag{10.14}$$

where, A_i and A_j are two log-ratio transformed vectors of the original sample vectors X_i and X_j. The naturally symmetric variant of ϕ, labeled as ϕ_s, defines the function phis() below:

$$\phi_s(A_i, A_j) = \frac{\text{var}(A_i - A_j)}{\text{var}(A_i + A_j)} \tag{10.15}$$

The centered log-ratio transformation (clr), $clr(X) = [\ln(\frac{x_1}{g_m(x)}), \ldots, \ln(\frac{x_i}{g_m(x)}), \ldots, \ln(\frac{x_D}{g_m(x)})]$ is used by default to transform the sample vectors of X_i and X_j to vectors of A_i and A_j. As an alternative, the transformation also can be implemented by the additive log-ratio transformation (alr), $alr(X) = [\ln(\frac{x_1}{x_D}), \ldots, \ln(\frac{x_i}{x_D}), \ldots, \ln(\frac{x_{D-1}}{x_D})]$.

In summary, proportionality borrowing compositional data analysis principals uses a log-ratio transformation of the original feature (e.g., taxon, OTU) vectors to transpose the data from a simplex into real Euclidean space; thus ensure the calculated variance of log-ratio (VLR). Through measuring proportionality does not change whether applied to relative values or to their absolute equivalent.

Through measuring proportionality, we can identify proportionally abundant taxa. Recently, a statistic for differential proportionality (called propd method) was proposed by Erb et al. (2017). It is equivalent to the squared t-statistic of one-way ANOVA for taxon ratios. To understand differential ratio expression, a change in the ratio of abundances between experimental groups, the new method takes a normalization-free approach, applies the techniques developed for the analysis of the differential expression of genes (Smyth 2004, 2005; Law et al. 2014) to the analysis of differential ratios. Although differential proportionality analysis was adopted from differential expression analysis, the interpretation of differential ratios differs considerably.

If a taxon ratio is detected to remain unchanged across all sample data, it means that the two taxa change in the same way (or otherwise remain both unchanged). In the case, the two taxa are correlated in both groups with a similar strength of correlation, but with different slopes, it suggests that the two taxa have differential proportionality. In other words, their proportionality factor is group-specific.

Assume n samples are partitioned into two conditions or groups of experimental replicates of sizes k and n − k, under the ANOVA framework, the variance of the log ratios of two vectors x, y can be decomposed into between-group variance and within-group variance. The propd method uses the VLR to test for differential proportionality. Here, we introduce two forms of differential proportionality: disjointed proportionality (denoted as θ_d) and emergent proportionality (denoted as θ_e).

Given two groups, sized k and $n - k$, the θ_d is defined as the pooled (weighted) VLR within the two groups divided by the total VLR:

$$\theta_d(X, Y) = \frac{(k - 1)VLR_1 + (n - k - 1)VLR_2}{(n - 1)VLR} \tag{10.16}$$

The disjointed proportionality considers the case where the proportionality of a pair holds in both groups, but the ratio between the partners changes between the groups (i.e., the *slope* of the proportionality changes).

Likewise, θ_e is defined as the fraction of variance that remains when subtracting the fraction of the dominating group variance:

$$\theta_e(X, Y) = 1 - \frac{\max[(k - 1)VLR_1, (n - k - 1)VLR_2]}{(n - 1)VLR}. \tag{10.17}$$

The emergent proportionality considers the case where there is proportionality in only one of the groups (i.e., the *strength* of the proportionality changes).

The propd method does not return a vector of p-values; however, we can estimate the false discovery rate (FDR) using permutations of the group assignments to generate an empiric distribution of θ values. To do this, specify each arbitrary cutoff of θ, then the FDR is calculated as the average random number of pairs with $\theta <$ cutoff divided by the observed number of pairs with $\theta <$ cutoff.

The relationship between θ_d and the F-statistic is defined by: $F = (n - 2)\frac{1-\theta_d}{\theta_d}$. We can also calculate an F-statistic via this relationship. After obtaining the F-statistic, we can calculate a moderated F-statistic through borrowing the technique from the limma package (Smyth 2005) and the use of precision weights (Law et al. 2014). We will cover more material on the borrow information approach in Chap. 11 when the over-dispersed models are introduced.

10.5.3 Illustrating Proportionality Analysis

In Sect. 10.4, the ALDEx2 package was used to compare differential abundances between two groups. However, the ALDEx2 package lacks capability for calculating proportionality or any other compositionally valid measure of association. The R package propr was designed for identifying proportionally abundant taxa using compositional data analysis (Lovell et al. 2015; Erb and Notredame 2016; Erb et al. 2017; Quinn et al. 2017). In this section, we use the propr package to determine which taxa are most correlated or compositionally associated in our "VdrFecalGenusCounts" data set. The data set has been used for illustrating exploratory compositional analysis in Sect. 10.3. We divide the proportionality analyses into four parts: proportionality calculation, identify proportionally abundant taxa, proportionality visualization, and differential proportionality analysis.

10.5.3.1 Calculating Proportionality

The proportionality metrics ϕ, ρ, and ϕ_s are calculated by the three principal functions, phit(), perb(), and phis(), respectively. By considering "strength" of proportionality (goodness-of-fit) rather than testing the hypothesis of proportionality, the three metrics measure proportionality in different ways and have different interpretations. First, the values of range are different: $\phi \in [0, \infty)$, $\rho \in [-1, 1]$ and $\phi_s \in [0, \infty)$. Second, the interpretations are different. The lower values of ϕ or ϕ_s indicates more proportionality (the closer ϕ is to zero, the stronger the proportionality), whereas the greater $|\rho|$ values indicates more proportionality with negative ρ values indicating inverse proportionality. We can consider the measure of ϕ as a dissimilarity metric (dissimilarity measure), ρ as a correlation metric. Third, ϕ lacks symmetry, while ϕ_s is a naturally symmetric variant version of ϕ; ρ is also symmetric. See the detail of their proportionality metrics below. We can force ϕ to be symmetry by specifying symmetrize = TRUE in the function phit() like this: phit

(X, symmetrize = TRUE). This forcing action reflects the lower left triangle of the matrix across the diagonal. Fourth, the variance corrections are different: ϕ corrects for just one of the taxa, whereas ρ and ϕ_s correct for the individual variance of each taxon in the pair. Readers can see above formulas of these metrics to get better understanding.

Overall Features of the Functions phit(), perb(), and phis().
The functions phit(), perb(), and phis() return the four proportionality matrix wrapped within an object of the propr class:

@counts—a matrix storing the original "count matrix" input.
@logratio—a matrix storing the log-ratio transformed "count matrix".
@matrix—a matrix storing the proportionality metrics.
@pairs—a vector indexing the proportionality of interest.

To illustrate these matrices, we load the data set, as we previously did. The original data set has the taxa (rows)–by–samples (columns) format. For proportionality analysis, the data set needs to be samples (rows)–by–taxa (columns) data frame. We transform the data set after loading.

```
> abund_table=read.csv("VdrFecalGenusCounts.csv",row.names=1,
check.names=FALSE)
> head(abund_table)
> abund_table_t<-t(abund_table)
```

We install and call propr package, then create the objects "phi", "rho" and "phs" using the functions phit(), perb(), and phis(), respectively. It returns an alert: Replacing 0 s in "count matrix" with 1. The propr package simply replaces 0 s with 1. The method of dealing zero values may be considered as a weakness of this package.

```
> library(propr)
> phi <- phit(abund_table_t, symmetrize = TRUE)
Alert: Replacing 0s in "count matrix" with 1.
> rho <- perb(abund_table_t, ivar = 0)
Alert: Replacing 0s in "count matrix" with 1.
> phs < phis(abund_table_t, ivar = 0)
Alert: Replacing 0s in "count matrix" with 1.
```

Returning the object "phi", "rho" or "phs" shows the summary of the four propr classes: counts, logratio, matrix and pairs.

```
> phi
@counts summary: 8 subjects by 248 features
@logratio summary: 8 subjects by 248 features
```

```
@matrix summary: 248 features by 248 features
@pairs summary: index with `[` method
```

Obtain the Original Count Matrix.

We can use head() function to either "phi", "rho" or "phs object to obtain count matrix formation or release these matrices directly by calling the objects.

```
> head(phi@counts)
             Tannerella Lactococcus Lactobacillus
5_15_dryST-28F       476         326            94
1_11_dryST-28F       549        2297           434
2_12_dryST-28F       578         548           719
3_13_dryST-28F       996        2378           322
             Lactobacillus::Lactococcus Parasutterella Helicobacter
5_15_dryST-28F                        1              1           89
1_11_dryST-28F                       25              1            1
2_12_dryST-28F                        5              4           13
3_13_dryST-28F                       17              2           24
```

Obtain the Log-Ratio Transformed Count Matrix.

We can call either of "phi", "rho" or "phs" object to obtain the log-ratio transformed matrix or review this matrix by the head() function.

```
> head(phi@logratio)
             Tannerella Lactococcus Lactobacillus
5_15_dryST-28F      5.810       5.431         4.188
1_11_dryST-28F      5.781       7.212         5.546
2_12_dryST-28F      5.790       5.737         6.009
3_13_dryST-28F      6.474       7.345         5.345
             Lactobacillus::Lactococcus Parasutterella Helicobacter
5_15_dryST-28F                   -0.3557        -0.3557       4.1330
1_11_dryST-28F                    2.6918        -0.5271      -0.5271
2_12_dryST-28F                    1.0402         0.8170       1.9957
3_13_dryST-28F                    2.4038         0.2637       2.7487
```

Obtain the Information About Pairs.

The following call releases the information about pairs.

```
> head(phi@pairs)
numeric(0)
```

Obtain the Proportionality Metrics.

The following call obtains and reviews the proportionality metric ϕ.

```
> head(phi@matrix)
                          Tannerella Lactococcus Lactobacillus
Tannerella                     0.000      6.8505       13.3980
Lactococcus                    6.850      0.0000        1.0599
Lactobacillus                 13.398      1.0599        0.0000
Lactobacillus::Lactococcus    18.035      0.6532·       0.9773
                          Lactobacillus::Lactococcus Parasutterella
Tannerella                                   18.0355          8.9163
Lactococcus                                   0.6532          1.9153
Lactobacillus                                 0.9773          0.7003
Lactobacillus::Lactococcus                    0.0000          1.2252
```

The following call obtains and reviews the proportionality metric ρ.

```
> head(rho@matrix)
                          Tannerella Lactococcus Lactobacillus
Tannerella                   1.00000      0.1975       -0.1451
Lactococcus                  0.19745      1.0000        0.5620
Lactobacillus               -0.14510      0.5620        1.0000
Lactobacillus::Lactococcus   0.07874      0.8115        0.6428
                          Lactobacillus::Lactococcus Parasutterella
Tannerella                                   0.07874         0.08694
Lactococcus                                  0.81150         0.11458
Lactobacillus                                0.64280         0.61507
Lactobacillus::Lactococcus                   1.00000         0.16756
```

The following call obtains and reviews the proportionality metric ϕ_s.

```
> head(phs@matrix)
                          Tannerella Lactococcus Lactobacillus
Tannerella                    0.0000      0.6702        1.3395
Lactococcus                   0.6702      0.0000        0.2804
Lactobacillus                 1.3395      0.2804        0.0000
Lactobacillus::Lactococcus    0.8540      0.1041        0.2174
                          Lactobacillus::Lactococcus Parasutterella
Tannerella                                   0.8540          0.8400
Lactococcus                                  0.1041          0.7944
Lactobacillus                                0.2174          0.2383
Lactobacillus::Lactococcus                   0.0000          0.7130
```

10.5.3.2   Identify Proportionally Abundant Taxa

Below we illustrate how to use the function perb() to identify proportionally abundant taxa step by step. The ϕ, ρ and ϕ_s metrics seek to identify those pairs of taxa that have a near constant ratio abundance across all samples in the given microbiome data sets. Given $\rho \in [-1, 1]$, its cutoff is easy to choose. Here, we perform proportionality analysis step by step using the function perb(). Reader can also try phit() and phs().

Step 1: Pre-filter to Remove Low Read Counts.

To minimize the number of lowly abundant taxa to be included in the final result, we subset the data table to include only those taxa with at least 10 counts in at least 5 samples.

```
> keep <- apply(abund_table_t, 2, function(x) sum(x >= 10) >= 5)
```

Step 2: Calculate Proportionality and Select the Highly Proportional Taxa.

The current version of the package lacks of hypothesis testing framework. Because the "highly proportion" has not been defined in literature, we arbitrarily select the "highly proportional" taxa with $\rho > 0.80$ for the purpose of illustration. By default, the propr package replaces all zero values with 1 when calculates proportionality.

```
> rho <- perb(abund_table_t, select = keep)
> best <- rho[">", 0.80]
> best
@counts summary: 8 subjects by 14 features
@logratio summary: 8 subjects by 14 features
@matrix summary: 14 features by 14 features
@pairs summary: 4 feature pairs
> best@pairs
[1]    18  92 108 123

> pirs_taxa<-row.names(abund_table[c(18,92,108,123),])
> pirs_taxa
[1] "Acholeplasma"        "Desulfotomaculum"
[3] "Blautia::Lactonifactor" "Ruminococcus::Blautia"
```

The results above showed that 14 abundant taxa are identified with 4 taxon pairs indexed with cutoff of $\rho > 0.80$. The 4 most compositionally associated taxa are *Acholeplasma*, *Desulfotomaculum*, *Blautia::Lactonifactor* and *Ruminococcus:: Blautia*.

Step 3: Release the Matrix with the Highly Proportional Taxa.

```
> taxa_best <- colnames(best@logratio)
> taxa_best
 [1] "Tannerella"          "Lactococcus"
 [3] "Lactobacillus"       "Lactobacillus::Lactococcus"
 [5] "Prevotella"          "Bacteroides"
 [7] "Eubacterium"         "Clostridium"
 [9] "Butyrivibrio"        "Alistipes"
[11] "Coprococcus"         "Parabacteroides"
[13] "Akkermansia"         "Turicibacter"
```

```
> head(best@matrix)
                             Tannerella Lactococcus Lactobacillus
Tannerella                      1.00000      0.1975       -0.1451
Lactococcus                     0.19745      1.0000        0.5620
Lactobacillus                  -0.14510      0.5620        1.0000
Lactobacillus::Lactococcus      0.07874      0.8115        0.6428
Prevotella                      0.54159      0.2666       -0.4314
Bacteroides                     0.43676      0.3317       -0.1135
                             Lactobacillus::Lactococcus Prevotella Bacteroides
Tannerella                                      0.07874     0.5416      0.4368
Lactococcus                                     0.81150     0.2666      0.3317
Lactobacillus                                   0.64280    -0.4314     -0.1135
Lactobacillus::Lactococcus                      1.00000     0.1422      0.2020
Prevotella                                      0.14218     1.0000      0.4889
Bacteroides                                     0.20205     0.4889      1.0000
                             Eubacterium Clostridium Butyrivibrio Alistipes
Tannerella                       0.24387     0.14110      0.13534   0.10694
Lactococcus                      0.23655    -0.09477      0.07611   0.08696
Lactobacillus                    0.10293    -0.19746     -0.07249   0.13124
Lactobacillus::Lactococcus       0.07585    -0.09046     -0.03532   0.25285
Prevotella                      -0.01065     0.15554      0.02341   0.03836
Bacteroides                      0.54784     0.61234      0.43019   0.52172
                             Coprococcus Parabacteroides Akkermansia
Tannerella                      0.063446          0.1318      0.3064
Lactococcus                    -0.035614         -0.1596      0.5975
Lactobacillus                  -0.036095         -0.6563      0.1382
Lactobacillus::Lactococcus     -0.042078         -0.3541      0.2978
Prevotella                      0.003815          0.4041      0.1970
Bacteroides                     0.577252          0.3865      0.2749
                             Turicibacter
Tannerella                        0.10257
Lactococcus                       0.12376
Lactobacillus                     0.01101
Lactobacillus::Lactococcus        0.15175
Prevotella                        0.22710
Bacteroides                       0.22721
```

10.5.3.3 Visualizing Proportionality

Three kinds of visualization can be done for better understanding proportionality in the data set: index-aware plots, index-naive plots, and down-stream plots.

Index-Aware Plots

Both functions plot() from the rlang package and dendrogram() from the ggdendro package are helpful for checking the indexed pairs. Here, we first use the plot() function to check the pairwise distribution of proportional pairs. It is useful to check whether the index cutoff has set too low or fine (Fig. 10.9).

```
> install packages("rlang")
> plot(best)
```

As an "index-aware" function, the plot() function only plots the 4 taxa pairs indexed with [. In above figure, the smear of straight diagonal lines shows that overall the 4 pairs are proportional: they all increases in log-ratio transformed

Fig. 10.9 Index-aware plot generated by the plot() function to check the pairwise distribution of proportional pairs

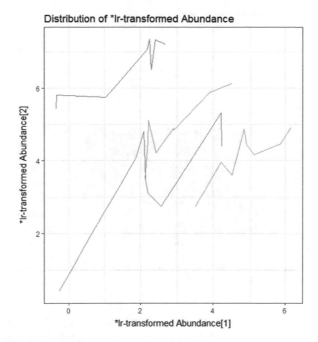

abundance. One line deviates considerably from the diagonal, so the index threshold maybe set low. However, the purpose here is just for illustration.

Next, we use the dendrogram() function to check how the indexed pairs cluster. The indexed pairs of taxa are clustered based on a hierarchical clustering of the proportionality matrix. In the propr package, the dissimilarity measure is defined as as.dist(1-abs(rho@matrix)). Only the indexed taxa pairs with [. method are plotted. If the used cutoff could not index any pairs, then the plot is generated using all taxon pairs (Fig. 10.10).

```
> install.packages('ggdendro')
> dendrogram(best)
Alert: Generating plot using indexed feature pairs.
'dendrogram' with 2 branches and 7 members total, at height 0.9647
```

Index-Naive Plots

Several index-naive plots, which incorporate all taxa in the propr object, can be conducted on proportionality analysis. They are the pca(), snapshot(), prism(), bokeh(), bucket() functions. Here, we illustrate two of them: the pca(), bucket(). Readers can try others by themselves.

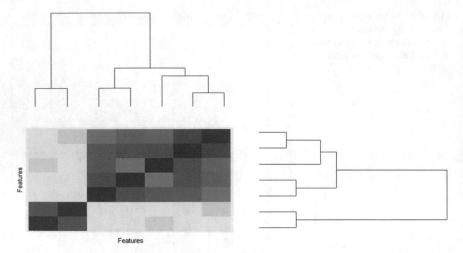

Fig. 10.10 Index-aware plot generated by the dendrogram() function to inspect how the indexed pairs cluster

First, we illustrate index-naive plots using the pca() function. Index-naive plots incorporate all taxa in the propr object. We use the simplify() function to keep those taxa that belong to an indexed taxa pair.

```
> best <- simplify(best)
```

In Sect. 10.3, we incorporate PCA to the log-ratio transformed data to generate the compositional Biplot. Same idea can be applied here. We can incorporate PCA to the indexed taxa pair of log-ratio transformed data. For using group membership to color the sample IDs, we create a group variable as we previously did (Fig. 10.11).

```
> grouping<-data.frame(row.names=rownames(abund_table_t),t(as.data.
frame(strsplit(rownames(abund_table_t),"_"))))
> grouping$Group <- with(grouping,ifelse(as.factor(X2)%in% c
(11,12,13,14,15),c("Vdr-/-"), c("WT")))

> pca(best, group = grouping$Group)
```

Next, we use the bucket() function to visualize the co-cluster of proportional taxa. The key features of bucket() function include: (1) it is "index-naive", plots all in the @matrix slot of the propr object; (2) identifies the taxa pairs where both constituents co-cluster (with the total number of clusters toggled by k); and (3) returns a vector of cluster memberships for all taxa in the propr object. The bucket() function is used to plot an estimation of the degree to which a taxon pair

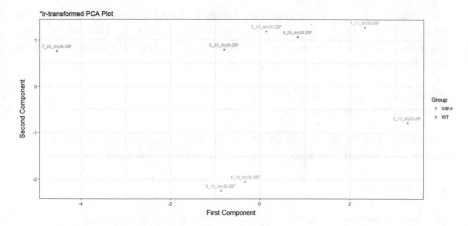

Fig. 10.11 Visualizing the samples based on log-ratio transformed data by PCA. This figure shows all samples projected across the first two components. This plot colors samples based on the genotype groups

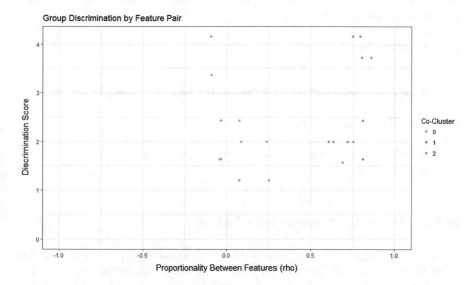

Fig. 10.12 Co-cluster analysis using the bucket() function

differentiates the genotype groups versus the proportionality between that pair. We specify the total number of clusters k = 2 as a try (Fig. 10.12).

```
> clusts <- bucket(best, group = grouping$Group, k = 2)
```

Reader can try prism() and bokeh() functions to visualize the co-clustering of proportional taxa. Both two share above key features with the bucket() function.

The differences are: the prism() plots the variance of the log-ratio (VLR) against the variances of log sum (VLS) on the log-ratio transformed taxa. The bokeh() plots pairs across the individual variances of the constituent log-ratio transformed taxa. The codes are given below:

```
> clusts <- prism(best, k = 2)
> clusts <- bokeh(best, k = 2)
```

Reader may also try the function snapshot() to visualize the density of the log-ratio transformed data across samples. The code is given below:

```
> snapshot(best)
```

Co-cluster analysis can help us to select the highly proportional module for down-stream analysis.

Down-Stream Plots
The following R codes extract co-cluster 2 from the propr object using the subset method and use the pca() function to check how well this cluster differentiates the two genotype groups (Fig. 10.13).

```
> sub <- subset(best, select = (clusts == 2))
> pca(sub, group = grouping$Group)
```

The following codes extract the names of the taxa that belong to this cluster.

```
> taxa <- colnames(sub@logratio)
> taxa
[1] "Eubacterium"  "Clostridium"  "Butyrivibrio" "Alistipes"
"Coprococcus"
```

10.5.3.4   Differential Proportionality Analysis

In this subsection, we will show how to perform differential proportionality analysis using the propd method. The propd() function estimates differential proportionality by calculating for all pairs of taxa and returns a propd object as a result. The syntax is given by:

$$propd(counts, group, alpha = NA, p = 1000)$$

where:

counts   a matrix of samples (as rows) and taxa (as columns);
group   experiment groups or conditions to label n-samples belong to;
alpha   an optional argument to trigger and guide transformation;

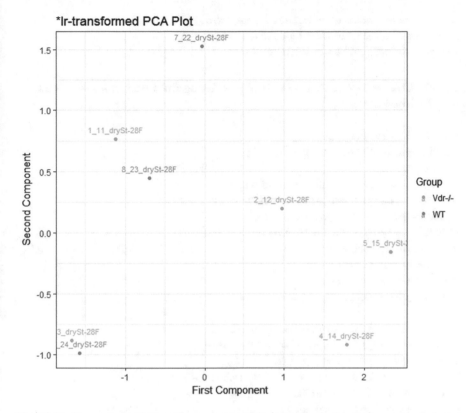

Fig. 10.13 Down-stream PCA with co-cluster analysis to check the performance of cluster differentiation between groups

p   the total number of permutations used to estimate the false discovery rate (FDR).

The resultant propd object contains both θ_d (by default) and θ_e metrics. Once a θ is active, we can conduct permutation testing (i.e., FDR estimation) and visualize log-ratio abundance. We illustrate differential proportionality analysis step by step as below.

Step 1: Estimate the Disjointed Proportionality and Emergent Proportionality Using the Function propd().

```
> library(propr)
> pd <- propd(abund_table_t, grouping$Group, alpha = NA, p = 1000)
Alert: Replacing 0s in "count matrix" with 1.
Alert: Replacing NaN theta values with 1.
Alert: Tabulating the presence of 0 counts.
```

Alert: Use 'setActive' to select a theta type.

Alert: Use 'updateCutoffs' to calculate FDR.

Alert: Use 'updateF' to calculate F-stat.

Step 2: Choose to Activate Which Metric Using the Functions setDisjointed() and setEmergent().

> theta_d <- setDisjointed(pd)

Alert: Update FDR or F-stat manually.

> theta_d

Not weighted and not alpha-transformed

@counts summary: 8 subjects by 248 features

@group summary: 2 unique groups (5 x 3)

@theta summary: 30628 feature pairs (theta_d)

@fdr summary: 1000 iterations

See ?propd for object methods

> theta_e <- setEmergent(pd)

Alert: Update FDR or F-stat manually.

> theta_e

Not weighted and not alpha-transformed

@counts summary: 8 subjects by 248 features

@group summary: 2 unique groups (5 x 3)

@theta summary: 30628 feature pairs (theta_e)

@fdr summary: 1000 iterations

See ?propd for object methods

Step 3: Estimate FDR Using the Function updateCutoffs().

```
> theta_d <- updateCutoffs(theta_d, cutoff = seq(0.05, 0.95,0.3))
|------------(25%)----------(50%)----------(75%)----------|
> theta_d
Not weighted and not alpha-transformed
@counts summary: 8 subjects by 248 features
@group summary: 2 unique groups ( 5 x 3 )
@theta summary: 30628 feature pairs ( theta_d )
@fdr summary: 1000 iterations
   cutoff randcounts truecounts      FDR
1   0.05      5.861          0      Inf
2   0.35    150.004         54   2.7779
3   0.65   1404.046       2117   0.6632
4   0.95  11927.995      14220   0.8388
See ?propd for object methods
```

```
> theta_e <- updateCutoffs(theta_e, cutoff = seq(0.05, 0.95,0.3))
|-----------(25%)----------(50%)----------(75%)----------|
> theta_e
Not weighted and not alpha-transformed
@counts summary: 8 subjects by 248 features
@group summary: 2 unique groups ( 5 x 3 )
@theta summary: 30628 feature pairs ( theta_e )
@fdr summary: 1000 iterations
   cutoff randcounts truecounts      FDR
1    0.05      388.7         253 1.5365
2    0.35    10960.1       10681 1.0261
3    0.65    16449.1       16152 1.0184
4    0.95    16916.9       16923 0.9996
See ?propd for object methods
```

Next, we illustrate how to calculate an F-statistic from θ_d and how to moderate the F-statistic using voom() function from the limma package.

Step 4: Calculate an F-statistic from θ_d.
The relationship between θ_d and the F-statistic is defined by:

$$F = (n - 2)\frac{1 - \theta_d}{\theta_d} \qquad (10.18)$$

In above calculation of differential proportionality, we specify alpha = NA in the propd() function without using the α transformation. Actually, we can calculate θ based on either using a weighted VLR or together a weighted with α-transformed approximation of the VLR. This defines four variant states of theta: weighted = FALSE, weighted = TRUE, weighted = FALSE, alpha = a positive value, and weighted = TRUE, alpha = a positive value.

Above, we use the updateCutoffs()function to calculate a FDR based on θ_d and θ_e. Actually, it applies to all types and variant states. In the following R codes, we specify pd_nn, pd_wn, pd_na, and pd_wa for weighted = FALSE & no alpha, weighted = TRUE & no alpha, weighted = FALSE & alpha = 0.05, and weighted = TRUE & alpha = 0.05, respectively.

```
> pd_nn <- propd(abund_table_t, grouping$Group, weighted = FALSE)
> pd_wn <- propd(abund_table_t, grouping$Group, weighted = TRUE)
> pd_na <- propd(abund_table_t, grouping$Group, weighted = FALSE,
alpha = 0.05)
> pd_wa <- propd(abund_table_t, grouping$Group, weighted = TRUE,
alpha = 0.05)
```

We can use the update() function to calculate the F-statistic from θ_d, which appends an "Fstat" column to the @theta slot.

```
> pd_nn<-updateF(pd_nn,moderated = FALSE)
> options(digits=4)
```

```
> head(pd_nn@theta$Fstat)
[1]  4.1628 13.4117 1.8338 3.3481 1.0797 0.1475

> pd_wa<-updateF(pd_wa,moderated = FALSE)
> options(digits=4)
> head(pd_wa@theta$Fstat)
[1]  3.0474 16.1341 2.0934 2.2976 0.5021 0.7706
```

Step 5: Moderate the *F*-statistic Using voom() Function from the Limma Package.

The *F*-statistic is not moderated. By borrowing from the limma package, we can calculate a moderated *F*-statistic for differential proportionality analysis, which is done by fitting the data to an empirical Bayes model through the eBayes() function with underlying mean-variance modeling through the voom() function.

The voom() function returns a matrix of the per-taxon weights for each sample. The weights of a taxon ratio can be calculated as the element-wise product of the per-taxon weights. The moderation and modeling are done for gene ratios. By applying the per-taxon moderation to ratios, a suitable reference must be selected and by default, the software uses the geometric mean of all taxa as the reference for each i-th composition (i.e., sample vector). By using this reference, the normalization becomes the corresponding log-ratio transformation (i.e., the clr transformation in the default case).

By changing the argument moderated = TRUE in the updateF() function, we calculate the moderated *F*-statistic:

```
> pd_nn<-updateF(pd_nn,moderated = TRUE, ivar = "clr")
> pd_wn<-updateF(pd_wn,moderated = TRUE, ivar = "clr")
> pd_na<-updateF(pd_na,moderated = TRUE, ivar = "clr")
> pd_wa<-updateF(pd_wa,moderated = TRUE, ivar = "clr")
```

Above the argument ivar = "clr" defines the clr transformation to use as the reference. We can check the appended "Fstat" and "theta_mod" column in the @theta slot.

```
> head(pd_nn@theta$Fstat)
[1] 0.8951 2.6591 0.6399 2.1382 0.8354 0.1123
> head(pd_nn@theta$theta_mod)
[1] 0.8702 0.6929 0.9036 0.7373 0.8778 0.9816
> head(pd_wa@theta$Fstat)
[1]  2.9061 15.8906 1.9659 2.0046 0.3025 0.6381
> head(pd_wa@theta$theta_mod)
[1] 0 0 0 0 0 0
```

10.6 Summary and Discussion

In this chapter, we introduced and illustrated the compositional analysis of microbiome data. The approach of compositional analysis with the development of the new statistical methods and accompanying packages provides a means to advance microbiome research. However, compositional analysis of microbiome data in general still has several main challenges as future research (Lovell et al. 2015; Quinn et al. 2017), including:

(1) Compositional analysis treats the really discrete count data as continuous (Bacon-Shone 2008) and relative. However, count data is not purely relative (Lovell, Pawlowsky-Glahn et al. 2015).
(2) Compositional analysis fails in the presence of zero values. The zero problem directly affects the application of the log-ratio transformations to modern genomics data sets because it is undefined to divide the zero (Zuur et al. 2009). Given currently there is no simple general remedy for the treatment of zeroes (Martín-Fernández et al. 2011), ALDEX package uses the cmultRepl() function to replace 0 values, while propr package by default replaces all zero values with 1. The appropriateness of this replacement is not guaranteed. We need carefully interpret the analysis results that contain zero values.
(3) Sparsity with excess zeros poses a unique challenge to microbiome data analysis. Compositional analysis cannot solve sparsity problem by replacing zero values with small non-zero counts, rather than makes the sparsity problem even more complicated.
(4) Biologically true compositional microbiome data do not exist. We treat microbiome data set as compositional when comparing to the features of compositional data. However, the 'compositional' in microbiome data is not in the sense as in the other fields, such as geology, petrology, sedimentology, and geochemistry.

Specifically, the main challenges of proportionality analysis include (1) it still lacks a hypothesis-testing framework, and (2) the values of ϕ and ρ are unstable in the setting of missing taxon data, unlike the VLR. More research are needed to solve these problems.

References

Aitchison, J. 1981. A new approach to null correlations of proportions. *Mathematical Geology* 13 (2): 175–189.

Aitchison, J. 1982. The statistical analysis of compositional data (with discussion). *Journal of the Royal Statistical Society, Series B (Statistical Methodology)* 44 (2): 139–177.

Aitchison, J. 1983. Principal component analysis of compositional data. *Biometrika* 70 (1): 57–65.

Aitchison, J. 1984. Reducing the dimensionality of compositional data sets. *Journal of the International Association for Mathematical Geology* 16 (6): 617–635.

Aitchison, J. 1986. *The statistical analysis of compositional data*. London: Chapman and Hall Ltd. Reprinted in 2003 with additional material by The Blackburn Press.

Aitchison, J. 1999. *A concise guide to compositional data analysis*. Posted by Vincent Granville on August 5, 2013 at 9:41am in New Books and Journals.

Aitchison, J. 2003. A concise guide to compositional data analysis. In *2nd Compositional Data Analysis Workshop*. Girona, Italy.

Aitchison, J., and J.A.C. Brown. 1969. The lognormal distribution with special reference to its uses in econometrics. Cambridge, UK: Cambridge University Press.

Aitchison, J., and J.J. Egozcue. 2005. Compositional data analysis: Where are we and where should we be heading? *Mathematical Geology* 37 (7): 829–850.

Aitchison, J., and M. Greenacre. 2002. Biplots of compositional data. *Journal of the Royal Statistical Society: Series C (Applied Statistics)* 51 (4): 375–392.

Aitchison, J., and J. Kay. 2003. Possible solution of some essential zero problems in compositional data analysis. In *Proceedings of CoDaWork'03, The 1st Compositional Data Analysis Workshop*. Girona, Spain: University of Girona. http://ima.ud.es/Activitats/CoDaWork03/.

Aitchison, J., C. Barceló-Vidal, et al. 2000. Logratio analysis and compositional distance. *Mathematical Geology* 32 (3): 271–275.

Altman, D.G., and J.M. Bland. 1983. Measurement in medicine: The analysis of method comparison studies. *Journal of the Royal Statistical Society. Series D (The Statistician)* 32 (3): 307–317.

Arumugam, M., J. Raes, et al. 2011. Enterotypes of the human gut microbiome. *Nature* 473 (7346): 174–180.

Bacon-Shone, J. 2003. Modelling structural zeros in compositional data. In *Proceedings of CoDaWork'03, The 1st Compositional Data Analysis Workshop*. Girona, Spain: University of Girona. http://ima.ud.es/Activitats/CoDaWork03/.

Bacon-Shone, J. 2008. Discrete and continuous compositions. In *Proceedings of CODAWORK'08, The 3rd Compositional Data Analysis Workshop*, ed. J. Daunis-i Estadella and J. Martín-Fernández. Girona: University of Girona.

Bacon-Shone, J. 2011. A short history of compositional data analysis. In *Compositional data analysis: Theory and applications*, ed. V. Pawlowsky-Glahn and A. Buccianti. Chichester, UK: Wiley.

Barceló-Vidal, C., J.A. Martín-Fernández, et al. 2001. Mathematical foundations of compositional data analysis. In *Proceedings of IAMG*.

Barnett, V. 1981. *Interpreting multivariate data*. New York: Wiley.

Bland, J.M., and D.G. Altman. 1999. Measuring agreement in method comparison studies. *Statistical Methods in Medical Research* 8 (2): 135–160.

Butte, A.J., and I.S. Kohane. 2000. Mutual information relevance networks: Functional genomic clustering using pairwise entropy measurements. In *Pacific Symposium on Biocomputing*, 418–429.

Cameron, A.C., and P.K. Trivedi. 1998. *Regression analysis of count data*. Cambridge, UK: Cambridge University Press.

Chen, E.Z., and H. Li. 2016. A two-part mixed-effects model for analyzing longitudinal microbiome compositional data. *Bioinformatics* 32 (17): 2611–2617.

Eaton, M.L. 1983. *Multivariate statistics. A vector space approach*, 512. New York: Wiley.

Egozcue, J.J. 2009. Reply to "On the Harker variation diagrams; …" by J.A. Cortés. *Mathematical Geosciences* 41 (7): 829–834.

Egozcue, J.J., and V. Pawlowsky-Glahn. 2005. Groups of parts and their balances in compositional data analysis. *Mathematical Geology* 37 (7): 795–828.

Egozcue, J.J., and V. Pawlowsky-Glahn. 2011. Basic concepts and procedures. In *Compositional data analysis: Theory and applications*, ed. V. Pawlowsky-Glahn and A. Buccianti. Chichester, UK: Wiley.

Egozcue, J.J., V. Pawlowsky-Glahn, et al. 2003. Isometric logratio transformations for compositional data analysis. *Mathematical Geology* 35 (3): 279–300.

Eisen, M.B., P.T. Spellman, et al. 1998. Cluster analysis and display of genome-wide expression patterns. *Proceedings of the National Academy of Sciences of the United States of America* 95 (25): 14863–14868.

Erb, I., and C. Notredame. 2016. How should we measure proportionality on relative gene expression data? *Theory in Biosciences* 135: 21–36.

Erb, I., T. Quinn, et al. 2017. Differential proportionality—A normalization-free approach to differential gene expression. bioRxiv.

Fernandes, A.D., J.M. Macklaim, et al. 2013. ANOVA-like differential expression (ALDEx) analysis for mixed population RNA-seq. *PLoS ONE* 8 (7): e67019.

Fernandes, A.D., J.N.S. Reid, et al. 2014. Unifying the analysis of high-throughput sequencing datasets: Characterizing RNA-seq, 16S rRNA gene sequencing and selective growth experiments by compositional data analysis. *Microbiome* 2 (1): 15.

Filzmoser, P., K. Hron, et al. 2012. Interpretation of multivariate outliers for compositional data. *Computers & Geosciences* 39: 77–85.

Finucane, M.M., T.J. Sharpton, et al. 2014. A taxonomic signature of obesity in the microbiome? Getting to the guts of the matter. *PLoS ONE* 9 (1): e84689.

Friedman, J., and E.J. Alm. 2012a. Inferring correlation networks from genomic survey data. *PLoS Computational Biology* 8 (9): 20.

Friedman, J., and E.J. Alm. 2012b. Inferring correlation networks from genomic survey data. *PLoS Computational Biology* 8 (9): e1002687.

Gabriel, K.R. 1971. The biplot graphic display of matrices with application to principal component analysis. *Biometrika* 58 (3): 453–467.

Gabriel, K.R. 1981. Biplot display of multivariate matrices for inspection of data and diagnosis. In *Interpreting multivariate data*, ed. V. Barnett. London: Wiley.

Gabriel, K.R., and C.L. Odoroff. 1990. Biplots in biomedical research. *Statistics in Medicine* 9 (5): 469–485.

Galton, F. 1879. The geometric mean, in vital and social statistics. *Proceedings of the Royal Society of London* 29: 365–366.

Gevers, D., S. Kugathasan, et al. 2014. The treatment-naïve microbiome in new-onset Crohn's disease. *Cell Host & Microbe* 15 (3): 382–392.

Gloor, G.B., and G. Reid. 2016. Compositional analysis: A valid approach to analyze microbiome high-throughput sequencing data. *Canadian Journal of Microbiology* 62 (8): 692–703.

Gloor, G.B., J.R. Wu, et al. 2016. It's all relative: Analyzing microbiome data as compositions. *Annals of Epidemiology* 26 (5): 322–329.

Gotelli, N.J. 2008. *A primer of ecology*. Sunderland, MA: Sinauer Associates Inc.

Greenacre, M.J. 1993. Biplots in correspondence analysis. *Journal of Applied Statistics* 20 (2): 251–269.

Hron, K., M. Templ, et al. 2010. Exploratory compositional data analysis using the R-package robCompositions. In *Proceedings 9th International Conference on Computer Data Analysis and Modeling*, vol. 1, ed. S. Aivazian, P. Filzmoser, and Y. Kharin, 179–186. Minsk: Belarusian State University.

Knights, D., E.K. Costello, et al. 2011. Supervised classification of human microbiota. *FEMS Microbiology Reviews* 35 (2): 343–359.

Kroonenberg, P.M. 2008. *Applied multiway data analysis*. Hoboken, NJ: Wiley.

Kurtz, Z.D., C.L. Müller, et al. 2015. Sparse and compositionally robust inference of microbial ecological networks. *PLoS Computational Biology* 11 (5): e1004226.

Law, C.W., Y. Chen, et al. 2014. Voom: Precision weights unlock linear model analysis tools for RNA-seq read counts. *Genome Biology* 15 (2): R29.

Ley, R.E., F. Bäckhed, et al. 2005. Obesity alters gut microbial ecology. *Proceedings of the National Academy of Sciences of the United States of America* 102 (31): 11070–11075.

Ley, R.E., P.J. Turnbaugh, et al. 2006. Microbial ecology: Human gut microbes associated with obesity. *Nature* 444 (7122): 1022–1023.

Li, H. 2015. Microbiome, metagenomics, and high-dimensional compositional data analysis. *Annual Review of Statistics and Its Application* 2: 73–94.

López-Kleine, L., L. Leal, et al. 2013. Biostatistical approaches for the reconstruction of gene co-expression networks based on transcriptomic data. *Briefings in Functional Genomics* 12 (5): 457–467.

Lovell, D., W. Müller, et al. 2011. Proportions, percentages, PPM: Do the molecular biosciences treat compositional data right? In *Compositional Data Anal: Theory and Applications*, ed. V. Pawlowsky-Glahn and A. Buccianti, 191–207. Chichester, UK: Wiley.

Lovell, D., V. Pawlowsky-Glahn, et al. 2015. Proportionality: A valid alternative to correlation for relative data. *PLoS Computational Biology* 11 (3): e1004075.

Mandal, S., W. Van Treuren, et al. 2015. Analysis of composition of microbiomes: A novel method for studying microbial composition. *Microbial Ecology in Health and Disease* 26: 27663.

Martin Bland, J., and D. Altman. 1986. Statistical methods for assessing agreement between two methods of clinical measurement. *The Lancet* 327 (8476): 307–310.

Martín-Fernández, J.A., C. Barceló-Vidal, et al. 2003. Dealing with zeros and missing values in compositional data sets using nonparametric imputation. *Mathematical Geology* 35 (3): 253–278.

Martín-Fernández, J.A., J. Palarea-Albaladejo, et al. 2011. Dealing with zeros. In *Compositional data analysis*, ed. V. Pawlowsky-Glahn and A. Buccianti, 43–58. Chichester, UK: Wiley.

Martín-Fernández, J.A., K. Hron, et al. 2012. Model-based replacement of rounded zeros in compositional data: Classical and robust approaches. *Computational Statistics & Data Analysis* 56: 2688–2704.

Martín-Fernández, J.-A., K. Hron, et al. 2015. Bayesian-multiplicative treatment of count zeros in compositional data sets. *Statistical Modelling* 15 (2): 134–158.

Mateu-Figueras, G., and V. Pawlowsky-Glahn. 2008. A critical approach to probability laws in geochemistry. *Mathematical Geosciences* 40 (5): 489–502.

Mateu-Figueras, G., V. Pawlowsky-Glahn, et al. 2011. The principle of working on coordinates. In *Compositional data analysis: Theory and applications*, ed. V. Pawlowsky-Glahn and A. Buccianti. Chichester, UK: Wiley.

McAlister, D. 1879. The law of the geometric mean. *Proceedings of the Royal Society of London* 29: 367–376.

McCullagh, P., and J.A. Nelder. 1989. *Generalized linear models*. Boca Raton, FL: Chapman and Hall/CRC.

Obayashi, T., and K. Kinoshita. 2011. COXPRESdb: A database to compare gene coexpression in seven model animals. *Nucleic Acids Research* 39 (Suppl 1): D1016–D1022.

Palarea-Albaladejo, J., and J.A. Martín-Fernández. 2008. A modified EM alr-algorithm for replacing rounded zeros in compositional data sets. *Computers & Geosciences* 34 (8): 902–917.

Palarea-Albaladejo, J., and J.A. Martín-Fernández. 2015. zCompositionsd—R package for multivariate imputation of left-censored data under a compositional approach. *Chemometrics and Intelligent Laboratory Systems* 143: 85–96.

Palarea-Albaladejo, J., J.A. Martín-Fernández, et al. 2007. A parametric approach for dealing with compositional rounded zeros. *Mathematical Geology* 39 (7): 625–645.

Pawlowsky-Glahn, V., and A. Buccianti. 2011. *Compositional data analysis: Theory and applications*. Chichester, UK: Wiley.

Pawlowsky-Glahn, V., J.J. Egozcue, et al. 2015. *Modeling and analysis of compositional data*. UK: Wiley.

Pearson, K. 1897. Mathematical contributions to the theory of evolution. On a form of spurious correlation which may arise when indices are used in the measurement of organs. *Proceedings of the Royal Society of London* LX: 489–502.

Quinn, T., M.F. Richardson, et al. 2017. Propr: An R-package for identifying proportionally abundant features using compositional data analysis. bioRxiv.

Shu, M., Y. Wang, et al. 2013. Fermentation of propionibacterium acnes, a commensal bacterium in the human skin microbiome, as skin probiotics against methicillin-resistant staphylococcus aureus. *PLoS ONE* 8 (2): e55380.

Smyth, G.K. 2004. Linear models and empirical Bayes methods for assessing differential expression in microarray experiments. *Statistical Applications in Genetics and Molecular Biology* 3 (1): 1–25.

Smyth, G.K. 2005. Limma: Linear models for microarray data. In *Bioinformatics and computational biology solutions using R and bioconductor*, ed. R. Gentleman, V. Carey, S. Dudoit, and W.H.R. Irizarry. New York: Springer.

Sweeney, T.E., and J.M. Morton. 2013. The human gut microbiome: A review of the effect of obesity and surgically induced weight loss. *JAMA Surgery* 148 (6): 563–569.

Sze, M.A., and P.D. Schloss. 2016. Looking for a signal in the noise: Revisiting obesity and the microbiome. *MBio* 7 (4): e01018–e01016.

Templ, M., K. Hron, et al. 2011. RobCompositions: An R-package for robust statistical analysis of compositional data. In *Compositional data analysis: Theory and applications*, ed. V. Pawlowsky-Glahn and A. Buccianti, 341–355. Chichester, UK: Wiley. https://doi.org/10.1002/9781119976462.ch25.

The Human Microbiome Project Consortium. 2012. Structure, function and diversity of the healthy human microbiome. *Nature* 486 (7402): 207–214.

Tsilimigras, M.C.B., and A.A. Fodor. 2016. Compositional data analysis of the microbiome: Fundamentals, tools, and challenges. *Annals of Epidemiology* 26 (5): 330–335.

Turnbaugh, P.J., R.E. Ley, et al. 2006. An obesity-associated gut microbiome with increased capacity for energy harvest. *Nature* 444 (7122): 1027–1031.

Turnbaugh, P.J., M. Hamady, et al. 2009. A core gut microbiome in obese and lean twins. *Nature* 457 (7228): 480–484.

van den Boogaart, K.G., and R. Tolosana-Delgado. 2008. "Compositions": A unified R package to analyze compositional data. *Computers & Geosciences* 34 (4): 320–338.

van den Boogaart, K.G., and R. Tolosana-Delgado. 2013. *Analyzing compositional data with R.* Berlin, Heidelberg: Springer.

van den Boogaart, K.G., R. Tolosana, et al. 2014. "Compositions: Compositional Data Analysis. R package version 1.40–1. http://CRAN.R-project.org/package=compositions.

Walters, W.A., Z. Xu, et al. 2014. Meta-analyses of human gut microbes associated with obesity and IBD. *FEBS Letters* 588 (22): 4223–4233.

Weiss, S.J., Z. Xu, et al. 2015. Effects of library size variance, sparsity, and compositionality on the analysis of microbiome data. *PeerJ Preprints* 3: e1157v1151.

Zhang, B., and S. Horvath. 2005. A general framework for weighted gene co-expression network analysis. *Statistical Applications in Genetics and Molecular Biology* 4: 12.

Zuur, A.F., E.N. Ieno, et al. 2009. *Mixed effects models and extensions in ecology with R.* New York, NY: Springer Science & Business Media, LLC.

Chapter 11
Modeling Over-Dispersed Microbiome Data

In Chap. 10, we treated microbiome abundance data as compositional. When doing so, we treated the "really discrete count data" as continuous (Bacon-Shone 2008). However, count data is not purely relative—the count pair (1, 2) carries different information than counts of (1000, 2000) even though the relative amounts of the two components are the same. Furthermore, simulation studies suggest that count models give more statistical power to detect differential expression than approximate normal models (Robinson and Oshlack 2010). Thus, the high-throughput sequencing datasets were advised to be treated as count data (Kuczynski et al. 2011; Anders et al. 2013); and the methods based on count distributions (e.g., logistic regression and other generalized linear models) or correspondence analysis (Greenacre 2011) were often used in the literature (Lovell et al. 2015).

In this chapter, we will describe Poisson, Negative Binomial (NB) models and the descriptive example in Sect. 11.1. In Sect. 11.2, we will review the methods for estimating dispersion and hypothesis testing in package edgeR, and in Sect. 11.3, we will discuss the associated implementation in edgeR. In Sect. 11.4, we will introduce the methods for estimating dispersion and hypothesis testing in package DESeq and DESeq2 and its implementation in DESeq2 in Sect. 11.5. Section 11.6 is summary and discussion.

11.1 Count-Based Differential Abundance Analysis of Microbiome Data

In microbiome study, after the composition of the microbiome is estimated at a given taxonomic level, researchers are often interested in identifying the taxa that show differential abundance between two or more groups. In the simplest case, the aim is to compare taxa differential abundance between two conditions, e.g., treated versus untreated or mutant versus wild type.

© Springer Nature Singapore Pte Ltd. 2018
Y. Xia et al., *Statistical Analysis of Microbiome Data with R*,
ICSA Book Series in Statistics, https://doi.org/10.1007/978-981-13-1534-3_11

This problem is similar with differential expression analysis for RNA-seq data (Li 2015). In RNA-Sequencing differential expression analysis, an initial and fundamental goal or task of data analysis is to differentiate gene expression, based on sequence count data between conditions. It is to determine whether there is evidence that sequence read counts for a gene are significantly different across experimental conditions. Like differentially expressed genes, a species/OTU is considered differentially abundant if its mean proportion is significantly different between two or more sample classes in the experimental design. DNA sequencing-based microbiome investigations not only have same questions to ask, but also use the same sequencing machines and represent the processed sequence data in the same manner as RNA-Seq analysis, a feature-by-sample contingency table where the features are OTUs instead of genes. Thus, the statistical tools that were originally developed for differential analysis of RNAseq data, such as the packages edgeR (Robinson et al. 2010) and DESeq, DESeq2 (Anders and Huber 2010; Love et al. 2014) were suggested for directly use to identify differentially abundant OTUs (McMurdie and Holmes 2014). In this Chapter, we adopt the methods and models originally used in RNA-Seq and other count data to analyze microbiome count data.

11.1.1   Biological and Technical Variations

Biological and technical variations are the two sources of variation or noise that may affect the analysis results in metagenomic analysis (including shotgun and 16S rRNA gene sequences) using DNA- or RNA-based profiling methods. Biological variation is intrinsic to all organisms. In contrast, technical variation is the uncertainty with which the abundance of each gene in each sample is estimated by the sequencing technology.

The design of a DNA- or RNA-based sequencing experiment can be considered as having three layers from top (biological replicate), to middle(library preparation and sample storage) and to bottom(sequence, samples/replicates). Many sources of variation can be partitioned along these three layers. But the two main sources of variation are biological variation and technical variation. Biological variation involves in the top layer, consisting of the experimental units. It occurs within the same specimen or within an individual over time and may be influenced by genetic or environmental factors, as well as by whether the samples are pooled or individual. Technical variation or shot noise is produced in the middle layer because various ligations of adaptors and PCR amplifications involves during the generation of libraries of cDNA fragments. It measures the variability in a sample subject, e.g., library preparation and sample storage. Except biological and technical variations, there still exists the third source of variation at the bottom layer, including other technology-specific effects, e.g., lane and flow cell effects. These technology-specific effects are beyond the library preparation effect. Among these sources of variation, biological effect is far larger than other effects, and library preparation effect is second largest, flow cell effect is third, while lane effect is smallest.

Generally, researchers repeatedly perform biological and technical replicates in each experiment to mitigate the effect of biological and technical variations.

Biological replicates refer to different biological samples. A biological replicate is where we perform the same test on multiple samples using the same material (e.g., same type of cells, tissue, et al.). Biological replicates are used to test the (biological) variations between samples within group, thus providing information that is necessary to make inferences between groups, and to generalize conclusions. A technical replicate refers to when we test the same sample multiple times or places. Its aim is to test the variation in the testing protocol itself. A typical example of technical replicate is the test of 21 representative DNA extraction protocols on the same fecal samples (Costea et al. 2017).

Technical variation in metagenomic analysis must be minimized to confidently assess the contributions of microbiota to human health (Costea et al. 2017). Using standards in sample processing may be helpful. However, to account for biological variation, we typically need a suitable statistical model. The count models have the advantage for separating biological from technical variation (Robinson and Smyth 2007, 2008).

11.1.2 Poisson Model

Application of Poisson Model in High-Throughput Sequencing Data
The high-throughput sequencing technologies measure gene expression by generating short reads or sequence tags. To evaluate differential expression (or abundance) between conditions, read counts are summarized at the genomic level of interest (e.g., genes or exons) or the taxonomic rank (e.g., genus, species/ OTU).

In high-throughput sequencing experiments, we can consider a DNA sample as a population of cDNA fragments, and consider each genomic feature (in the case of 16s RNA-sequencing, taxon or OTU) as a very large pool of DNA fragments for which the population size is to be estimated. Thus, we can think sequencing a DNA sample as random sampling (repeated draws) of each of these cDNA fragments, with the aim of estimating the relative abundance of each species in the population (McCarthy et al. 2012).

If each cDNA fragment has the same chance of being selected for sequencing, and the fragments are selected independently, then the number of read counts for a given genomic feature or taxon (OTU) should follow a Poisson distribution.

Poisson model is the most popular regression model for count data. It assumes that each observed count Y_i is sampled from a Poisson distribution with the conditional mean μ_i given a vector of covariates/predictors X_i for each i th subject. The Poisson distribution, derived based on modeling the number of independent events from a memory-less Poisson process with a constant event rate, has the following density function:

$$P(Y_i = y | X_i) = \frac{\exp(-\mu_i)\mu_i^y}{y_i!}, \tag{11.1}$$

where Y_i is the number of read counts and $\mu_i = \exp(X_i^T \beta)$ is a real number which expects from cDNA fragments. We briefly derive it as below.

Consider Y_i as a random variable. Suppose the proportion of cDNA fragments arising from the genomic feature or taxon (OTU) i is p then we can derive the probability function of Y_i. Assume that the total number of sequenced reads is n. We are interested in the probability that Y_i takes a particular value y. If there are y aligned reads to feature i (successes), then there must be $n - y$ not aligned reads to feature i (failures). Given y successes and $n - y$ failures, each outcome has the individual probability $p^y(1 - p)^{n-y}$. Since there are total $\binom{n}{y}$ possible ways of arranging y successes in n trials, thus the total probability of y successes in n independent trials is:

$$P(Y_i = y) = \binom{n}{y} p^y (1 - p)^{n-y}, \quad \text{for } y = 0, 1, 2, \ldots, n \tag{11.2}$$

This is the binomial distribution with parameters n and p.

Now, suppose that the number of sequenced reads becomes large and the probability p shrinks.

We consider splitting the pool of DNA fragments into a greater number n of subintervals, the probability p of one accident in one of these shorter subintervals will decrease. Let $\mu_i = np$, then above (11.2) become:

$$P(Y_i = y) = \binom{n}{y} p^y (1 - p)^{n-y} = \binom{n}{y} \left(\frac{\mu_i}{n}\right)^y \left(1 - \frac{\mu_i}{n}\right)^{n-y} \tag{11.3}$$

Take the limit of the binomial probability as $n \to \infty$, then the binomial distribution approximates to the Poisson distribution with parameter μ_i as above.

If we assume the RNA sequencing experiments as random samplings of reads distribution, the Poisson distribution provides a flexible and convenient model for analyzing the gene (or taxon, OTU) counts from a fixed pool of genes (or taxa, OTUs). Comparing to biological replicates (Robinson et al. 2010), technical replicates have low variation (Marioni et al. 2008; Wang et al. 2010), and the variation in the read counts of features across technical replicates can be adequately modeled by a Poisson distribution (Marioni et al. 2008). For example, the Poisson distribution has been used to test differential expression in early RNA-seq studies, using a single source of RNA (Marioni et al. 2008; Wang et al. 2010).

The Biases of Between-Samples and Within-Sample

Related to biological and technical variations, two biases exist in an RNA-seq experiment: one is "between-samples" and another is "within-sample". For example, the sequencing depths or library sizes (the total number of mapped reads) are typically different among samples; the observed counts are not directly comparable between samples (Soneson and Delorenzi 2013). Thus, the between-samples biases occur. The within-sample biases also occur because the genes (here gene is a general term, which can refer to taxon at any level in microbiome study) are usually tested individually for expression (abundance) differences between conditions. However, researchers usually ignore this factor and assume that all samples affect similarly (Oshlack et al. 2010).

Poisson Model Has No Capability of Modeling Overdispersed Data

There are several possible causes of overdispersion: correlated gene counts, clustering of subjects, and within group heterogeneity. For example, within RNA sequencing data context, both biological replicates (e.g., RNA from different individuals) and technical replicates (e.g., same source of RNA) are often correlated and/or highly sparse, resulting in a conditional variance $Var(Y_i|X_i)$ much large than the mean $\mu_i = \exp(X_i^T \beta)$, a phenomenon known as overdispersion. In other words, RNA-Seq data are overdispersed due to between and within library variation (Robinson et al. 2010; Robinson and Oshlack 2010). The variance of sequence counts tends to be larger than expected for multinomial or Poisson distribution. Thus, it is difficult to use Poisson model for analyzing the genomic count data.

A distinctive feature of the Poisson is the equality of the variance and mean, $Var(Y_i|X_i) = \mu_i$, which unfortunately also becomes a major limitation of this model in applications to the genomic (including microbiome) count data. Biological replication of an experiment implies that a new pool of DNA fragments is generated. It indicates that an identical probability p from feature (taxon) i of the genome for biological replicates does not exist. Also, when there are biological replicates (i.e., given an independent sample of biological replicates), overdispersion in the observed gene counts is most likely due to within group variation (i.e., within group heterogeneity). Under this situation, the assumption of Poisson distribution is too restrictive (Robinson and Smyth 2007; Nagalakshmi et al. 2008), and Poisson model predicts smaller variations than what is seen in the data (Anders and Huber 2010). Thus, the Poisson model does not take account of biological variation or any technical sources that might cause the relative abundance of different genes to vary between different RNA samples (McCarthy et al. 2012).

Therefore, when overdispersion is an issue, the estimates based on Poisson regression will be inefficient (Cameron and Trivedi 1998; Xia et al. 2012) and be prone to high false positive rates resulting from underestimation of sampling error (Kvam et al. 2012).

Some software packages, such as SAS, permit estimation of a dispersion parameter to accommodate overdispersion. For example, the SAS GENMOD and GLIMMIX procedures allow the modification of the Poisson model by including a dispersion parameter ϕ to account for such overdispersion. With this technique,

$Var(\mu_i) = \phi\mu_i$ (where $\phi > 0$), when $\phi < 1$, the variance is less than its mean, indicating underdispersion, while for $\phi > 1$, the variance is large than its mean, implying overdispersion in the data. This approach is ad hoc in the sense that it addresses overdispersed Poisson distribution at the "back end" estimation stage, rather than at the "front end" by explicitly modeling the overdispersion such as the negative binomial (NB) model we discuss next.

11.1.3 Negative Binomial Model

As the most common alternative to Poisson regression, NB regression model addresses overdispersion by explicitly modeling the correlated and sparse events via a latent variable. Specifically, NB extends the Poisson by positing that the conditional mean μ_i of Y_i is not only determined by X_i but also by a heterogeneity (latent) component e_i independent of X_i. If we assume that $\exp(e_i)$ is distributed with a gamma $\left(\frac{1}{\phi}, \frac{1}{\phi}\right)$, we obtain the NB model with the following density function:

$$P(Y_i|X_i) = \frac{\Gamma(Y_i + 1/\phi)}{\Gamma(Y_i + 1)\Gamma(1/\phi)} \left(\frac{1/\phi}{1/\phi + \mu_i}\right)^{\frac{1}{\phi}} \left(\frac{\mu_i}{1/\phi + \mu_i}\right)^{Y_i}, \quad (11.4)$$

where $\mu_i = \exp(X_i^T\beta + e_i) = \exp(X_i^T\beta)\exp(e_i)$.

Since $E(\exp(e_i)) = 1$, $E(\exp(X_i^T\beta + e_i)) = E(\exp(X_i^T\beta))$, i.e., whether we assume a Poisson or a negative binomial distribution, the expect value of μ_i does not change. Because $\phi > 0$, under the NB distribution, $Var(Y_i|X_i) = \mu_i(1 + \phi\mu_i) > \mu_i$, the variance of the NB is greater than its mean, making provision for overdispersion. Note that NB and Poisson models may be viewed as nested because as ϕ approaches 0, NB approaches the Poisson.

The NB model outperforms the Poisson model in analyzing overdispersed data by using the overdispersion parameter (Xia et al. 2012) and is commonly used to model count data when overdispersion presents (Cameron and Trivedi 1998).

11.2 NB Model in edgeR

11.2.1 Development of NB in the Setting of Genomic Count Data

The NB model has been shown to be a good fit to RNA-seq data (McCarthy et al. 2012). Compared to Poisson regression with only one parameter for mean, NB has an additional dispersion parameter ϕ. The benefit of NB overdispersion parameter is to provide more refined possibilities for separating biological variation from technical variation (Robinson and Smyth 2007, 2008), which is flexible enough to account for biological variation. Therefore, NB model can facilitate our understanding the variation of features (taxa) among biological replicates to make inferences that are relevant to the corresponding population. Furthermore, the simulation studies show that an assumption of a NB distribution can be robust even if the data are not truly negative binomially distributed (Lu et al. 2005). Thus, the NB model should provide a powerful framework (e.g., via GLMs) for analyzing arbitrarily complex experimental designs and a more flexible statistical framework for real data.

In recent years, many statistical methods have been developed to examine differential expression of replicated count data through different statistical models based on the NB distribution. Here, we briefly describe NB models in the setting of genomic count data. Assume the genomic count data can be summarized into a table of counts, with rows corresponding to genes (or taxa, OTUs) and columns to samples; let Y_{ij} denote the observed number of reads for gene i and sample j, then for gene i and sample j in experimental group k, the data can be modeled by NB model:

$$Y_{ij} \sim NB(m_j p_{ik}, \phi_i), \tag{11.5}$$

where m_j is the library size (total number of reads), ϕ_i is the dispersion with $\phi_i > 0$ representing overdispersion relative to the Poisson distribution (Robinson and Smyth 2007). When $\phi_i = 0$, the NB distribution reduces to Poisson, and p_{ik} is the true relative abundance of gene i in experimental group k to which sample j belongs. By using the NB parameterization, the mean and variance are given:

$$E(Y_{ij}) = \mu_{ij} = m_j p_{ik}, \; Var(Y_{ij}) = \mu_{ij}(1 + \mu_{ij}\phi_i). \tag{11.6}$$

The mean parameters μ_{ij} depend on the sequencing depth for sample j as well as on the amount of RNA from gene i in the sample. For RNA-seq data analysis, the parameters of interest are the relative abundance of gene p_{ik}. Statistical models can be formulated to test for the differences of relative abundance or changes in expression level between experimental conditions, possibly adjusting for covariates, and to estimate the log-fold changes in expression.

11.2.2   Dispersion Estimators of NB in edgeR

For reliable statistical testing, it is critical to obtain good estimates of each gene's dispersion (Anders et al. 2013). Many methods for modeling RNA-Seq data by NB regression are available now, mainly differ in their approach to model dispersion across genes (Yu et al. 2013).

To address the over-dispersion problem, both edgeR and DESeq use the related NB distribution as statistical framework to develop a dispersion estimator through the mean-variance relationship of $Var(Y_{ij}) = \mu_{ij}(1 + \mu_{ij}\phi_i)$. The consistent (though non-linear) relationship between variance and mean indicates that parameters of a NB model, especially ϕ_i can be adequately estimated among biological replicates of microbiome data (McMurdie and Holmes 2014).

Conditional and Common Dispersion Estimators

A small number of biological libraries replicates (samples) cause the uncertainty in estimating the dispersion parameter for every gene. With this in mind, Robinson and Smyth originally developed a conditional maximum likelihood (CML) estimator (Robinson and Smyth 2008) with small-sample estimation of NB dispersion for serial analysis of gene expression (SAGE), and is now applied to RNA-seq data analysis (Robinson and Smyth 2007). Given a single gene counts Y_{ij} distributed as NB: $Y_{ij} \sim NB(m_j p_{ij}, \phi_i)$, now assume that all n libraries have the same size (i.e., $m_i \equiv m$), then the sum of identically distributed NB random variables is also NB.

We write as:

$$Z = Y_1 + Y_2 \cdots + Y_n \sim NB(nmp, \phi n^{-1}). \tag{11.7}$$

An exact conditional maximum likelihood for ϕ that is independent of p is given as below (Robinson and Smyth 2008):

$$
\begin{aligned}
l_{Y|Z} &= z(\phi) \\
&= \left[\sum_{i=1}^{n} \log \Gamma(y_i + \phi^{-1}) \right] + \log \Gamma(n\phi^{-1}) - \log \Gamma(z + n\phi^{-1}) - n \log \Gamma(\phi^{-1}).
\end{aligned}
\tag{11.8}
$$

If the assumption that all genes had the same dispersion parameter is true (that is, the dispersion parameter is the same across all genes), then the common dispersion parameter could be estimated very accurately from all the available data using a conditional maximum likelihood approach. The common dispersion estimator maximizes the common likelihood:

$l_C(\phi) = \sum_{i=1}^{G} l_i(\phi_i)$, where G is the number of genes.

Quantile-Adjusted Dispersion Estimators

When the library sizes are unequal, the counts are not identically distributed, and the conditioning argument does not hold exactly. A quantile adjusted conditional maximum likelihood (qCML) was devised to adjust the observed counts up or down depending on whether the corresponding library sizes are below or above the geometric mean (Robinson and Smyth 2008). This creates the quantile-adjusted "pseudodata" for allowing the use of the CML machinery to achieve an accurate estimate of ϕ.

Gene-Wise Dispersion Estimator

A common dispersion for all genes may be a too restrictive assumption and be rare in practice. Thus, methods of estimating the gene-wise dispersion have received considerable attention (Anders et al. 2013). It has been shown that borrowing information across genes could provide better estimate the variance (Smyth 2004; Cui et al. 2005).

A moderated test was proposed for RNA-seq data to allow different genes to have different dispersion parameters, and by using a weighted likelihood approach to borrow information across genes to average the variability across all genes (Robinson and Smyth 2008; Anders et al. 2013), the individual gene-wise dispersion (ϕ_i) were squeezed towards the common value (ϕ) (Robinson and Smyth 2007). The weighted conditional log-likelihood is given by:

$$WL(\phi) = l_i(\phi_i) + \alpha l_C(\phi_i), \tag{11.9}$$

where α is the weight given to the common likelihood. In general, ϕ_i represents the coefficient of variation of biological variation between the samples. Initially the methods worked only for a two-group comparison. Later, the capabilities of estimating and moderating the dispersion have been extended for multiple-groups comparison.

11.2.3 Hypothesis Testing in edgeR

The Wald test and Fisher's exact test are two main statistical tests in edgeR to detect differentially expressed (or abundant) genes (taxa, OTUs) between conditions.

11.2.3.1 The Wald Test

Consider each single gene i, let Y_{ij} denote the observed count for class k and library j for a particular gene. Here, $j = 1, \ldots, n_k$ and for simplicity, assume just a two-group comparison so that k = 1, 2. This analysis specially requires only one of n_1 or n_2 to be greater than 1.

Under the NB statistical framework, for the gene counts Y_{ij}, $Y_{ij} \sim NB(\mu_{ij}, \phi)$, where ϕ is the dispersion. It exists the following mean-variance relationship: $Var(Y_{ij}) = \mu_{ij} + \phi_i\mu_{ij}^2$, making $\phi = 0$ the Poisson distribution. When parametrized in terms of its mean μ_{ij} and variance $Var(Y_{ij})$, we get $p_i = \frac{\mu_{ij}}{Var(Y_{ij})}$ and $\phi_i = \frac{Var(Y_{ij}) - \mu_{ij}}{\mu_{ij}^2}$.

Now let p_{ik} be the true relative abundance of this gene in RNA of class k, then $\mu_{ij} = m_{ij}p_{ik}$, where m_{ij} is the library size for sample j. To assess differences in relative abundance, the null hypothesis $H_0 : P_{i1} = P_{i2}$ is proposed to test against the two-sided alternative; and the test is repeated for each gene.

The default test statistic in edgeR is the Wald test used in Lu et al. (2005), which is based on the beta-binomial model (Baggerly et al. 2003). The test statistic simply divides the difference of the two estimated proportions $P_{i2} - P_{i1}$ by its estimated standard error. Actually, this is the classical two-sample Welch's t-test.

11.2.3.2 NB-Based Exact Test

For a 2×2 contingency table with the columns representing different treatment groups, the rows presenting different outcomes, the null hypothesis of Fisher's exact test is that treatments do not affect outcomes. The null hypothesis could be interpreted as the probability of having a particular outcome not being influenced by the treatment group, and the test is to evaluate whether the two treatment groups differ in the proportions with each outcome.

Under the null hypothesis of no association, Fisher showed that the probability of obtaining the frequencies a, b, c and d in Table 11.1 is given by the hypergeometric distribution:

$$\frac{\binom{a+b}{a}\binom{c+d}{c}}{\binom{n}{a+c}} = \frac{(a+b)!(c+d)!(a+c)!(b+d)!}{a!b!c!d!n!} \tag{11.10}$$

To calculate the significance of the observed data, Fisher showed that we need only calculating the total probability of observing data as extreme or more extreme if the null hypothesis is true. Two-sided test is to compute the p-value by summing the probabilities for all tables with probabilities less than or equal to that of the observed table. However, similar as Poisson model, Fisher's exact test only deals with the technical variation and fails to take into account the variation between libraries (Robinson et al. 2010).

A variation of the Fisher's exact test is developed for contingency tables, but replacing the hypergeometric probabilities with NB, using quantile adjustment (Robinson and Smyth 2008).

Table 11.1 A design 2×2 contingency table

	Group A	Group B	Row total
outcome 1	a	b	a + b
outcome 2	c	d	c + d
Column total	a + c	b + d	a + b + c + d (= n)

Where n represent the grand total

For the 2-sample test, let Z_{tA} and Z_{tB} be the sum of pseudocounts for class A and class B, respectively, over the number of libraries, n_A and n_B. Then under the null hypothesis,

$$Z_{tk} \sim NB(n_k m^* p_t, \phi n_k^{-1}), \quad k \in A, B. \tag{11.11}$$

where $m^* = \left(\prod_{j=1}^{n_k} m_j\right)^{\frac{1}{n}}$, p_t represents the proportion of the sum library. $n_k = n_A + n_B$.

This approach showed improvements in accuracy compared with the overdispersed logistic and log-linear approaches, but the methods initially were limited to pairwise comparisons and worked only for a two-group comparison; later, the capabilities of estimating and moderating the dispersion have been extended for multiple-groups comparison. For the more complex experimental designs, edgeR needs a generalized linear model. The multiple hypothesis correction is adjusted by the standard statistical methods (e.g., Benjamini-Hochberg method).

11.3 The edgeR Package

The edgeR and DESeq2 are R packages for differential expression analysis of RNA-Seq, SAGE-Seq, ChIP-Seq or HiC count data. The simulation studies show that edgeR and DESeq2 remain among the top performers (Soneson and Delorenzi 2013; McMurdie and Holmes 2014) and widely enjoyed success for highly similar RNA-Seq data. The edgeR and DESeq2 were recommended for performing analysis of differential abundance in microbiome experiment data (McMurdie and Holmes 2014).

11.3.1 Introduction

The package edgeR, is an implementation of the methodology developed by Robinson and Smyth (Robinson and Smyth 2007, 2008; Robinson et al. 2010). It was reviewed as one of most popular implementations of variance stabilization technique currently used in RNA-Seq analysis and can be adapted for microbiome count data (McMurdie and Holmes 2014). This approach allows valid comparison across OTUs (features) while substantially improving both power and accuracy in the detection of differential abundance.

As a penalized approach to identify differences, the current version of package edgeR has a variety of penalized overdispersion approaches to commonly penalize dispersion, shrink individual genes/tags, or use the tag-wise procedure with a trend as a function of expression level. The edgeR package implements an exact binomial test, which generalized for overdispersed counts via the function exactTest().

The total number of aligned reads is very different in RNA- and DNA-sequencing. Thus, normalization is one of the key issues in analysis of gene differential expression in RNA-seq and differential abundance of taxa in microbiome. The common method of normalization is to divide read count by the total number of aligned reads in the sample. However, the edgeR deals with normalization in a different way. The authors of edgeR argued that normalization issues arise only to the extent that technical factors have sample-specific effects (Chen et al. 2017) because edgeR concerns the differential expression analysis rather than the quantification of expression levels. The edgeR estimates relative changes in expression levels between conditions, but not directly estimates absolute expression levels. Thus, the aim of normalization is to identify and remove systematic technical differences among samples occurring in the data to ensure the minimal impact of technical bias on the results.

In edgeR package, the overall strategy of normalization is to choose an appropriate baseline, and then express sample counts relative to that baseline. The normalization methods associated with edgeR and DESeq2 have been shown to outperform other methods, particularly in the cases of expressed RNA varying across biological conditions or in the presence of highly expressed genes. There are several approaches of normalization implemented in edgeR package. We briefly describe them below.

(1) Total read count normalization implemented by the function: cpm(..., normalized.lib.sizes = TRUE) (Robinson et al. 2010)

This approach assumes that read counts are proportional to expression level and sequencing depth. Its calculation is to divide the read count by total number of reads and then rescale the factors to counts per million: $C_j = \frac{10^6}{D_j}$, where, C_j is the normalization factor associated with sample j, D_j is the total number of reads for sample j.

(2) Upper quantile normalization implemented by the function calcNormFactors (..., method = "upperquartile", $p = 0.75$) (Bullard et al. 2010)

Due to the preponderance of zero and low-count genes, the median is uninformative for the different levels of sequencing effort. Thus, this method uses the per-sample upper-quartile (75-th percentile) to scale counts within samples. The formula of calculation is given below:

$$C_j = \frac{\exp\left\{\frac{1}{N}\sum_{l=1}^{N}\log\left(D_l Q_l^{(p)}\right)\right\}}{D_j Q_j^{(p)}},$$ where, $Q_j^{(p)}$ is the upper quantile (p-th percentile) of

sample j after of library-size scaling the reads count; $D_j Q_j^{(p)}$ is the re-scale of the upper quantile by the total reads count; $C_j = \frac{1}{D_j Q_j^{(p)}}$ is the correction multiplicative factor; $p = 0.75$ upper quartile normalization; and factors should multiple to one

$$C_j = \frac{\exp\left\{\frac{1}{N}\sum_{l=1}^{N}\log\left(D_l Q_l^{(p)}\right)\right\}}{D_j Q_j^{(p)}}.$$

(3) Relative Log Expression (RLE) implemented in the function calcNormFactors (..., method = "RLE") (Anders and Huber 2010)

In this method, each size factor estimate C_j is computed as the median of the ratios of the j-th sample's counts to those of a pseudo-reference sample—the geometric mean across samples:

$$C_j = median_i\left\{\frac{Y_{ij}}{\left(\prod_{l=1}^{N} Y_{il}\right)^{1/N}}\right\}, \text{ where, } C_j \text{ is the correction factor: the median}$$

across genes for each sample; Y_{ij} is counts for i-th gene in j-th sample; $\left(\prod_{l=1}^{N} Y_{il}\right)^{1/N}$ is the geometric mean across samples, the pseudo-reference sample; $\frac{Y_{ij}}{\left(\prod_{l=1}^{N} Y_{il}\right)^{1/N}}$ is centering samples with rapport to the pseudo-reference sample. To normalized counts, the factors should multiple to one $C_j = \frac{\exp\left\{\sum_{l=1}^{N}\log(C_l)\right\}}{C_j}$.

(4) Trimmed Mean of M-values (TMM) implemented by the function calcNormFactors (..., method = "TMM") (Robinson and Oshlack 2010)

If the most genes are not differentially expressed, the total read count is strongly dependent on a few highly expressed transcripts. The method of a trimmed mean is the average after removing the upper and lower percentages of the data. The TMM procedure is doubly trimmed, by log-fold-changes $M_i(j, r)$ (sample j relative to sample r for gene i) and by absolute intensity:

$$M_i(j, r) = \log_2 Y_{ij}/D_j - \log_2(Y_{ir}/D_r)$$

and $A_i(k, r) = \frac{1}{2}\left(\log_2(Y_{ij}/D_j) + \log_2(Y_{ir}/D_r)\right)$.

By default, the method trims the M_i values by 30% and the A_i values by 5%, but these settings can be tailored to a given experiment. The weighted mean of M_i is given:

$$TMM(j, r) = \frac{\sum_{i \in G} w_i(j,r)M_i(j,r)}{\sum_{i \in G} w_i(j,r)}, \text{ where G represents the set of genes with valid } M_i$$

and A_i values.

11.3.2   Step-by-Step Implementing edgeR

In this section, we illustrate the edgeR package using a human microbiome data. The analysis process consists of three main procedures, namely normalization, dispersion estimation, and test for differential expression.

Cigarette Smokers Data Set

This data set was used in Chap. 7. It was collected to study on the effect of smoking on the upper respiratory tract microbiome (Charlson et al. 2010). This data set consists of 60 subjects (32 non-smokers and 28 smokers). Bacterial communities were profiled using 454 pyrosequencing of 16S sequence tags. The original paper analyzed the microbiome from the right and left throat and nose to assess microbiome composition and effects of cigarette smoking. Here we use a subset of throat samples from left side of body to illustrate the overdispersion which is typical of such datasets. The packages edgeR was one of the recommended differential (abundant) analysis tools for RNA-seq data and microbiome data to identify differentially represent genes or abundant OTUs (McMurdie and Holmes 2014). We here directly use the otu-table from this study.

Step-by-Step Implementing edgeR

The edgeR requires two types of input files: count data files containing raw counts or OTUs, and sample or meta data containing group and covariate information. The edgeR works on a specific feature (taxa)-by-sample matrix, a table of integer read counts, with rows corresponding to a unique feature identifier (e.g., the gene ids) and columns to independent libraries (e.g., the sample ids). The edgeR also needs an experimental design matrix to process the specific designed study. A typical bioinformatics workflow for identifying differentially expressed genes (DEGs) in RNA-seq and differentially abundant taxa (DAT) in DNA-seq data includes mapping short reads, quantification of gene expression (taxon abundance), normalization, and DEG and DAT identification. The statistical analysis of RNA-seq and DNA-seq data is considered more to focus on last two stages and consist of several steps for data management, exploration and statistical hypothesis testing. We illustrate the implementation of the edgeR package by the following steps:

Step 1: Load Datasets and Setting Up the Count Matrix

We use the left-side throat data from the GUniFrac package, we first install the package and load datasets.

```
> install.packages("GUniFrac")
> library(GUniFrac)
> data(throat.otu.tab)
> head(throat.otu.tab)
```

The original format of OTU-table is samples-by-OTUs, we transpose it to OUTs-by-samples format to meet the edgeR input data requirement.

```
> throat<-t(throat.otu.tab)
> counts<-throat
> head(counts)
```

Step 2: Build the edgeR Object
We install Bioconductor package edgeR by issuing the command R in a terminal window and type:

Source ("http://www.Bioconductor.org/biocLite.R")

biocLite(c(edgeR))

This retrieves an automatic installation tool (*biocLite*) to install the version-matched packages, and automatically download and install all other pre-requisite packages.

The edgeR stores data in a simple list-based data object called a DGEList. This type of object can be manipulated like any list in R, thus, it is easy to use. To cover the count matrix into an edgeR object in R, we first create a group variable or extract group information from meta-table: tell the edgeR which samples belong to which group, and then specify the count matrix and the groups in the function DGEList(). However, before make edgeR object, we need to check to make sure the dimension of counts table is equal to the length of group. If these two numbers are not matched, it indicates something wrong in the data processing and the edgeR object can not be built. Extract group information from meta-table and assign group variable.

```
> data(throat.meta)
> group <- throat.meta$SmokingStatus
> head(group)
[1] NonSmoker
Smoker        Smoker        Smoker        Smoker        Smoker
Levels: NonSmoker Smoker
> dim(counts)
[1] 856 60
> length(groups)
[1] 60
```

The following codes build the edgeR object:

```
> library(edgeR)
> y <- DGEList(counts=counts,group=group)
```

We can use the names() function to look at the elements that the object contains.

```
> names(y)
[1] "counts"  "samples"
```

These elements can be accessed using the $ symbol:

```
> head(y$counts)        # original count matrix
> y$samples             # contains a summary of samples
> sum(y$all.zeros)      # How many genes have 0 counts across all samples
[1] 0
```

Step 3: Filter the Data

Typically, several thousand genes or taxa are expressed or abundant in all samples in a DNA/RNA-Seq experiment. Too low count reads suggest something wrong with samples or the sequencing. To effectively detect truly differentially expressed genes or abundant taxa and conduct downstream analysis, it usually removes very low expressed genes or abundant taxa in the any of experimental conditions in the early stage, before processing the normalization and differential abundance testing. This is called filtering. Filtering increases sensitivity and precision to identify the differentially expressed genes or abundant taxa (Sha et al. 2015). However, the critical thing is to choose an optimal filtering threshold.

Filtering can be done by many ways (Rau et al. 2013; Sha et al. 2015). Such as independent data filtering, in which the filter is independent from the subsequent test (Bourgon et al. 2010). But most data filters belong to ad hoc data filters, including filtering genes or taxa with a total read count or average counts smaller than or below an empirical threshold (Sultan et al. 2008; Anders and Huber 2010; Robinson et al. 2010; Law et al. 2014; Love et al. 2014), or with at least one zero count in each experimental condition (Bottomly et al. 2011).

For ad hoc data filters, it is critical to choose an appropriate filtering threshold. Obviously selecting an arbitrary threshold value as filtering criterion is not a good way. Thus, in practice, most proposed and routinely used data filters have some algorithms considered, such as, using the distribution (Harati et al. 2014), linking to normalization in some way, based on external controls (Munro et al. 2014), rather than directly to the raw counts.

The mean-based filters and maximum-based filters are the two broad categories of filters for DNA-and RNA-seq data (Rau et al. 2013). The mean-based and maximum-based filters remove those genes (taxa) with mean or maximum normalized counts across all samples less than or equal to a pre-specified cutoff from the analysis, respectively.

CPM filter used in the edgeR actually is a generalized version of the maximum-based filter. It is based on counts per million (CPM), calculated as the raw counts divided by the library sizes and multiplied by one million. For example, we choose a cutoff, such as, at least 100 counts per million (calculated with cpm() in R) in more number of samples (i.e., 10) to remove those genes (taxa) with a CPM value less than this cutoff from the analysis. When we choose the number of samples, the group labels are ignored, but the number should be larger than the size of the smallest group. The example count data have been filtered. To show the procedure, we keep an OTU with a cpm of 100 in greater at least two samples.

```
> dim(y)
[1] 856   60
> y_full <- y                 # keep the old one in case we mess up
> head(y$counts)
> apply(y$counts, 2, sum)   # total OTU counts per sample
> keep <- rowSums(cpm(y)>100) >= 2
> y <- y[keep,]
> dim(y)
[1] 616   60
```

This reduces the dataset from 856 OTUs to 616. The filtered OTUs is very little power to detect differential expression (abundance), so little information is lost by filtering. Now we reset the library sizes:

```
> y$samples$lib.size <- colSums(y$counts)
> y$samples
```

Step 4: Normalize the Data
Normalization is often used to ensure that parameters are comparable because different libraries are sequenced to different depths. After filtering, we start to normalize the data. First, calculate the normalization factors to correct for the different compositions of the samples. In edgeR, RNA or DNA composition is normalized by finding a set of scaling factors for the library sizes that minimize the log-fold changes between the samples for most genes (OTUs in this case). The calcNormaFactors() function is used to a set of scaling factors. The default method for calculating these scale factors uses the TMM method (Trimmed Mean of M-values) to calculate normalization factors between samples. The method of total read count normalization has been shown to perform equally well (Dillies et al. 2013). It should be noted that the raw read counts are not actually altered after normalization. Here, we use the default normalization method.

```
> y <- calcNormFactors(y)
> y
> y$samples
                group lib.size norm.factors
ESC_1.1_OPL   NonSmoker     1053      0.5461
ESC_1.3_OPL      Smoker     1060      2.2958
ESC_1.4_OPL      Smoker     1281      1.2167
ESC_1.5_OPL      Smoker     1212      1.4487
ESC_1.6_OPL      Smoker      922      1.6580
ESC_1.10_OPL     Smoker     1264      2.3956
ESC_1.11_OPL  NonSmoker     1512      0.8739
ESC_1.12_OPL  NonSmoker     1095      0.8154
ESC_1.13_OPL  NonSmoker      897      2.1827
ESC_1.14_OPL  NonSmoker     1016      1.2246
ESC_1.15_OPL     Smoker      792      2.1339
ESC_1.18_OPL  NonSmoker     1420      1.4727
ESC_1.19_OPL  NonSmoker     3733      0.5375
ESC_1.20_OPL     Smoker     1530      0.6201
......
```

The effective library size is the product of the original library size and the scaling factor. In all downsteam analyses, the effective library size replaces the original library size.

```
> # effective library sizes
> y$samples$lib.size*y$samples$norm.factors
 [1]  575.0 2433.5 1558.6 1755.8 1528.7 3028.0 1321.3  892.8
 [9] 1957.9 1244.2 1690.1 2091.3 2006.4  948.7  839.3 4353.3
[17]  666.7 1497.9  887.4 2524.1 2214.9  685.2  853.8 1787.3
[25]  969.5  533.9 1904.0  535.1 2129.8 2776.1 3614.0 1487.8
[33] 2613.0 2119.7 2342.6 1687.5  896.4 2375.8 1424.7  800.2
[41] 1452.5 1550.9 2131.5 1080.7 1202.6 1081.9 1123.1 2047.1
[49] 2865.9 1599.1 1140.0 1089.5 1816.4 2120.3  654.4 1049.6
[57] 1849.9 2560.0 2815.2  333.2
```

Without the replacement, the default value is 1 for all values in y$samples$ norm.factors.

Step 5: Explore the Data by Multi-dimensional Scaling (MDS) Plot
An MDS plot measures the similarity of the samples and projects this measure into 2-dimensions.

In the plot, the samples, which are similar, are near to each other while samples that are dissimilar are far from each other. The following R codes create the MDS plot (Fig. 11.1):

```
> plotMDS(y, method="bcv", main = "MDS Plot for throat Count Data",
+             col=as.numeric(y$samples$group), labels = colnames(y$-
counts))
> legend("topright", as.character(unique(y$samples$-
group)), col=1:2, cex=0.8, pch=16)
```

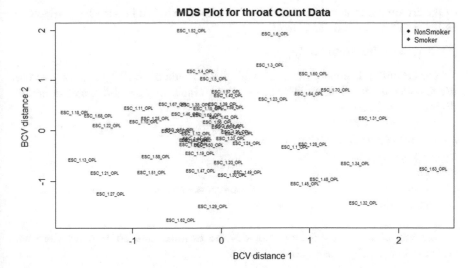

Fig. 11.1 Multi-dimensional scaling (MDS) plot to show sample similarity and dissimilarity between groups. This plot shows that most samples are dissimilar by non-smokers and smokers

To create a pdf format file, use following R codes:

```
> # Output plot as a pdf
> pdf("MDS_plot.pdf", width = 7, height = 7 ) # in inches
> plotMDS(y, method="bcv", main = "MDS Plot for throat Count Data",
+            col=as.numeric(y$samples$group), cex=0.8, labels = colnames
             (y$counts))
> legend("topright", as.character(unique(y$samples$-
group)), col=1:2, cex=0.8, pch=16)
> dev.off() # tells R to turn off device and writing to the pdf.
```

If the plots are created in R, we can also save plots as pdf's, png's, etc. (see ? pdf).

Step 6: Estimate the Dispersions
The first major step in the analyses of RNA-seq differential expression and microbiome abundance count data using the NB model is to estimate the dispersion parameter for each gene or taxon (OTU). The dispersion measures the biological variability of within-group variability, i.e., variability between replicates (or called inter-library variation) for that gene (taxon, OTU). For strongly abundant genes, the dispersion can be understood as a squared coefficient of variation: that is, a dispersion value of 0.01 indicates that the gene's expression tends to differ usually by $\sqrt{0.01} = 10\%$ between samples of the same treatment group. Typically, the shape

of the dispersion fit is an exponentially decaying curve. We fit a model in edgeR to estimate the dispersions as below:

(1) Estimate the common dispersion.

The common dispersion measure will give an idea of overall variability across the genome for the dataset. We rename the variable to y1 and estimate common dispersion as below:

```
> y1 <- estimateCommonDisp(y, verbose=T)
Disp = 5.61103 , BCV = 2.3688
> names(y1)
[1] "counts"        "samples"       "common.dispersion"     "pseudo.counts"
[5] "pseudo.lib.size"     "AveLogCPM"
```

The output of the estimation includes the estimate and some other elements added to the edgeR object, y1.

(2) Fit a trended model to get a tag/taxon wise dispersion.

In steep 2, we fit a trended model. If a trend model is not fit, edgeR by default uses the common dispersion as a trend. Once the trend model is fitted, we can estimate the tag-wise (in term of microbiome data, taxa-wise) dispersions, which is a function of this model. In this scenario, each gene will get its own unique dispersion estimate. But the common dispersion is still used in the calculation. The tag-wise dispersions are squeezed toward the common value: a trended estimate computed by the "moving average" approach.

```
> #estimate the tag-wise dispersion
> y1 <- estimateTagwiseDisp(y1)
> names(y1)

[1] "counts"            "samples"       "common.dispersion"   "pseudo.counts"
[5] "pseudo.lib.size"   "AveLogCPM"     "prior.df"            "prior.n"
[9] "tagwise.dispersion" "span"
```

We can use the plotBCV() function to plot the tag-wise biological coefficient of variation (square root of dispersions) against log2-CPM (Fig. 11.2).

```
> plotBCV(y1)
```

(3) Fit a generalized linear model to estimate the genewise dispersion.

We can also fit a generalized linear model (GLM) using edgeR to estimate the genewise dispersion. Before fitting GLMs, we need to define the design matrix. In this case, the design matrix is created as:

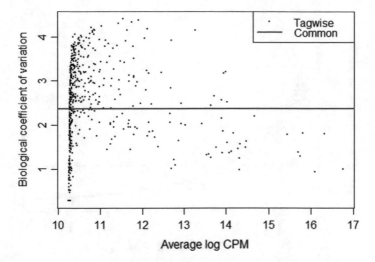

Fig. 11.2 Plot of gene (taxon)-wise biological coefficient of variation (BCV) against gene abundance (in $\log_2$ counts per million). The BCV is the square root of the negative binomial dispersion

```
> #use a generalized linear model to estimate the dispersion
> design <- model.matrix(~group)
> rownames(design) <- colnames(y)
> design
               (Intercept) groupSmoker
ESC_1.1_OPL              1           0
ESC_1.3_OPL              1           1
ESC_1.4_OPL              1           1
ESC_1.5_OPL              1           1
ESC_1.6_OPL              1           1
ESC_1.10_OPL            1           1
......

attr(,"assign")
[1] 0 1
attr(,"contrasts")
attr(,"contrasts")$group
[1] "contr.treatment"
```

attr(,"assign")

[1] 0 1

attr(,"contrasts")

attr(,"contrasts")$group

[1] "contr.treatment"

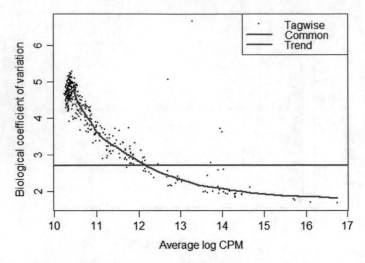

Fig. 11.3 Plot of gene (taxon)-wise biological coefficient of variation (BCV) against gene abundance (in $\log_2$ counts per million) based on fitted GLM

Now we can estimate the genewise dispersion over all genes /OTUs, allowing for a possible abundance trend. The estimation is also robust against potential outlier genes/OTUs.

```
> library(statmod)
> y2 <- estimateDisp(y, design, robust=TRUE)
> y2$common.dispersion
[1] 7.348
```

Again we plot the tagwise biological coefficient of variation (square root of dispersions) against log2-CPM (Fig. 11.3).

```
> plotBCV(y2)
```

The coefficient of biological variation (BCV) is the square root of dispersion. The plot shows that the trended dispersion decreases with expression level. At low logCPM, the dispersions are very large indeed.

Note that only the trended dispersion is used under the quasi-likelihood (QL) pipeline, whereas the tagwise and common estimates are not. The following R codes estimate the QL dispersions using the glmQLFit() function, and then visualize them with the plotQLDisp () function (Fig. 11.4).

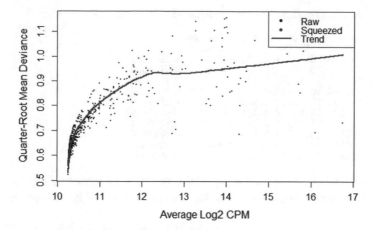

Fig. 11.4 Plot of quarter-root mean deviance against gene abundance (in $\log_2$ counts per million) based on fitted the quasi-likelihood GLM

```
> fit <- glmQLFit(y2, design, robust=TRUE)
> plotQLDisp(fit)
```

Step 7: Test the Differential Abundance
Once NB models are fitted and dispersion estimates are obtained for each gene, we can test the differentially expressed (abundant) genes (OTUs) between conditions either using the function exactTest () or GLM approach.

The exactTest() Approach
The classic edgeR approach uses the function exactTest() to make the pairwise comparisons between the groups. The output of exactTest() is a list of elements, one of which is a table of the results.

The null hypothesis of this example study is that there is no effect of the smoking on the OTUs: the observed difference between Smoker and NonSmoker was merely caused by experimental variability, i.e., the type of variability that we can just as well expect between different samples in the same group. The hypothesis testing for each OTU is to find whether there is a sufficient evidence to decide against the null hypothesis. The codes below find differential abundance of the OTUs in Smoker versus NonSmoker.

```
> et <- exactTest(y1,pair = c( "NonSmoker", "Smoker" ))
> topTags(et)
Comparison of groups:  Smoker-NonSmoker
         logFC   logCPM        PValue          FDR
411    6.582714 12.14801 1.844586e-06 0.001136265
1280  -3.914412 10.79061 1.325503e-04 0.039145889
3538   1.903514 13.59133 2.126347e-04 0.039145889
4363   3.505148 10.61836 2.541941e-04 0.039145889
4357  -4.064894 11.95855 3.373681e-04 0.041563749
2621  -3.961877 13.89518 4.753634e-04 0.048803980
1437  -4.917752 11.21345 7.964182e-04 0.062239716
1490   1.181922 16.09314 8.083080e-04 0.062239716
444   -2.290007 11.34563 1.116190e-03 0.076396983
4036   1.685491 13.91434 1.348299e-03 0.079674392
```

The test statistic is reported as a *p*-value, which is the probability that a log fold change as strong or even stronger as the observed one would be seen under the null hypothesis.

edgeR uses the Benjamini-Hochberg(BH) method for adjusting the false discovery rate (FDR). The BH-adjusted *p*-values are given in the column FDR of the test object.

Alternatively, we can specify the number to compare the smoking status. The pair = c (1, 2) is equivalent to pair = c ("NonSmoker", "Smoker"). By default the levels of group are in alphabetical order; in this case, the alphabetical order is same as the numerical order.

```
> et1 <- exactTest(y1, pair=c(1,2))
```

Below we use the function topTags () to tabulate the top differentially expressed (abundant) genes (or taxa or OTUs, etc.).

```
> topTags(et1)
Comparison of groups:  Smoker-NonSmoker
         logFC   logCPM        PValue          FDR
411    6.582714 12.14801 1.844586e-06 0.001136265
1280  -3.914412 10.79061 1.325503e-04 0.039145889
3538   1.903514 13.59133 2.126347e-04 0.039145889
4363   3.505148 10.61836 2.541941e-04 0.039145889
4357  -4.064894 11.95855 3.373681e-04 0.041563749
2621  -3.961877 13.89518 4.753634e-04 0.048803980
1437  -4.917752 11.21345 7.964182e-04 0.062239716
1490   1.181922 16.09314 8.083080e-04 0.062239716
444   -2.290007 11.34563 1.116190e-03 0.076396983
4036   1.685491 13.91434 1.348299e-03 0.079674392
```

We can use the function relevel () to relevel "Smoker" as the control or reference level.

```
> y3 <- y

> y3$samples$group <- relevel(y3$samples$group, ref="Smoker")

> levels(y3$samples$group)

[1] "Smoker"       "NonSmoker"
```

When pair is not specified, the default is to compare the first two group levels, so following two lines of R codes both compare Smoker versus NonSkoker.

```
> et <- exactTest(y1)
> et <- exactTest(y1,pair = c("NonSmoker", "Smoker"))
```

GLM Approach

GLM approach of differential abundance analysis is similar to the exactTest () approach, but is more feasible. This approach requires a design matrix to describe the treatment conditions. We use the function model.matrix () to construct the design matrix.

```
> design <- model.matrix(~group)
> rownames(design) <- colnames(y)
> design
             (Intercept) groupSmoker
ESC_1.1_OPL           1            0
ESC_1.3_OPL           1            1
ESC_1.4_OPL           1            1
ESC_1.5_OPL           1            1
ESC_1.6_OPL           1            1
ESC_1.10_OPL          1            1
......

attr(,"assign")
[1] 0 1
attr(,"contrasts")
attr(,"contrasts")$group
[1] "contr.treatment"
```

As shown below, we first conduct GLM F test and likelihood ratio test using this design as one argument. Then we use the glmQLFTest() function with the contrast argument to compare smokers versus non-smokers.

```
> fit <- glmQLFit(y1, design)
> qlf <- glmQLFTest(fit, contrast=c(-1,1))
> topTags(qlf)
Coefficient:  -1*(Intercept) 1*groupSmoker
        logFC    logCPM         F        PValue           FDR
328  14.78231  10.27672  189.2938  7.599979e-25  3.211365e-22
1583 14.90000  10.28153  181.9246  1.042651e-24  3.211365e-22
4817 14.77254  10.33648  140.5660  9.779248e-23  2.008006e-20
3336 14.47977  10.32503  138.9352  1.467443e-22  2.259861e-20
4116 14.68436  10.32269  137.2099  2.260429e-22  2.784848e-20
5682 14.22083  10.32289  132.1039  8.252121e-22  8.472178e-20
1039 14.64245  10.27005  199.6868  2.257737e-21  1.218636e-19
1592 14.71278  10.27451  191.2489  2.257881e-21  1.218636e-19
2053 14.76317  10.27667  186.3259  2.257943e-21  1.218636e-19
4365 15.07973  10.30524  152.8595  2.258943e-21  1.218636e-19
```

```
> FDR <- p.adjust(qlf$table$PValue, method="BH")
> sum(FDR < 0.05)
[1] 514

> topTags(qlf,n=15)
Coefficient:  -1*(Intercept) 1*groupSmoker
         logFC    logCPM        F       PValue          FDR
328   14.78231  10.27672  189.2938  7.599979e-25  3.211365e-22
1583  14.90000  10.28153  181.9246  1.042651e-24  3.211365e-22
4817  14.77254  10.33648  140.5660  9.779248e-23  2.008006e-20
3336  14.47977  10.32503  138.9352  1.467443e-22  2.259861e-20
4116  14.68436  10.32269  137.2099  2.260429e-22  2.784848e-20
5682  14.22083  10.32289  132.1039  8.252121e-22  8.472178e-20
1039  14.64245  10.27005  199.6868  2.257737e-21  1.218636e-19
1592  14.71278  10.27451  191.2489  2.257881e-21  1.218636e-19
2053  14.76317  10.27667  186.3259  2.257943e-21  1.218636e-19
4365  15.07973  10.30524  152.8595  2.258943e-21  1.218636e-19
1947  15.19313  10.31343  142.9830  2.372648e-21  1.218636e-19
4859  14.01220  10.31780  128.0090  2.373967e-21  1.218636e-19
589   15.09218  10.36253  125.0654  5.126725e-21  2.429279e-19
5603  15.32280  10.32720  136.0716  1.062377e-20  4.674457e-19
4164  15.30893  10.32517  132.2279  2.492027e-20  1.023393e-18
```

The following R codes use the glmLRT() function with the contrast argument to compare smokers versus non-smokers.

```
> qlf_lrt <- glmLRT(fit, contrast=c(-1,1))
> topTags(qlf_lrt)
Coefficient:  -1*(Intercept) 1*groupSmoker
         logFC    logCPM        LR       PValue          FDR
411   20.27118  12.14801  73.23177  1.152849e-17  7.101551e-15
5227  18.24855  10.97486  64.71055  8.674936e-16  2.671880e-13
330   17.93663  10.85406  63.48383  1.616884e-15  3.002041e-13
1724  17.85291  10.82525  63.11546  1.949377e-15  3.002041e-13
4363  17.19547  10.61836  60.40577  7.718646e-15  9.509372e-13
4816  17.07590  10.59608  59.72834  1.088973e-14  1.118013e-12
2047  17.33654  10.85711  58.56713  1.964718e-14  1.722583e-12
913   16.82513  10.55138  58.31168  2.237121e-14  1.722583e-12
2775  16.62499  10.50933  57.38676  3.580098e-14  2.450378e-12
4697  16.52253  10.47702  57.16818  4.000920e-14  2.464567e-12
```

Below we illustrate an alternative way to define a coefficient for each level of groups using the model.matrix() function. The argument "0+ group" tells the function: not to include an intercept column, instead to include a column for each group.

```
> #another design
> design1 <- model.matrix(~0+group, data=y$samples)
> colnames(design1) <- levels(y1$samples$group)
> design1
             NonSmoker Smoker
ESC_1.1_OPL          1       0
ESC_1.3_OPL          0       1
ESC_1.4_OPL          0       1
ESC_1.5_OPL          0       1
ESC_1.6_OPL          0       1
ESC_1.10_OPL         0       1
......

attr(,"assign")
[1] 1 1
attr(,"contrasts")
attr(,"contrasts")$group
[1] "contr.treatment"
```

We conduct the same tests but use an alternative design.

```
> fit1 <- glmQLFit(y1, design1)
> qlf1 <- glmQLFTest(fit1, contrast=c(-1,1))
> topTags(qlf1)
Coefficient:  -1*NonSmoker 1*Smoker
          logFC    logCPM        F       PValue          FDR
411    6.581023 12.14801 41.83656 3.163184e-09 1.948521e-06
898   -5.831264 12.11934 31.54269 1.051140e-07 2.224466e-05
2047   3.960646 10.85711 30.34414 1.738782e-07 2.224466e-05
5227   4.558393 10.97486 31.14861 1.863529e-07 2.224466e-05
5661  -5.829844 11.74643 30.59848 2.181289e-07 2.224466e-05
4363   3.505305 10.61836 29.98538 2.965998e-07 2.224466e-05
330    4.246471 10.85406 29.87519 3.100209e-07 2.224466e-05
1437  -4.904218 11.21345 29.54856 3.335261e-07 2.224466e-05
1280  -3.916511 10.79061 29.36615 3.591945e-07 2.224466e-05
1724   4.162745 10.82525 29.49614 3.611146e-07 2.224466e-05

> FDR1 <- p.adjust(qlf1$table$PValue, method="BH")
> sum(FDR1 < 0.05)
[1] 106

> topTags(qlf1,n=15)
Coefficient:  -1*NonSmoker 1*Smoker
          logFC    logCPM        F       PValue          FDR
411    6.581023 12.14801 41.83656 3.163184e-09 1.948521e-06
898   -5.831264 12.11934 31.54269 1.051140e-07 2.224466e-05
2047   3.960646 10.85711 30.34414 1.738782e-07 2.224466e-05
5227   4.558393 10.97486 31.14861 1.863529e-07 2.224466e-05
5661  -5.829844 11.74643 30.59848 2.181289e-07 2.224466e-05
4363   3.505305 10.61836 29.98538 2.965998e-07 2.224466e-05
330    4.246471 10.85406 29.87519 3.100209e-07 2.224466e-05
1437  -4.904218 11.21345 29.54856 3.335261e-07 2.224466e-05
1280  -3.916511 10.79061 29.36615 3.591945e-07 2.224466e-05
1724   4.162745 10.82525 29.49614 3.611146e-07 2.224466e-05
3427  -5.304055 11.42595 29.11452 3.979515e-07 2.228528e-05
4816   3.385737 10.59608 26.99928 9.986558e-07 5.126433e-05
292   -3.660121 10.71986 24.57597 2.622920e-06 1.158191e-04
990   -4.061853 11.02059 24.04396 2.632253e-06 1.158191e-04
1840  -3.814417 10.78399 23.87888 3.527299e-06 1.387900e-04

> qlf1_lrt <- glmLRT(fit1, contrast=c(-1,1))
> topTags(qlf1_lrt)
Coefficient:  -1*NonSmoker 1*Smoker
          logFC    logCPM       LR       PValue          FDR
411    6.581023 12.14801 41.89863 9.613021e-11 5.921621e-08
5661  -5.829844 11.74643 32.12473 1.445855e-08 4.453233e-06
898   -5.831264 12.11934 28.88847 7.666809e-08 1.417283e-05
3427  -5.304055 11.42595 28.53476 9.203134e-08 1.417283e-05
1437  -4.904218 11.21345 26.08075 3.274322e-07 3.871834e-05
5227   4.558393 10.97486 25.80798 3.771267e-07 3.871834e-05
330    4.246471 10.85406 23.82571 1.054646e-06 9.280885e-05
1724   4.162745 10.82525 23.20645 1.455082e-06 1.120413e-04
1280  -3.916511 10.79061 19.88884 8.207813e-06 5.519126e-04
2047   3.960646 10.85711 19.72132 8.959620e-06 5.519126e-04
```

Step 8: Interpret the Results of Differential Expression Analysis with Diagnostic Plots

Once the data have been processed and the dispersion estimates are moderated, we can use diagnostic plots to help interpreting the results of differential abundance analysis. In Chap. 10, we introduced the volcano plot to illustrate relationship between effect size and *p*-value in compositional data analysis. Here, we use MA-plot and volcano plot to help interpret the results of differential expression analysis.

MA-Plot Using the plotSmear()

MA plots is used to visualize high-throughput sequencing analysis. It is a plot of log-fold change (M-values, i.e., the log of the ratio of level counts for each OTU between two samples) against the log-average (A-values, i.e., the average level counts for each OTU across the two samples). In edgeR, the function plotSmear() can visualize the differential abundance data to provide a useful overview for an experiment with a two-group comparison. For illustration, we use the result in the et1 object from above exact test (Fig. 11.5).

```
> da = decideTestsDGE(et1 , p.value = 0.1)
> da_OTUs = rownames(y1)[as.logical(da)]
> plotSmear(et1 , de.tags = da_OTUs, cex = 0.5)
> abline(h = c(-2, 2), col = "blue")
```

Volcano Plot

The "volcano plot" is an effective way to summarize both fold-change and a measure of statistical test, usually with a *p*-value. It is a scatter-plot of the negative $\log_{10}$-transformed p-values from the gene-specific test (on the y-axis) against the $\log_2$ fold change (on the x-axis).

To graph a volcano plot, we first construct a table containing the $\log_2$ fold change and the negative $\log_{10}$-transformed *p*-values:

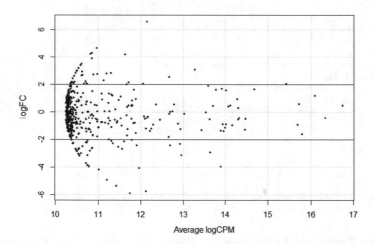

Fig. 11.5 MA-plot generated by the function plotSmear () in edgeR. Red points present those taxa with the adjusted *p*-value less than 0.1. The horizontal blue lines show 4-fold changes

```
> tab = data.frame(logFC = et1$table[, 1], negLogPval = -log10(et1$table[, 3]
))
> head(tab)
    logFC negLogPval
1  0.8494    0.3418
2  0.9128    0.6619
3  0.5919    0.2681
4 -0.1413    0.0000
5 -1.4131    0.5129
6 -5.8721    2.7097
```

Then we use the functions par () and plot () to generate the volcano plot.

```
> par(mar = c(5, 4, 4, 4))
> plot(tab, pch = 16, cex = 0.6, xlab = expression(log[2] ~ fold ~ change),
+       ylab = expression(-log[10] ~ pvalue))
```

Finally, we identify OTUs (points) in the two regions of interest on the plot: dots with large magnitude fold changes (being left- or right-of center) and points with high statistical significance (being towards the top) (Fig. 11.6).

```
> # Log2 fold change and p-value cutoffs
> lfc = 2
> pval = 0.1
```

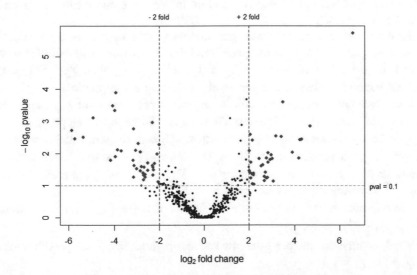

Fig. 11.6 Volcano plot. The red points indicate OTUs of interest that display both large-magnitude fold-changes (x-axis) as well as high statistical significance ($-\log_{10}$ of p-value, y-axis). The dashed green-line shows the p-value cutoff ($pval = 0.1$) with points above the line having p-value < 0.1 and points below the line having p-value > 0.1. The vertical dashed blue lines shows 2-fold changes

```
> # Selecting interest OTUs
> sig_OTUs = (abs(tab$logFC) > lfc & tab$negLogPval > -log10(pval))
> # Identifying the selected OTUs
> points(tab[sig_OTUs, ], pch = 16, cex = 0.8, col = "red")
> abline(h = -log10(pval), col = "green3", lty = 2)
> abline(v = c(-lfc, lfc), col = "blue", lty = 2)
> mtext(paste("pval =", pval), side = 4, at = -log10(pval), cex = 0.8,
line = 0.5, las = 1)
> mtext(c(paste("-", lfc, "fold"), paste("+", lfc, "fold")), side = 3,
at = c(-lfc, lfc),
+         cex = 0.8, line = 0.5)
```

11.4   NB Model in DESeq and DESeq2

11.4.1   NB Model in DESeq

Similar in edgeR, Anders and Huber (2010) proposed a NB model to account for biological variations for high-throughput sequencing count data via the relationship of mean and variance:$Var(Y_{ij}) = \mu_{ij}(1 + \mu_{ij}\phi_i)$. Instead of using a single proportionality constant ϕ_i that is the same throughout the experiment and can be estimated from the data in edgeR, DESeq extends this model by allowing more general, data-driven relationships of variance and mean. Variance and mean are linked by local linear regression.

As the above NB model under genomic data, let's Y_{ij} present the number of reads in sample j that assigned to gene i, and the expectation value of the observed counts for gene i in sample j is μ_{ij} and $Var(Y_{ij}) = \sigma_{ij}^2$, then $Y_{ij} \sim NB(\mu_{ij}, \sigma_{ij}^2)$. The NB method in DESeq is based on the following assumptions:

First, decompose μ_{ij} into a condition-dependent per-gene value $q_{i,\rho(j)}$ and a size factor s_j and assume that μ_{ij} is the product of a condition-dependent per-gene value $q_{i,\rho(j)}$ and a size factor s_j: $\mu_{ij} = q_{i,\rho(j)}s_j$, where $\rho(j)$ is the experimental condition of sample j, $q_{i,\rho(j)}$ is proportional to the expectation value of the true concentration of fragments from gene i under condition $\rho(j)$. The size factor s_j represents the coverage, or sampling depth, of library j.

Second, decompose the variance σ_{ij}^2 into shot noise (μ_{ij}) and raw variance $(s_j^2 v_{i,\rho(j)})$: $\sigma_{ij}^2 = \mu_{ij} + s_j^2 v_{i,\rho(j)}$.

Third, assume that the per-gene raw variance parameter $v_{i,\rho}$ is a smooth function of $q_i, \rho : v_{i,\rho(j)} = v_\rho(q_{i,\rho(j)})$.

After decomposition of NB parameters in genomic data setting, the model has three sets of parameters: size factors s_j, strength parameters $q_{i\rho}$ and the smooth functions v_ρ, which are estimated from the data. Especially, each size factor estimate s_j is computed as the median of the ratios of the j-th sample's counts to those of the pseudo-reference sample obtained by taking the geometric mean across samples. $q_{i\rho}$ is estimated by averaging the counts from the samples j corresponding to condition ρ, then transforms it to the common scale. The smooth function v_ρ is obtained by using a local regression. The approach of statistical testing for differential expression (abundance) is similar as in edgeR and is analogous to what is taken by other conditioned tests (e.g., Fisher's exact test).

In summary, both DESeq and edgeR assume a NB distribution and incorporate information sharing in the dispersion estimation. However, there are two main distinctions of DESeq from edgeR: (1) DESeq adds the assumption of a locally linear relationship between over-dispersion and mean expression levels of the data; and (2) the way of the information sharing in the dispersion estimation accounts for the main difference between the two methods. Compared to edgeR, DESeq first uses either parametric or local regression to estimate the dispersion by modeling the observed mean variance relationship for the genes in the data set. The dispersion of a gene is conservatively defined as the largest of the fitted values and the individual dispersion estimate for the gene.

11.4.2 NB Model in DESeq2

Love, Huber and Anders proposed the DESeq2 NB model for differential analysis of count data (Love et al. 2014). This method is a successor to DESeq and uses shrinkage estimation for dispersions and fold changes to improve stability and interpretability of estimates. The authors emphasized that the DESeq2 method is focused on the strength rather than the mere presence of differential expression, thus it enables to assess quantitative differences across groups of samples.

11.4.2.1 Model and Normalization

With the same count matrix, one row for each gene i and one column for each sample j, as DESeq and edgeR, let us Y_{ij} present the number of reads in sample j that assigned to gene i, then

$$Y_{ij} \sim NB(\mu_{ij}, \phi_i \mu_{ij}^2), \tag{11.12}$$

where μ_{ij} is fitted mean, is taken as a quantity q_{ij}, proportional to the concentration of cDNA fragments from the gene in the sample, scaled by a normalization factor (library size factor) s_{ij}, i.e., $\mu_{ij} = s_{ij} q_{ij}$.

If we assume all genes in a sample having the same constant s_j, which accounts for differences in sequencing depth between samples, then these size factors can be estimated by the median-of-ratios method already used in DESeq. However, it is better to calculate gene-specific normalization factors s_{ij} to account for sources of technical biases, such as differing dependence on GC content or gene length. DESeq2 fits the data by a generalized linear model (GLM) (McCullagh and Nelder 1989). With a logarithmic link, q_{ij} is modeled as $\log_2(q_{ij}) = x_{j.}\beta_i$, where $x_{j.}$ is model matrix column for sample j, β_i is moderated log-fold change for gene i.

11.4.2.2 Estimation of Dispersions

The gene-specific dispersion parameter ϕ_i in $Var(Y_{ij}) = \mu_{ij}(1 + \mu_{ij}\phi_i)$ is to estimate the within-group variability, i.e., the variability between replicates. DESeq2 assumes that genes of similar average expression strength have the similar dispersion and fits the gene-specific dispersion towards the average dispersion, using an empirical Bayes approach. It estimates the width of the prior distribution from data and automatically controls the amount of shrinkage, based on the observed properties of data.

The details of formula for estimating dispersions are beyond the book. For simplicity, first, the dispersion parameter ϕ_i is assumed to follow a lognormal prior distribution that is centered around a trend that depends on the gene's mean normalized read count. Next, for a gene i, a negative binomial GLM without an logarithmic fold change (LFC) prior for the design matrix X to the gene's count data is fitted to get a gene-wise dispersion estimate. Then, the final dispersion estimate is obtained by forming a logarithmic posterior for the dispersion from the Cox-Reid adjusted logarithmic likelihood and the logarithmic prior (Love et al. 2014).

11.4.2.3 Shrinkage Estimation of Logarithmic Fold Changes

A common difficulty in analyzing high-throughput sequencing data is the strong variance of the LFC estimation for genes with low read count. DESeq2 overcomes this issue by shrinking LFC estimates toward zero in a manner so that shrinkage is stronger when the available information for a gene is low due to lower counts, possible higher dispersion, or fewer degrees of freedom.

To incorporate empirical Bayes shrinkage of LFCs, DESeq2 postulates a zero-centered normal prior for the coefficients β_i of model $\log_2(q_{ij}) = x_{j.}\beta_i$ that represent LFCs (i.e., typically, all coefficients except for the intercept β_{i0}): $\beta_i \sim N(0, \sigma^2)$. Here, σ is for the empirical prior widths. The shrunken LFCs and their standard errors are used in the Wald tests for differential expression or abundance.

11.4.2.4 Hypothesis Testing in DESeq2

After GLMs are fitted for each gene, DESeq2 uses a Wald test for significance of differential expression or abundance. This is the default inference method in the package DESeq2 and one of main changes compared to the (older) version DESeq. The Wald test compares the beta estimate β_i (the shrunken estimate of LFC) divided by its estimated standard error SE (β_i), resulting in a z-statistic, which is compared to a standard normal distribution. It allows testing of individual coefficients and contrasts of coefficients. The p-values from the subset of genes are adjusted for multiple testing, using the Benjamini and Hochberg method.

11.5 The DESeq and DESeq2 Packages

11.5.1 Introduction

DESeq is another variance stabilization technique based on a NB model that was recommended and adapted for microbiome count data (McMurdie and Holmes 2014). With the variance stabilization technique, the DESeq and DESeq2 packages have the capability to model overdispersed microbiome data from 16S rRNA gene sequencing.

The differential abundance analysis in DESeq and DESeq2 needs raw counts as input. Generally, homoskedastic data works best for exploratory statistical methods for multidimensional data, especially methods for data visualization (e.g., clustering and ordination). However, microbiome data and other DNA-and RNA gene sequencing data are sparse with many zero values. It is challenging to use standard statistical methods to analyze these data. To avoid the issue, a simple strategy is to take the logarithm of the normalized count values plus a small pseudocount. DESeq2 offers three transformation methods to transform count data. One method is to use the pseudocounts to transform count data, i.e., in the form $y = \log 2(n + n_0)$, where n represents the count values and n_0 is a positive constant.

The genes or taxa with low counts often show the strongest relative differences between samples, and tend to dominate the analysis results. DESeq2 has offered two alternative approaches, the regularized logarithm (rlog) and variance stabilizing transformations (VST), to solve to the potential problems. These approaches also offer more theoretical justification and rationale of choosing the parameter to plug in n_0 above. For genes (taxa) with high counts, the rlog transformation differs not much from an ordinary $\log_2$ transformation. For genes with lower counts, however, the values are shrunken towards the genes' averages across all samples. The algorithm is implemented via an empirical Bayesian prior in the form of a ridge penalty to ensure the rlog-transformed data being approximately homoscedastic.

The nbinomTest() in DESeq and the nbinomWaldTest() in DESeq2 are two main functions implement the NB methods. The nbinomTest() is a NB conditioned test similar to the edgeR test above. The nbinomWaldTest is a NB Wald Test using standard maximum likelihood estimates for GLM coefficients assuming a zero-mean normal prior distribution. DESeq and DESeq2 use the relative log expression (RLE) normalization method (Anders and Huber 2010), which is implemented via the function estimateSizeFactors().

11.5.2   Step-by-Step Implementing DESeq2

The DESeq2 needs count data in the form of a rectangular table (matrix) of integer values as input data. The table cell in the i-th row and the j-th column of the table tells how many reads have been mapped to gene (OTU) i in sample j. The count tables typically generated from RNA-Seq or other high-throughput sequencing experiments. Like in the edgeR, the DESeq2 also need several procedures to conduct differential abundance analysis of microbiome data. Here, we use the same data set implemented in the edgeR package and conduct the analysis step-by-step, using the DESeq2:

Step 1: Create the Count Table
The example data sets consist of two parts: otu-table and meta-table. Below, we show how to build a DESeqDataSet object from these two tables. The object is needed for analysis using the DESeq2 package.

First, load the package GUniFrac and bring otu-table to R workplace.

```
> library("DESeq2")
> library(GUniFrac)
> data(throat.otu.tab)
> otu_tab<-throat.otu.tab
> head(otu_tab)
             4695 2983 2554 3315 879 1313 5661 4125 2115 3309
ESC_1.1_OPL     1    0    0    0    0    0    0    0    0    0
ESC_1.3_OPL     0    0    0    0    0    0    0    0    0    0
ESC_1.4_OPL     0    0    0    0    0    0    0    0    0    0
ESC_1.5_OPL     1    0    0    0    0    0    0    0    0    0
ESC_1.6_OPL     0    0    0    0    0    0    0    0    0    0
ESC_1.10_OPL    0    0    0    0    0    0    0    0    0    0
......
```

Then, convert the countData object to a matrix in order to use the function DESeqDataSetFromMatrix() to create a DESeq object.

```
> countData<-as(otu_tab, "matrix")
> head(countData)
             4695 2983 2554 3315 879 1313 5661 4125 2115 3309
ESC_1.1_OPL     1    0    0    0    0    0    0    0    0    0
ESC_1.3_OPL     0    0    0    0    0    0    0    0    0    0
ESC_1.4_OPL     0    0    0    0    0    0    0    0    0    0
ESC_1.5_OPL     1    0    0    0    0    0    0    0    0    0
ESC_1.6_OPL     0    0    0    0    0    0    0    0    0    0
ESC_1.10_OPL    0    0    0    0    0    0    0    0    0    0
```

```
> countData<-(t(countData))#DESeq2 need taxa(genes=rows) by samples(=columns)
format
> head(countData)
      ESC_1.1_OPL ESC_1.3_OPL ESC_1.4_OPL ESC_1.5_OPL ESC_1.6_OPL
4695            1           0           0           1           0
2983            0           0           0           0           0
2554            0           0           0           0           0
3315            0           0           0           0           0
879             0           0           0           0           0
1313            0           0           0           0           0
......
```

In this count table, each row represents a gene (OTU), each column represents a sequenced RNA library, and the values give the raw numbers of sequencing reads that were mapped to the respective gene (OTU) in each library.

Step 2: Create the Sample Metadata Table

```
> data(throat.meta)
> head(throat.meta)
             BarcodeSequence LinkerPrimerSequence SmokingStatus
ESC_1.1_OPL        ACGTCATG      CTGCTGCCTYCCGTA      NonSmoker
ESC_1.3_OPL        ACTCGTGA      CTGCTGCCTYCCGTA         Smoker
ESC_1.4_OPL        ACTGCTGA      CTGCTGCCTYCCGTA         Smoker
ESC_1.5_OPL        AGACTGTC      CTGCTGCCTYCCGTA         Smoker
ESC_1.6_OPL        AGCTGATC      CTGCTGCCTYCCGTA         Smoker
ESC_1.10_OPL       ATGCGCTA      CTGCTGCCTYCCGTA         Smoker
......
```

The metadata mainly consist of the sample information of our interest, here the smoking status. We extract it from meta-table.

```
> group<-throat.meta$SmokingStatus
> head(group)
[1] NonSmoker Smoker     Smoker     Smoker     Smoker     Smoker
Levels: NonSmoker Smoker
```

Step 3: Build the DESeq2 Object
In the sequencing experiment, the bioinformatics tools produce the count tables, called count files, count matrix or SummarizedExperiment, depending on the used tools. Different kinds of outputs need different DESeq2 functions to input to R workplace. For example, both packages GenomicAlignments (Bioc) and easyRNASeq (Bioc) generate SummarizedExperiment output, which needs the DESeqDataSet() input function to read. The HTSeq (Python) package produces count files, the function DESeqDataSetFromHTSeq() is required, whereas the output of Rsubread (Bioc) is a count matrix, needing the function DESeqDataSetFromMatrix(). Count matrix is easy to understand. Here, we briefly introduce the output SummarizedExperiment.

A SummarizedExperiment is an object. One of its subclasses is the DESeqDataSet, the data object of the DESeq2. The object SummarizedExperiment has three components: the assay(s) (e.g., counts), the rowData and the colData. The assay(s) contains the matrix (or matrices) of summarized values, the rowData contains information about the genomic ranges, and the colData contains information about the samples or experiments. The first row of each data table represents the ids. The first row of colData (ids) lines up with the first column of the assay.

The DESeqDataSet object is built on the SummarizedExperiment object. It must have an associated design formula to tell which variables in the column metadata table (colData) specify the experimental design and how these factors should be used in the analysis. The formula is like a typical "lm" formula in R: a tilde ($\sim$) followed by the variables with plus signs between them. To effectively use the default settings of the package, for two or more variables, put the variable of interest at the end of the formula and the control level at the first level. The DESeqDataSet can be constructed either from a SummarizedExperiment object or more generally, from a count table (i.e., matrix) and a column metadata table which have been loaded into R.

After both count table and sample metadata table are created, it is critical to make the row names of metadata dataframe to equal to the column names of the countData, which makes the i-th gene (OTU) to match the j sample.

```
> metaData<-data.frame(row.names=colnames(countData),group=group)
> head(metaData)
                     group
ESC_1.1_OPL   NonSmoker
ESC_1.3_OPL     Smoker
ESC_1.4_OPL     Smoker
ESC_1.5_OPL     Smoker
ESC_1.6_OPL     Smoker
ESC_1.10_OPL    Smoker
```

We now have both "countdata" (a table with the read counts) and "coldata" (a table with metadata on the count table's columns). These are all the ingredients what we need for our data object in a form that is suitable for analysis, To construct the data object from the matrix of counts and the metadata table, we call library DESeq2 and use the function DESeqDataSetFromMatrix() as below:

```
> library("DESeq2")
> dds <- DESeqDataSetFromMatrix(countData = countData,
+                                colData = metaData,
+                                design = ~ group)
```

Step 4: Filter the Data
We have already created a count table and fed it into a DESeq2 object, the next step is to filter the data. The datasets have passed the quality control, so we do not expect this procedure conducted below will affect the data. The codes are just for illustration.

```
> dds <- dds[rowSums(counts(dds)) > 0,]
> dds
```

```
class: DESeqDataSet
dim: 856 60
metadata(1): version
assays(5): counts mu cooks replaceCounts replaceCooks
rownames(856): 4695 2983 ... 434 3447
rowData names(22): baseMean baseVar ... maxCooks replace
colnames(60): ESC_1.1_OPL ESC_1.3_OPL ... ESC_1.69_OPL
    ESC_1.70_OPL
colData names(3): group sizeFactor replaceable
```

Step 5: Normalize the Count Data

DESeq2 uses the "median ratio method" described in Anders and Huber (2010) to estimate the size factors. It first defines a virtual reference sample by taking the median of each gene's values across samples and then computes size factors as the median of ratios of each sample to the reference sample (Anders and Huber 2010). An offset is built in the statistical model of DESeq2.

Generally, the ratios of size factors roughly match those of the library sizes. Thus, the size factors are considered as a measure of library. It suggests that the libraries have been sequenced equally deeply if all size factors are roughly equal to one.

The codes below compute the size factors:

```
> dds <- estimateSizeFactors(dds)
```

The estimated size factors can be accessed using the accessor function sizeFactors().

```
> sizeFactors(dds)
  ESC_1.1_OPL   ESC_1.3_OPL   ESC_1.4_OPL   ESC_1.5_OPL   ESC_1.6_OPL
    0.0569773     1.8232736     1.5953644     1.6523417     0.4558184
 ESC_1.10_OPL  ESC_1.11_OPL  ESC_1.12_OPL  ESC_1.13_OPL  ESC_1.14_OPL
    2.3360693     2.9058423     1.5953644     0.3418638     1.3104779
 ESC_1.15_OPL  ESC_1.18_OPL  ESC_1.19_OPL  ESC_1.20_OPL  ESC_1.21_OPL
    0.3988411     4.1023656     2.5070012     0.5697730     1.0825687
 ESC_1.22_OPL  ESC_1.23_OPL  ESC_1.24_OPL  ESC_1.25_OPL  ESC_1.26_OPL
    2.3360693     0.5697730     1.2535006     3.5895699     3.8744564
 ESC_1.27_OPL  ESC_1.28_OPL  ESC_1.29_OPL  ESC_1.30_OPL  ESC_1.31_OPL
    0.4558184     0.5127957     0.1139546     0.5697730     0.4558184
 ESC_1.32_OPL  ESC_1.33_OPL  ESC_1.34_OPL  ESC_1.35_OPL  ESC_1.36_OPL
    0.0569773     5.1849343     0.7976822     0.9686141     0.6267503
 ESC_1.37_OPL  ESC_1.39_OPL  ESC_1.40_OPL  ESC_1.42_OPL  ESC_1.43_OPL
    3.5325926     3.3616607     1.5383871     1.7093190     1.8802509
 ESC_1.44_OPL  ESC_1.45_OPL  ESC_1.46_OPL  ESC_1.47_OPL  ESC_1.48_OPL
    3.8744564     5.7547073     0.6837276     1.8232736     0.1139546
 ESC_1.49_OPL  ESC_1.50_OPL  ESC_1.51_OPL  ESC_1.52_OPL  ESC_1.53_OPL
    0.6837276     2.1651374     3.6465472     0.1709319     0.7407049
 ESC_1.55_OPL  ESC_1.56_OPL  ESC_1.57_OPL  ESC_1.58_OPL  ESC_1.59_OPL
    0.8546595     2.9628196     4.5012067     1.7093190     1.3674552
 ESC_1.60_OPL  ESC_1.61_OPL  ESC_1.62_OPL  ESC_1.63_OPL  ESC_1.64_OPL
    0.2848865     1.8232736     0.0569773     0.4558184     2.2221147
 ESC_1.65_OPL  ESC_1.67_OPL  ESC_1.68_OPL  ESC_1.69_OPL  ESC_1.70_OPL
    1.0255914     2.1081601     0.7976822     1.4244325     0.1139546
```

You can obtain the normalized count values by dividing each column of the count table by the corresponding size factor. Then you can re-scale it to give a counts-per million interpretation.

Step 6: Estimate the Dispersion

DESeq2 also uses the NB model. The first task in the analysis of abundance microbiome data is to estimate the dispersion parameter for each OTU. When a NB model is fitted, within-group variability, i.e., the variability between replicates, is modeled by the dispersion parameter ϕ_i. The dispersion parameters are estimated using the function estimateDispersions():

```
> dds<- estimateDispersions(dds)
```

Step 7: Test the Differential Abundance

In DESeq2, we can make a single call using the function DESeq() to estimate the size factors, the dispersion for each gene, to fit a generalized linear model and among others. The returned results table contains all the fitted information and can be extracted out.

DESeq2 conducts the differential expression analysis based on the NB distribution. It performs a default analysis through the following steps:

1. estimation of size factors: estimateSizeFactors
2. estimation of dispersion: estimateDispersions
3. Negative Binomial GLM fitting and Wald statistics: nbinomWaldTest

After the DESeq function returns a DESeqDataSet object, results tables ($\log_2$ fold changes and p-values) can be generated using the results() function. An independent filtering and p-value adjustment for multiple test correction also can be performed. One sample of use is as below:

DESeq(object, test = c("Wald", "LRT"), fitType = c("parametric", "local", "mean"))

where,

object = a DESeqDataSet object.

test = either "Wald" or "LRT", which will then use either Wald significance tests (defined by nbinomWaldTest()) , or the likelihood ratio test on the difference in deviance between a full and reduced model formula (defined by nbinomLRT()).

fitType either = "parametric", "local", or "mean" for the type of fitting of dispersions to the mean intensity.

Run the Function DESeq()

Before run the DESeq(), make sure that "NonSmoker" is the first level in the condition factor, so that the default $\log_2$ fold changes are calculated as "Smoker" over "NonSmoker" and not the other way around. We can use the following two ways to set the factor levels to make sure to get fold change Smoker-NonSmoker: either by

```
> dds$group <- relevel(dds$group, "NonSmoker") or by
> dds$group <- factor(dds$group, levels = c("NonSmoker", "Smoker"))
```

Now we are ready to run the abundance analysis by making a single call to the function DESeq():

```
> dds <- DESeq(dds)
```

Extract the Results Table

The following R codes call the results () function to generate and extract the results tables including the results with $\log_2$ fold changes, p-values and adjusted p-values. Other results, adjusted p-values according to the Benjamini-Hochberg rule to control the FDR, also can be extracted. Without providing any arguments, this function will extract the estimated $\log_2$ fold changes and p-values for the last variable in the design formula.

```
> res <- results(dds)
> res
log2 fold change (MLE): group Smoker vs NonSmoker
Wald test p-value: group Smoker vs NonSmoker
DataFrame with 856 rows and 6 columns
          baseMean log2FoldChange     lfcSE       stat    pvalue      padj
         <numeric>      <numeric> <numeric>  <numeric> <numeric> <numeric>
4695    0.40826356     0.81077907  1.964026 0.412814755 0.6797423        NA
2983    0.07751625     0.66023009  2.935580 0.224906156 0.8220523        NA
2554    0.09788960     0.50406423  2.812641 0.179213864 0.8577698        NA
3315    0.05745814     0.25158195  2.936180 0.085683412 0.9317181        NA
879     0.01290504     0.01563854  2.936103 0.005326293 0.9957503        NA
...            ...            ...       ...         ...       ...       ...
596    75.26585401     0.2175720 0.5196639   0.4186783 0.6754513 0.8384913
4225    0.01125054     0.4340144 2.9364195   0.1478039 0.8824975        NA
3675    0.01470834     0.2816641 2.9362770   0.0959256 0.9235797        NA
434     0.40220696    -0.4274031 2.9346973  -0.1456379 0.8842073        NA
3447    0.01500073     0.4864376 2.9362344   0.1656671 0.8684189        NA
```

More information on results columns, such as which variables and tests were used, can be found by calling the function mcols() on the results object. All row-wise calculated values (intermediate dispersion calculations, coefficients, standard errors, etc.) are stored in the DESeqDataSet object, e.g., dds in this case. These values are accessible by calling the mcols () function on dds. Descriptions of the columns are accessible by two calls to the mcols().

```
> mcols(res, use.names=TRUE)
DataFrame with 6 rows and 2 columns
                           type
                      <character>
baseMean           intermediate
log2FoldChange          results
lfcSE                   results
stat                    results
pvalue                  results
padj                    results

                                                    description
                                                    <character>
baseMean                        mean of normalized counts for all samples
log2FoldChange log2 fold change (MLE): group Smoker vs NonSmoker
lfcSE                            standard error: group Smoker vs NonSmoker
stat                             Wald statistic: group Smoker vs NonSmoker
pvalue                    Wald test p-value: group Smoker vs NonSmoker
padj                                                BH adjusted p-values
```

The first column, baseMean, is just the average of the normalized count values, dividing by size factors, taken over all samples. The remaining four columns refer to a specific contrast: the comparison of the levels Smoker versus NonSmoker of the factor variable group.

The column log2FoldChange is the effect size estimate. It tells us how much the OTU's abundance seems to be different due to group with Smoker in comparison to NonSmoker. This value is reported on a logarithmic scale to base 2. Thus, for example, a $\log_2$ fold change of 2 means that the OTU's abundance is increased by a multiplicative factor of $2^2 = 4$.

We extract some results of interest as below.

```
> mcols(dds,use.names=TRUE)[1:4,1:4]
DataFrame with 4 rows and 4 columns
         baseMean    baseVar   allZero dispGeneEst
        <numeric>  <numeric> <logical>   <numeric>
4695  0.40826356  5.2748513     FALSE 19.64448160
2983  0.07751625  0.1360280     FALSE  0.00000001
2554  0.09788960  0.1639122     FALSE  0.00000001
3315  0.05745814  0.1048561     FALSE  0.00000001


> substr(names(mcols(dds)),1,10)
 [1] "baseMean"    "baseVar"     "allZero"     "dispGeneEs"  "dispFit"
 [6] "dispersion"  "dispIter"    "dispOutlie"  "dispMAP"     "Intercept"
[11] "group_Smok"  "SE_Interce"  "SE_group_S"  "WaldStatis"  "WaldStatis"
[16] "WaldPvalue"  "WaldPvalue"  "betaConv"    "betaIter"    "deviance"
[21] "maxCooks"    "replace"


> head(assays(dds)[["mu"]])
       ESC_1.1_OPL ESC_1.3_OPL ESC_1.4_OPL ESC_1.5_OPL ESC_1.6_OPL
4695    0.01229007   0.6898793   0.6036444   0.6252031  0.17246982
2983    0.01037213   0.5245259   0.4589601   0.4753516  0.13113147
2554    0.01134357   0.5147996   0.4504496   0.4665371  0.12869989
3315    0.01134877   0.4323469   0.3783035   0.3918144  0.10808672
879     0.01226195   0.3966589   0.3470765   0.3594721  0.09916472
1313    0.01505693   0.4323476   0.3783041   0.3918150  0.10808690
```

```
> head(dispersions(dds))
[1] 25.98183 60.00000 54.94283 60.00000 60.00000 60.00000
> head(mcols(dds)$dispersion)
[1] 25.98183 60.00000 54.94283 60.00000 60.00000 60.00000

> sizeFactors(dds)
  ESC_1.1_OPL   ESC_1.3_OPL   ESC_1.4_OPL   ESC_1.5_OPL   ESC_1.6_OPL
    0.0569773     1.8232736     1.5953644     1.6523417     0.4558184
 ESC_1.10_OPL  ESC_1.11_OPL  ESC_1.12_OPL  ESC_1.13_OPL  ESC_1.14_OPL
    2.3360693     2.9058423     1.5953644     0.3418638     1.3104779
 ESC_1.15_OPL  ESC_1.18_OPL  ESC_1.19_OPL  ESC_1.20_OPL  ESC_1.21_OPL
    0.3988411     4.1023656     2.5070012     0.5697730     1.0825687
 ESC_1.22_OPL  ESC_1.23_OPL  ESC_1.24_OPL  ESC_1.25_OPL  ESC_1.26_OPL
    2.3360693     0.5697730     1.2535006     3.5895699     3.8744564
 ESC_1.27_OPL  ESC_1.28_OPL  ESC_1.29_OPL  ESC_1.30_OPL  ESC_1.31_OPL
    0.4558184     0.5127957     0.1139546     0.5697730     0.4558184
 ESC_1.32_OPL  ESC_1.33_OPL  ESC_1.34_OPL  ESC_1.35_OPL  ESC_1.36_OPL
    0.0569773     5.1849343     0.7976822     0.9686141     0.6267503
 ESC_1.37_OPL  ESC_1.39_OPL  ESC_1.40_OPL  ESC_1.42_OPL  ESC_1.43_OPL
    3.5325926     3.3616607     1.5383871     1.7093190     1.8802509
 ESC_1.44_OPL  ESC_1.45_OPL  ESC_1.46_OPL  ESC_1.47_OPL  ESC_1.48_OPL
    3.8744564     5.7547073     0.6837276     1.8232736     0.1139546
 ESC_1.49_OPL  ESC_1.50_OPL  ESC_1.51_OPL  ESC_1.52_OPL  ESC_1.53_OPL
    0.6837276     2.1651374     3.6465472     0.1709319     0.7407049
 ESC_1.55_OPL  ESC_1.56_OPL  ESC_1.57_OPL  ESC_1.58_OPL  ESC_1.59_OPL
    0.8546595     2.9628196     4.5012067     1.7093190     1.3674552
 ESC_1.60_OPL  ESC_1.61_OPL  ESC_1.62_OPL  ESC_1.63_OPL  ESC_1.64_OPL
    0.2848865     1.8232736     0.0569773     0.4558184     2.2221147
 ESC_1.65_OPL  ESC_1.67_OPL  ESC_1.68_OPL  ESC_1.69_OPL  ESC_1.70_OPL
    1.0255914     2.1081601     0.7976822     1.4244325     0.1139546


> head(coef(dds))
      Intercept group_Smoker_vs_NonSmoker
4695 -2.212894                0.81077907
2983 -2.457675                0.66023009
2554 -2.328513                0.50406423
3315 -2.327852                0.25158195
879  -2.216199                0.01563854
1313 -1.919960               -0.15630774
```

Compare Differential Abundance Between Groups Using Contrast

We can compare any two levels of a variable by specifying three values: the variable name, the numerator name, and the denominator name. The contrast results can be extracted using the function results(). The following results show the $\log_2$ of the fold change of Smoker over NonSmoker. The extracted results are same as those extracted by using res <- results(dds) because these two ways are actually same.

```
> res <- results(dds, contrast = c("group", "Smoker", "NonSmoker") )
> res
log2 fold change (MLE): group Smoker vs NonSmoker
Wald test p-value: group Smoker vs NonSmoker
DataFrame with 856 rows and 6 columns
          baseMean log2FoldChange     lfcSE         stat    pvalue      padj
         <numeric>      <numeric> <numeric>    <numeric> <numeric> <numeric>
    4695 0.40826356     0.81077907  1.964026 0.412814755 0.6797423        NA
    2983 0.07751625     0.66023009  2.935580 0.224906156 0.8220523        NA
    2554 0.09788960     0.50406423  2.812641 0.179213864 0.8577698        NA
    3315 0.05745814     0.25158195  2.936180 0.085683412 0.9317181        NA
     879 0.01290504     0.01563854  2.936103 0.005326293 0.9957503        NA
     ...        ...            ...       ...          ...       ...       ...
     596 75.26585401     0.2175720 0.5196639    0.4186783 0.6754513 0.8384913
    4225 0.01125054     0.4340144 2.9364195    0.1478039 0.8824975        NA
    3675 0.01470834     0.2816641 2.9362770    0.0959256 0.9235797        NA
     434 0.40220696    -0.4274031 2.9346973   -0.1456379 0.8842073        NA
    3447 0.01500073     0.4864376 2.9362344    0.1656671 0.8684189        NA
```

Adjust *p*-Values Using FDR

Let's check how many OTUs that have a *p*-value below and greater than 0.01.

```
> sum(res$pvalue < 0.01, na.rm=TRUE )
[1] 17
> table(is.na(res$pvalue))
FALSE
  856
```

As edgeR, DESeq2 uses the Benjamini-Hochberg(HB) method to adjust FDR. In hypothesis testing, we usually set up a small value, say, 0.01, as threshold. Briefly, the FDR method calculates for each OTU an adjusted *p*-value which answers the following question: if one called significant all OTUs with a *p*-value less than or equal to this OTU's *p*-value threshold, what would be the fraction of false positives (FDR) among them? The BH-adjusted *p*-values are given in the column FDR of the test object.

Now, if the null hypothesis is true for all OTUs, i.e., no OTU is affected by smoking. Then, by the definition of *p*-value, we expect up to 1% of the OTU to have a *p*-value below 0.01. This amounts to 8.56 OTUs. Thus, if we consider these 17 OTUs with *p*-value less than 0.01 as differentially being abundant, then there should be 8.56/17 = 50% false positives.

Now we consider a fraction of 10% false positives acceptable, that is, all OTUs with an adjusted *p*-value below 0.1 as significant, let's check haw many OTUs there.

```
> table(res[,"padj"] < 0.1)
FALSE TRUE
   85    23
```

In publications, we often report the significant OTUs with the strongest down-regulation and upregulation. We sort the results by the $\log_2$ fold change estimate. Then, head the order to get the significant OTUs with the strongest down-regulation; tail the order to get the significant OTUs with the strongest upregulation.

```
> res_Sig <- res[which(res$padj < 0.1 ),]
> head(res_Sig[order(res_Sig$log2FoldChange),])
log2 fold change (MLE): group Smoker vs NonSmoker
Wald test p-value: group Smoker vs NonSmoker
DataFrame with 6 rows and 6 columns
        baseMean log2FoldChange     lfcSE      stat      pvalue
       <numeric>      <numeric> <numeric> <numeric>   <numeric>
2621   24.466720      -4.375709  1.195949 -3.658775 0.0002534236
797     3.761548      -3.847800  1.555247 -2.474076 0.0133581159
2300   11.930517      -3.791208  1.150284 -3.295889 0.0009811082
4551    5.637375      -3.670423  1.574858 -2.330638 0.0197724787
4357    3.603393      -3.650119  1.278209 -2.855650 0.0042948785
444     3.250048      -2.797241  0.981123 -2.851060 0.0043573687
              padj
         <numeric>
2621   0.005473949
797    0.072735125
2300   0.010595968
4551   0.092844682
4357   0.033613987
444    0.033613987


> tail(res_Sig[order( res_Sig$log2FoldChange ),])
log2 fold change (MLE): group Smoker vs NonSmoker
Wald test p-value: group Smoker vs NonSmoker
DataFrame with 6 rows and 6 columns
        baseMean log2FoldChange     lfcSE      stat      pvalue
       <numeric>      <numeric> <numeric> <numeric>   <numeric>
2831   42.999603       3.164360 0.8879625  3.563619 3.657762e-04
1633    4.202140       3.175464 0.9448628  3.360768 7.772617e-04
2434   76.272020       3.181675 0.7098175  4.482384 7.381376e-06
2893    5.182641       3.431377 0.9893132  3.468444 5.234820e-04
171     2.476577       4.257418 1.7694243  2.406103 1.612371e-02
411     4.561144       5.746783 2.1643727  2.655172 7.926787e-03
              padj
         <numeric>
2831   0.0056434045
1633   0.0093271403
2434   0.0007971886
2893   0.0070670066
171    0.0829219216
411    0.0503584097
```

Step 8: Diagnose and Improve the Testing Results

Data visualization and clustering can diagnose and help interpreting the results of differential abundance analysis. Here, we introduce several different plots that are associated with diagnostics, clustering, interpretation of differential abundance analysis.

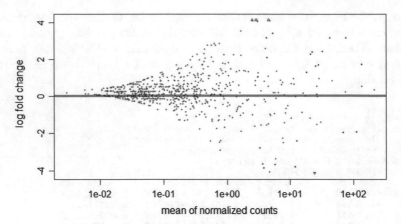

Fig. 11.7 The MA-plot shows the log$_2$ fold changes from the smoking status over the mean of normalized counts, i.e., the average of counts normalized by size factor. Points represent the OTUs. The red points indicate those OTUs with the adjusted *p*-value below a threshold (here 0.1, the default). Points that fall out of the window are plotted as open triangles pointing either up or down. The x axis is the average abundance over all samples, the y axis the log$_2$ fold change between smoker and non smoker

Diagnostic Plot Using the plotMA()
In Sect. 11.3.2, when we implement the edgeR package, a MA-plot is done by the function plotSmear() to visualize the differential abundance data. Here, we use the function plotMA() to review the analysis results. It first transforms the data onto M (log ratio) and A (mean average) scales, then overview the differences of values for comparing the OTUs between Smokers versus Non-smokers (Fig. 11.7).

```
> plotMA(res)
```

Diagnostic Plot Using the plotDispEsts()
The dispersion of a gene (taxon, OTU) measures a gene (taxon, OTU)'s variance. In DESeq2, it is used to model the overall variance of a gene (taxon, OTU)'s count values. The dispersion can be interpreted as the square of the coefficient of biological variation. The DESeq2's dispersion estimates can be plotted by the function plotDispEsts(). The function visualizes DESeq2's dispersion estimates in this way: plots the per-gene dispersion estimates together with the fitted mean-dispersion relationship (Fig. 11.8).

```
> plotDispEsts(dds, ylim = c(1e-2, 1e3))
```

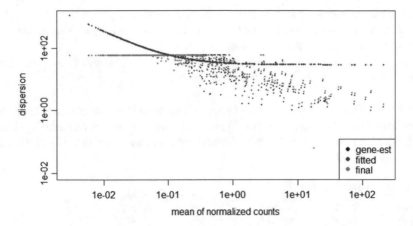

Fig. 11.8 Plot of dispersion estimates. The black points are the dispersion estimates for each OTU as obtained by considering the information from each gene separately. Usually these values fluctuate strongly around their true values. Blue points present the final estimated values. The red trend line is fitted to show how the dispersions dependence on the mean, and then shrink each OTU's estimate towards the red line to obtain the final estimates (blue points). The final estimated values are used in the hypothesis test. Blue circles present the dispersion outliers above the main "cloud" of points. They are OTUs which have high otu-wise dispersion estimates and are therefore not shrunk toward the fitted trend line and therefore are not used for the hypothesis test. We did not see in this case

Clustering with Heatmap

Heatmap is often used to explore the degrees of similarity and more distant relationships among groups of closely related genes (taxa, OTUs in this case). It combines clustering methods with a graphical representation of the count table. In Chap. 7, we illustrate heatmap using the phyloseq package. Here, we use heatmap to cluster OTUs via the DESeq2 package.

The first step to make a heatmap with 16S RNA-seq data is to transform the raw counts of reads to approximately homoskedastic data. The transformation can be done either by the rlog()or varianceStabilizingTransformation(). The latter is recommended by the DESeq2. Below we do rlog and variance stabilizing transformations to transform the data.

```
> rld <- rlog(dds)
> vst <-varianceStabilizingTransformation(dds)
```

To show the effect of the transformation, we do three plots: (1) the first sample against the second by using the log2 () function (after adding 1, to avoid taking the log of zero); (2) rlog-transformed values; and (3) variance-stabilizing transformed values.

```
> par(mfrow = c(1, 3))
> plot(log2( 1+counts(dds, normalized=TRUE)[,1:2] ), main="Ordinary log2
```

```
transformation",col="#00000020", pch=20, cex=0.3 )
>   plot(assay(rld)[,1:2],  main="regularized-logarithm  transformation
(rlog)", col="#00000020", pch=20, cex=0.3 )
>   plot(assay(vst)[,1:2],  main="Variance  stabilizing  transformations
(VST). ",col="#00000020", pch=20, cex=0.3 )
```

The plot shows that sample 1 and sample 2 are positively correlated after the rlog transformation. The function rlogTransform() returns a SummarizedExperiment object which contains the rlog-transformed values in its assay slot. We check these values (Fig. 11.9):

```
> head(assay(rld))[,1-3]
      ESC_1.1_OPL ESC_1.4_OPL ESC_1.5_OPL ESC_1.6_OPL
4695       -1.406      -1.958      -1.755      -1.828
2983       -1.999      -2.194      -2.196      -2.121
2554       -1.923      -2.143      -2.145      -2.060
3315       -2.079      -2.243      -2.245      -2.181
879        -2.172      -2.225      -2.226      -2.205
1313       -1.860      -2.077      -2.079      -1.995
```

Finally, we cluster the OTUs with heatmap below. Several packages are required for completing a high quality of plot. Load these packages before call the heatmap.2 () function. The clustering is only relevant to OTUs that actually are differentially abundant. Here, we select the 10 OTUs with the highest variance across samples for demonstration (Fig. 11.10).

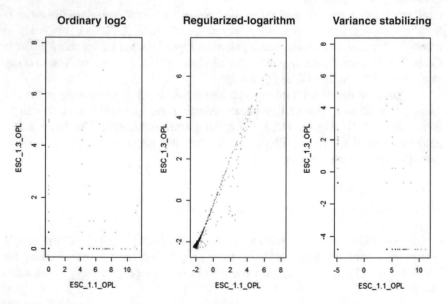

Fig. 11.9 Scatter plot of sample 2 versus sample 1. Left: using an ordinary $\log_2$ transformation. Middle: using regularized-logarithm transformation. Right: using variance stabilizing transformations

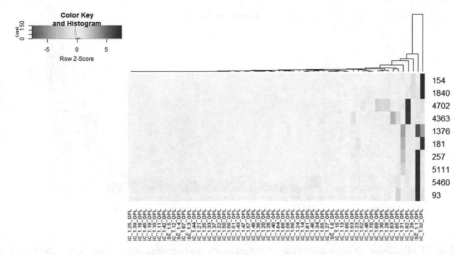

Fig. 11.10 Heatmap with OTU clustering. The dendrogram at the top shows us a hierarchical clustering of the samples. Red-blue and white in cells reflect high and low abundance levels, respectively, as indicated in the color key bar (rlog-transformed value). Hierarchical clustering was derived using the Euclidean distance as the similarity measure and the Ward clustering as agglomeration method. On the heatmap, the blocks of OTUs covary across subjects. Heatmap with clustering is often insightful because we can see the OTUs–subjects covarying effects between groups

```
> library("gplots")
> library("RColorBrewer")
> library("genefilter")
> library(SummarizedExperiment)
> topVarGenes <- head(order(rowVars(assay(rld)), decreasing=TRUE ),10)
> heatmap.2(assay(rld)[topVarGenes,], scale="row",
+            trace="none", dendrogram="column",
+            col = colorRampPalette(rev(brewer.pal(9, "RdBu")))(255))
```

Histogram of *p*-Values
We can also plot the histogram of the *p*-values to diagnose the distribution of the *p*-values. *P*-values are uniformly distributed under the null hypothesis: the histogram of *p*-values looks flat and uniformly distributed over the interval [0, 1] (Murdoch et al. 2008). Significant *p*-values thus become visible as an enrichment of *p*-values near zero in the histogram. In other words, if the *p*-values are computed correctly, then the histogram of the *p*-values will have a rectangular shape with a

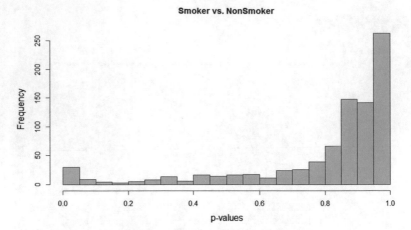

Fig. 11.11 Histogram of the *p*-values returned by the test for differential abundance. The figure indicates a wrong null distribution of *p*-values

peak at zero. To check whether *p*-values have been computed correctly here, we plot the histogram of *p*-values as below (Fig. 11.11):

```
> hist(res$pvalue, breaks=20, col="grey",
+        main = "Smoker vs. NonSmoker", xlab = "p-values")
```

Clearly the *p*-values returned by DESeq2 are not correctly computed, which suggest something wrong with the assumed variance of the null distribution. Thus, the Wald test is not appropriate for the data here. Before finally correct the wrongly computed *p*-values, we first introduce the independent filtering because the correction of the *p*-values needs this procedure.

Independent Filtering
DESeq2 automatically performs independent filtering to filter out weakly differential OTUs. Although these weak OTUs are tested as non-significant; however, they affect the multiple testing procedure. Thus, it is better to remove them for the analysis. The independent filtering is performed to maximize the number of OTUs that will have a BH-adjusted *p*-value less than a critical value (by default, alpha is set to 0.1). The adjusted *p*-values for the OTUs that do not pass the filter threshold are set to NA. The filter threshold value and the number of rejections at each quantile of the filter statistic are stored as metadata of the object returned by results.

```
> metadata(res)
$filterThreshold
87.48%
 1.191

$filterTheta
[1] 0.8748

$filterNumRej
          theta numRej
2.921% 0.02921     10
4.8%   0.04800     10
6.679% 0.06679     10
8.558% 0.08558     10
10.44% 0.10437     10
12.32% 0.12316     11
14.2%  0.14196     11
16.07% 0.16075     11
17.95% 0.17954     11
19.83% 0.19833     11
21.71% 0.21712     11
23.59% 0.23591     11
25.47% 0.25471     11
27.35% 0.27350     11
29.23% 0.29229     11
31.11% 0.31108     11
32.99% 0.32987     11
34.87% 0.34866     11
36.75% 0.36746     11
38.62% 0.38625     11
40.5%  0.40504     11
42.38% 0.42383     11
44.26% 0.44262     11
46.14% 0.46142     11
48.02% 0.48021     11
49.9%  0.49900     12
51.78% 0.51779     12
53.66% 0.53658     12
55.54% 0.55537     12
57.42% 0.57417     12
59.3%  0.59296     12
61.17% 0.61175     12
63.05% 0.63054     14
64.93% 0.64933     14
66.81% 0.66812     14
68.69% 0.68692     16
70.57% 0.70571     16
72.45% 0.72450     16
74.33% 0.74329     16
76.21% 0.76208     17
78.09% 0.78087     17
79.97% 0.79967     17
81.85% 0.81846     17
83.72% 0.83725     20
85.6%  0.85604     21
87.48% 0.87483     23
89.36% 0.89362     23
91.24% 0.91242     27
93.12% 0.93121     22
95%    0.95000     18
```

```
$lo.fit
$lo.fit$x
 [1] 0.02921 0.04800 0.06679 0.08558 0.10437 0.12316 0.14196
 [8] 0.16075 0.17954 0.19833 0.21712 0.23591 0.25471 0.27350
[15] 0.29229 0.31108 0.32987 0.34866 0.36746 0.38625 0.40504
[22] 0.42383 0.44262 0.46142 0.48021 0.49900 0.51779 0.53658
[29] 0.55537 0.57417 0.59296 0.61175 0.63054 0.64933 0.66812
[36] 0.68692 0.70571 0.72450 0.74329 0.76208 0.78087 0.79967
[43] 0.81846 0.83725 0.85604 0.87483 0.89362 0.91242 0.93121
[50] 0.95000

$lo.fit$y
 [1]  9.811  9.952 10.104 10.262 10.418 10.582 10.749 10.899
 [9] 10.983 11.000 11.000 11.000 11.000 11.000 11.000 11.000
[17] 11.000 11.000 11.000 11.000 11.000 11.017 11.101 11.252
[25] 11.418 11.584 11.761 11.924 12.061 12.392 12.765 13.113
[33] 13.527 14.043 14.558 15.006 15.450 15.933 16.388 16.916
[41] 17.687 18.437 19.218 20.044 20.653 21.007 21.351 21.696
[49] 22.035 22.368


$alpha
[1] 0.1
```

We can extract them by using following codes:

```
> metadata(res)$alpha
[1] 0.1
> metadata(res)$filterThreshold
87.48%
 1.191
```

As seen in Fig. 11.12, we can plot the filterNumRej attribute of the results object to see how the number of rejections changes for various cutoffs based on mean normalized count.

```
> plot(metadata(res)$filterNumRej,
+       type="b", ylab="number of rejections",
+       xlab="quantiles of filter")
> lines(metadata(res)$lo.fit, col="red")
> abline(v=metadata(res)$filterTheta)
```

Re-estimate the *p*-Values.

After performing the independent filtering, we can re-estimate the *p*-values via the fdrtool package. For a convenient reference, we reprint the partial result output below:

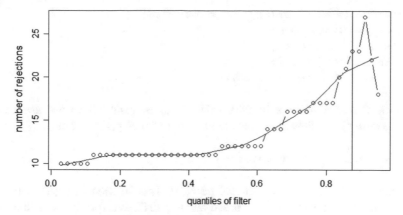

Fig. 11.12 Plot of independent filtering. The figure plots the number of rejections (adjusted *p*-value less than a significance level) against the quantiles of a filter statistic (the mean of normalized counts). The number of rejections is maximized by the function results(). The vertical line presents the threshold chosen

```
> res
log2 fold change (MLE): group Smoker vs NonSmoker
Wald test p-value: group Smoker vs NonSmoker
DataFrame with 856 rows and 6 columns
        baseMean log2FoldChange    lfcSE      stat    pvalue
       <numeric>      <numeric> <numeric> <numeric> <numeric>
4695    0.40826        0.81078     1.964  0.412815    0.6797
2983    0.07752        0.66023     2.936  0.224906    0.8221
2554    0.09789        0.50406     2.813  0.179214    0.8578
3315    0.05746        0.25158     2.936  0.085683    0.9317
879     0.01291        0.01564     2.936  0.005326    0.9958
...         ...            ...       ...       ...       ...
596    75.26585         0.2176    0.5197   0.41868    0.6755
4225    0.01125         0.4340    2.9364   0.14780    0.8825
3675    0.01471         0.2817    2.9363   0.09593    0.9236
434     0.40221        -0.4274    2.9347  -0.14564    0.8842
3447    0.01500         0.4864    2.9362   0.16567    0.8684
          padj
       <numeric>
4695        NA
2983        NA
2554        NA
3315        NA
879         NA
...        ...
596     0.8385
4225        NA
3675        NA
434         NA
3447        NA
```

The filtered out OTUs by independent filtering are set to NA, let's remove them by the function !is.na() with the padj object.

```
> # remove filtered out OTUs by independent filtering
> # they have NA adj. pvals
> res <- res[ !is.na(res$padj),]
> # with NA pvals (outliers)
> res <- res[ !is.na(res$pvalue),]
```

Now, let's remove the adjusted *p*-values from the result object because we will add the correct *p*-values based on the results of fdrtool package later.

```
> res <- res[, -which(names(res) == "padj")]
```

Below we install and call fdrtool package. The function fdrtool() is used to re-estimate the adjusted *p*-values based on "res$stat". We specify statistic = "normal" for using z-scores as input to fdrtool() to re-estimate the *p*-value (Fig. 11.13).

```
> install.packages("fdrtool")
> library(fdrtool)
> res_fdr <- fdrtool(res$stat, statistic= "normal", plot = T)
```

We can check the parameters of the fdrtool output using the head () function, and then print the parameters of interest.

```
> head(res_fdr)
```

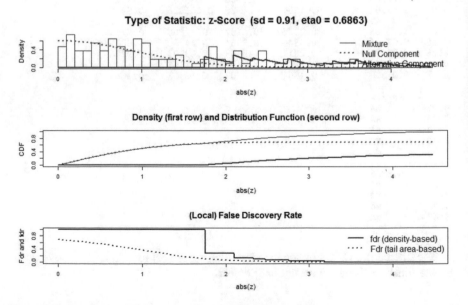

Fig. 11.13 Plot of false discovery rate from the fdrtool package

The estimated parameters in the output include: 'pval', 'qval', 'lfdr', 'statistic' from 'normal' and 'param' ('cutoff', 'N.cens', 'eta0', 'eta0.SE', 'sd', 'sd.SE'). They can be printed using $ sign. For example, to print the estimated null model standard deviation, use the codes:

```
> res_fdr$param[1, "sd"]
   sd
0.9102
> sd
standardGeneric for "sd" defined from package "BiocGenerics"
```

The null model 'sd' estimated by the fdrtool package is 0.91, which is less than the theoretical 'sd' of 1, as expected from the *p*-value histogram. The re-estimated values and the new BH-adjusted *p*-values can be added to the previous result dataframe using below codes:

```
> res[,"padj"] <- p.adjust(res_fdr$pval, method = "BH")
```

The updated result dataframe can be used for downstream analysis and reporting. Let's check the distribution of the 'correct' *p*-values (Fig. 11.14).

```
> hist(res_fdr$pval, col = "gray", main = "Smoker vs. NonSkoer, correct
null model", xlab = "Corrected p-values")
```

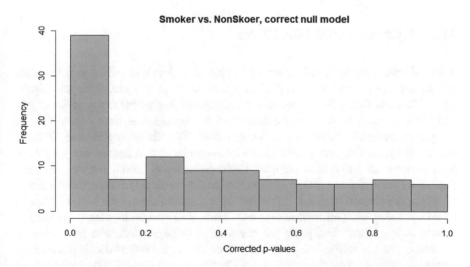

Fig. 11.14 Histogram of the *p*-values re-estimated by the fdrtool package. The figure indicates a 'correct' null distribution of *p*-values. The histogram of the *p*-values has a rectangular shape with a peak at zero

Step 9: Extract Differentially Abundant OTUs and Export Results Table
Now we are ready to extract the number of differential abundant OTUs from the result dataframe.

```
# Now, table the adjusted p-values to see how many
> table(res[,"padj"] < 0.1)
FALSE    TRUE
   79      29
```

Before removing the weakly abundant OTUs from the input to the BH-FDR procedure, 23 significant OTUs are identified; now the significant OTUs increase to 29 at an FDR of 0.1. Thus, removing the weakly abundant OTUs improves the power of test.

Finally, we save the results table in a CSV format, which can be easily loaded with a spreadsheet program such as Excel.

```
> res[1:2,]
log2 fold change (MLE): group Smoker vs NonSmoker
Wald test p-value: group Smoker vs NonSmoker
DataFrame with 2 rows and 6 columns
       baseMean log2FoldChange      lfcSE      stat     pvalue       padj
      <numeric>      <numeric>  <numeric> <numeric>  <numeric>  <numeric>
4194     1.631         -1.899     1.4916    -1.273   0.202922    0.38476
3227    69.083         -1.968     0.7154    -2.751   0.005934    0.01691
> write.csv( as.data.frame(res), file="results.csv" )
```

11.6 Summary and Discussion

In this chapter, we reviewed differential expression data analysis in genomic data setting, especially presented the statistical framework of NB models in the edgeR, and DESeq and DESeq2 approaches. We illustrated implementations of the edgeR and DESeq2 with human microbiome data to demonstrate their capabilities to analyze differential abundant microbiome data. We chose edgeR and DESeq2 because they are frequently used in the RNA-sequencing literature and they have been demonstrated that their methods based on negative binomial modeling have improved specificity and sensitivities as well as good control of false positive errors with comparable performance. It does not indicate that they are the best methods to be used for analyzing all microbiome data. Each study is specific; the users need to choose their methods and packages based on the design, data, and preference or combining several methods in their study since no single method dominates another across all settings (Nookaew et al. 2012; Rapaport et al. 2013; Soneson and Delorenzi 2013).

We noticed the differences in several important areas between the methods implemented in the edgeR and DESeq(2), for example, the data structures, their default normalization, the dispersion estimation (Anders et al. 2013). But we have no intention to compare these two methods. Effective comparisons of different statistical methods need not only apply them to real data, but also more statistical tools, such as simulation studies. Several studies in RNA-sequencing data literature have done comprehensive comparisons of edgeR and DESeq(2) among methods (Harris et al. 2010; Nookaew et al. 2012; Rapaport et al. 2013; Soneson and Delorenzi 2013). However, the comparisons with application to microbiome data are still limited.

The packages edgeR and DESeq were recommended to identify differentially abundant OTUs (McMurdie and Holmes 2014). However, these methods may not perform well in identifying the differential abundant OTUs, as the counts at the OTU level are very sparse and the models cannot account for many zeros observed (Li 2015). Although the NB formulations in edgeR and DESeq are adjusted to ensure the over-dispersion parameter α_i locally to fit the unobserved heterogeneity of RNA sequence data, these approaches may not be appropriate if the over-dispersion is due to excess zeros because they underestimate the probability of zeros and consequently underestimate the variability present in the outcome. In such situations, alternative methods and models with the capability to incorporate excess zeros, such as zero inflated/hurdle models that account for over-dispersion due to excess zeros, are useful and necessary. Chapter 12 will present the models which have the parameters to dealing with the zero-inflated and over-dispersed data.

References

Anders, S., and W. Huber. 2010. Differential expression analysis for sequence count data. *Genome Biology* 11 (10): R106.

Anders, S., D.J. McCarthy, et al. 2013. Count-based differential expression analysis of RNA sequencing data using R and Bioconductor. *Nature Protocols* 8 (9): 1765–1786.

Bacon-Shone, J. 2008. Discrete and continuous compositions. In *Proceedings of CODAWORK'08, The 3rd Compositional Data Analysis Workshop*, ed. J. Daunis-i Estadella and J. E. Fernández. Girona: University of Girona.

Baggerly, K.A., L. Deng, et al. 2003. Differential expression in SAGE: Accounting for normal between-library variation. *Bioinformatics* 19 (12): 1477–1483.

Bottomly, D., N.A.R. Walter, et al. 2011. Evaluating gene expression in C57BL/6 J and DBA/2 J mouse striatum using RNA-seq and microarrays. *PLoS ONE* 6 (3): e17820.

Bourgon, R., R. Gentleman, et al. 2010. Independent filtering increases detection power for high-throughput experiments. *Proceedings of the National Academy of Sciences* 107 (21): 9546–9551.

Bullard, J.H., E. Purdom, et al. 2010. Evaluation of statistical methods for normalization and differential expression in mRNA-seq experiments. *BMC Bioinformatics* 11 (1): 94.

Cameron, A.C., and P.K. Trivedi. 1998. *Regression analysis of count data*. Cambridge, UK: Cambridge University Press.

Charlson, E.S., J. Chen, et al. 2010. Disordered microbial communities in the upper respiratory tract of cigarette smokers. *PLoS ONE* 5 (12): e15216.

Chen, Y., D. McCarthy, et al. 2017. *edgeR: Differential expression analysis of digital gene expression data User's Guide.* (Last revised September 15, 2017): 1–115.

Costea, P. I., G. Zeller, et al. 2017. Towards standards for human fecal sample processing in metagenomic studies. *Nature Biotechnology* (advance online publication).

Cui, X., J.T. Hwang, et al. 2005. Improved statistical tests for differential gene expression by shrinking variance components estimates. *Biostatistics* 6 (1): 59–75.

Dillies, M.-A., A. Rau, et al. 2013. A comprehensive evaluation of normalization methods for illumina high-throughput RNA sequencing data analysis. *Briefings in Bioinformatics* 14 (6): 671–683.

Greenacre, M. 2011. Compositional data and correspondence analysis. In *Compositional data analysis: Theory and applications*, ed. V. Pawlowsky-Glahn, and A. Buccianti, 104–113. Chichester, UK: Wiley.

Harati, S., J.H. Phan, et al. 2014. Investigation of factors affecting RNA-seq gene expression calls. *Proceedings of Conference of IEEE Engineering in Medicine and Biology Society* 5 (10): 6944805.

Harris, R. A., T. Wang, et al. 2010. Comparison of sequencing-based methods to profile DNA methylation and identification of monoallelic epigenetic modifications. *Nat Biotechnol* 28.

Kuczynski, J., C.L. Lauber, et al. 2011. Experimental and analytical tools for studying the human microbiome. *Nature Reviews Genetics* 13 (1): 47–58.

Kvam, V.M., P. Liu, et al. 2012. A comparison of statistical methods for detecting differentially expressed genes from RNA-seq data. *American Journal of Botany* 99 (2): 248–256.

Law, C.W., Y. Chen, et al. 2014. voom: Precision weights unlock linear model analysis tools for RNA-seq read counts. *Genome Biology* 15 (2): R29.

Li, H. 2015. Microbiome, metagenomics, and high-dimensional compositional data analysis. *Annual Review of Statistics and Its Application* 2: 73–94.

Love, M.I., W. Huber, et al. 2014. Moderated estimation of fold change and dispersion for RNA-seq data with DESeq2. *Genome Biology* 15 (12): 550.

Lovell, D., V. Pawlowsky-Glahn, et al. 2015. Proportionality: A valid alternative to correlation for relative data. *PLoS Computational Biology* 11 (3): e1004075.

Lu, J., J. K. Tomfohr, et al. 2005. Identifying differential expression in multiple SAGE libraries: an overdispersed log-linear model approach. *BMC Bioinformatics* 6.

Marioni, J.C., C.E. Mason, et al. 2008. RNA-seq: An assessment of technical reproducibility and comparison with gene expression arrays. *Genome Research* 18 (9): 1509–1517.

McCarthy, D.J., Y. Chen, et al. 2012. Differential expression analysis of multifactor RNA-Seq experiments with respect to biological variation. *Nucleic Acids Research* 40 (10): 4288–4297.

McCullagh, P., and J. Nelder. 1989. *Generalized linearmodels.* London, UK: Chapman & Hall/ CRC.

McMurdie, P.J., and S. Holmes. 2014. Waste not, want not: Why rarefying microbiome data is inadmissible. *PLoS Computational Biology* 10 (4): e1003531.

Munro, S.A., S.P. Lund, et al. 2014. Assessing technical performance in differential gene expression experiments with external spike-in RNA control ratio mixtures. *Nature Communications* 5: 5125.

Murdoch, D.J., Y.-L. Tsai, et al. 2008. P-values are random variables. *The American Statistician* 62 (3): 242–245.

Nagalakshmi, U., Z. Wang, et al. 2008. The transcriptional landscape of the yeast genome defined by RNA sequencing. *Science* 320.

Nookaew, I., M. Papini, et al. 2012. A comprehensive comparison of RNA-seq-based transcriptome analysis from reads to differential gene expression and cross-comparison with microarrays: A case study in Saccharomyces cerevisiae. *Nucleic Acids Research* 40 (20): 10084–10097.

Oshlack, A., M.D. Robinson, et al. 2010. From RNA-seq reads to differential expression results. *Genome Biology* 11 (12): 220.

Rapaport, F., R. Khanin, et al. 2013. Comprehensive evaluation of differential gene expression analysis methods for RNA-seq data. *Genome Biology* 14 (9): R95–R95.

Rau, A., M. Gallopin, et al. 2013. Data-based filtering for replicated high-throughput transcriptome sequencing experiments. *Bioinformatics* 29 (17): 2146–2152.

Robinson, M.D., D.J. McCarthy, et al. 2010. edgeR: A bioconductor package for differential expression analysis of digital gene expression data. *Bioinformatics* 26 (1): 139–140.

Robinson, M.D., and A. Oshlack. 2010. A scaling normalization method for differential expression analysis of RNA-seq data. *Genome Biology* 11 (3): R25–R25.

Robinson, M.D., and G.K. Smyth. 2007. Moderated statistical tests for assessing differences in tag abundance. *Bioinformatics* 23 (21): 2881–2887.

Robinson, M.D., and G.K. Smyth. 2008. Small-sample estimation of negative binomial dispersion, with applications to SAGE data. *Biostatistics* 9 (2): 321–332.

Sha, Y., J. H. Phan, et al. 2015. Effect of low-expression gene filtering on detection of differentially expressed genes in RNA-seq data. *Conference Proceedings: 2015 37th Annual International Conference of the IEEE Engineering in Medicine and Biology Society*, 6461–6464.

Smyth, G.K. 2004. Linear models and empirical bayes methods for assessing differential expression in microarray experiments. *Statistical Applications in Genetics and Molecular Biology* 3: 12.

Soneson, C., and M. Delorenzi. 2013. A comparison of methods for differential expression analysis of RNA-seq data. *BMC Bioinformatics* 14 (91): 1471–2105.

Sultan, M., M.H. Schulz, et al. 2008. A global view of gene activity and alternative splicing by deep sequencing of the human transcriptome. *Science* 321 (5891): 956–960.

Wang, L., Z. Feng, et al. 2010. DEGseq: An R package for identifying differentially expressed genes from RNA-seq data. *Bioinformatics* 26 (1): 136–138.

Xia, Y., D. Morrison-Beedy, et al. 2012. Modeling count outcomes from HIV risk reduction interventions: A comparison of competing statistical models for count responses. *AIDS Research and Treatment* 2012: 11 pages.

Yu, D., W. Huber, et al. 2013. Shrinkage estimation of dispersion in negative binomial models for RNA-seq experiments with small sample size. *Bioinformatics* 29 (10): 1275–1282.

Chapter 12
Modeling Zero-Inflated Microbiome Data

In this chapter, we introduce and illustrate how to model zero-inflated microbiome data. In Sect. 12.1, we briefly introduce modeling zero-inflated data. The remaining of this chapter is organized as follows: Sect. 12.2 introduce zero-inflated Poisson (ZIP) and negative binomial model (ZINB) and their implementations in real microbiome data. Section 12.3 introduce zero-hurdle Poisson (ZHP) and zero-hurdle negative binomial (ZHNB) and implement them with the same data set. The zero-inflated beta regression model with random-effects (ZIBR) is covered and illustrated in Sect. 12.4. We conclude this chapter by a summary and discussion in Sect. 12.5.

12.1   Introduction

In microbiome study, identifying the significantly differentially abundant taxa among groups or different conditions is the main interest for microbiome researchers, after estimating a given level of taxonomic microbiome composition. Two general approaches can reach the goal: either consider the taxa as compositional components in the whole ecosystem and use compositional data analysis, or directly use count data-based models. In Chap. 11, we introduced two negative-binomial (NB) count data-based models and their implementation via the edgeR and DESeq2 packages.

Microbiome data typically is overdispersed and sparse with many zeros. When the number of zeros is excess than the standard distributions (e.g., normal, Poisson, binomial, NB, beta or gamma) can be readily fit, the data set is considered as 'zero inflated' (Heilbron 1994; Martin et al. 2005; Tu and Liu 2014).

The zero-inflated data may reduce overdispersion due to two sources: 'zero-driven overdispersion' and 'Poisson overdispersion'. In zero-driven overdispersion, preponderance of zeros drives the variance greater than the mean.

© Springer Nature Singapore Pte Ltd. 2018

Y. Xia et al., *Statistical Analysis of Microbiome Data with R*,

ICSA Book Series in Statistics, https://doi.org/10.1007/978-981-13-1534-3_12

And in Poisson overdispersion, overdispersion is caused by the unobserved heterogeneity in the event stage.

In omics, the zero issues are more complicated. Dealing with zeros is one of the biggest challenges in microbiome research. The available approaches and tools for compositional data analysis have not fully addressed the data complexity, including sparsity issue. Under the framework of compositional data analysis, the zeros are treated as different categories: rounded, sampling, or structural zeros. Compositional data analysis typically takes log-ratio approach. However, the zero problem directly affects the application of the log-ratio transformations to modern genomics data sets because it is undefined to divide the zero (Zuur et al. 2009). Generally, to ensure log-ratio approach appropriate, zero is either replaced by a small value generated by a function, or directly replaced by a small value, i.e., one, although the zero issue is handled according to the differentiating zero sources. This simple general remedy faces many difficulties, problems, and challenges, especially in the field of omics research. NB methods are appropriate for dealing with generally overdispersed data, but may not perform well in identifying the OTUs with differential abundances when many zeros are observed. Currently, microbiome researchers including compositional data analysts, especially biostatisticians, prefer to using the mixture models to analyze the excessive zeros jointly or two-part models to analyze zeros and non-zeros as two steps.

The difference between the mixture and two-part models is how to deal with the different types of zeros (Zuur et al. 2009). Mixture models consist of two distributions. In mixture models, the rounded zeros are explicitly modeled with a distribution, i.e., the binomial distribution. The structural zeros are modeled as the probability of expecting a zero under the considered distribution, i.e., the negative binomial or the Poisson distribution; and the nonzero values are analyzed as the rest of the data. As suggested by the names, the two-part models consist of two parts: first, the data are considered as zeros versus non-zeros and the probability of a zero value is modeled by a binomial distribution; and second, the non-zero values are analyzed via a truncated Poisson or truncated negative binomial models.

In summary, the overdispersed and sparse microbiome data pose a big challenge for microbiome researchers and biostatisticians to choose an appropriate model to analyze.

12.2 Zero-Inflated Models: ZIP and ZINB

Although NB is capable of addressing overdispersion, it is not appropriate for modeling the data with a high percentage of zero counts. To model such excess of zeros, zero-inflated regression (e.g., ZIP or ZINB) may be applied. There is a long history of using ZIP and ZINB to fit data (Cohen 1963), but the early application of ZIP and ZINB have without covariates. ZIP regression models originated in the econometrics literature (Mullahy 1986), but until 1992, Lambert provided the general form of ZIP regression with covariates to model defects in a manufacturing process (Lambert 1992). Since this publication, the general application of zero-inflated models has become widespread in a wide range of disciplines, including econometrics (Freund et al. 1999), epidemiology (Bohning et al. 1999; Lewsey and Thomson 2004), occupational health (Lee et al. 2002; Yau et al. 2004), medicine including aging (Campbell et al. 1991; Bin 2002; Yusuf et al. 2017), ecology (Martin et al. 2005), and currently microbiome (Xu et al. 2015; Wang et al. 2016).

12.2.1   ZIP Model

ZIP is a mixture of two statistical processes: one always generating zero counts and the other with both zero and nonzero counts. ZIP assumes that each observation comes from one of two potential distributions, with one (group 1) consisting of a constant zero while the other (group 2) following Poisson. In a ZIP model, a logit model is typically used to analyze the probability of the constant zero or structural zero, whereas the count data is analyzed by the Poisson regression. Thus, two kinds of zeros are modeled by this mixture model: the sampling zeros due to sampling variability under Poisson and the structural zeros above and beyond the expected zero frequency under Poisson. In other words, an observed zero is generated by either the logistic process or the Poisson process.

Specifically, let $p_i = \Pr(i \in \text{group 1 (structural zero)}|Z_i)$, and $1 - p_i = \Pr(i \in \text{group 2 (sampling zero)}|Z_i)$. Then, ZIP has the following distribution:

$$P(Y_i|X_i, Z_i) = p_i + (1 - p_i)\exp(-\mu_i) \quad \text{for } Y_i = 0, \tag{12.1}$$

$$P(Y_i|X_i, Z_i) = (1 - p_i)\frac{\exp(-\mu_i)(\mu_i)^{Y_i}}{Y_i!} \quad \text{for } Y_i > 0, \tag{12.2}$$

where Z_i and X_i are two sets of covariates linked to the logit and count data modules by $\text{Log}\left(\frac{p_i}{1-p_i}\right) = Z_i\gamma$, and $\text{Log}(\mu_i) = X_i\beta$. It is clear from (12.1) that the observed zeros arise from both the zero-component distribution and the Poisson distribution. i.e., the two sources of structural and sampling zeros. Therefore, the zero-component distribution provides the capability to model the 'excess' or 'inflated' zeros that are observed in addition to the zeros that are expected to be observed under the assumed Poisson distribution. The mean and variance of a ZIP model are given by:

$$E(Y_i|X_i, Z_i) = p_i 0 + \mu_i(1 - p_i) = \mu_i(1 - p_i), \tag{12.3}$$

$$Var(Y_i|X_i, Z_i) = \mu_i(1 - p_i)(1 + \mu_i p_i). \tag{12.4}$$

By (12.3) and (12.4), $Var(Y_i|X_i, Z_i) / E(Y_i|X_i, Z_i) = 1 + \mu_i p_i = 1 + [p_i / (1 - p_i)]E(Y_i|X_i, Z_i)$. Therefore, if p_i approaches zero, that is, the amount of structural zeros decreases to zero, ZIP reduces to Poisson.

12.2.2 ZINB Model

By replacing the Poisson distribution for the count data in ZIP with the negative binomial distribution, we obtain the zero-inflated negative binomial distribution, or ZINB. Thus, a ZINB has the general form:

$$P(Y_i|X_i, Z_i) = p_i + (1 - p_i)g(\mu_i), \quad \text{if } Y_i = 0, \tag{12.5}$$

$$P(Y_i|X_i, Z_i) = (1 - p_i)f(\mu_i), \quad Y_i > 0, \tag{12.6}$$

where $g(\mu_i) = P(Y_i = 0|X_i) = \left(\frac{\alpha^{-1}}{\mu_i + \alpha^{-1}}\right)^{1/\alpha}$ in the count data model, and $f(\mu_i)$ is the density of the negative binomial distribution. $f(\mu_i) = \frac{\Gamma(y_i + \alpha^{-1})}{y_i!\Gamma(\alpha^{-1})}\left(\frac{1}{1 + \alpha\mu_i}\right)^{1/\alpha} \left(\frac{\alpha\mu_i}{1 + \alpha\mu_i}\right)^{y_i}$, for $\alpha > 0$, $y_i \geq 0$.

The binary process can be modeled using either logit or probit or other models for binary outcomes. The mean and variance of the ZINB are

$$E(Y_i|X_i, Z_i) = \mu_i(1 - p_i), \tag{12.7}$$

$$Var(Y_i|X_i, Z_i) = \mu_i(1 - p_i)(1 + \mu_i(p_i + \alpha)), \tag{12.8}$$

where, α is the dispersion parameter. It follows from (12.7) and (12.8) that

$$\frac{Var(Y_i|X_i, Z_i)}{E(Y_i|X_i, Z_i)} = 1 + \mu_i(p_i + \alpha) = 1 + \left[\frac{p_i + \alpha}{1 - p_i}\right]E(Y_i|X_i, Z_i)$$

For ZINB, $Var(Y_i|X_i, Z_i) > E(Y_i|X_i, Z_i)$, demonstrating that ZINB has the capability to model overdispersion. Because $\frac{(p_i + \alpha)}{(1 - p_i)}$ is a function of both zero-inflated parameter p and dispersion parameter α, ZINB accounts for both population heterogeneity (mixture) and overdispersion in the distribution of the NB component of ZINB. Thus, NB is capable to model overdispersion due to unobserved heterogeneity; ZIP focuses on the violation of the Poisson by the population heterogeneity in the presence of structural zeros, while ZINB addresses both sources of heterogeneity. Both ZIP and ZINB models demonstrate $Var(Y_i|X_i, Z_i) > E(Y_i|X_i, Z_i)$, thereby accounting for overdispersion resulting from structural zeros. As Poisson is nested within NB, ZIP is nested within ZINB. ZINB can be viewed as an extension of ZIP in analogous to NB being an extension of Poisson.

12.2.3 Modeling Using ZIP and ZINB

12.2.3.1 Vaginal Microbiota Data

The data are from a published study (Romero et al. 2014), which included non-pregnant women (n = 32) and pregnant women who delivered at term (38–42 weeks) without complications (n = 22). The purpose of this study is to analyze whether the composition and stability of the vaginal microbiota of normal pregnant women is different from that of non-pregnant women. For statistical methods, briefly, the linear mixed-effects models including Poisson, NB, ZINB were used to identify the phenotypes, whose relative abundance was different between the non-pregnant and pregnant women for each OTU. The statistical analyses were carried out using SAS. Here, we conduct the analyses with ZIP, ZINB, PH and NBH in R using the sequence counts data called 'allTD_long'. The data structure and format are presented in Table 12.1.

In Table 12.1, the ID represents the identifier of a given subject; nReads is the total number of reads in the sample, DX is the group indicator (0 = non-pregnant; 1 = pregnant); Y is the number of sequences (count); Spec gives the name of the OTU; and Ind is a numeric indicator for the OTU (1,…, 28).

As shown in the histogram of Fig. 12.1, the sequencing count data are characterized by many zero-valued observations and the variance is much larger than its mean. It indicates overdispersion in the data. This histogram shows that the marginal distribution does not resemble a typical Poisson distribution.

12.2.3.2 Analyzing Data with Excess Zeros and Overdispersion

Count data are typically modeled via Poisson regression. However, due to the limitation of the Poisson, its application is problematic in the presence of excess zeros. Failure to account for the extra zeros may result in biased parameter estimation and misleading inference. In the Poisson model, the $Var(Y) = E(Y)$, overdispersion is said to occur when this ratio is greater than 1. If overdispersion is ignored, the standard errors for the parameter estimates will be seriously underestimated, resulting in overly optimistic standard errors, smaller p-values and lack of fit from deviance tests (Hinde and Demétrio 1998; Hall 2000; Agresti 2002; Yau et al. 2003; Atkins and Gallop 2007; Xia et al. 2012; Desjardins 2016).

Table 12.1 The first three rows of the sequence counts data

ID	nReads	DX	Y	Spec	Ind
432	2209	0	4	*Lactobacillus iners*	1
424	4485	0	7	*Lactobacillus iners*	1
439	2447	0	175	*Lactobacillus iners*	1

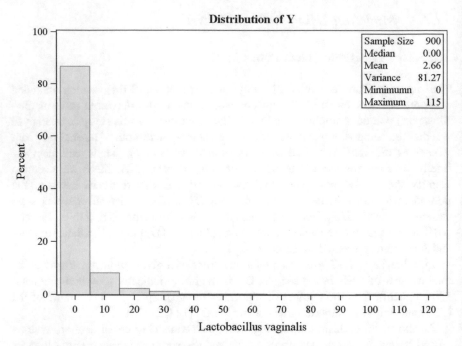

Fig. 12.1 The observed distribution of number of sequencing count for OTU *Lactobacillus vaginalis*. This figure shows the right-skewed distribution of the number of OTU (species) *Lactobacillus vaginalis*, with a preponderance of zeros.

The abundance of all bacteria species (OTUs) have their variances greater than their means, as shown in Fig. 12.1 here, and Table 2.6 in Chap. 2. Particularly, the abundance data of species have many zeros (average 58.57% of all 28 species) with the lowest *Lactobacillus* having 14.44% zeros, the highest *Streptococcus anginosus* having 73.78% zeros. The large percent of zeros in each of these outcomes, coupled with overdispersion, does not allow the analysis of these data using the traditional model Poisson log-linear model.

In Chap. 11, we analyzed bacteria OTUs via packages edgeR and DESeq2 implementing NB regression. As mentioned, NB is an extension of Poisson to address overdispersion and may be the best fitting of the count distributions without zero-inflation. However, the NB models were used to describe the distribution assuming that overdispersion is only due to unobserved heterogeneity and/or clustering, but not due to excess zeros. Therefore, if the abundance data involve overdispersion due to unobserved heterogeneity and/or clustering, as well as the preponderance of zero frequency (absent species or OTU in the case of vaginal microbiota), Poisson and NB models likely lead to underestimating the probability of absent species (Yan et al. 2013) status and misleading results.

Zero inflated regression addresses excess zeros with increasing predictability in situations with excess zeros. It models structural zeros separately from the sampling zeros and the positive counts. ZIP or ZINB regression employs a mixture of a logistic regression for modeling structural zeros, and a log-linear regression for modeling the remaining count data. In the example data set, *Lactobacillus* is a keystone genus in the vagina. *Lactobacillus* spp. are described as being part of the gastrointestinal endogenous flora and as a regulator of the vaginal ecosystem in women in their reproductive age (Shopova 2001). It is important in human health as well. In women of European ancestry, *Lactobacillus* species including *Lactobacillus vaginalis, Lactobacillus jensenii, Lactobacillus crispatus* and *Lactobacillus gasseri,* are normally a major part of the vaginal microbiota (Ma et al. 2012; Fettweis et al. 2014; Petrova et al. 2015). Thus, the presence of *Lactobacillus species* is a biomarker of vaginal health and may protect reproductive age women from non-indigenous pathogens (Romero et al. 2014).

Within our context, p models the at-risk subgroup of bacteria species as represented by the structural zeros, while μ models the non-risk subgroup comprised of the positive abundance and sampling zeros (in this case, absence of *Lactobacillus species* is thought as 'risk'). ZIP and ZINB both use a logistic model to model the at-risk p, but they use different regressions to model the non-risk subgroup: ZIP uses Poisson, whereas ZINB uses NB to account for overdispersion.

12.2.3.3   Conceptual Adjustment for Using ZIP and ZINB

ZIP and ZINB are conceptually appropriate for analyzing microbiome data. For example, within our context, it is plausible to assume that the bacteria species belong to one of the two groups of women, with one consisting of abstinent *Lactobacillus species*, and the other with presence of *Lactobacillus species*. The subjects in the first group had absence of *Lactobacillus species* during the pregnant period because of the nature of their abstinence. Those in the second group also had absence of *Lactobacillus species* in pregnancy, but happened to have no *Lactobacillus species* present. Thus, the number of observed zeros is inflated by the structural zeros representing the abstinent pregnant women in the first group, which could not be explained in the same manner as the sampling zeros from the pregnant women with presence of *Lactobacillus species*. In concept, NB does not have two types of zeros, whereas ZIP and ZINB do distinguish two types of zero observation.

Within the context of the example, the subjects continually abstinent from *Lactobacillus species* during the pregnant period would have structural zeros as their outcomes. These subjects formed the at-risk subgroup for the medical outcome under consideration, while the remaining subjects with either sampling zeros or positive count outcomes constituted the non-risk subgroup. The logistic regression module of ZIP models the probability of structural zeros, allowing us to assess whether the pregnancy had triggered abstinence from the non-risky medical condition under the examined example. The Poisson module models the mean frequency of the count outcome for the non-risk subgroup, providing information on the effect of the pregnancy for maintaining the frequency of the medical condition for these subjects. Thus, we obtain two sets of estimates: one contains information about the effect of the pregnancy for triggering abstinence, while the other for maintaining the frequency of the medical condition for those who continued to be at non-risk.

12.2.3.4 Step-by-Step Implementing ZIP and ZINB

Both zero-inflated and hurdle models are readily fit in most major statistical software. The pscl package in R (Zeileis et al. 2008) is capable of fitting a variety of zero-inflated and hurdle models. Here, we illustrate zero-inflated models: ZIP and ZINB. In Sect. 12.3, we illustrate zero-hurdle models: ZHP and ZHNB.

There are 28 bacteria species in the example data set. We choose the last one "*Lactobacillus vaginalis*" for illustration. The response variable is the number of sequences (count) Y, the explanatory variable of interest is DX (group), the offset is the total number of reads (nReads). The analysis will be performed by each species.

Step 1: Load Abundance Data and Prepare Analysis Dataset
Load abundance data and check first few lines:

```
> abund_table=read.csv("allTD_long.csv",header=TRUE)
> head(abund_table)
   ID nReads DX    Y          Spec Ind
1 432   2209  0    4 Lactobacillus.iners   1
2 424   4485  0    7 Lactobacillus.iners   1
3 439   2447  0  175 Lactobacillus.iners   1
4 410   2679  0 2040 Lactobacillus.iners   1
5 410   3383  0 2879 Lactobacillus.iners   1
6 403   3024  0   36 Lactobacillus.iners   1
> tail(abund_table)
         ID nReads DX Y              Spec Ind
25195 412   2912  0 0 Lactobacillus.vaginalis   28
25196 407   2468  0 0 Lactobacillus.vaginalis   28
25197 432   3332  0 0 Lactobacillus.vaginalis   28
25198 442   3044  0 0 Lactobacillus.vaginalis   28
25199 442   2844  0 0 Lactobacillus.vaginalis   28
25200 405   3398  0 0 Lactobacillus.vaginalis   28

> library(dplyr)
> abund_table_28 <- filter(abund_table, Ind == 28)
> head(abund_table_28)
   ID nReads DX Y              Spec Ind
1 432   2209  0 0 Lactobacillus.vaginalis   28
2 424   4485  0 0 Lactobacillus.vaginalis   28
3 439   2447  0 0 Lactobacillus.vaginalis   28
4 410   2679  0 0 Lactobacillus.vaginalis   28
5 410   3383  0 0 Lactobacillus.vaginalis   28
6 403   3024  0 0 Lactobacillus.vaginalis   28
```

The following R codes create the group variable "x", and define it as a factor:

```
> abund_table_28$x<- with(abund_table_28,ifelse(as.factor(DX)%in% "0",0, 1))
> head(abund_table_28)
   ID nReads DX Y           Spec Ind x
1 432   2209  0 0 Lactobacillus.vaginalis  28 0
2 424   4485  0 0 Lactobacillus.vaginalis  28 0
3 439   2447  0 0 Lactobacillus.vaginalis  28 0
4 410   2679  0 0 Lactobacillus.vaginalis  28 0
5 410   3383  0 0 Lactobacillus.vaginalis  28 0
6 403   3024  0 0 Lactobacillus.vaginalis  28 0
> names(abund_table_28)
[1] "ID"     "nReads" "DX"     "Y"       "Spec"  "Ind"
[7] "x"
> abund_table_28$fx <- factor(abund_table_28$x)
> names(abund_table_28)
[1] "ID"     "nReads" "DX"     "Y"       "Spec"  "Ind"
[7] "x"      "fx"
```

Removing missing values is not really necessary, but it makes model validation easier.

```
> I = is.na(abund_table_28$Y) | is.na(abund_table_28$fx)|is.na(abund_-
table_28$nReads)
> abund_table_28a < - abund_table_28[!I,]
```

Step 2: Check Outcome Distribution and Zeros
The following R codes are used to check outcome distribution and zeros (Fig. 12.2):

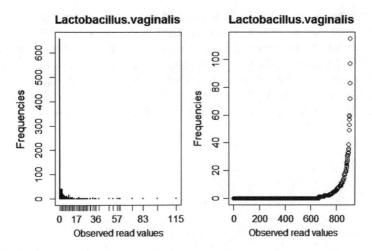

Fig. 12.2 Distribution of outcome *Lactobacillus vaginalis*

```
> par(mfrow = c(1,2))
> plot(table(abund_table_28a$Y),ylab = "Frequencies",main =
"Lactobacillus.vaginalis", xlab = "Observed read values")
> plot(sort(abund_table_28a$Y),ylab = "Frequencies",main =
"Lactobacillus.vaginalis", xlab = "Observed read values")
```

Step 3: Create the Offset

The total count read is used to create the offset. The offset will be adjusted as a covariate in the model later to ensure microbiome response is relative abundance instead of count data. This step is critical for fitting linear mixed effects models in microbiome study.

```
> abund_table_28a$Offset < - log(abund_table_28a$nReads);
> head(abund_table_28a$Offset)
[1] 7.700 8.408 7.803 7.893 8.127 8.014
```

Step 4: Create a Formula for Fitting ZIP and ZINB

The formula can be used to specify both components of the model. If a formula of type $y \sim x1 + x2$ is supplied, then the same covariates (independent variables) are employed in both components. This is equivalent to $y \sim x1 + x2|\ x1 + x2$. Of course, a different set of covariates could be specified for the structural zero component, e.g., $y \sim x1 + x2|\ z1 + z2 + z3$ giving the count data model $y \sim x1 + x2$ conditional on (|) the structural zero model $y \sim z1 + z2 + z3$.

```
> f28 < - formula(Y ~  fx + offset(Offset)|1)
```

Offsets can be specified in both parts of the model pertaining to count and structural zero models: $y \sim x1 + offset(x2)|\ z1 + z2 + offset(z3)$, where x2 is used as an offset (i.e., with coefficient fixed to 1) in the count part and z3 analogously in the structural zero part. The $y \sim x1 + offset(x2)$ is equivalent to $y \sim x1 + offset$ $(x2)|\ x1 + offset(x2)$. The offset() can be wrapped within the formula, or the zeroinfl () function as below Zip28 <- zeroinfl(f28, dist = "poisson", link = "logit", offset = Offset, data = abund_table_28a). The offset argument can also be set only for the count model as above, such as, formula = y ~ x1 + offset(x2)|x1. The formula Y ~ fx|1 specifies the following link functions for the count and the binomial data, respectively:

$$\mu_i = \exp(\alpha + \beta \times fx_i) \text{ and } p_i = \frac{\exp(v)}{1 + \exp(v)}$$

The mean μ_i for the Poisson count data is modeled in terms of the covariate fx and the probability p_i for the binomial distribution with a constant. The above fitting is actually based on the study design of the example data. In the formula, the random effect is allowed only on the non-zero inflation component (Poisson mean for the ZIP model, negative binomial mean for the ZINB model).

If we think that based on biology the probability of structural zeros is also a function of fx, then use the formula Y ~ fx|fx, which specifies the following link functions for the count and the binomial data, respectively:

$$\mu_i = \exp(\alpha + \beta \times fx_i) \text{ and } p_i = \frac{\exp(v + \gamma fx_i)}{1 + \exp(v + \gamma fx_i)}$$

The mean μ_i for the Poisson count data is modeled in terms of the covariate fx and the probability p_i for the binomial distribution with a same covariate fx. The set of covariates for the Poisson count data and the binomial data can be different. To illustrate more features of zero-inflated and zero-hurdle models and to compare these features, in this chapter, we choose the same covariate for both count and binomial distributions, but only set offset argument to count component:

```
> f28 < - formula(Y ~ fx + offset(Offset) | fx)
```

Step 5: Fit ZIP and ZINB.

The following R codes load the "pscl" package and use its function zeroinfl() to fit a zero-inflated Poisson model for response variable *Lactobacillus vaginalis* with main effect for the group (fx), indicating pregnant women versus non-pregnant women:

```
> library(pscl)
> ZIP28 < - zeroinfl(formula = f28, dist = "poisson",
link = "logit", data = abund_table_28a)
```

In above formula, the *dist* option specifies the distribution for the count data. Currently Poisson, negative binomial, and geometric distributions are available in this package. The *link = logit* option specifies the logistic link for the structural zeros versus the non-structural zeros (the sampling zeros plus the positive counts).

A binomial distribution is always used to model the distinction. The offset term (the log of the total number of reads in a given sample) is used here to allow for a comparison in the relative abundance (and not absolute counts) between groups.

```
> summary(ZIP28)
Call:

zeroinfl(formula = f28, data = abund_table_28a, dist = "poisson",
    link = "logit")

Pearson residuals:
    Min     1Q  Median      3Q     Max
 -1.013 -0.485 -0.472 -0.447  34.683

Count model coefficients (poisson with log link):
             Estimate Std. Error z value Pr(>|z|)
(Intercept)   -6.2729     0.0304  -206.1   <2e-16 ***
fx1            0.8080     0.0412    19.6   <2e-16 ***

Zero-inflation model coefficients (binomial with logit link):
             Estimate Std. Error z value Pr(>|z|)
(Intercept)   1.2594     0.0878    14.35  < 2e-16 ***
fx1          -1.3601     0.1912    -7.11  1.1e-12 ***
---
Signif. codes:  0 '***' 0.001 '**' 0.01 '*' 0.05 '.' 0.1 ' ' 1

Number of iterations in BFGS optimization: 13
Log-likelihood: -2.28e+03 on 4 Df
```

The row with BFGS optimization refers to the number of optimal iterations. The group variable (fx1) is significant for log-link function. However, the ZIP model is fitted here for assuming no overdispersion in the non-zero count data. Recall that ZIP model only deal with overdispersion caused by the excessive number of zeros, but not directly with overdispersion in the non-zero count data. We can fit ZINB model and check the overdispersion parameter. The comprehensive model comparisons will be presented in Sect. 12.3.4. The following codes fit a ZINB using the same function zeroinfl() and predictor variable as ZIP:

```
> ZINB28 < - zeroinfl(formula = f28, dist = "negbin",
link = "logit", data = abund_table_28a)
```

The ZINB outputs are printed below.

```
> summary(ZINB28)

Call:
zeroinfl(formula = f28, data = abund_table_28a, dist = "negbin",
    link = "logit")

Pearson residuals:
   Min     1Q Median     3Q    Max
-0.483 -0.327 -0.323 -0.232 23.302

Count model coefficients (negbin with log link):
            Estimate Std. Error z value Pr(>|z|)
(Intercept)   -6.835      0.186  -36.80  < 2e-16 ***
fx1            1.101      0.218    5.05  4.3e-07 ***
Log(theta)    -1.024      0.276   -3.70  0.00021 ***

Zero-inflation model coefficients (binomial with logit link):
            Estimate Std. Error z value Pr(>|z|)
(Intercept)    0.431      0.268    1.61  0.10771
fx1           -1.399      0.373   -3.75  0.00017 ***
---
Signif. codes:  0 '***' 0.001 '**' 0.01 '*' 0.05 '.' 0.1 ' ' 1

Theta = 0.359
Number of iterations in BFGS optimization: 54
Log-likelihood: -1.22e+03 on 5 Df
```

The theta value indicates that the data are overdispersed.

12.3 Zero-Hurdle Models: ZHP and ZHNB

Closely related to the Zero-inflated models, are the zero-hurdle (hurdle-at-zero) models. Hurdle models were first proposed and applied for continuous data by Cragg (1971). In principle, the hurdle could be set at any value, but the hurdle-at-zero models are most useful. The term "with-zeros" was used by Johnson and Kotz when they discussed the discrete distributions (count data) (Johnson and Kotz 1969). Thus, the hurdle models are getting particularly popular by addressing the frequently observed "too many" or "too few" zero counts, compared to the Poisson model. The zero-hurdle models were further developed by Mullahy in the econometrics context in 1986, where the econometric treatment was first allowed for regression effects (Mullahy 1986). Hurdle models were popularized by Cameron and Trivedi (2013) in order to deal with count data sets having more zero counts than allowed for by the Poisson and NB models. They are more commonly used as an alternative class of mixture models in various fields, such as econometrics (Cameron and Trivedi 2013), ecology (Welsh et al. 1996; Sileshi et al. 2009), public health (Rose et al. 2006; Hu et al. 2011) and cancer research (Dwivedi et al. 2010). Recently, Xu et al. assessed their suitability for use to model microbiome data (Xu et al. 2015). Wang et al. applied them to analyze bacteria species (OTUs) in the vitamin D receptor and gut microbiota study (Wang et al. 2016). The zero-hurdle models can be expressed as the zero-hurdle Poisson (ZHP) model and zero-hurdle negative Binomial (ZHNB) model.

12.3.1   ZHP Model

ZHP model is a two-component model: a hurdle component models the zero versus the non-zero counts, and a truncated Poisson count component is employed for the non-zero counts:

$$P(Y_i|X_i, Z_i) = p_i \quad \text{for } Y_i = 0, \tag{12.9}$$

$$P(Y_i|X_i, Z_i) = (1 - p_i) \frac{\exp(-\mu_i)(\mu_i)^{Y_i}}{Y_i!(1 - \exp(-\mu_i))} \quad \text{for } Y_i \geq 0. \tag{12.10}$$

In contrast to the zero-inflated model, the zero and non-zero counts are separated in the hurdle model. The first component is a binomial probability model to determine whether a zero or non-zero outcome occurs; and the second being count data truncated-at-zero to analyze the positive counts.

Specifically, zero-hurdle models do not make the distinction between structural and sampling zeros and handle them identically: unlike p_i in the zero-inflated model (12.1), the p_i in (12.9) does not model the *excess* zeros, but *all* zeros. The mean and variance of Y_i for the ZHP model are given by:

$$E(Y_i|X_i, Z_i) = \frac{(1 - p_i)\mu_i}{1 - \exp(-\mu_i)}, \tag{12.11}$$

$$Var(Y_i|X_i, Z_i) = \frac{(1 - p_i)\mu_i}{1 - \exp(-\mu_i)}(1 + \mu_i) - \left(\frac{(1 - p_i)\mu_i}{1 - \exp(-\mu_i)}\right)^2, \tag{12.12}$$

By (12.11) and (12.12), we can obtain $\frac{Var(Y_i|X_i, Z_i)}{E(Y_i|X_i, Z_i)} = 1 + \mu - \frac{(1-p_i)\mu_i}{1-\exp(-\mu_i)}$. Thus, the model can be used to analyze over or underdispersed data, depending on the values of μ_i.

It is not straightforward to show ZHP and ZHNB have the capability to analyze over-dispersed and under-dispersed data by comparing above $Var(Y_i|X_i, Z_i)/E(Y_i|X_i, Z_i)$. However, we can compare $Var(Y)/E(Y)$ in a general hurdle formulation to show that the hurdle models naturally admit overdispersion or underdispersion (Mullahy 1986). Given any two probability distribution functions for nonnegative integers f_1 and f_2, presenting the hurdle part and the parent process, the hurdle-at-zero model has the probability distribution:

$$P(Y = 0) = f_1(0) \tag{12.13}$$

$$P(Y = y) = f_2(y)\frac{1 - f_1(0)}{1 - f_2(0)} = \Phi f_2(y), \quad y = 1, 2, \dots \tag{12.14}$$

where $\Phi = \frac{1-f_1(0)}{1-f_2(0)}$. The numerator of Φ can be interpreted as the probability of crossing the hurdle (or more precisely in case of bacteria species (OTU), the probability to present at least one read) and the denominator is a normalization for f_2. It follows immediately that the hurdle model collapses to the parent model if $f_1 = f_2$, $\Phi = 1$. The corresponding mean and variance are given by:

$$E(Y) = \Phi\mu_2 = \sum_{y=1}^{\infty} y f_2(y)\Phi. \tag{12.15}$$

$$Var(Y) = P(Y > 0)Var(Y|Y > 0) + P(Y = 0)E(Y|Y > 0)$$
$$= \sum_{y=1}^{\infty} y^2 f_2(y)\Phi - \left[\Phi \sum_{y=1}^{\infty} y f_2(y)\right]^2 . \tag{12.16}$$

where μ_2 is the expected value associated with the probability distribution function f_2. By (12.15) and (12.16),

$$\frac{Var(Y)}{E(Y)} = \frac{\sum_{y=1}^{\infty} y^2 f_2(y)\Phi - \left[\Phi \sum_{y=1}^{\infty} y f_2(y)\right]^2}{\sum_{y=1}^{\infty} y f_2(y)\Phi}. \tag{12.17}$$

Consequently, the model can be over or underdispersed, depending on the values of the parent processes f_1 and f_2. For example, for $\Phi = 1$, (12.17) reduces to the variance-mean ratio of the parent model. If f_2 is a Poisson distribution, this is case of equidispersion with $Var(Y)/E(Y) = 1$. For f_2 Poisson and $\Phi \neq 1$, (12.13) and (12.14) define a hurdle Poisson model. $0 < \Phi < 1$ yields overdispersion, $1 < \Phi < c$ underdispersion. You can find those also in the other paper (Winkelmann and Zimmermann 1995). Thus, from a statistical point of view, the hurdle-at-zero-models have ability to address either more or less zeros in the data than predicted by the Poisson and NB models. The first situation leads to handle overdispersion (zero inflation) compared to the Poisson or NB model, the second to underdispersion (zero deflation).

The variance of the hurdle model can be written as:

$$Var(Y_i|X_i) = E(Y_i|X_i) + \sigma_i^2 [E(Y_i|X_i)]^2. \tag{12.18}$$

where $E(Y_i|X_i)$ is given in (12.17) and $\sigma_i^2 = (1 - \Phi_i)/\Phi_i$.

12.3.2 ZHNB Model

The ZHNB is obtained by replacing the zero-truncated Poisson with a truncated NB model to analyze the truncated-at-zero count.

$$P(Y_i|X_i, Z_i) = p_i \quad \text{for} \ \ Y_i = 0, \tag{12.9}$$

$P(Y_i|X_i, Z_i)$

$$= (1 - p_i) \frac{\Gamma(y_i + \alpha^{-1})}{\left(1 - \left(\frac{\alpha^{-1}}{\alpha^{-1} + \mu_i}\right)^{1/\alpha}\right) \Gamma(y_i + 1) \Gamma(\alpha^{-1})} \left(\frac{\alpha^{-1}}{\alpha^{-1} + \mu_i}\right)^{1/\alpha} \left(\frac{\mu_i}{\alpha^{-1} + \mu_i}\right)^{y_i} \quad \text{for} \ \ Y_i > 0,$$

$$\tag{12.19}$$

where $\alpha \ (\geq 0)$ is a dispersion parameter that is assumed not to depend on covariates. It can be seen in Eq. 12.19 (and noted above), that the positive count is governed by a truncated-at-zero negative binomial as the probability function for the positive count is divided by 1 minus the probability function of a negative binomial evaluated at zero. The mean and variance of NHNB are given by:

$$E(Y_i|X_i, Z_i) = \frac{(1 - p_i)\mu_i}{1 - p_0}, \quad \text{where} \quad p_0 = \left(\frac{\alpha^{-1}}{\mu_i + \alpha^{-1}}\right)^{1/\alpha}, \tag{12.20}$$

$$\begin{aligned} Var(Y_i|X_i, Z_i) &= \frac{(1 - p_i)\mu_i}{1 - p_0}(1 + \mu_i + \alpha\mu_i) - \left(\frac{(1 - p_i)\mu_i}{1 - p_0}\right)^2 \\ &= \frac{(1 - p_i)\mu_i}{1 - p_0}\left[1 + \mu_i + \alpha\mu_i - \frac{(1 - p_i)\mu_i}{1 - p_0}\right] \end{aligned} \tag{12.21}$$

By (12.20) and (12.21), we obtain that $\frac{Var(Y_i|X_i, Z_i)}{E(Y_i|X_i, Z_i)} = 1 + \mu_i + \alpha\mu_i - \frac{(1 - p_i)\mu_i}{1 - p_0}$. Thus, the model can be over or underdispersed, depending on the values of α and μ_i.

12.3.3   Modeling ZHP and ZHNB

12.3.3.1   Zero Hurdle Models Deal with Excess Zeros

Except zero inflated models, Zero hurdle models can also be used to model count data in situations with excess zeros. In medical and health fields, researchers preferred the zero-hurdle models when only at-risk zeros are present in the population and in epidemiologic studies, researchers thought the hurdle models not only may satisfactorily account for excess zeros, but also perhaps even as good as zero-inflated models (Dwivedi et al. 2010). However, the zero-hurdle regressions model the zeros by different ways. The hurdle models have two-components: a hurdle component for zeros versus non-zeros and a truncated count component for positive counts. Thus, they model zeros separately from the positive counts: treat the data as a presence and absence level and analyze the presence data with a count model.

The zero-hurdle models do not make the distinction between structural and sampling zeros, and assume all zeros to come from a single population. The zero values are either considered as structural zeros (Potts and Elith 2006) or sampling zeros (Dwivedi et al. 2010) regardless of the single population or source of zeros. Actually, the formulation of the zero-hurdle models does not tell us the source of zeros.

12.3.3.2 Conceptual Adjustment for Using Zero-Hurdle Models

In the example data set, the zero-hurdle models could be employed to estimate the Lactobacillus species frequency among pregnant women. The theoretical ground for using zero-hurdle models is: all the pregnant women are indeed at some risk of having absence of *Lactobacillus species*. The risk of pregnant women could be estimated by a two-stage process within the framework of zero hurdle models. In a first stage, the individual's risk is evaluated on whether or not the *Lactobacillus species* present in pregnancy and conditional on an absence, in a second stage how large of the risk is assessed. The zero-hurdle models also possess a natural interpretation for the positive counts (presence of *Lactobacillus species*). It is reasonable to believe that the women who have presence of *Lactobacillus species* in pregnancy have different risks compared to those who are absent of the species.

The assumption of single source of zeros is considered as a weaknesses of the zero-hurdle models (Chipeta et al. 2014). Actually, if the existence of a distinct structural-zero class does not seem to be justified, a hurdle model should be used (Desjardins 2016). Such situation exists in real studies: multiple data-generating processes are at play, but without first-hand knowledge of the data collection process and response variable measure and the data generating mechanism of the zeros. In microbiome data, another reason to use the zero-hurdle models is that sometime it is difficult to differentiate zeros into structural and sampling zeros from conceptual and data generating perspectives.

For example, it is unclear to what extent a structural-zero class of women who are never at a risk for being absent of *Lactobacillus species*. Instead, researchers are more likely interested in understanding predictors of pregnant women who are not absent of *Lactobacillus species* and predictors that put pregnant women at a high risk for a high number of *Lactobacillus species* absent. Thus, in this context, zero-hurdle models would be the more conceptually and theoretically intriguing model.

To illustrate zero-hurdle models, we fit the ZPH and ZHNB models, using the same data set as the ZIP and ZINB models. Please remember, the probability that modeled by the binomial regression are different between ZIP and ZINB, and ZHP and ZHNB models. In ZIP and ZINB, the binomial regression models the probability of a structural zero versus other types of data, whereas in ZHP and ZHNB, it models the probability of presence versus absence of a taxon.

Hence, the estimated regression parameters obtained by ZHP and ZHNB have opposite signs from those obtained by ZIP and ZINB due to the different definition of p_i. In the illustrating example, the binomial distribution is used to model the absence (zero) versus presence (positive counts) of *Lactobacillus species*, and a Poisson (for ZHP) or negative binomial (for ZHNB) distribution for the counts.

We use same formula and offset as fitting ZIP and ZINB models above to fit ZHP and ZHNB models using the function hurdle() from the "pscl" package.

```
> ZHP28 <- hurdle(formula = f28, dist= "poisson", data = abund_table_28)
> summary(ZHP28)

Call:
hurdle(formula = f28, data = abund_table_28, dist = "poisson")

Pearson residuals:
   Min     1Q Median     3Q    Max
-1.014 -0.484 -0.473 -0.448 34.655

Count model coefficients (truncated poisson with log link):
            Estimate Std. Error z value Pr(>|z|)
(Intercept)  -6.2715     0.0303  -206.7   <2e-16 ***
fx1           0.8066     0.0412    19.6   <2e-16 ***
Zero hurdle model coefficients (binomial with logit link):
            Estimate Std. Error z value Pr(>|z|)
(Intercept)  -1.2689     0.0876  -14.49  < 2e-16 ***
fx1           1.3697     0.1911    7.17  7.7e-13 ***
---
Signif. codes:  0 '***' 0.001 '**' 0.01 '*' 0.05 '.' 0.1 ' ' 1

Number of iterations in BFGS optimization: 11
Log-likelihood: -2.28e+03 on 4 Df

> ZHNB28 <- hurdle(formula = f28, dist= "negbin", data = abund_table_28)
```

The ZHNB modeling results are printed using the summary() function as follow:

```
> summary(ZHNB28)

Call:
hurdle(formula = f28, data = abund_table_28, dist = "negbin")

Pearson residuals:
   Min     1Q  Median     3Q     Max
-0.510 -0.334  -0.328  -0.240  22.839

Count model coefficients (truncated negbin with log link):
            Estimate Std. Error z value Pr(>|z|)
(Intercept)   -6.760      0.169  -40.00  < 2e-16 ***
fx1            1.069      0.212    5.05  4.5e-07 ***
Log(theta)    -0.927      0.255   -3.63  0.00028 ***
Zero hurdle model coefficients (binomial with logit link):
            Estimate Std. Error z value Pr(>|z|)
(Intercept)  -1.2689     0.0876  -14.49  < 2e-16 ***
fx1           1.3697     0.1911    7.17  7.7e-13 ***
---
Signif. codes:  0 '***' 0.001 '**' 0.01 '*' 0.05 '.' 0.1 ' ' 1

Theta: count = 0.396
Number of iterations in BFGS optimization: 20
Log-likelihood: -1.23e+03 on 5 Df
```

12.3.4   Comparing Zero-Inflated and Zero-Hurdle Models

So far, we describe and differentiate between zero-inflated models and hurdle models from modeling and concepts. In general, ZIP versus ZHP, ZINB vs ZHNB, respectively, give similar model fit and predicted values, but different estimated parameters. These two models differ from their interpretation of model parameters, conceptualization of the zeros, and their ability to deal with zero-deflation (fewer zeros than would be expected by the data-generating process). Particularly, it is difficult to tell whether they are the appropriate choice for the data at hand, although ZIP and ZINB address structural zeros. Such zeros are latent and not directly observed. Thus, it is important to apply goodness of fit statistics to help guide the selection of models appropriate and optimal for the data. Here, we compare ZIP, ZINB, ZHP, and ZHNB models using likelihood ratio test in Sect. 12.3.4.1, Akaike's information criterion (AIC) in Sect. 12.3.4.2, Bayesian information criterion (BIC) in Sect. 12.3.4.3, Vuong test in Sect. 12.3.4.4.

12.3.4.1   Using Likelihood Ratio Test

In general, nested models are compared using likelihood or score test, while non-nested models are evaluated using AIC and/or the Vuong test (Vuong 1989; Long 1997). For the models considered, ZIP is nested within ZINB, ZHP nested within ZHNB. The function lrtest() from the package "lmtest" perform likelihood ratio test. The package "lmtest" is not part of the base installation, let us install it now and conduct the test.

```
> library(lmtest)
> lrtest(ZIP28,ZINB28)
Likelihood ratio test

Model 1: Y ~ fx + offset(Offset) | fx
Model 2: Y ~ fx + offset(Offset) | fx
   #Df LogLik Df Chisq Pr(> Chisq)
1    4  -2284
2    5  -1224  1  2121    < 2e-16 ***
---
Signif. codes:  0 '***' 0.001 '**' 0.01 '*' 0.05 '.' 0.1 ' ' 1
```

The likelihood ratio test is used to test whether or not the Poisson variance equals the NB variance, i.e., the variance structure of the Poisson of $var(Y_i) = \mu_i$ is same as that of the NB of $var(Y_i) = \mu_i(1 + \alpha\mu_i)$. The testing results show that these two variances are very significant, thus the ZIP model is not appropriate. ZINB model should be chosen.

```
> lrtest(ZHP28,ZHNB28)
Likelihood ratio test

Model 1: Y ~ fx + offset(Offset) | fx.
Model 2: Y ~ fx + offset(Offset) | fx
   #Df LogLik Df Chisq Pr(> Chisq)
1    4  -2285
2    5  -1229  1  2111    < 2e-16 ***
---
Signif. codes:  0 '***' 0.001 '**' 0.01 '*' 0.05 '.' 0.1 ' ' 1
```

The likelihood ratio test is conducted by running the function lrtest(), which produces a χ^2 statistic of 2111. It provides an overwhelming evidence to support the negative binomial model and hence the ZHNB model.

12.3.4.2 Using AIC

Akaike's information criterion (AIC) (Akaike 1973, 1974; Burnham and Anderson 2004; Aho et al. 2014) is one of the traditional model-comparison criteria; can be used for comparing non-nested models. Here, we use AIC to choose between non-nested mixture models (e.g., ZHNB vs. ZINB). This statistic takes into consideration model parsimony penalizing for the number of predictors in the model; the AIC is defined as $-2 \log(L) + 2k$, where L is the likelihood of the estimated model and k is the number of parameters. The first term is essentially the deviance and the second a penalty for the number of parameters. The smaller the AIC value, the better the model fit. The following R codes call the AIC() function to obtain the AIC values for each fitted model and then use the t() function to transpose the matrix.

```
> #lower is better
> t(AIC(ZIP28, ZINB28, ZHP28, ZHNB28))
     ZIP28 ZINB28 ZHP28 ZHNB28
df       4      5     4      5
AIC   4576   2458  4577   2468
```

In the four fitted models, the AIC of the corresponding zero-inflated models and zero-hurdle models is very close. The lowest AIC is observed with the ZINB and ZHNB is second lowest model.

The AIC values from these four fitted models suggest that overdispersion of the data is not only caused by the excess zero observations, but also due to non-zero count frequencies. The ZIP and ZHP models can address the lack of fit for the zero observations, but fail to capture the nonzero frequencies correctly, whereas the ZINB and ZHNB fit the data best.

12.3.4.3   Using BIC

It turns out that there is no or little difference in AIC between the according zero-hurdle and zero-inflated models, although we could rely on the AIC to select between non-nested mixture models (e.g., ZHNB vs. ZINB) (Cameron and Trivedi 2013). Indeed, for a single binary predictor, the ZHNB model and the ZINB model can be seen as re-parametrization of each other. This provides evidence that, it is difficult to use AIC to differentiate the zero-hurdle and zero-inflated models in some situations. Thus, other indices, such as BIC (Schwarz 1978) and Vuong test, may be the competing alternatives. Furthermore, the simulation study showed that if unobserved heterogeneity is large, the relative predictive performance of BIC often perform better than AIC (Brewer et al. 2016).

The BIC is defined as $-2\log L + \log(N) \times k$, where L is the likelihood of the estimated model, N is the number of case, and k is the number of parameters. As in AIC, the penalties are there to reduce the effects of overfitting, and note that the penalty is stronger for BIC than AIC for any reasonable sample size. As BIC imposes a harsher penalty for the estimation of each additional covariate, it often yields oversimplified models. When the data have large heterogeneity, it is just due to the stronger penalty that afforded the BIC performs better than AIC (Brewer et al. 2016). Although the simulation study is under the framework of linear models, we need further confirm whether the general principles can extend to all classes of model. However, large heterogeneity often presents in microbiome and ecology data. Thus, we use BIC as an alternative AIC to compare the models.

Currently, the "pscl" package had no function to calculate BIC values. Therefore, we use the "nonnest2" package here. Package "nonnest2" was developed to test non-nested models via theory supplied by Vuong test. This package has the capabilities to test model distinguishability and model fit for both nested and non-nested models. It also includes functionality to calculate AIC and BIC and associated confidence intervals. The syntax is given:

icci(object1, object2, conf.level = 0.95)

where, object1 = a model object, object2 = a model object, and conf.level = confidence level of the interval. Note: if models are nested or if the "variance test" from vuongtest() indicates models are indistinguishable, then the intervals returned from icci() will be incorrect.

```
> library(nonnest2)
> #lower is better
> icci(ZIP28,ZINB28)

Model 1
  Class: zeroinfl
  Call: zeroinfl(formula = f28, data = abund_table_28a, dist =
"poisson")
  AIC: 4576.392
  BIC: 4595.602

Model 2
  Class: zeroinfl
  Call: zeroinfl(formula = f28, data = abund_table_28a, dist =
"negbin")
  AIC: 2457.649
  BIC: 2481.661

95% Confidence Interval of AIC difference (AICdiff = AIC1 - AIC2)
  1074.887 < AICdiff < 3162.601

95% Confidence Interval of BIC difference (BICdiff = BIC1 - BIC2)
  1070.084 < BICdiff < 3157.798

> icci(ZHP28,ZHNB28)

Model 1
  Class: hurdle
  Call: hurdle(formula = f28, data = abund_table_28a, dist = "poisson")
  AIC: 4577.106
  BIC: 4596.316
```

```
Model 2
  Class: hurdle
  Call: hurdle(formula = f28, data = abund_table_28a, dist = "negbin")
  AIC: 2467.693
  BIC: 2491.705

95% Confidence Interval of AIC difference (AICdiff = AIC1 - AIC2)
  1067.104 < AICdiff < 3151.721

95% Confidence Interval of BIC difference (BICdiff = BIC1 - BIC2)
  1062.302 < BICdiff < 3146.919
```

The BIC results are consistent with those of AIC. ZINB is the best model, followed by ZHNB model.

12.3.4.4   Using Vuong Test

Vuong proposes a general model selection approach to test whether the competing models are nested, overlapping, or non-nested, or whether the models are correctly specified. Especially, in the context of zero-inflated and zero-hurdle models, Vuong test is associated to test for overdispersion and zero-inflation. Vuong's statistic is the average log-likelihood ratio suitably normalized so that it can be compared to a standard normal. The test statistic is defined by:

$$V = \frac{\sqrt{n}\,\bar{m}}{S_m},$$

(12.22)

where n is the sample size, S_m is the standard error of the test statistic, $\bar{m} = \left(\frac{1}{n}\right) \sum_{i=1}^{n} m_i$ and $S_m^2 = \left(\frac{1}{n-1}\right) \sum_{i=1}^{n} (m_i - \bar{m})^2$, and $m_i = \log\left[\frac{f_1(y_i)}{f_2(y_i)}\right]$, f_1 and f_2 are two competing probability models such as ZIP versus ZHP within our context. The statistic has an asymptotically standard normal distribution and the test is directional, with a large positive (negative) value favoring $f_1(f_2)$, and a value close to zero indicating that neither model fits the data well (Vuong 1989; Long 1997; Xia et al. 2012). In practice, we need to choose a critical value, c, for a significance level (often 1.96 to correspond to $\alpha = 0.05$). When $V > c$, the statistic favors the model in the numerator, when $V < -c$, the statistic favors the model in the denominator, and when $V \in (-c, c)$ neither model is favored. Here, c is set as 1.96 to be consistent with standard convention.

```
> # compare ZIP vs. ZHP
> vuong(ZIP28, ZHP28)
Vuong Non-Nested Hypothesis Test-Statistic:
(test-statistic is asymptotically distributed N(0,1) under the
 null that the models are indistinguishible)
--------------------------------------------------------------
              Vuong z-statistic              H_A p-value
Raw                         1.425 model1 > model2   0.077
AIC-corrected               1.425 model1 > model2   0.077
BIC-corrected               1.425 model1 > model2   0.077


> # compare ZIP vs. ZHNB
> vuong(ZIP28, ZHNB28)
Vuong Non-Nested Hypothesis Test-Statistic:
(test-statistic is asymptotically distributed N(0,1) under the
 null that the models are indistinguishible)
--------------------------------------------------------------
              Vuong z-statistic              H_A p-value
Raw                        -3.964 model2 > model1 3.7e-05
AIC-corrected              -3.964 model2 > model1 3.7e-05
BIC-corrected              -3.964 model2 > model1 3.7e-05

> # compare ZINB vs. ZHP
> vuong(ZINB28, ZHP28)
Vuong Non-Nested Hypothesis Test-Statistic:
(test-statistic is asymptotically distributed N(0,1) under the
 null that the models are indistinguishible)
--------------------------------------------------------------
              Vuong z-statistic              H_A p-value
Raw                         3.984 model1 > model2 3.4e-05
AIC-corrected               3.984 model1 > model2 3.4e-05
BIC-corrected               3.984 model1 > model2 3.4e-05

> # compare ZINB vs. ZHNB
> vuong(ZINB28, ZHNB28)
Vuong Non-Nested Hypothesis Test-Statistic:
(test-statistic is asymptotically distributed N(0,1) under the
 null that the models are indistinguishible)
--------------------------------------------------------------
              Vuong z-statistic              H_A p-value
Raw                         3.985 model1 > model2 3.4e-05
AIC-corrected               3.985 model1 > model2 3.4e-05
BIC-corrected               3.985 model1 > model2 3.4e-05


> # compare ZHNB vs. ZHP
> vuong(ZHNB28, ZHP28)
Vuong Non-Nested Hypothesis Test-Statistic:
(test-statistic is asymptotically distributed N(0,1) under the
 null that the models are indistinguishible)
------------------------------------------- -----------------
              Vuong z-statistic              H_A p-value
Raw                         3.968 model1 > model2 3.6e-05
AIC-corrected               3.968 model1 > model2 3.6e-05
BIC-corrected               3.968 model1 > model2 3.6e-05
```

Table 12.2 Model comparison based on likelihood ratio, AIC, BIC and Vuong Test

Model	LRT	AIC	BIC	Ranking based on Vuong test
ZIP	ZINB	4576	4595.6	3
ZINB		2458	2481.7	1
ZHP	ZHNB	4577	4596.3	4
ZHNB		2468	2491.7	2

Results from the model comparison using the AIC, BIC and Vuong's statistic are presented in Table 12.2. These statistics simultaneously test for overdispersion and zero-inflation.

Please note, LRT: the Likelihood Ratio test, AIC: Akaike's Information Criterion; BIC: Bayesian information criterion; ZIP: the zero-inflated Poisson model; ZINB: zero-inflated negative binomial model; ZHP: zero-hurdle Poisson model; ZHNB: zero-hurdle negative binomial model; and the Vuong test ranking corresponds to the order of the best fitting models.

Table 12.2 shows overwhelming support for the ZINB model best on the AIC, BIC. The ZINB model is ranked first, fitting significantly better than the ZHNB, ZIP, and ZHP models ($V > 3.9$, $p < 0.001$ for three comparisons); the ZHNB is ranked second, fitting significantly better than the ZIP and the ZHP models ($V > 3.9$, $p < 0.001$ for both comparisons).

12.3.5   Interpreting Main Effects of Modeling Results

In this example, we fit the models including only group variable (pregnant vs. non-pregnant women) as main effect. The coefficient represents the difference in mean log relative abundance between samples from pregnant and non-pregnant women.

We extract the most important output from the fitted ZINB model as follows:

```
Count model coefficients (negbin with log link):
            Estimate Std. Error z value Pr(>|z|)
(Intercept)   -6.835     0.186  -36.80  < 2e-16 ***
fx1            1.101     0.218    5.05  4.3e-07 ***
Log(theta)    -1.024     0.276   -3.70  0.00021 ***

Zero-inflation model coefficients (binomial with logit link):
            Estimate Std. Error z value Pr(>|z|)
(Intercept)    0.431     0.268    1.61  0.10771
fx1           -1.399     0.373   -3.75  0.00017 ***
```

For the fitted ZHNB model we obtain the following:

```
Count model coefficients (truncated negbin with log link):
            Estimate Std. Error z value Pr(>|z|)
(Intercept)   -6.760      0.169  -40.00  < 2e-16 ***
fx1            1.069      0.212    5.05  4.5e-07 ***
Log(theta)    -0.927      0.255   -3.63  0.00028 ***
Zero hurdle model coefficients (binomial with logit link):
            Estimate Std. Error z value Pr(>|z|)
(Intercept)  -1.2689     0.0876  -14.49  < 2e-16 ***
fx1           1.3697     0.1911    7.17  7.7e-13 ***
```

By default, the output shows estimated coefficients, standard errors, values for the Wald test and associated *p*-values, but no confidence intervals. Two main observations can be made here. First, both models yield similar results for the count component. Second, the zero component has not only the estimated parameters different in magnitude, but also their signs reversed. The difference in signs between ZINB and ZHNB is due to the hurdle() function(binomial regression) in the "pscl" package modeling the probability of a non-zero count, instead of the probability of a zero count.

We further convert the estimated log odds of coefficients into the odds of coefficients for convenient interpretation. The following R codes use the exponential function to convert the coefficients from the fitted ZINB model:

```
> expZINB28Coef <- exp(coef((ZINB28)))
> expZINB28Coef <- matrix(expZINB28Coef, ncol = 2)
> expZINB28Coef
         [,1]    [,2]
[1,] 0.001075 1.5388
[2,] 3.008239 0.2469
> colnames(expZINB28Coef) <- c("Count_model","Zero_inflation_model")
> expZINB28Coef
     Count_model Zero_inflation_model
[1,]    0.001075               1.5388
[2,]    3.008239               0.2469
```

The following R codes use the exponential function to convert the coefficients from the fitted ZHNB model:

```
> expZHNB28Coef <- exp(coef((ZHNB28)))
> expZHNB28Coef <- matrix(expZHNB28Coef, ncol = 2)
> colnames(expZHNB28Coef) <- c("Count_model","Zero_hurdle_model")
> expZHNB28Coef
     Count_model Zero_hurdle_model
[1,]     0.00116            0.2811
[2,]     2.91183            3.9341
```

It is very important to carefully interpret the zero-count parameters from zero-inflated and hurdle models. The correct parameter interpretation should be based on the model definitions. As defined, the logistic component in the zero-inflated models corresponds to inferences about the structural zero group; in contrast, the logistic component in the hurdle corresponds to inferences about the zeros, in general.

From the ZINB model we can derive that the estimated odds of observing an *excess zero* in pregnant women is $\exp(-1.399) = 0.2469$ times the odds in non-pregnant women ($p = 0.00017$).

It is not correct if we interpret that the odds of observing no *Lactobacillus vaginalis* is significantly smaller in pregnant women than that in non-pregnant women. Actually, we could not make such conclusion based on above odds from ZIP and ZINB. Remember in the zero-inflated model, structural zeros belong to latent class; it cannot be directly verified from the data, and hence it is difficult to intuitively interpret the notion of 'excess' zeros in the these models(ZIP and ZINB). However, we could interpret the odds of *excess zero* as the odds of membership in the 'always zero' group (i.e., the group of women who would never have present of any *Lactobacillus vaginalis*) is estimated to be 0.2469 lower in pregnant women than in non-pregnant women, based on the literature (Karazsia and van Dulmen 2008; Xia et al. 2012). The baseline odds of being among those who never have present of any *Lactobacillus vaginalis* is 1.5388.

In contrast to zero-inflated models, the zero-component has an intuitive interpretation in the zero-hurdle models. By definition, the zero component of ZHNB model clearly separates the non-zero count and zeros. The results from the zero component can be interpreted: the expected odds of a pregnant woman having positive *Lactobacillus vaginalis* are $\exp(1.3697) = 3.9341$ times the expected odds for a non-pregnant woman, holding the other variables constant with $p < 0.00001$. Thus, the odds of observing *Lactobacillus vaginalis* is significantly larger in pregnant women than that in non-pregnant women. We can reverse the odds to compare the zeros and non-zeros, equals $\exp(-1.3697) = 0.2542$, which supports the conclusion: the odds of no observing *Lactobacillus vaginalis* is significantly smaller in pregnant women than in non-pregnant women. The baseline odds of having a positive count versus zero is 0.2811.

Next, the parameters from the count component can be elaborated this way. For the log-linear component in the zero-inflated model, parameters are interpreted with respect to the non-structural zero group, whereas for the hurdle model they are interpreted with respect to the non-zero group. In ZINB, we find that the mean frequency of *Lactobacillus vaginalis* is $\mu_i = \exp(-6.835) = 0.0011$ in the non-pregnant women and $\exp(-6.835 + 1.101) = 0.0032$ in the pregnant women. This is only correct in the 'not always zero' group (i.e., the women who are at non-risk of presenting *Lactobacillus vaginalis*). However, the mean frequency of all subjects under the ZINB model is not μ_i, but is given by $(1 - p_i)\mu_i$. Thus, the mean frequency of *Lactobacillus vaginalis* for non-pregnant women is $\exp(-6.835)/(1 + \exp(0.431)) = 0.00042$, and the mean frequency of this outcome for pregnant women is $\exp(-6.835 + 1.101)/(1 + \exp(0.431 - 1.399)) = 0.0023$. The increase of this outcome in pregnant women is $(0.0023 - 0.00042)/0.0023 = 81.7\%$.

For the count component from ZHNB model—that is, parameter estimates conditional on a woman having positive *Lactobacillus vaginalis*—the mean frequency of *Lactobacillus vaginalis* for a pregnant woman are $\exp(1.069) = 2.91$ times the mean frequency of *Lactobacillus vaginalis* for a non-pregnant woman holding the other variables constant.

In summary, we compared zero-inflated and zero-hurdle models based on LRT, AIC, BIC and Vuong's statistic. The best model is ZINB; the second best model is ZHNB. There was clear evidence of overdispersion based on the estimated dispersion parameter from the ZINB and ZHNB models. There was also strong support of zero-inflation as the zero-inflated counterparts from ZIP, ZINB, ZHP and ZHNB, although we did not explicitly compare them with the models not accounting for zero-inflation such as Poisson and NB.

Overall ZINB outperforms ZHNB to fit the data for this specific outcome (*Lactobacillus vaginalis*). However, the zero-inflated models assume the existence of a latent structural-zero class. If such a class does not seem justified, a hurdle model should be preferred to use for the easier interpretation of zeros. For example, it is difficult to know the data-generating mechanism of zeros in microbiome study. Additionally, hurdle models can handle zero-deflation, whereas zero-inflated models are not able to do.

We suggest that model section should be based on (1) model fitting (to choose better-fitted models); (2) conceptual appropriateness (the chosen models should be conceptually interpretable); and (3) parsimony (i.e., Occam's razor, given all the criteria met, the simplest is selected as the best model).

12.3.6   Multiple Testing Issue and Adjusting **P-Values**

In this illustrating example, there are 28 vaginal bacteria defined at the genus and the species levels. We fit one of them (*Lactobacillus vaginalis*). The interested reader can analyze and compare the relative abundance of the 27 remaining bacteria using the codes and procedures above. Because we are making 28 tests on the same sample, an adjustment for multiple testing is needed. We can convert the *p*-values into q-values using the formula provided in Sect. 8.4.4.3. As noted, the q-value is an adjusted *p*-value, taking into account the false discovery rate (FDR). A q-value of 0.05 implies that we are willing to accept 5% of the tests found to be statistically significant (e.g., by *p*-value) being false positives. In microbiome studies, the final significance level is usually defined by fold change of the outcome variable and q-value. For example, a q-value < 0.1 and fold change >1.5 is used to claim significance.

12.4 Zero-Inflated Beta Regression Model with Random Effects

12.4.1 Introduction

Longitudinal study designs have become increasingly common now in microbiome studies, because they capture both between-individual differences and within subject dynamics. It offers the opportunity to study how microbial abundance changes across time and its association with treatments, clinical conditions or other covariates. For example, we can use a longitudinal study design to identify the bacterial taxa that change their differential abundances under different treatments across time.

Chen and Li (2016) developed a two-part zero-inflated Beta regression model with random-effects (ZIBR) for testing the association between microbial abundance and clinical covariates for longitudinal microbiome data. The development of ZIBR was motivated by the zero-inflated beta regression model (Peng et al. 2015) and zero-or-one inflated beta regression model (Ospina and Ferrari 2012) for proportion data in order to provide statistical methods to handle longitudinal or repeatedly measured proportion data. ZIBR includes a logistic regression component to model presence/absence of the taxon in the samples and a Beta regression component to model non-zero abundance of the taxon. Each component has a random effect to account for the correlations among the repeated measurements on the same subject. ZIBR includes two random intercept terms in order to model the dependency of the data measured over time and allows modeling multiple sources of variance that cannot be accounted for by the observed covariates.

12.4.2 ZIBR Model

The model considers each taxon separately. For each given bacterial taxon, let Y_{it} ($i = 1, 2, \ldots, N, t = 1, 2, \ldots, T$) be its relative abundance for subject i at time t, where $0 \leq Y_{it} < 1$. Assume that:

$$Y_{it} \sim 0 \text{ with probability } 1 - p_{it} \tag{12.23}$$

$$Y_{it} \sim Beta(\mu_{it}\phi, (1 - \mu_{it})\phi) \text{ with probability } p_{it}, \tag{12.24}$$

where the density function of the Beta distribution is parameterized as

$$f(y_{it}; \mu_{it}, \phi) = \frac{\Gamma(\phi)}{\Gamma(\mu_{it}\phi)\Gamma((1 - \mu_{it})\phi)} y_{it}^{\mu_{it}\phi - 1} (1 - y_{it})^{(1 - \mu_{it})\phi - 1}$$

with μ_{it} ($0 < \mu_{it} < 1$) and ϕ ($\phi > 0$) being the mean and dispersion parameters of the Beta distribution, respectively. The parameter p_{it} is the probability that the observation Y_{it} is generated from the Beta component.

Under the statistical framework, both the probability p_{it} of the logistic component and the mean of the Beta component μ_{it} depend on the covariates through the logit link functions:

$$\log it(p_{it}) = \log\left(\frac{p_{it}}{1 - p_{it}}\right) = \alpha_0 + X_{it}^T \alpha + \alpha_i, \tag{12.25}$$

$$\log it(\mu_{it}) = \log\left(\frac{\mu_{it}}{1 - \mu_{it}}\right) = \beta_0 + Z_{it}^T \beta + b_i, \tag{12.26}$$

where α_0 and β_0 are intercepts, a_i and b_i are the individual-specific random intercepts, X_i and Z_i are the covariates that can be time dependent and are not necessarily the same, and α and β are the corresponding vectors of the regression coefficients.

This model is considered as a two-part model with a logistic component and a Beta component. The logistic component models the presence/absence of the taxon in the samples and the Beta component models the non-zero abundance of the taxon. The data observed are from a mixture of these two models. The model is flexible to allow that the covariates can affect the microbiome composition in two different ways: affecting either the presence/absence of the taxon in the samples, or the relative abundance when the taxon presents in the samples.

To capture correlations and to account for multiple sources of variance, ZIBR model allows the repeated measures $Y_{it}(t = 1, \ldots, T)$ on the same subject i to share the same individual-specific random effects of a_i and b_i across different time points. In practice, for accommodating often adequate to capture the longitudinal correlations, the model only includes the random intercepts.

The random effects are assumed to follow an independent normal distribution: $a_i \sim N(0, \sigma_1^2)$, $b_i \sim N(0, \sigma_2^2)$. The parameters can be estimated by the standard maximum likelihood estimation.

12.4.3 Hypothesis Testing of ZIBR

Three statistical hypotheses proposed in ZIBR model are as below:

$H_0 : \alpha_j = 0$; $H_0 : \beta_j = 0$; $H_0 : \alpha_j = 0$ and $\beta_j = 0$ for each covariate X_j and Z_j.

They are used to test the following three biologically relevant null hypotheses by the likelihood ratio test, respectively: (1) the covariates associated with the bacterial taxon affect the bacterial taxon presence or absence; (2) the taxon associated with the covariates show different abundances; and (3) the covariates affect the taxon in terms of both presence/absence and its abundance.

The p-value can be obtained for each of these hypotheses. If the covariate X and Z are the same, the joint null (3) is $H_0 : \alpha_j = 0$ and $\beta_j = 0$, which tests the overall association between the covariate and the taxon abundance.

The setting of the proposed model is similar to the zero-inflated Poisson, binomial and negative binomial regression with random effects (Hall 2000; Min and Agresti 2005). It allows subject-specific random effect to be included in the model in order to model the dependency of the observations across time. Furthermore, ZIBR equips two components to have different individual-specific random effects to allow possible different dependency structures for the zero and non-zero parts of the data.

12.4.4   Modeling Using ZIBR

12.4.4.1   Pediatric IBD Patients

The illustrating data sets are from a real microbiome study (Lee et al. 2015; Lewis et al. 2015; Chen and Li 2016), which compared different therapies for pediatric IBD patients. The study collected 90 children with IBD who received one of the three study therapies: anti-TNF (N = 52), exclusive enteral nutrition (EEN) (N = 22) and partial enteral nutrition with ad lib diet (PEN) (N = 16). The taxa abundance data are generated by shotgun metagenomic analysis. Gut microbiome samples were collected at four time points: baseline, 1 week, 4 weeks and 8 weeks into the therapy. The bacterial abundances at genus level were used. The purpose of this study was to identify the bacterial genera comparing overall different abundances between EEN and anti-TNF treatments over three time points, adjusting covariates (treatment, week and baseline abundance).

12.4.4.2   Step-by-Step Implementing ZIBR

The ZIBR model and its associated likelihood ratio tests are implemented via the zibr() function in ZIBR package. The syntax of zibr() function is as follows:

zibr(logistic.cov = logistic.cov,beta.cov = beta.cov,Y = Y,subject.ind = subject.ind,time.ind = time.ind)

where, logistic.cov = covariates for the logistic component with format of samples (= rows) by covariates (= columns); beta.cov = covariates for the beta component with format of samples (= rows) by covariates (= columns); time.ind = the variable with time points. The ordering of the samples in the above matrix or vectors must be consistent. Y = response variable, it can be any level of taxa depending which level of taxa we choose to fit. From scientific point, species or genus is often used; subject.ind = subject or sample id indicator.

The zibr() function will return the following results:

(1) logistic.est.table: the estimated coefficients for logistic component;
(2) logistic.s1.est: the estimated standard deviation for the random effect in the logistic component;

(3) beta.est.table: the estimated coefficients for beta component;
(4) beta.s2.est: the estimated standard deviation for the random effect in the beta component;
(5) beta.v.est: the estimated dispersion parameter in the beta component;
(6) joint.p: the *p*-values for jointly testing each covariate in both logistic and beta component.

In order to fit ZIBR model by using the ZIBR package, we need to install and make it available to R workplace first. We install the ZIBR package from Github website and set R work directory folder.

```
> install.packages("devtools")
> devtools::install_github("chvlyl/ZIBR")
> library(ZIBR)
> setwd("E:/Home/MicrobiomeStatR/Analysis")
```

The ZIBR example from the authors of this package is an excellent sample for illustrating ZIBR model. We promote this method and its application. Here, we modify the programs and illustrate and explain its application step by step.

Step 1: Import Taxa Abundance Data and Meta Data

As fitting regression in microbiome study, ZIBR regression needs two kinds of data: taxa abundance data and meta data. The response variable (abundance read counts) is typically stored in taxa file, covariates including group and sample information in meta file. Abundance read counts are either or not included in the taxa file depending on the data generating pipelines. In this example, these data files are separately stored, thus need to import them into R workplace, and merge them together before fitting the model.

The following R codes import the raw taxa data and name the object as 'taxa_table', then check the first few rows of data.

```
> rawfile<-
"https://raw.githubusercontent.com/chvlyl/PLEASE/master/1_Data/Raw_Data/MetaP
hlAn/PLEASE/G_Remove_unclassfied_Renormalized_Merge_Rel_MetaPhlAn_Result.xls"
> taxa_table <- read.table(rawfile,sep='\t',header=TRUE,row.names = 1,
+                          check.names=FALSE,stringsAsFactors=FALSE)
> head(taxa_table)
                5001-01 5001-02  5001-03   5001-04 5002-01
g__Bacteroides   0.4272  0.2319  0.02041  0.00533 72.3830
g__Ruminococcus  0.0000  0.0000  0.00613  0.00000  4.9632
                5002-02 5002-03 5002-04   5003-01 5003-02
g__Bacteroides   58.558  6.7429   4.247 20.98819 24.2252
g__Ruminococcus   4.528 17.5592   5.952  1.29717  1.8270
                5003-03 5003-04 5004-01 5004-02 5004 03
g__Bacteroides  58.72660 55.1687 83.0756 44.8019 61.7801
g__Ruminococcus  0.46149  0.8113  2.8420  0.3798 17.6647
```

The original taxa data have the format of taxa (in rows)-by-samples (in columns). Below the data are converted to samples (in rows)-by-taxa (in columns) data table.

```
> taxa_table_t <- t(taxa_table)
> head(taxa_table_t)
          g__Bacteroides g__Ruminococcus g__Faecalibacterium
5001-01          0.42722         0.00000               0.000
5001-02          0.23188         0.00000               0.000
5001-03          0.02041         0.00613               0.000
5001-04          0.00533         0.00000               0.000
5002-01         72.38299         4.96320               8.471
5002-02         58.55836         4.52818              20.786
```

Check the data table dimensions to make sure the data loaded correctly. There are total 335 samples and 105 bacteria taxa in the taxa table.

```
> cat('samples','taxa',dim(taxa_table_t),'\n')
samples taxa 335 105
> taxa_table_t[1:3,1:3]
          g__Bacteroides g__Ruminococcus g__Faecalibacterium
5001-01          0.42722         0.00000                   0
5001-02          0.23188         0.00000                   0
5001-03          0.02041         0.00613                   0
```

Below load total read counts data and name the object as 'abund_table', then check the first few rows of data.

```
> totalreadfile <-
'https://raw.githubusercontent.com/chvlyl/PLEASE/master/1_Data/Raw_Data/MetaP
hlAn/Human_Reads/please_combo_human_reads.xls'
> abund_table <- read.table(totalreadfile,sep='\t',header=TRUE,
+                          row.names=1,stringsAsFactors=FALSE)
> head(abund_table)
     NonHumanReads TotalReads HumanReads HumanPer GroupFcp GroupPcdai
4000      17525422   19515697    1990275 10.19833    Combo      Combo
4001      18089762   18185930      96168  0.52880    Combo      Combo
4002      27311061   27338002      26941  0.09855    Combo      Combo
4004      11051439   11092808      41369  0.37294    Combo      Combo
4005       9434025    9492196      58171  0.61283    Combo      Combo
4006      23327496   23634581     307085  1.29930    Combo      Combo
```

You can see that the data are already in the format of samples (in rows)-by-taxa (in columns).

Now, load meta data and name the object as 'meta_table', then check the first or last few rows of data to check the dataset format and treatment information.

```
> samplefile <-
'https://raw.githubusercontent.com/chvlyl/PLEASE/master/1_Data/Processed_Data
/Sample_Information/2015_02_13_Processed_Sample_Information.csv'
> meta_table <- read.csv(samplefile,row.names=1)
> head(meta_table)
> tail(meta_table)
        Subject Species.Cluster   Cluster Treatment FCPResponse      Type
7014-03    7014       cluster 1 cluster 1      Diet          0 PLEASE-T3
7014-04    7014       cluster 1 cluster 1      Diet          0 PLEASE-T4
7015-01    7015       cluster 1 cluster 1      Diet          1 PLEASE-T1
7015-02    7015       cluster 1 cluster 1      Diet          1 PLEASE-T2
7015-03    7015       cluster 1 cluster 1      Diet          1 PLEASE-T3
7015-04    7015       cluster 1 cluster 1      Diet          1 PLEASE-T4
        Time BristolScore  FCP PCDAI PUCAI log.FCP  Group      Response
7014-03    3            6 1123    NA    25   7.024 PLEASE Non.Response
7014-04    4           NA   NA    15    15      NA PLEASE Non.Response
7015-01    1            4 1968    40    35   7.585 PLEASE     Response
7015-02    2            4 1003    NA    25   6.911 PLEASE     Response
7015-03    3            4  459    NA    25   6.129 PLEASE     Response
7015-04    4            5  202    10    20   5.308 PLEASE     Response
        Antibiotics.visit Steroids Treatment.Specific Disease NonHumanReads
7014-03           Not.Use  Not.Use                EEN   Crohn        480246
7014-04             <NA>   Not.Use                EEN   Crohn            NA
7015-01               Use  Not.Use                EEN   Crohn       7191073
7015-02               Use  Not.Use                EEN   Crohn        207572
7015-03               Use  Not.Use                EEN   Crohn      14681706
7015-04               Use  Not.Use                EEN   Crohn       1339882
        Human.Per Fungi.Per Distance Bact.Div Species.Distance
7014-03    3.9754 0.0004165   0.6667    87.66           0.6889
7014-04        NA        NA       NA       NA               NA
7015-01   10.0875 0.0132386   0.3333   130.55           0.4066
7015-02    0.3677 0.0289056   0.7619   109.03           0.7640
7015-03    0.2664 0.0002861   0.3571    93.35           0.3556
7015-04    1.8486 0.0053736   0.5238    94.42           0.5556
```

The data have the format of samples (in rows)-by-covariates (in columns). The column 'Treatment.Specific' includes the treatment information.

Step 2: Filter Low Abundant Taxa Data
To filter low read counts from abundance data table, you need define one cutoff of low depth. It is often based researcher's experience or literature. Here, it is based low non-human reads (NonHumanReads < 10000).

```
> low_samples <- subset(abund_table,NonHumanReads<10000)
> low_samples[,1:5]
        NonHumanReads TotalReads HumanReads HumanPer GroupFcp
5010-02          1014       1104         90  8.15217    TNF.N
5018-03          6101       6121         20  0.32674   Diet.R
5023-04          1954       2679        725 27.06234    TNF.R
6007-01          1809       4249       2440 57.42528    TNF.R
7001-02          9965       9971          6  0.06017   Diet.N
7001-03           566        613         47  7.66721   Diet.N
7001-04           626        637         11  1.72684   Diet.N
7002-04           683        696         13  1.86782   Diet.N
7003-02          4681       5719       1038 18.15003  Diet.NR
7003-03          4935       5049        114  2.25787  Diet.NR
7009-02          1895       1916         21  1.09603   Diet.N
7009-03          5319       5361         42  0.78344   Diet.N
7010-02          2375       2400         25  1.04167   Diet.N
7010-03          6312       6495        183  2.81755   Diet.N
```

There are 14 samples with NonHumanReads < 10,000 in abundance table. You can check how many taxa with low depth counts in the raw taxa data using following R codes.

```
> rownames(taxa_table_t)[which(rownames(taxa_table_t) %in% rownames
(low_samples))]
[1] "5018-03" "7001-02" "7003-02" "7003-03" "7009-03" "7010-03"
```

There are 6 taxa with NonHumanReads < 10,000 in the raw taxa data. Now, you can use the which() function with negative sign '−' to delete these 6 low depth samples from the taxa table:

```
> taxa_table_t < - taxa_table_t[-which(rownames(taxa_table_t) %in%
rownames(low_samples)),]
```

As recall, before deletion, there are 335 samples with 105 bacteria taxa. After deletion the updated taxa table now has 329 samples with 105 bacteria taxa.

```
> # Before deletion
> dim(taxa_table_t)
[1] 335 105
> # After deletion
> dim(taxa_table_t)
[1] 329 105
```

For effectively modeling, we need further filter and remove the low abundant taxa data. In this case, the authors of this example use both sum () and quantile() functions to process further filtering. You can apply the double criteria to remove the low sequencing depth samples and low abundant taxa.

```
> filter_index1 <- apply(taxa_table_t,2,function(X){sum(X>0)>0.4*length(X)})
> filter_index2 <- apply(taxa_table_t,2,function(X){quantile(X,0.9)>1})
> taxa_filter <- taxa_table_t[,filter_index1 & filter_index2]
> head(taxa_filter)
        g__Bacteroides g__Ruminococcus g__Faecalibacterium
5001-01        0.42722         0.00000               0.000
5001-02        0.23188         0.00000               0.000
5001-03        0.02041         0.00613               0.000
5001-04        0.00533         0.00000               0.000
5002-01       72.38299         4.96320               8.471
5002-02       58.55836         4.52818              20.786
        g__Bifidobacterium g__Escherichia g__Clostridium
5001-01             0.3757        38.3172         0.2228
5001-02             2.0725        21.4206        21.0454
5001-03             1.0331        41.2590        20.4835
5001-04             0.6021        36.0904        12.0391
5002-01             1.3608         0.8564         4.1348
5002-02             3.7974         1.0430         3.0277
```

Now, create a taxa data table for ZIBR modeling. The following R codes re-sum the bacteria by samples (rows) and time 100 to make sure the sum of row is 100.

```
> taxa_filter <- 100*sweep(taxa_filter, 1, rowSums(taxa_filter), FUN="/")
> head(taxa_filter)
        g__Bacteroides g__Ruminococcus g__Faecalibacterium g__Bifidobacterium
5001-01       0.451461        0.000000               0.000             0.3970
5001-02       0.234517        0.000000               0.000             2.0961
5001-03       0.020862        0.006266               0.000             1.0559
5001-04       0.007695        0.000000               0.000             0.8692
5002-01      73.264555        5.023647               8.574             1.3774
5002-02      59.815023        4.625356              21.232             3.8789

> cat('after filter:','samples','taxa',dim(taxa_filter),'\n')
after filter: samples taxa 329 18
```

After filter, there remains 18 bacteria in the taxa table. The following R codes check which taxa remain:

```
> cat(colnames(taxa_filter),'\n')
g__Bacteroides  g__Ruminococcus  g__Faecalibacterium  g__Bifidobacterium
g__Escherichia g__Clostridium g__Dialister g__Eubacterium g__Roseburia
g__Streptococcus g__Dorea g__Parabacteroides
g__Lactobacillus g__Veillonella g__Haemophilus
g__Alistipes g__Collinsella g__Coprobacillus
```

Check to see if the row sum is 100.

```
> head(rowSums(taxa_filter))
5001-01 5001-02 5001-03 5001-04 5002-01 5002-02
    100     100     100     100     100     100
```

We rename the filtered taxa table as 'taxa_data' for analysis later.

```
> taxa_data <- taxa_filter
> head(taxa_data)
        g__Bacteroides g__Ruminococcus g__Faecalibacterium g__Bifidobacterium
5001-01       0.451461        0.000000               0.000             0.3970
5001-02       0.234517        0.000000               0.000             2.0961
5001-03       0.020862        0.006266               0.000             1.0559
5001-04       0.007695        0.000000               0.000             0.8692
5002-01      73.264555        5.023647               8.574             1.3774
5002-02      59.815023        4.625356              21.232             3.8789

> dim(taxa_data)
[1] 329  18
```

Step 3: Create Covariates for Meta Table

Any randomized longitudinal study setting should have a treatment variable and a time variable for testing the dynamic variability between treatments over time. The following R codes are used to create covariates: Time, Treat(antiTNF + EEN) and Time by Treatment interaction term.

```
> library(dplyr)
> # create covariates:Time, antiTNF+EEN
> reg_cov <-
+    data.frame(Sample=rownames(taxa_data),stringsAsFactors = FALSE) %>%
+    left_join(add_rownames(meta_table,var = 'Sample'),by='Sample')%>%
+    # exclude PEN, just keep antiTNF and EEN
+    dplyr::filter(Treatment.Specific!='PEN') %>%
+    # subset meta table
+    dplyr::select(Sample,Time,Subject,Response,Treatment.Specific) %>%#
+    group_by(Subject) %>% summarise(count = n()) %>% dplyr::filter(count==4)
%>%
+    dplyr::select(Subject) %>%
+    left_join(add_rownames(meta_table,var = 'Sample'),by='Subject') %>%
+    # create treatment variable Treat and code antiTNF as 1, EEN as 0
+    mutate(Treat=ifelse(Treatment.Specific=='antiTNF',1,0)) %>%
+    dplyr::select(Sample,Subject,Time,Response,Treat) %>%
+    dplyr::mutate(Subject=paste('S',Subject,sep='')) %>%
+    # recode Time variable
+
dplyr::mutate(Time=ifelse(Time=='1',0,ifelse(Time=='2',1,ifelse(Time=='3',4,
ifelse(Time=='4',8,NA))))) %>%
+    # create Time by Treatment interaction term
+    dplyr::mutate(Time.X.Treatment=Time*Treat) %>%
+    as.data.frame
> # take out first time point
> reg_cov_t1   <-   subset(reg_cov,Time==0)
> rownames(reg_cov_t1) <- reg_cov_t1$Subject
> reg_cov_t234 <-   subset(reg_cov,Time!=0)
> reg_cov_t234 <- data.frame(
+    baseline_sample=reg_cov_t1[reg_cov_t234$Subject,'Sample'],
+    baseline_subject=reg_cov_t1[reg_cov_t234$Subject,'Subject'],
+    reg_cov_t234,
+    stringsAsFactors = FALSE)

> head(reg_cov_t234)
  baseline_sample baseline_subject  Sample Subject Time     Response Treat
2          5001-01           S5001 5001-02   S5001    1 Non.Response     1
3          5001-01           S5001 5001-03   S5001    4 Non.Response     1
4          5001-01           S5001 5001-04   S5001    8 Non.Response     1
6          5002-01           S5002 5002-02   S5002    1 Non.Response     1
7          5002-01           S5002 5002-03   S5002    4 Non.Response     1
8          5002-01           S5002 5002-04   S5002    8 Non.Response     1
  Time.X.Treatment
2                1
3                4
4                8
6                1
7                4
8                8
```

Step 4: Fit ZIBR Model

The following R codes fit ZIBR model on the example data using the zibr() function from the ZIBR package. ZIBR considers each taxon separately and independently analyzes each taxon. As we fit all 18 taxa together, before fitting we need create a matrix to hold these taxa and list to hold the *p*-values. This is done by calling the Matrix package.

```
> library(Matrix)
> library(ZIBR)
> # create a matrix to hold taxa
> taxa_all <- colnames(taxa_data)
> taxa_all
 [1] "g__Bacteroides"        "g__Ruminococcus"      "g__Faecalibacterium"
 [4] "g__Bifidobacterium"    "g__Escherichia"       "g__Clostridium"
 [7] "g__Dialister"          "g__Eubacterium"       "g__Roseburia"
[10] "g__Streptococcus"      "g__Dorea"             "g__Parabacteroides"
[13] "g__Lactobacillus"      "g__Veillonella"       "g__Haemophilus"
[16] "g__Alistipes"          "g__Collinsella"       "g__Coprobacillus"
> # create a list to hold p-values
> p_taxa_list_zibr <- list()
> p_taxa_list_zibr
list()
> #ZIBR independently fit each taxon.
> for (taxa in taxa_all){
+   #for example,taxa = "g__Bacteroides"
+   ###create covariates
+   X <- data.frame(
+     Baseline=taxa_data[reg_cov_t234$baseline_sample, taxa]/100,
+     reg_cov_t234[,c('Time','Treat')]
+   )
+   rownames(X) <- reg_cov_t234$Sample
+   Z <- X
+   subject_ind <- reg_cov_t234$Subject
+   time_ind    <- reg_cov_t234$Time
+   ###create a table to summarize statistics
+   cat(taxa,'\n')
+   Y <- taxa_data[reg_cov_t234$Sample, taxa]/100
+   cat('Zeros/All',sum(Y==0),'/',length(Y),'\n')
+   if (sum(Y>0)<10 | sum(Y==0) <10 | max(Y)<0.01){
+     print('skip')
+     next
+   }else{
+     est <- zibr(logistic.cov=X,beta.cov=Z,Y=Y,
+                 subject.ind=subject_ind,
+                 time.ind=time_ind,
+                 quad.n=30,verbose=TRUE)
+     p_taxa_list_zibr[[taxa]] <- est$joint.p
+
+   }
+ }
```

The following are the summarized statistics from fitting ZIBR.

```
g__Bacteroides
Zeros/All 3 / 177
[1] "skip"
g__Ruminococcus
Zeros/All 18 / 177
g__Faecalibacterium
Zeros/All 27 / 177
g__Bifidobacterium
Zeros/All 35 / 177
g__Escherichia
Zeros/All 34 / 177
g__Clostridium
Zeros/All 19 / 177
g__Dialister
Zeros/All 83 / 177
g__Eubacterium
Zeros/All 42 / 177
g__Roseburia
Zeros/All 61 / 177
g__Streptococcus
Zeros/All 24 / 177
g__Dorea
Zeros/All 83 / 177
g__Parabacteroides
Zeros/All 74 / 177
g__Lactobacillus
Zeros/All 94 / 177
g__Veillonella
Zeros/All 61 / 177
g__Haemophilus
Zeros/All 77 / 177
g__Alistipes
Zeros/All 23 / 177
g__Collinsella
Zeros/All 106 / 177
g__Coprobacillus
Zeros/All 89 / 177
```

Step 5: Adjust *p*-Values

We print the unadjusted *p*-values:

```
> # unadjusted p values
> p_taxa_zibr <- t(as.data.frame(p_taxa_list_zibr))
> p_taxa_zibr
                      Baseline     Time      Treat
g__Ruminococcus      1.303e-03 0.220442 6.135e-03
g__Faecalibacterium  1.042e-06 0.639001 1.791e-03
g__Bifidobacterium   1.249e-04 0.495912 1.452e-03
g__Escherichia       1.099e-12 0.060012 5.520e-02
g__Clostridium       5.517e-04 0.864729 2.035e-01
g__Dialister         1.314e-03 0.345004 6.046e-03
g__Eubacterium       1.184e-02 0.026991 1.631e-02
g__Roseburia         3.834e-05 0.250054 1.300e-01
g__Streptococcus     1.162e-02 0.238892 9.931e-05
g__Dorea             2.974e-07 0.795932 1.050e-01
g__Parabacteroides   7.027e-08 0.099298 1.722e-01
g__Lactobacillus     9.565e-08 0.358874 3.136e-03
g__Veillonella       2.138e-07 0.989408 9.800e-03
g__Haemophilus       2.883e-08 0.346125 3.654e-05
g__Alistipes         1.508e-12 0.003998 3.036e-08
g__Collinsella       1.887e-09 0.604587 1.348e-02
g__Coprobacillus     2.970e-06 0.818501 5.358e-01
```

In Chap. 8, we illustrated how to adjust *p*-values for multiple comparisons using various approaches, here we nest the p.adjust() function in the mutate_each() function to make FDR correction.

```
> library(dplyr)
> p_taxa_zibr_adj < -
+ add_rownames(as.data.frame
(p_taxa_zibr),var = 'Taxa') % > % mutate_each(funs(p.adjust(.,'fdr')),
-Taxa)
```

We print the FDR-adjusted *p*-values as below:

```
> p_taxa_zibr_adj
# A tibble: 17 x 4
                   Taxa  Baseline     Time      Treat
                  <chr>     <dbl>    <dbl>      <dbl>
1       g__Ruminococcus 1.489e-03 0.60727 1.304e-02
2   g__Faecalibacterium 1.969e-06 0.83562 6.090e-03
3    g__Bifidobacterium 1.770e-04 0.76641 6.090e-03
4        g__Escherichia 1.282e-11 0.34007 7.819e-02
5        g__Clostridium 7.215e-04 0.91877 2.163e-01
6          g__Dialister 1.489e-03 0.61009 1.304e-02
7        g__Eubacterium 1.184e-02 0.22942 2.521e-02
8          g__Roseburia 5.925e-05 0.60727 1.579e-01
9      g__Streptococcus 1.184e-02 0.60727 5.627e-04
10             g__Dorea 6.319e-07 0.91877 1.373e-01
11   g__Parabacteroides 2.389e-07 0.42202 1.951e-01
12     g__Lactobacillus 2.710e-07 0.61009 8.886e-03
13       g__Veillonella 5.193e-07 0.98941 1.851e-02
14       g__Haemophilus 1.225e-07 0.61009 3.106e-04
15         g__Alistipes 1.282e-11 0.06797 5.161e-07
16       g__Collinsella 1.069e-08 0.83562 2.291e-02
17     g__Coprobacillus 5.049e-06 0.91877 5.358e-01
```

Step 6: Write Results Table

We print the results table with html format and write the results table to file called "Results_antiTNF_EEN_ZIBR.csv" in the R directory folder "E:/Home/MicrobiomeStatR/Analysis".

```
> # make the table
> library(xtable)
> table < -xtable
(p_taxa_zibr_adj, caption = "Table of significant taxa", digits = 3,
label = "sig_taxa_table")
> print.xtable(table, type = "html", file = "IBD_Table.html")
> write.csv(p_taxa_zibr_adj,file = paste('Results_antiTNF_PEN_ZIBR.csv',
sep = "))
```

For the detail of interpretation of fitting ZIBR using this example, readers can reference the original research paper. Briefly ZIBR identified 11 genera, including *Ruminococcus, Faecalibacterium, Bifidobacterium, Dialister, Eubacterium, Streptococcus, Lactobacillus, Veillonella, Haemophilus, Alistipes, Collinsella*. The results show that the baseline abundance of these taxa had large effects on their abundance of the treatment and these taxa were relatively stable during the 8 weeks of treatments (see Table 12.3).

Table 12.3 Result from fitted ZIBR on dataset of pediatric IBD patients

	Taxa	Baseline	Time	Treat
1	g__Ruminococcus	0.001	0.607	0.013
2	g__Faecalibacterium	0.000	0.836	0.006
3	g__Bifidobacterium	0.000	0.766	0.006
4	g__Escherichia	0.000	0.340	0.078
5	g__Clostridium	0.001	0.919	0.216
6	g__Dialister	0.001	0.610	0.013
7	g__Eubacterium	0.012	0.229	0.025
8	g__Roseburia	0.000	0.607	0.158
9	g__Streptococcus	0.012	0.607	0.001
10	g__Dorea	0.000	0.919	0.137
11	g__Parabacteroides	0.000	0.422	0.195
12	g__Lactobacillus	0.000	0.610	0.009
13	g__Veillonella	0.000	0.989	0.019
14	g__Haemophilus	0.000	0.610	0.000
15	g__Alistipes	0.000	0.068	0.000
16	g__Collinsella	0.000	0.836	0.023
17	g__Coprobacillus	0.000	0.919	0.536

Table of significant taxa

12.5   Summary and Discussion

In this chapter, we first introduced zero-inflated and zero hurdle models for dealing with excess zeros. Then, we illustrated step-by-step implementing two zero-inflated (ZIP and ZINB), and two zero hurdle (ZHP and ZHNB) models in a real microbiome data set. We interpreted model fitting results of these four models and compared them using various methods. Furthermore, we introduced the zero-inflated beta regression model with random-effects (ZIBR). The advantages of ZIBR include extension of zero-inflated regressions to longitudinal setting, jointly modeling the covariates that affect the taxon in terms of both presence/absence (via a logistic regression component) and its abundance (via a Beta regression component). We also highlighted ZIBR's joint modeling capability by step-by-step implementing ZIBR using a real data set.

In the context of zero-inflated models, two recently developed models and packages drew our attention: one is the general framework of differential distribution analysis of microbiome data based on a ZINB regression model and the "MicrobiomeDDA" package for implementing the proposed methods. Another is the "metamicrobiomeR" package, which was designed to perform meta-analysis across microbiome studies using random effect models based on zero-inflated beta GAMLSS. We have reviewed and briefly introduced these two methods and packages in Chap. 3.

References

Agresti, A. 2002. *Categorical data analysis*. Hoboken, New Jersey, Sons, Inc., Publication.

Aho, K., D. Derryberry, et al. 2014. Model selection for ecologists: The worldviews of AIC and BIC. *Ecology* 95 (3): 631–636.

Akaike, H. 1973. *Information theory and an extension of the maximum likelihood principle*. 2nd international symposium on information theory, Budapest: Akademiai Kiado.

Akaike, H. 1974. A new look at the statistical model identification. *IEEE Transactions on Automatic Control* 19 (6): 716–723.

Atkins, D., and R. Gallop. 2007. Rethinking how family researchers model infrequent outcomes: A tutorial on count regression and zero-inflated models. *Journal of Family Psychology* 21 (4): 726.

Bin, C.Y. 2002. Zero-inflated models for regression analysis of count data: A study of growth and development. *Statistics in Medicine* 21 (10): 1461–1469.

Bohning, D., E. Dietz, et al. 1999. The zero-inflated poisson model and the decayed, missing and filled teeth index in dental epidemiology. *Journal of the Royal Statistical Society. Series A (Statistics in Society)* 162 (2): 195–209.

Brewer, M.J., A. Butler, et al. 2016. The relative performance of AIC, AICC and BIC in the presence of unobserved heterogeneity. *Methods in Ecology and Evolution* 7 (6): 679–692.

Burnham, K.P., and D.R. Anderson. 2004. Multimodel inference: Understanding AIC and BIC in model selection. *Sociological Methods & Research* 33 (2): 261–304.

Cameron, A.C., and P.K. Trivedi. 2013. *Regression analysis of count data*. New York: Cambridge University Press.

Campbell, M.J., D. Machin, et al. 1991. Coping with extra Poisson variability in the analysis of factors influencing vaginal ring expulsions. *Statistics in Medicine* 10 (2): 241–254.

Chen, E.Z., and H. Li. 2016. A two-part mixed-effects model for analyzing longitudinal microbiome compositional data. *Bioinformatics* 32 (17): 2611–2617.

Chipeta, M.G., B.M. Ngwira, et al. 2014. Zero adjusted models with applications to analysing helminths count data. *BMC Research Notes* 7: 856.

Cohen, A.C. 1963. *Estimation in mixtures of discrete distributions*. Proceedings of the international symposium on discrete distributions, Montreal, Quebec.

Cragg, J.G. 1971. Some statistical models for limited dependent variables with application to the demand for durable goods. *Econometrica* 39 (5): 829–844.

Desjardins, C.D. 2016. Modeling zero-inflated and overdispersed count data: An empirical study of school suspensions. *The Journal of Experimental Education* 84 (3): 449–472.

Dwivedi, A.K., S.N. Dwivedi, et al. 2010. Statistical models for predicting number of involved nodes in breast cancer patients. *Health* 2 (7): 641–651.

Fettweis, J.M., J.P. Brooks, et al. 2014. Differences in vaginal microbiome in African American women versus women of European ancestry. *Microbiology* 160 (Pt 10): 2272–2282.

Freund, D.A., T.J. Kniesner, et al. 1999. Dealing with the common econometric problems of count data with excess zeros, endogenous treatment effects, and attrition bias. *Economics Letters* 62 (1): 7–12.

Gonzalez, A., A. King, et al. 2012. Characterizing microbial communities through space and time. *Current Opinion in Biotechnology* 23 (3): 431–436.

Graveley, B.R., and A.N. Brooks, et al. 2011. The developmental transcriptome of Drosophila melanogaster. *Nature* 471.

Hall, D.B. 2000. Zero-inflated Poisson and binomial regression with random effects: A case study. *Biometrics* 56 (4): 1030–1039.

Heilbron, D.C. 1994. Zero-altered and other regression models for count data with added zeros. *Biometrical Journal* 36 (5): 531–547.

Hinde, J., and C. Demétrio. 1998. Overdispersion: Models and estimation. *Computational Statistics & Data Analysis* 27 (2): 151.

Hu, M.-C., M. Pavlicova, et al. 2011. Zero-inflated and hurdle models of count data with extra zeros: Examples from an HIV-risk reduction intervention trial. *The American Journal of Drug and Alcohol Abuse* 37 (5): 367–375.

Johnson, N.L., and S. Kotz. 1969. *Distributions in statistics: Discrete distributions*. Boston, MA: Haughton Mifflin.

Karazsia, B.T., and M.H.M. van Dulmen. 2008. Regression models for count data: Illustrations using longitudinal predictors of childhood injury*. *Journal of Pediatric Psychology* 33 (10): 1076–1084.

Lambert, D. 1992. Zero-inflated poisson regression, with an application to defects in manufacturing. *Technometrics* 34 (1): 1–14.

Lee, A.H., M.R. Stevenson, et al. 2002. Modeling young driver motor vehicle crashes: Data with extra zeros. *Accident Analysis and Prevention* 34 (4): 515–521.

Lee, D., R.N. Baldassano, et al. 2015. Comparative effectiveness of nutritional and biological therapy in North American children with active Crohn's Disease. *Inflammatory Bowel Diseases* 21 (8): 1786–1793.

Lewis, J.D., E.Z. Chen, et al. 2015. Inflammation, antibiotics, and diet as environmental stressors of the gut microbiome in pediatric Crohn's Disease. *Cell Host & Microbe* 18 (4): 489–500.

Lewsey, J.D., and W.M. Thomson. 2004. The utility of the zero-inflated Poisson and zero-inflated negative binomial models: A case study of cross-sectional and longitudinal DMF data examining the effect of socio-economic status. *Community Dentistry and Oral Epidemiology* 32 (3): 183–189.

Long, J.S. 1997. *Regression models for categorical and limited dependent variables*. Thousand Oaks, CA, USA: Sage Publications.

Ma, B., L.J. Forney, et al. 2012. Vaginal microbiome: Rethinking health and disease. *Annual Review of Microbiology* 66 (1): 371–389.

Martin, T.G., B.A. Wintle, et al. 2005. Zero tolerance ecology: Improving ecological inference by modelling the source of zero observations. *Ecology Letters* 8 (11): 1235–1246.

Min, Y., and A. Agresti. 2005. Random effect models for repeated measures of zero-inflated count data. *Statistical Modelling* 5 (1): 1–19.

Mullahy, J. 1986. Specification and testing of some modified count data models. *Journal of Econometrics* 33 (3): 341–365.

Ospina, R., and S.L.P. Ferrari. 2012. A general class of zero-or-one inflated beta regression models. *Computational Statistics & Data Analysis* 56 (6): 1609–1623.

Peng, X., G. Li, et al. 2015. Zero-inflated beta regression for differential abundance analysis with metagenomics data. *Journal of Computational Biology* 16: 16.

Petrova, M.I., E. Lievens, et al. 2015. Lactobacillus species as biomarkers and agents that can promote various aspects of vaginal health. *Frontiers in Physiology* 6 (81).

Potts, J.M., and J. Elith. 2006. Comparing species abundance models. *Ecological Modelling* 199 (2): 153–163.

Romero, R., S.S. Hassan, et al. 2014. The composition and stability of the vaginal microbiota of normal pregnant women is different from that of non-pregnant women. *Microbiome* 2: 4.

Rose, C.E., S.W. Martin, et al. 2006. On the use of zero-inflated and hurdle models for modeling vaccine adverse event count data. *Journal of Biopharmaceutical Statistics* 16 (4): 463–481.

Schwarz, G. 1978. Estimating the dimension of a model. *The Annals of Statistics* 6 (2): 461–464.

Shopova, E. 2001. Lactobacillus spp. as part of the normal microflora and as pathogens in humans. *Akush Ginekol* 42 (2): 22–25.

Sileshi, G., G. Hailu, et al. 2009. Traditional occupancy–abundance models are inadequate for zero-inflated ecological count data. *Ecological Modelling* 220 (15): 1764–1775.

Tu, W., and H. Liu. 2014. Zero-inflated data. *Wiley StatsRef: statistics reference online*. Chichester: Wiley.

Vuong, Q.H. 1989. Likelihood ratio tests for model selection and non-nested hypotheses. *Econometrica* 57 (2): 307–333.

Wang, J., L.B. Thingholm, et al. 2016. Genome-wide association analysis identifies variation in vitamin D receptor and other host factors influencing the gut microbiota. *Nature Genetics* 48 (11): 1396–1406.

Welsh, A.H., R.B. Cunningham, et al. 1996. Modelling the abundance of rare species: Statistical models for counts with extra zeros. *Ecological Modelling* 88 (1): 297–308.

Winkelmann, R., and K.F. Zimmermann. 1995. Recent developments in count data modelling: Theory and application. *Journal of Economic Surveys* 9 (1): 1–24.

Xia, Y., D. Morrison-Beedy, et al. 2012. Modeling count outcomes from HIV risk reduction interventions: A comparison of competing statistical models for count responses. *AIDS Research and Treatment* 2012: 11 pages.

Xu, L., A.D. Paterson, et al. 2015. Assessment and selection of competing models for zero-inflated microbiome data. *PLoS ONE* 10 (7): e0129606.

Yan, H., R. Potu, et al. 2013. Dietary fat content and fiber type modulate hind gut microbial community and metabolic markers in the pig. *PLoS One* 8: e59581.

Yau, K., K. Wang, et al. 2003. Zero-inflated negative binomial mixed regression modeling of over-dispersed count data with extra zeros. *Biometrical Journal* 45 (4): 437.

Yau, K.K.W., A.H. Lee, et al. 2004. Modeling zero-inflated count series with application to occupational health. *Computer Methods and Programs in Biomedicine* 74 (1): 47–52.

Yusuf, O., T. Bello, et al. 2017. Zero inflated poisson and zero inflated negative binomial models with application to number of falls in the elderly. *Biostatistics and Biometrics Open Access Journal* 1 (4): 555566.

Zeileis, A., C. Kleiber, et al. 2008. Regression models for count data in R. *Journal of Statistical Software* 27 (8): 1–25.

Zuur, A.F., E.N. Ieno, et al. 2009. *Mixed effects models and extensions in ecology with R*. New York, NY: Springer Science & Business Media, LLC.

Index

© Springer Nature Singapore Pte Ltd. 2018
Y. Xia et al., *Statistical Analysis of Microbiome Data with R*,
ICSA Book Series in Statistics, https://doi.org/10.1007/978-981-13-1534-3

Printed in the United States
By Bookmasters